Very little is known about the aut
he is a retired Government of
apparently hoary, but healthy. Wh
back:

> ...The real author of the *Original Yoga* is the
> world, Patañjali is the prime propagator of yoga. Any other claim to authorship, therefore, cannot but be spurious.
>
> ...It is Truth that matters, not the utterer of the Truth. No Truth ever becomes a bit truer even when repeated by the most distinguished person.
>
> ...Hence all genuine aspirants of yoga should be content to remain unknown and unnoticed by others.

His other published work is *Hindu Concept of Life and Death.*

They also do a separate package called "Amplifier" that takes amp modelling to a whole new level, allowing you to switch tubes, transformers and change parameters that I didn't know existed.

Backblaze

This is a paid subscription cloud backup software. It's under $10 a month and creates automatic cloud backups of your data. Having a backup solution is vital because, at some point, something will fail... and you don't want to lose all your tabs, scores, recording projects or masters of your songs.

It runs in the background and is fairly easy to use. I strongly recommend you use their service!

Torpedo Wall of sound

This is an AU/VST plugin that models impulse responses from speaker cabinets. It's free software that comes with a range of cabinets and microphones. You can also pay to get additional cabinets from their website at a very reasonable price.

You can use this with amp simulators to get a more realistic tone. It works nicely in conjunction with Positive Grid BIAS.

The software tends to be a bit slow and unresponsive when editing, but it does the job.

About the Author

Sam Russell has been playing electric guitar and composing for 18 years. He has released two albums:

- Impetuous Desire - a heavy metal album of original songs
- Bach's 1st and 2nd Cello Suites for Electric Guitar

and numerous classical compositions, including an album of string quartets and an album of duets for electric guitar and cello (performed, but not yet released).

He writes articles at www.study-guitar.com.

The Original Yoga

The concept of yoga is exclusively an Indian product. Yoga appears in history for the first time as estimated between the third and second centuries BC. At this time, though still without a definite date, there flourished a person called Patañjali, who is believed moulded the extant knowledge of yoga and wrote *Yogasūtra.*

The author of this book once replied against some requests:

> . . . The real author of the *Original Yoga* is the Lord Śiva. In the mundane world, Patañjali is the prime propagator of yoga. Any other claim to authorship, therefore, cannot but be spurious.
>
> . . . It is Truth that matters, not the utterer of the Truth. No Truth ever becomes a bit truer even when repeated by the most distinguished person.
>
> . . . Hence all genuine aspirants of yoga should be content to remain unknown and unnoticed by others.

Shyam Ghosh (1904–2000) was a Vedic research scholar. He studied other Hindu scriptures as well, some of which he translated and published, including an exhaustive commentary on Patañjali's *Yogasūtra.*

Having boycotted his school at the call of Mahatma Gandhi in 1920, Shyam Ghosh joined Freedom Movement and participated in meetings and rallies organized by Pt. Jawaharlal Nehru and other leaders. Later, after a few years of self-education, he worked his way to the editorial staff of three national daily newspapers before being selected as the editor of the AIR journals—*The Indian Listener, Awaz,* and *Sarang* (now defunct).

After a few years he was shifted to the Publications Division of the same Ministry as Deputy Director, and then on to the Finance Ministry, where he worked as Financial Advisor to the Director-General of Supply and Disposal.

He had always been averse to personal publicity. "An author should be judged by his work, and not by his personal qualifications," was his firm view.

Some of his other works are: *Ṛgveda for the Layman* (2002) and *Hindu Concept of Life and Death* (1989; repr., 2002).

The Original Yoga

as expounded in Śivasaṃhitā, Gheraṇḍasaṃhitā, and Pātañjala Yogasūtra

Original Text in Sanskrit
Translated, Edited, and Annotated with an Introduction by

Shyam Ghosh

MUNSHIRAM MANOHARLAL

Munshiram Manoharlal Publishers Pvt. Ltd.

ISBN 978-81-215-0892-6 (PB)
ISBN 978-81-215-0891-9 (HB)
Reprinted 1999, 2003, 2009, **2017**
First published 1980

PRINTED IN INDIA
Published by
Munshiram Manoharlal Publishers Pvt. Ltd.
PO Box 5715, 54 Rani Jhansi Road, New Delhi 110 055, INDIA

www.mrmlbooks.com

To
my grandchildren
Soumi, Devyani, Joydeep, Jayanta, Shilpi, and
all other grandchildren of the world
so that
"they may gain the right knowledge and an undistracted mind."

A yogi is more than one who practises austerities; he is more than one who performs deeds without seeking the fruits thereof. In my view he is better than even one who possesses knowledge. Therefore, O Arjuna, be thou a yogi.

—*The Bhagavadgītā*, VI.46

Contents

CONTENTS

Preface to the Second Edition

Since the first edition of this book was published, further research into Vedic literature has revealed that the concept of yoga did originate in the minds of the Vedic *ṛṣis.* In various hymns the sages did refer to the benefits to be derived from proper breathing and also its effect on the brain-cells when the breath is held inside for sometime. (This is now known as *prāṇāyāma.*) They referred to the twin respiration as Aśvins and designated these two as "divine physicians".

The concept of yoga is thus an exclusively Indian product, and it is this concept that later proliferated into the different branches of Haṭhayoga and Rājayoga.

SHYAM GHOSH

New Delhi
25 July 1998

Introduction

When we speak of the original yoga the question naturally arises, what exactly is the original yoga? For it is well-known that originally the yoga that we know of today did not exist: it was not in its present form anyhow. The form in which it might have existed in the earliest of times can only be imagined today as some stray and nebulous ideas then prevailing about the need to discipline the body and mind. Indeed a very, very long and indeterminable period must have elapsed before those ideas could synthetize into any recognizable shape. The exact origin of yoga, therefore, may be said today to have got lost in the mists of prehistory.

According to some authorities, however, the earliest historical evidence of yoga is provided by a terracotta seal excavated in the beginning of the present century at Mohenjo-Daro in Sind, now in Pakistan. This seal depicts the Hindu god Śiva sitting in yogic posture, with a hooded serpent standing over him. Archaeologists and historians have assessed this seal to be a product of the third millennium BC. But, apparently, no supporting material is available to justify a conclusion that the knowledge of yoga did prevail at that period.

Nor, unfortunately, is there any reference to the practice of yoga found in that treasure trove of Hindu wisdom—the Vedas—whose own existence, according to some constricted western view, goes back to the second millennium BC but which perhaps actually flourished much anterior to that period.

As a single collected, coordinated and systematized science, however, yoga appears in history for the first time at a period now estimated as between the second and the third century BC. At this time—though still without a definite date—there flourished a person called Patañjali, reputed even then as a *muni* (sage) and a *ṛṣi* (conveyer of knowledge), who is believed to have moulded into shape all the extant knowledge of yoga and reduced the same into pithy aphorisms in a compilation entitled the *Yogasūtra.* Before that time no mention of yoga as a compact science is found anywhere, even though the word "yoga" does appear sporadically in several ethical writings of the period, notably the Upaniṣads (cf. *Kaṭha,* VI.11, 18; *Śvetāśvatara,* VI.13) ascribed to the sixth century BC.

All this may lead some to infer that yoga perhaps is really non-Hindu by birth, adopted and reared by a people who later on came to be known as Hindus. It is of course an idea that can be neither accepted nor rejected. For we have also on record that Hindus in fact emerged as a race only in *circa* 1000 BC: prior to that the land was peopled apparently by a conglomerate of races—Austrics, Proto-Nordics, Eurasians, Eurafricans, Negritos and Mongoloids—who had successively streamed into the land from all corners of the earth. Indeed, viewed against this backdrop, yoga today may well appear to be the heritage of all mankind!

However, *Śivasaṃhitā,* a fundamental work on yoga though itself undated, indicates that the first yoga instructions emanated direct from the mouth of Lord Śiva, regarded by Hindus as *Mahāyogī* or the Supreme Yogi. Its opening verses contain the following:

> Now the Lord Śiva, bestower of deliverance upon all beings, expoundeth for the benefit of His devotees the Discipline of Yoga so that, forsaking the views of those who are inclined to disputations resulting from wrong knowledge, they may gain the right knowledge and an undistracted mind. (*SS,** I.2–3)

Although *Gheraṇḍasaṃhitā,* presumably a later work, corroborates this view by recording that "the secret of this science has been described in detail by the Lord Śiva" (*GS,*** VII.22), no concrete evidence is found in any other work to substantiate this origin of yoga. On the contrary distinct signs are noticed in several works of that period of a tendency to ascribe the origin of all words of wisdom to some popular personage or deity of the time. As a matter of fact many learned scribes then going by the name of Vyāsa preferred not to project their own personality when recording gems of knowledge that emanated from the spiritual giants of the day. In this respect the two Saṃhitās perhaps belong to the same class as the venerated *Bhagavadgītā* where, too, the essence of Hindu *dharma* comes direct from the mouth of Lord Kṛṣṇa, despite the

**SS* abbreviated for *Śivasaṃhitā.*
***GS* abbreviated for *Gheraṇḍasaṃhitā.*

fact that the Epic of which it forms part is known to have been composed by a sage called Kṛṣṇa-Dvaipāyana.

At any rate it is clear now that the knowledge of yoga, in one form or another, did prevail in Hindu-land as long ago as the seventh century BC—that is, a hundred years or so before the birth of Goutama the Buddha. This period bears indisputable proof of the practice of yoga, as now found corroborated by the Buddhist lore of the time. There is, for instance, a specific mention of the names of two yogis, Ālāṛha Kālāma and Uddaka Rāmaputta, who are said to have taught yoga to the young Goutama. The name of Vardhamāna Mahāvīra, the last apostle of the Jains, can also be traced to this momentous period. However, as an historically identified practitioner of yoga, Buddha remains to this day one of the earliest and greatest of yogis that ever lived in this land.

As a matter of fact the entire mass of Buddhist literature subsisting today is sprinkled with yogic terminology, mostly written of course in the prevalent Pāli and Prākṛta languages of the time. Thus we have accounts of yogic disciplines observed by the Buddha himself, and preached by him to his disciples, well preserved in such eminent books as *Buddhacarita* (by Aśvaghoṣa), *Lalitavistara*, *Nidānakathā*, and the *Majjhimanikāya*. In the last one, the Buddha's own words are recorded thus:

> O *Bhikkhus!* when I had not attained *sambodhi* (full knowledge), when I had not been bestowed with complete knowledge, I was subject to the law of *jāti* (birth and death) and sought only birth and death; I was subject to the law of *jarā* (decay) and yet sought decay; I was subject to *vyādhi* (disease) and yet sought disease; I was subject to *śoka* (grief) and yet sought grief; I was subject to *samkleśa* (sorrow) and yet sought sorrow. Then the thought came into my mind: why am I seeking these births, deaths, disease, decay, griefs and sorrows? When being subject to the laws of birth and death etc. brings (ultimate) sorrow, I must really seek the supreme *ajāta* (non-birth) and *nirvāṇa* (emancipation) through *yoga-kṣema* (fruits of *yoga*). . . .—*Majjhimanikāya Ariyapariyesanasutta* (Author's translation)

Again, in the *Mahāsaccakasutta* of the same, the Buddha describes his yogic experience as follows:

> Gritting my teeth and pressing the tongue against the palate (cf. *SS*, III.80, 88; *GS*, V.55) I controlled my thoughts with all the

force at my command, so much so that sweat trickled down from arm pits. (Author's translation)

In the *Saṃyuttanikāya* the Buddha says:

I have gained Insight, I have gained Knowledge, I have gained *Prajñā* (Highest Wisdom) and I have gained the Light. (Author's translation)

The Buddha acknowledged all these to be the "Ancient Way" and emphasized that he was saying nothing new, other (earlier) Buddhas had already mentioned these!

From the above it would appear that the knowledge and practice of yoga were prevalent in this land at least quite a few centuries before the appearance of Goutama the Buddha. As a compact science, however, the birth of yoga can be attributed only to Patañjali in the second/third century BC.

As of present the two Saṃhitās, together with the *Yogasūtra* of Patañjali, hold all the essential knowledge of yoga coming down from the very earliest of times although it must be admitted that similar knowledge, dispensed in other words and with varied emphasis, can also be had from some other treatises as well. Among these latter, particular mention may be made of *Brahmasaṃhitā, Aṣṭāvakrasaṃhitā, Ṣaṭacakra-nirūpaṇam, Triśikha Brāhmaṇa, Dhyānabindu Upaniṣad*, and the *Yogatattva Upaniṣad*. However, out of all the above, the *Yogasūtra* of Patañjali alone seems to have attracted the most attention, having been translated, along with commentaries by eminent scholars and spiritual luminaries like the late Swami Vivekananda, into several Indian and foreign languages. In it is to be found the essence of all yogic knowledge.

Contrary to some popular belief, however, yoga is not a mere keep-fit device. *Āsanas* and *prāṇāyāma* are no doubt a good means for achieving a perfect physiological condition. But these surely are not the be-all and end-all of yoga. As a matter of fact these, when practised without the ground being prepared by the other two "limbs of yoga," viz., *yama* and *niyama*, may well deprive one of the full benefits expected of them. Also, in some cases—*prāṇāyāma*, for instance—the absence of *yama* enjoined in the practice of continence can even result in positive harm. Yet it is noticed that yogic exercises are often propagated indiscriminately, with scant regard for such fundamentals of yoga.

Equally erroneous is the view that yoga is a philosophy which can be practised only by a highly evolved intellectual or spiritual person. Needless to say, it is nothing of the kind. Yoga in fact is beneficial for both the high and the low; if anything, it is indicated more for the common man. As a complete scientific guide, yoga is designed for all who seek a full, happy and purposeful life. It is indeed the rational man's creed! For it is the rational man who soon recognizes that he is in an adverse world—a plaything of his circumstances. While seeking Peace and Happiness he often misses both, mainly because his mind and body are ill-equipped to withstand the buffets of his circumstances. He is dismayed too when he observes that many others like him simply disappear from the scene without ever reaching the fringe of either, with only unaccountable tensions figuring in the balance-sheet of their life! To such a person yoga brings hope. Helped by yoga he can confidently master his circumstances, and soon be back on the true track of Peace and Happiness.

Nor is yoga the training of mind and body alone. The complete yoga in fact envisages the establishment of that fine rapport between the mind and spirit which alone releases man from his own trap of sorrows. For, in the final analysis—so the apostles of yoga discovered—physical and mental happiness are but transient and do not subsist unless they are truly pegged down to the spirit. Hence abiding Happiness or Bliss is to be sought only in the state of superconsciousness when the individual soul dwells in ecstatic harmony with the Universal Soul—a grace that comes as the supreme gift of yoga!

The discipline of yoga therefore embraces all three fields—the body, the mind and the spirit, i.e., the training of all three in this order. The principle underlying this training is that, first, the perfection of the body helps in the perfection of the mind, and then, when mental efficiency has been gained, the same is used to attain the higher spiritual perfection. Individually and collectively the three planes of perfection connote Happiness or Bliss. Yoga merely teaches how one may graduate through all three stages.

Accordingly, practical yoga stresses the need for graded, regular and diligent practice. Indeed *abhyāsa* (practice) is the keynote of the entire science of yoga. It is through assiduous practice that the seemingly-impossible postures (*āsanas*) and exercises (*mudrās**)

**Mudrā*, lit. a symbol or sign; also an aperitif. Esoterically, however, it signifies a posture adopted as an earnest of the desired union of Śakti (Force) and Śiva (Consciousness).

are mastered and performed with ease within a reasonable period of time. Nor are all of these to be undertaken at once, or performed one after another. Each exercise is devised to serve a particular purpose only, viz. to make some limb or organ of the body more efficient.

In this connection it is interesting to recall an incident, reported not long ago, when a young prisoner in Louiseville, USA, baffled his prison guards and the trying judge by sliding off in open view the heavy chains that clamped his ankles. That was no magical performance, of course—only manipulation made easy by *constant practice* and, possibly, some natural talent too!

For purposes of yoga, however, the kind of practice needed to achieve an optimum of physical and mental efficiency is listed in the two Saṃhitās. There is, to begin with, a phased programme of internal and external purification (*dhauti-śuddhi*) involving both wet and dry treatment of the mouth, throat, the nasal passage, the oesophagus, the bowels and the lower intestines down to the rectum. (*GS*, I.12–60). Such preliminaries are considered essential in so far as they condition the body for the more intricate exercises that follow. Next come *āsanas* (correct posture), *mudrās* (mystic exercises), *prāṇāyāma* (breath-control)—mainly for the purpose of cleansing the *nāḍīs* (by which term is meant both physical and psychic channels within the body)—and, finally, the technique of concentration, meditation and ecstasy.

The philosophy of yoga conceives of the Cosmos within the body, revolving on its axis the *meru-daṇḍa* (spinal column) and invested with the sun, the moon and stars—all floating in the Void within the body. (*SS*, II.1–12). In this manner macrocosm has been compressed into microcosm. Then, within this cosmic miniature the *prāṇa*, most vital of the ten airs pervading the body (*SS*, III.4–8; *GS*, V.59–64), is sought to be regulated by a systematic control of the breathing process which, incidentally, happens to be the principal motive power within. For this purpose again, clear instructions are available regarding the appropriate time, place, diet and the technique of *kumbhaka* or breath-retension. (*GS*, V.3–31 and 45 et seq.). The total number of inspiration and expiration in the course of 24 hours, their range and frequency during, for instance, sleep, meals, walking, singing, coitus and exercises—all are set down for the information of the neophyte. (*GS*, IV.83–86)

Yoga is broadly divided into two parts—Haṭhayoga and Rājayoga.

Haṭhayoga is also known as Kriyāyoga. Mantrayoga, Karmayoga, Jñānayoga, Bhaktiyoga, and Layayoga are intermediate and complementary disciplines, each designed to take the yogi to his cherished goal. Haṭhayoga is primarily concerned with building up the body, so that it may become immune to disease and decay. Hence we find at the end to each excercise a repeated assurance that successful completion of the exercise would ensure "robust health and freedom from decay and death."

Death? No doubt many would feel inclined to dismiss this as a somewhat tall claim. Yet it happens that modern science has already accepted such a possibility, at least in theory. Biologists in fact have experimented extensively with metazoan (multicelled) tissues in their laboratories—culturing them, feeding them with appropriate nutrition and removing the harmful products of their metabolism—and then found to their surprise that the tissues showed indubitable signs of life *for an indefinite period!* Death, thus, is defined as a consequence of the disorganized *ideal condition* of the body. Normally this disorganization is preceded by a period of senescence or decay, a condition medically described as "protoplasmic hysteresis."* Such a condition yoga seeks to combat, thereby ensuring freedom from "decay and death."

With the body made inviolable, yoga proceeds to master the mind. The mind, it has been observed, does not function apart from the breathing process: the two in fact are correlated. Thus it is possible to synchronize the modifications of thought with the rhythm of the breath we breathe. Hence, says yoga, a correct and regulated rhythm of the breath is imperative for proper control of the propensities of the mind. To this end the practice of *prāṇāyāma* is directed. *Prāṇāyāma* not only regulates the breathing process but it also brings about the much-needed order and onepointedness in the thinking process. In a way it transmutes the mind into Pure Intelligence and Reason.

When the yogi rises to the psychic plane he deals with psychic forces within him—forces that lie concentrated in what are esoterically termed *cakras* (lotuses) placed at five specific points alongside the spinal column, and two in the head. These seven *cakras*** are:

*Cf. R. Pearl, *The Biology of Death*; T.S.P. Strangeways, *Technique of Tissue Culture in Vitro.*

**Actually the first six are *cakras* proper (*ṣaṭacakra*) and the seventh, viz., Sahasrāra is the abode of Consciousness or the Self.

(i) Mūlādhāra, placed against the sacrum as root-support of the spinal column, (ii) Swādhiṣṭhāna, about four centimetres above, at the sex centre, (iii) Maṇipura, next above, near the navel, (iv) Anāhata, inside the heart, (v) Viśuddha, inside the throat, (vi) Ājñā, between the eyebrows, and (vii) Sahasrāra in the brain-centre. Both *Śivasaṃhitā* and the *Yogasūtra* emphasize the special role of these *cakras* and the kind of supernormal power that may be expected through intensive concentration upon each. (*SS*, V.63–74, 92–99 et seq. and *PY*,* III.21–35). The supernormal powers include the power to become infinitely small (invisibility), power to become excessively large (pervasion), power to float in the air (leviation) and the power to bewitch (fascination).

Before, however, the yogi may aspire for such powers he must first discipline himself with *pratyāhāra*, or control of his sense faculties. Even as *āsana* and *prāṇāyāma* (control of breath) counter the infirmities of the body, and *dhāraṇā* and *dhyāna* (meditation) those of the mind, in a similar manner *pratyāhāra* (abnegation) counters the infirmities of the heart, i.e. controls the cravings of the senses. (*GS*, IV.3–7). *Pratyāhāra* assists both *dhāraṇā* and *dhyāna*, which involve visualization of and concentration upon objects (i) concrete, (ii) effulgent and (iii) subtle in a prescribed order. Competency in these three disciplines, viz., *pratyāhāra, dhāraṇā* and *dhyāna*, qualifies the yogi to enter the highest psychic plane where *samādhi* or transcendental ecstasy is experienced.

Samādhi, thus, is the climax of a full course of physical, sensual and mental control gained through assiduous practice of *āsanas, mudrās, mantras, kumbhaka, pratyāhāra, dhāraṇā*, and *dhyāna* and, as the *Gheraṇḍasaṃhitā* aptly points out, it is "a superb yogic state reached by great good luck," (*GS*, VII.1). *Mantras* of course are abbreviated prayers, often reduced to single syllables, which, when intoned in the correct manner, produce sound-waves and vibration in the psychic field within, awakening in the process the dormant Kuṇḍalinī (Serpent Power) and forcing the same upward to the brain-centre called Sahasrāra.

Kuṇḍalinī, then, is the key to success in yoga. This highly concentrated psychic force, esoterically described as *nāda-bindu*** or the quintessence of cosmic energy, remains dormant "asleep like

**PY* abbreviated for *Pātañjala Yogasūtra.*

***Nāda-bindu* is the subtle *anāhata* (unstruck) sound-wave which manifests itself as consciousness in every living creature. It represents Cosmic Energy and is believed to got "recorded" in a creature the moment *nāda* (sound) and *bindu* (particle a coiled serpent" (*SS*, V.80–83)—at the sacrum (the triangular bone at the nether end of the spinal column). In yoga the Kuṇḍalinī is identified as the goddess Śakti (Force) abiding in a micro form. Thus, once aroused with the aid of *prāṇāyāma, mantras* and *mudrās* the goddess aspires to meet her spouse Śiva (identified as the *Puruṣa* or Self) dwelling in the thousand-petalled lotus Sahasrāra at the summit. She then takes the path of the Brahmarandhra (Passage of Knowledge), identified as the median nerve (Suṣumnā *nāḍī*) threading through the spinal column and opening (via medulla oblongata) into the Sahasrāra placed in the causal region of the brain, or seat of man's consciousness. (*SS*, II.23–27; IV.2–8; V.161–62; *GS*, III.47–49). When the goddess Śakti arrives at her coveted place the yogi experiences a transcendental trance called Samprajñāta, or *samādhi* "with consciousness." He is then able to recall from the Unconscious all his past, including earlier lives—his psychic heritage, in short. He is now in complete Ecstatic Bliss, and has reached his journey's end!

And yet it is not the real End. For, in this *samādhi*, the yogi is still conscious of his transcendental bliss. In other words his experience in this state of *samādhi* is that of a quality-endowed bliss. Hence, longing to shed the last vestige of consciousness, he now strives for a quality-*less* bliss (*nirguṇa kaivalya*) or oneness with the Universal Soul—the yogi's ultimate goal of Emancipation or Limitlessness.

The superior stages of *samādhi* are dealt with in greater detail in the *Yogasūtra*. The *Yogasūtra* in fact distinguishes itself by its deep analysis of man's mind in all its aspects, including the peculiar character of propensities in the mind and the way to curb them. The comprehensive knowledge of mind revealed in this work would seem to humble much of modern psychology and psychophysics: it is indeed mental science *par excellence.* In it Patañjali, using precise and succinct language, identifies Cognition, Intelligence, Reason, Will, Discrimination, and the Highest Wisdom (*Prajña*). He discusses the varied conditions of the mind, the causes of modification of thoughts, the methods for their control including observance of mental hygiene, the "Great Vows," countering of negative thoughts by positive ones, limiting the mind's "field" through concentration, forcing it into onepointedness, and finally establishing that supercontrol over it which alone makes man the master of himself.

of matter) unite. The *nāda-bindu* is normally indicated by the sign (ँ) placed over the mystic symbol of the Supreme, thus—ॐ (*Aum*).

The *Yogasūtra* sweeps over the widest range of natural science. It defines the character of Matter, both gross as well as fine, the nature of Time and Space, the Law of Cause and Effect (and how the two could be de-linked), the Law of Continuity ("nothing is abrupt in nature"), the Law of Evolution (natural selection in the psychic field), the Law of *Karma* (past impressions in the Unconscious transmuting into *kleśa*, a term denoting both pleasure and pain), and finally dwells on the concept of Infinity and the operation of the three primal Qualities (*guṇas*) of Nature before leading the yogi on to the end-product of all this knowledge, namely, superconsciousness and thence Emancipation.

In amassing all this knowledge and bringing it within the compass of a system, Patañjali's task was evidently lightened by the preachings and practical demonstrations of yoga by the Buddha, who had preceded him by some three hundred years. The *Majjhimanikāya*, for example, mentions some methods of mind-control such as counter-thoughts and mentally "looking away" (*dvedha-vitakkasutta*) the substance of which is also found in the *Yogasūtra* (*PY*, I.32–39). Similarly, the classification of the Eight Limbs of yoga (*PY*, II.29) could perhaps be compared to the Eight-fold Path preached by the Śākya *muni*. In any case, yogic methods analogous to the Buddha's *samyaka dṛṣṭi* (clear insight and equipoise), *samyaka saṅkalpa* (complete non-attachment and non-hostility), *samyaka vāka* (complete control of speech and strict practice of truth), *samyaka karmānta* (complete rejection of evil thoughts, non-craving and non-acceptance), *samyaka ājīva* (right living and right means of livelihood), *samyaka vyāyāma* (conation or constant endeavour to maintain the path), *samyaka smṛti* (constant mental alertness and continence); and *samyaka samādhi* (complete *samādhi*)—can be easily distinguished in the various *sūtras* of Patañjali.

Of course much of the non-Buddhist knowledge of yoga also must have gone into the *Yogasūtra*. Even so the terminological similarity found in both Buddhist and Hindu works on yoga cannot perhaps be totally ignored. It is notable, for instance, that words like *nirvāṇa*—variously referred to in Buddhist literature as *pāra* (crossing over), *anta* (the end), *layana* (merging), and *śaraṇa* (the refuge)—as also *śuddhi* (purity) and *śivam* (emancipation) used as alternatives to *nirvāṇa* (cf. *Saṃyuttanikāya*, 16, 26) signify exactly the same idea as is sought to be conveyed by Patañjali by his *sattva* (purity) and *Puruṣa* (Self) merging into oneness (*kaivalya*) or Emancipation. The nine forms of *dhyāna* preached by the Buddha also fall within the purview of the various types of *samādhi* culminating in Samprajñāta and A-samprajñāta *samādhis* advised by Patañjali. (*PY*, I.17–18). Perhaps the analogy need not be pursued if only because of the fact that Buddhist yoga, anyhow, was born in Hindu-land.

The spiritual nuances of Hindu yoga find greater expression in the *Bhagavadgītā* where the Yogeśvara (Lord of Yoga) himself initiates a deluded and distracted Arjuna into the mysteries of yoga. Kṛṣṇa was well aware that Arjuna had many divine qualities (*sampadam daivīmabhijāto-si. BG*, XVI.5) such as truth, non-violence, forgiveness, patience, compassion, selflessness, etc., and yet he found Arjuna lacking in the supreme quality of yoga which alone could help him to understand and face a very critical situation. Therefore, himself defining yoga as that high state of equanimity (*samattvam yoga uccyate, BG*, II.48), Kṛṣṇa revealed to him how that could be achieved by rising above the conflicting dualities of life such as success and failure, praise and blame, desire and aversion, happiness and sorrow, etc. and performing actions, regardless of the fruits thereof, in pursuance of the infallible dictates of one's inner Self. For, as Kṛṣṇa explained, although the senses are very strong and stronger than the senses is the mind, and stronger than the mind is intelligence—it is That (the Self) which is the strongest of all. (*BG*, III.42). Hence *karma-saṃnyāsa* yoga, which calls for bold action—and not inaction, lukewarmness or despondency (*na niragnir na cākriyaḥ, BG*, VI.1)—was commended as the only rational way of life.

Both Saṃhitās, it will be noted, repeatedly emphasize the need for a guru. A guru in fact has been declared indispensable for any aspirant of yoga and no yoga may be practised without his personal direction and blessings. A similar note of warning is struck against the proliferation of this "secret" knowledge. On the other hand, the *Yogasūtra* does not impose any such restrictions: its priceless knowledge would appear to be free for one and all and apparently needs no assistance from a guru for processing it. As such it would not be unreasonable to infer that a guru is perhaps not a *sine qua non* for purposes of learning yoga—certainly not Rājayoga. When followed intelligently and practised with due care, yoga would seem to be as safe as the knowledge and practice of any other science.

The two bans inscribed in the Saṃhitās—however relevant at a time when knowledge as a rule passed direct by word of mouth from the adept to the neophyte—cannot therefore be considered pertinent for modern times. However, a really competent guru, if available, should be a welcome help any time.

For obvious reasons the three treatises—*Śivasaṃhitā, Gheraṇḍa-saṃhitā* and the *Yogasūtra* presented here under one cover—do not appear in their chronological order. All the same the knowledge contained in these do constitute the sum and substance of the science of yoga known in this land from time immemorial. This knowledge also represents the true character of culture prevailing in this part of the world—a culture whose pre-eminence becomes all the more apparent when it is juxtaposed against what is sometimes portrayed by a few "researchers" who choose to underscore some corrupt religious practices or the erotic contents of temple architecture. The latter perhaps represent the real East as much as the real West of today would, were it to be judged solely by the legacy of some present-day "popular" art, music, literature, dress and customs found, say, in the 40th century AD! As Sir John Woodroffe (Arthur Avalon) aptly puts it:

> All evil and ignorance is so much by its nature on the surface and affords so apt a subject for adverse judgement that it is readily seized upon and the more so that it is convenient material for religious polemic. Nevertheless I repeat that we must do credit both to our intelligence and sense of justice by endeavouring to understand any religion in its highest and truest aspect.—*Śrīcakra-sambhāra Tantra*, Foreword, p. vii

The original texts of all three treatises are in Sanskrit. Their translation into English has been attempted here with the full consciousness of the present writer's own limitations in both these languages. Hence scholars of these two languages will probably detect many errors committed in an overzealous but honest attempt to interpret ideas so punctiliously put in an ancient language and now translated into a modern one. It is needless therefore to add that any omission or commission pointed out in this respect will be gratefully acknowledged and dutifully rectified in a subsequent edition.

ACKNOWLEDGEMENTS

The explanatory notes given under the translated texts have been prepared with the help of various reference books in English, Sanskrit and Bengali. Comments appearing under each *sūtra* are based on *Rājamārtaṇḍa*, otherwise known as *Bhojavṛtti*, a commentary on Pātañjala-Darśana in Sanskrit by Rājā Bhoja. Rājā Bhoja, besides being the ruler of Dhārā (Mālwā), was also an eminent Sanskrit scholar and a poet who flourished in the eleventh century AD. His versatility—comparable perhaps to that of the Italian genius of the fifteenth century AD. Leonardo da Vinci—may be judged from his *Samarāṅgaṇa Sūtradhāra*, a work in Sanskrit in which he discusses mechanics of a new type found nowadays in elevators and aircraft. His other works include *Amaraṭīkā, Campū Rāmāyaṇa, Saraswatī Kaṇṭhābharaṇa, Rājavārtika*, and *Cāru-caryā*.

References to Buddhist literature made in this Introduction have been compiled largely with the aid of *2500 Years of Buddhism*, a Government of India publication, and *Buddha-prasaṅga* (in Bengali) by the late Mahesh Chandra Ghosh, published by Visvabharati.

My grateful thanks are due also to Dr. Manju Sen, M.Sc., Ph.D., for the valuable assistance given by her in identifying many rare Indian plants and trees (along with their botanical names) mentioned in the two Saṃhitās; to Dr. Tejomitra, M.A., Ph.D., of the DAV Post-Graduate College, Dehra Dun, for kindly translating a portion of *Bhojavṛtti* into Hindi to enable me to comprehend the correct significance of the same; to Mr. Hiren Gupta, formerly of the UNICEF, for the generous loan of many reference books from his select library; to Mr. S.R. Sethi, formerly Manager, Government of India Press, for his invaluable technical help in the printing and production of this book, and, last but not least, to Mr. H.P. Gautam for his unremitting friendly advice and encouragement during the preparation of this book.

SHYAM GHOSH

Rudralaya
Dehra Dun

Book I

Śivasaṃhitā

CHAPTER I

The Path of Harmony

एकं ज्ञानं नित्यमाद्यन्तशून्यं नान्यत् किञ्चिद्वर्त्तते वस्तु सत्यम्।
यद्भेदोस्मिन्निन्द्रियोपाधिना वै ज्ञानस्यायं भासते नान्यथैव।। १।।

There is but One Knowledge, and that is Eternal—without beginning and without end. Than it naught exists that is true. Whatsoever else seem different (in this world) are but the attributes of the senses. Those are reflected by that Knowledge, not otherwise.—1

अथ भक्तानुरक्तो हि वक्ति योगानुशासनम्।
ईश्वरः सर्वभूतानामात्ममुक्तिप्रदायकः।। २।।
त्यक्त्वा विवादशीलानां मतं दुर्ज्ञानहेतुकम्।
आत्मज्ञानाय भूतानामनन्यगति चेतसाम्।। ३।।

Now the Lord (Śiva), bestower of deliverance upon all beings, expoundeth for the benefit of His devotees the discipline of yoga, so that they may, forsaking the views of those inclined to disputations resulting from wrong knowledge, gain the right knowledge and an undistracted mind.—2–3

सत्यं केचित् प्रशंसन्ति तपः शौचं तथापरे।
क्षमा केचित् प्रशंसन्ति तथैव सममार्जवम्।। ४।।

Some eulogize truth (*satya*); others austerity (*tapas*) and purity (*śauca*); still others praise forgiveness (*kṣamā*), equanimity (*sama*) and humility (*ārjava*).—4

केचिद्दानं प्रशंसन्ति पितृकर्म तथापरे।
केचित् कर्म प्रशंसन्ति केचिद्वैराग्यमुत्तमम्।। ५।।

Some praise charity (*dāna*), others offerings to forefathers (*pitṛ-karma*); some eulogize action (*karma*) and some regard non-attachment (*vairāgya*) as the best.—5

केचिद्गृहस्थकर्मणि प्रशंसन्ति विचक्षणाः।
अग्निहोत्रादिकं कर्म तथा केचित् परं विदुः।। ६।।

Some wise persons praise the deeds of family life (*grhastha*), while others consider fire-offerings (*agnihotra* rites) etc. to be the best.—6

मन्त्रयोगं प्रशंसन्ति केचित्तीर्थानुसेवनम्।
एवं बहूनुपायांस्तु प्रवदन्ति हि मुक्तये।। ७।।

(Similarly) the yoga of *mantras* (prayers) is praised by some and some (reckon) the path of pilgrimage (*tīrtha*) as best. In this manner numerous are the ways that have been spoken of for (attaining) *mukti.*—7

एवं व्यवसिता लोके कृत्याकृत्यविदो जनाः।
व्यामोहमेव गच्छन्ति विमुक्ताः पापकर्मभिः।। ८।।

Thus placed in this world betwixt do-able and not do-able actions men, even though freed from evil deeds, drift into disorder.—8

एतन्मतावलम्बी यो लब्ध्वा दुरितपुण्यके।
भ्रमतीत्यवशः सोऽत्र जन्ममृत्यु परम्पराम्।। ९।।

Those who hold such views, gather (the fruits of) good and bad deeds, and due to that wander aimlessly in a cycle of births and deaths.—9

अन्यैर्मतिमतां श्रेष्ठैर्गुप्तालोकानतत्परैः।
आत्मानो बहवः प्रोक्ता नित्याः सर्वगतास्तथा।। १०।।

Others who are wise, perfect, deep in thinking and alert, describe the *Ātman* (Self) as boundless, eternal and all-pervading.—10

यद्यत् प्रत्यक्षविषयं तदन्यन्नास्ति चक्षते।
कुतः स्वर्गादयः सन्तीत्यन्ये निश्चित-मानसाः।। ११।।

"Whatever (things) are apparent, exist; those not apparent, do not exist. Where are the heavens, etc.?"—such are the confident views of some.—11

ज्ञानप्रवाह इत्यन्ये शून्य कौचित् परं विदुः।
द्वावेव तत्वं मन्यन्तेऽपरे प्रकृतिपुरुषौ।। १२।।

Yet others know it to be Radiant Knowledge, or as void (*śūnya*);

still others regard it as a dual entity (quintessence) of *Prakṛti* and *Puruṣa*.—12

अत्यन्तभिन्नमतयः परमार्थ पराङ्मुखाः।
एवमन्ये तु संचिन्त्य यथामति यथाश्रुतम्।
निरीश्वरमिदं प्राह सेश्वरञ्च तथापरे।। १३।।
वदन्ति विविधैर्भेदैः सुयुक्त्या स्थितिकातराः।। १४।।

Entirely different are the views of those who are apathetic to the Reality; also of those who have (merely) collected whatever was heard or thought of. These say, there is no God. Yet others—eager to know the correct position—dissolve all contradictions by sound logic and declare: There *is* God.—13–14

एते चान्ये च मुनयः संज्ञाभेदाः पृथग्विधाः।
शास्त्रेषु कथित ह्येते लोकव्यामोहकारकाः।। १५।।

These (latter) and many other sages—as is also stated in the *śāstras* (scriptures)—confirm that the cause of man's delusion is fragmentations and disputations (in the mind).—15

एतद्विवादशीलानां मतं वक्तुं न शक्यते।
भ्रमन्त्यस्मिन् जनाः सर्वे मुक्तिमार्गवहिष्कृताः।। १६।।

The various views of all disputing persons I am unable to relate. All such people wander aimlessly, driven away from the Path of Salvation.—16

आलोक्य सर्वशास्त्राणि विचार्य च पुनः पुनः।
इदमेकं सुनिष्पन्नं योगशास्त्रं मतं परम्।। १७।।

(However) after consulting all the *śāstras*, and after pondering over them again and again, it has been found that the views of the Yogaśāstra are the best.—17

यस्मिन् ज्ञाते सर्वमिदं ज्ञातं भवति निश्चितम्।
तस्मिन् परिश्रमः कार्यः किमन्यत् शास्त्रभाषितम्।। १८।।

When by knowing this (Yogaśāstra) all others are clearly known, of what profit can it be to labour and find out what the other *śāstras* say?—18

योगशास्त्रमिदं गोप्यमस्माभिः परिभाषितम्।
सुभक्ताय प्रदातव्यं त्रैलोक्ये च महात्मने।। १९।।

This Yogaśāstra, as related by Mc. is secret. It may be passed on only to the most devoted and great souls in all three worlds.—19

कर्मकाण्डो ज्ञानकाण्ड: इति भेदौ द्विधामत:।
भवति द्विविधो भेदौ ज्ञानकाण्डस्य कर्मण:।। २०।।

Now, there are two paths: the *karma* (action) way, and the *jñāna* (knowledge) way. Again, action performed in the course of knowledge-way is twofold.—20

द्विविध: कर्मकाण्ड: स्यान्निषेधविधिपूर्वक:।। २१।।

Pursuit and control of the action-way is also twofold.—21

निषिद्धकर्मकरणे पापं भवति निश्चितम्।
विधानकर्मकरणे पुण्यं भवति निश्चितम्।। २२।।

It is positively unrighteous to perform forbidden actions (*karma*). It is positively righteous to perform the commended actions.—22

त्रिविधो विधिकूट: स्यान्नित्यनैमित्यकाम्यत:।
नित्ये कृतेऽकिल्विषं स्यात् काम्ये नैमित्तिके फलम्।। २३।।

(Actions are) of three complex character: the ordinary, the particular and the desired ones. The ordinary (not premeditated) do not attract sin. The particular and the desired (premeditated) ones bear fruit.—23

द्विविधन्तु फलं ज्ञेयं स्वर्गं नरकमेव च।
स्वर्गे नानाविधञ्चैव नरकेऽपि तथा भवेत्।। २४।।

The fruits (of particular and desired actions) are also twofold—both here and hereafter. In heaven (the fruits or pleasures) are manifold; so are they (the fruits or suffereings) in hell.—24

पुण्यकर्मणि वै स्वर्गो नरकं पापकर्मणि।
कर्मबन्धमयी सृष्टिर्नान्यथा भवति ध्रुवम्।। २५।।

To Heaven through pious deeds and to Hell through impious deeds—this is the way how creation is *karma*-bound. This is positive, and cannot be otherwise.—25

जन्तुभिश्चानुसूयन्ते स्वर्गे नानासुखानि च।
नानाविधानि दु:खानि नरके दु:सहानि वै।। २६।।

In heaven too people experience *asūya* (anger, hatred, jealousy, etc.) as well as many pleasures. In hell (they suffer) many kinds of unbearable pains.—26

पापकर्मवशाद्दुःखं पुण्यकर्मवशात् सुखम्।
तस्मात् सुखार्थी विविधं पुण्यं प्रकुरुते भृशम्।। २७।।

Suffering comes from impious deeds (even as) pleasure is the outcome of pious deeds. Hence he who is desirous of pleasure performs pious deeds only.—27

पापभोगावसाने तु पुनर्जन्म भवेद्वहुः।
पुण्यभोगावसाने तु नान्यथा भवति ध्रुवम्।। २८।।

After the expiation of sins, follow several re-births (according to *karma*). Nor is it otherwise when virtues are expended. This is certain.—28

स्वर्गेऽपि दुःखसम्भोगः परस्त्रीदर्शनादिषु।
ततो दुःखमिदं सर्वं भवेन्नास्त्यत्र संशयः।। २९।।

(Despite all the virtues) even the mere coveting of another's wife brings sorrow in heaven. Hence all such things in this world are undoubtedly (the cause of) sorrow.—29

तत्कर्म कल्पकैः प्रोक्तं पुण्यपापमिति द्विधा।
पुण्यपापमयो बन्धो देहिनां भवति क्रमः।।३०।।

The thinkers (sages) have described *karma* as twofold: righteous and unrighteous. In course of time the creatures get bound to their virtue and vice.—30

इहामुत्र फलद्वेषी सफलं कर्म संत्यजेत्।
नित्ये नैमित्तिके संगं त्यक्त्वा योगे प्रवर्त्तते।। ३१।।

Those who are averse to the fruits (of actions) shed all fruitful actions (*karma*) in this very world. Renouncing attachment to ordinary as well as particular actions, they engage themselves in the practice of yoga.—31

कर्मकाण्डस्य माहात्म्यं बुध्वा योगी त्यजेत् सुधीः।
पुण्यपापद्वयं त्यक्त्वा ज्ञानकाण्डे प्रवर्त्तते।। ३२।।

(Hence) having understood the real character (importance) of the *karma*-method, the wise yogi forsakes that and turns to the *knowledge*-method, abandoning both virtue and vice.—32

आत्मावारे तु द्रष्टव्यः श्रोतव्येत्यादिका श्रुतिः।
सा सेव्या तु प्रयत्नेन मुक्तिदाहेतुदायिनी।। ३३।।

That the *Ātman* can be seen (realized) on this shore (i.e.

in this very life) is learnt from the ancient Śrutis (scriptures). The same (knowledge) must be nursed as the means and harbinger of *mukti*.—33

दुरितेषु च पुण्येषु यो धीवृत्तिं प्रचोदयात्।
सोऽहं प्रवर्त्तते मत्तो जगत्सर्वं चराचरम्।
सर्वञ्च दृश्यते मत्तः सर्वञ्च मयि लीयते।
न तद्भिन्नोऽस्मिन् न मद्भिन्नो न तु किञ्चन।। ३४।।

That which directs the propensity of mind towards virtue and vice is Me. The entire moving and unmoving universe is born in Me, is seen (stays) in Me, and merges in Me. I am not apart from that, nor anything is apart from Me.—34

जलपूर्णेष्वसंख्येषु शरावेषु यथा भवेत्।
एकस्य भात्यसंख्यत्वं तद्भेदोऽत्र न दृश्यते।
उपाधिषु शरावेषु या संख्या वर्त्तते परम्।
सा संख्या भवति यथा रवौ चात्मनि सा तथा।। ३५।।

Just as the reflection of the sun in a number of saucers filled with water appears numerous irrespective of the fact that the sun is one and the quality of the saucers the same, even so is the case with the *Ātman*.—35

यथैकः कल्पकः स्वप्ने नानाविधतयेष्यते।
जागरेऽपि तथाप्येकस्तथैव वहुधा जगत्।। ३६।।

Just as in a dream one thing is imagined in many forms and the same on awakening becomes one again, in a similar manner the world appears manifold (to the person in illusion).—36

रार्गबुद्धिर्यथा रज्जौ शुक्तौ वा रजतभ्रमः।
तद्वदेवमिदं विश्वं विवृतं परमात्मनि।। ३७।।

Just as a piece of rope is (sometimes) mistaken for a serpent and a mother-of-pearl is taken for silver, in a similar manner the world phenomena disguise the Supreme *Ātman*.—37

रज्जुज्ञानाद्यथा सर्पो मिथ्यारूपो निवर्त्तते।
आत्मज्ञानात्तथा याति मिथ्याभूतमिदं जगत्।। ३८।।

Even as a correct knowledge of the rope dispels the illusion of the snake, a right knowledge of the Self (*Ātman*) dispels the illusion of world phenomena.—38

रौप्यभ्रान्तिरियं याति शुक्तिज्ञानाद्यथा खलु।
जगद्भ्रान्तिरियं याति चात्मज्ञानात् सदा तथा।। ३९।।

Just as the illusion of silver disappears upon recognizing the mother-of-pearl, so does the illusion of the world disappear upon realization of the Self.—39

यथा वंशोरगभ्रान्तिर्भवेद्भेकवसाञ्जनात्।
तथा जगदिदं भ्रान्तिरध्यासकल्पनाञ्जनात्।। ४०।।

Just as a piece of bamboo, when seen after applying kohl to the eyes, is mistaken for a snake because of clouded vision, so is this world clouded with the "kohl" of imagination.—40

आत्मज्ञानाद्यथा नास्ति रज्जुज्ञानादभुजङ्गमः।
यथा दोषवशात् शुक्लः पीतं भवति नान्यथा।
अज्ञानदोषादात्मापि जगद्भवति दुस्त्यजम्।। ४१।।

Even as the snake disappears when the rope is recognized, all illusions disappear with the knowledge of the Self. Because of ignorance it is difficult for the Self to discard the world (phenomena) even as due to debility (of a person suffering from jaundice) all things appear yellow.—41

दोषनाशे यथा शुक्लः गृह्यते रोगिणा स्वयम्।
शुद्धज्ञानात् तथाज्ञाननाशादात्मतया क्रिया।। ४२।।

Just as the patient recovers his natural state when the flaw is removed, similar is the process in respect of the *Ātman* when ignorance is removed and pure knowledge is gained.—42

कालत्रयेऽपि न यथा रज्जुः सर्पो भवेदिति।
तथात्मा न भवेद्विश्वं गुणातीतो निरञ्जनः।। ४३।।

Even as the rope does not become a snake in all three divisions of Time (past, present and future), the *Ātman*, which is quality-less and faultless (i.e. without ignorance), can never become world phenomena.—43

आगमापायिनोऽनित्या नाश्यत्वादीश्वरादयः।
आत्मबोधेन केनापि शास्त्रादेतद्विनिश्चितम्।। ४४।।

Without Self-realisation even the gods would be nowhere, being then a mere subject of births and deaths and impermanence. This is the positive conclusion of the *śāstras*.—44

यथा वातवशात् सिन्धौ व्युत्पन्नाः फेनबुद्बुदाः।
तथात्मनि समुद्भूतः संसारः क्षणभंगुरः।। ४५।।

Even as the foam and bubbles in the ocean caused by wind are (short-lived), in a similar manner the world phenomena appear transient to the (knowledge-endowed) *Ātman.*—45

अभेदो भासते नित्यं वस्तुभेदो न भासते।
द्विधा-त्रिधादिभेदोयं भ्रमत्वे पर्यवस्यति।। ४६।।

(Then) the Eternal shines forth in full glory and no diversity is seen. It is due to illusion that these appear double, treble, etc.—46

यद्भूतं यच्च भाव्यं वै मूर्तामूर्त्तं तथैव च।
सर्वमेव जगदिदं विवृतं परमात्मनि।। ४७।।

Whatever has become and whatever shall be, also all form and formless—everything in this world is pervaded by the *Paramātman* (Supreme Self).—47

कल्पकैः कल्पिता विद्या मिथ्याजाता मृषात्मिका।
एतन्मूलं जगदिदं कथं सत्यं भविष्यति।। ४८।।

(This world) is the product of imagination, falsely created, and is as paralyzing as hypnosis. With such a base how can this world be true?—48

चैतन्यात् सर्वमुत्पन्नं जगदेतच्चराचरम्।
तस्मात् सर्वं परित्यज्य चैतन्यन्तु समाश्रयेत।। ४९।।

Out of consciousness is born all the animate and inanimate objects of this world. Hence, abandoning all these one should abide in consciousness itself.—49

घटस्याभ्यन्तरे वाह्ये यथाकाशं प्रवर्त्तते।
तथात्माभ्यन्तरे वाह्ये कार्यवर्गेषु नित्यशः।। ५०।।

Even as space pervades both inside and outside a pot, so is the *Ātman* constantly inside and outside as necessary.—50

असंलग्नं यथाकाशं मिथ्याभूतेषु पञ्चसु।
असंलग्नस्तथा ह्यात्मा कार्यवर्गेषु नान्यथा।। ५१।।

Just as space does not attach itself falsely to the five Elements, in a similar way the *Atman* remains unattached to the various actions. It is never otherwise.—51

ईश्वरादि जगत् सर्वमात्मा व्याप्य समन्ततः।
एकोऽस्ति सच्चिदानन्दः पूर्णोऽद्वैतविवर्जितः।। ५२।।

Everything in this world is permeated with the Supreme Being. It is one (Brahman), *Saccidānanda* (Being-Knowledge-Bliss), perfect and without duality.—52

यस्मात् प्रकाशको नास्ति स्वप्रकाशो भवेत्ततः।
स्वप्रकाशो यतस्तस्मादात्मा ज्योतिः स्वरूपकः।। ५३।।

That which receives no light (from anything) is self-illuminated. Through self-illumination the *Ātman* takes on the form of light (becomes effulgent).—53

परिच्छेदो यतो नास्ति देशकालस्वरूपतः।
आत्मनः सर्वथा तस्मादात्मा पूर्णो भवेत् किल।। ५४।।

Indivisible like Time and Space, the *Ātman* in its natural state is always truly complete (whole).—54

यस्मान्न विद्यते नाशो पञ्चभूतैर्मृषात्मकैः।
आत्मा तस्माद्भवेन्नित्यः तन्नाशो न भवेत् खलु।। ५५।।

That which is not destroyed like the false phenomena of five Elements—is the *Ātman*. It is eternal and is never annihilated.—55

यस्मात्तदन्यो नास्तीह तस्मादेकोऽस्ति सर्वदा।
यस्मात्तदन्यो मिथ्या स्यादात्मा सत्यो भवेत्ततः।। ५६।।

Than which nothing else exists, is the One that always exists. When everything else turns false the *Ātman* alone remains true.—56

अविद्याभूतसंसारे दुःखनाशः सुखं यतः।
ज्ञानादत्यन्तशून्यं स्यात् तस्मादात्मा भवेत् सुखम्।। ५७।।

In a world full of ignorancc and with cxtrcmc paucity of knowledge, happiness comes only when sorrow is removed (destroyed). The *Ātman*, however, is ever happy.—57

यस्मान्नाशितमज्ञानं ज्ञानेन विश्वकारणम्।
तस्मादात्मा भवेज्ज्ञानं ज्ञानं तस्मात् सनातनम्।। ५८।।

When ignorance is dispelled by knowledge, and that knowledge removes the cause of world phenomena, the *Ātman* itself becomes knowledge, and that knowledge is everlasting.—58

कालतो विविधं विश्वं यदा चैव भवेदिदम्।
तदेकोऽस्ति स एवात्मा कल्पनापथवर्जितः।। ५९।।

Just as the universe is one, although it appears different in the course of time, in the same manner the *Ātman* is one when it is withdrawn from the path of (deluded) imagination.—59

न खं वायुर्न चाग्निश्च न जलं पृथिवी न च।
नैतत्कार्यं नेश्वरादि पूर्णैकात्मा भवेत् किल।। ६०।।

Neither the sky, air, fire, water and earth nor their work, nor even the gods are perfect. The *Ātman* alone is (perfect).—60

बाह्यानि सर्वभूतानि विनाशं यान्ति कालतः।
यतो वाचो निवर्त्तन्ते आत्मा द्वैतविवर्जितः।। ६१।।

All the externally seen things are destroyed in course of time. The *Ātman* alone is without duality and beyond words.—61

आत्मानमात्मनो योगी पश्यत्यात्मनि निश्चितम्।
सर्वसंकल्पसंन्यासी त्यक्त्वामिथ्याभवग्रहः।। ६२।।

Divested of all desires and abandoning the false world phenomena, the yogi clearly perceives his own Self as the *Ātman*.—62

आत्मनात्मनि चात्मानं दृष्ट्वानन्तं सुखात्मकम्।
विस्मृत्य विश्वं रमते समाधेस्तीव्रतस्तथा।। ६३।।

Having perceived his own Self as the *Ātman*, which bestows eternal bliss, he dwells in intense ecstasy (*samādhi*) and is oblivious of the world.—63

मायैव विश्वजननी नान्या तत्वधिया परा।
यया नाशं समायाति विश्वं नास्ति तदा खलु।। ६४।।

Māyā (illusion) is the mother of world phenomena. There is nothing truer than this. When this (*māyā*) is removed, the world phenomena cease to exist.—64

हेयं सर्वमिदं यत्तु मायाविलसितं यतः।
ततो न प्रीतिविषयस्तनुवित्त सुखात्मकः।। ६५।।

All these that are invested with *māyā* are to be rejected (by the yogi). Hence pleasurable things like the body (senses) and wealth cannot be the harbinger of (real) happiness.—65

अरिमित्रमुदासीनं त्रिविधं स्यादिदं जगत्।
व्यवहारेषु नियतं दृश्यते नान्यथा पुनः।। ६६।।

प्रियाप्रियाभेदस्तु वस्तुषु नियतस्फुटम्।
आत्मोपाधि वशादेवं भवेत् पुत्रोऽपि नान्यथा।। ६७।।

This world is of three kinds: adverse, friendly and indifferent. Only through dealings do they appear as such, not otherwise. They are agreeable or disagreeable according to one's own reflected ego. Even in the case of one's own son it is not otherwise.—66 and 67

मायाविलसितं विश्वं ज्ञात्वैव श्रुतियुक्तितः।
अध्यारोपापवादाभ्यां लयं कुर्वन्ति योगिनः।। ६८।।

Recognizing the world as one invested with *māyā*, the yogi rids himself of all aberrations and fallacies in accordance with the directions of the Śrutis.—68

कर्मजन्यमिदं विश्वं मत्त्वा कर्माणि वेदतः।
निखिलोपाधिविजितो यदा भवति पुरुषः।
तदा विवक्षतेऽखण्ड ज्ञानरूपी निरञ्जनः।। ६९।।

When the Self has triumphed over all attributes of Nature—i.e. after realizing that the world phenomena are the product of *karma* and the character of those *karma*—only then does it shine fully as the Clear Light of Knowledge.—69

सो कामयतः पुरुषः सृजते च प्रजा स्वयम्।
अविद्या भासते यस्मात् तस्मान्मिथ्या स्वभाविनी।। ७०।।

That Self, moved by volition, creates its own offsprings (in the mind). Wherever ignorance prevails, the same is bound to be false.—70

शुद्धब्रह्मत्वसम्बन्धो विद्यया सहितो भवेत्।
ब्रह्म तेन सती याति यत आभासते नभः।। ७१।।

Pure (attributeless) Brahman is ever associated with knowledge (consciousness). When that (consciousness) is immanent, Brahman appears as Void (space).—71

तस्मात् प्रकाशते वायुर्वायोरग्निस्ततो जलम्।
प्रकाशते ततः पृथ्वी कल्पनेयं स्थिताऽसती।। ७२।।

From that (space) appears air, and from air fire, from fire water, and from that earth. These remain non-activated and rooted in the imagination.—72

आकाशाद्वायुराकाशपवनादग्नि सम्भव:।
खं-वाताग्नेर्जलं व्योमवाताग्निवारितो मही।। ७३।।

From space is born air; space and air produce fire; then space, air and fire (produce) water, while earth is formed by space, air, fire and water.—73

खं शब्दलक्षणं वायुश्चञ्चल: स्पर्शलक्षण:।
स्याद्रूपलक्षणन्तेज: सलिलं रसलक्षणम्।। ७४।।
गन्धलाक्षणिका पृथ्वी नान्यथा भवति ध्रुवम्।
विशेषणो गुणस्फूर्त्तिर्यत: शास्त्राद्विनिर्णय:।। ७५।।

Sound is the character of space; touch the character of air in motion; form is the character of fire; succulence of water, and smell of earth. This is always so, and this does not change. The *śāstras* have determined that the character of a quality is its effect.—74 and 75

स्यादेकगुणमाकाशं द्विगुणो वायुरुच्यते।
तथैव त्रिगुणं तेजो भवन्त्यापश्चतुर्गुणा:।। ७६।।
शब्द: स्पर्शश्च रूपञ्च रसोगन्धस्तथैव च।
एतत् पञ्चगुणा पृथ्वी कल्पकै: कल्प्यतेऽधुना।। ७७।।

Space has one quality (viz., sound), the air two (sound+touch), fire three (sound + touch + form), water four (sound + touch + form + succulence), and earth five (sound + touch + form + succulence + smell). Such a five-elemental world has now been determined by the sages.—76 and 77

चक्षुषा गृह्यते रूपं गन्धो घ्राणेन गृह्यते।
रसो रसनया स्पर्शस्त्वचा सगृह्यते परम्।। ७८।।
श्रोत्रेण गृह्यते शब्दो नियतं भाति नान्यथा।। ७९।।

Form is perceived by eyes, smell by the nose, succulence by tongue, touch by the skin and sound by the ears. These are the conclusions (of the sages) and can never be otherwise.—78 and 79

चैतन्यात् सर्वमुत्पन्नं जगदेतच्चराचरम्।
अस्ति चेत् कल्पनेयं स्यान्नास्ति चेदस्ति चिन्मय:।। ८०।।

Out of consciousness is born all the moving and non-moving world. When imagined, those (world phenomena) exist; when not, they are but Pure Knowledge.—80

पृथ्वी शीर्णा जलेमग्ना जलं मग्नञ्च तेजसि।
लीनं वायौ तथा तेजो व्योम्नि वातोलयं ययौ।
अविद्यायां महाकाशो लीयते परमे पदे।। ८१।।

When the earth dissolves into water, and water into fire, fire into air and air into sky, then through illusion the entire space is withdrawn into the Supreme.—81

विक्षेपावरणा शक्तिर्दुरन्ता सुखरूपिणी।
जड़रूपा महामाया रजःसत्वतमो गुणाः।। ८२।।

The Great Illusion has powers of manifestation (expansion), mystery (concealment), irresistible force and bliss, as well as the material qualities of purity (*sattva*), motion (*rajas*) and inertia (*tamas*).—82

सा मायावरणाशक्त्यावृता विज्ञानरूपिणी।
दर्शयेज्जगदाकारं तं विक्षेपस्वभावतः।। ८३।।

That mystic veil of *māyā* (illusion), when invested with force (*śakti*) and knowledge (*vijñāna*), appears in the shape of this world and is manifested naturally.—83

तमोगुणाधिका विद्या सा दुर्गा भवेत् स्वयम्।
ईश्वरस्तदुपहितं चैतन्यं तदभूद् ध्रुवम्।। ८४।।
रजोगुणाधिका विद्या ज्ञेया वै सा सरस्वती।
यच्चित्स्वरूपी भवति ब्रह्मा तदुपधायिका।। ८५।।
सत्वाधिका च या विद्या लक्ष्मीः दिव्यरूपिणी।
चैतन्यं तदुपहितं विष्णुर्भवति नान्यथा।। ८६।।

The knowledge that has more of *tamas* (inertia) in it takes the form of Durgā (Pārvatī), while that which is invested with consciousness is the Supreme (Śiva). A knowledge that has more of *rajas* (forcc) in it should be known as Saraswatī, the mind form created by Brahmā, while the one that has an excess of *sattva* (purity) in it is Lakṣmī, endowed with the attribute of intelligence of Viṣṇu.—84–86

ईशाद्याः सकला देवा दृश्यन्ते परमात्मनि।
शरीरादि जड़ं सर्वं सा विद्या तत्तथा तथा।। ८७।।

(In this way) Śiva and the other gods are all seen in the Paramātman (Supreme), and all material objects, like the physical body, etc., are known accordingly.—87

एतं रूपेण कल्पन्ते कल्पकाः विश्वसम्भवम्।
तत्वातत्वं भवन्तीह कल्पनान्योन्यचोदिता।। ८८।।

In this manner the visualizers (sages) have visualized the possibility (creation) of the universe. It is the sequence of imagination that turns these into actuality or otherwise.—88

प्रमेयत्वादि रूपेण सर्ववस्तु प्रकाशते।
तथैव वस्तु नास्त्यैव भासको वर्त्तते परम्।। ८९।।
स्वरूपत्वेन रूपेण स्वरूपं वस्तु भास्यते।
विशेषशब्दोपादाने भेदो भवति नान्यथा।। ९०।।

All things become apparent when they are cognized. Hence there is nothing that really exists. The Supreme alone exists; He is the illuminator of all things. Objects appear in their own form because of the form in which they are imagined and the particular words that are assigned to them.—89 and 90

एकः सत्तापूरितानन्दरूपः पूर्णो व्यापी वर्त्तते नास्ति किञ्चित्।
एतज्ज्ञानं यः करोत्येव नित्यं मुक्तः स स्यान्मृत्युसंसारदुःखात्।। ९१।।

He who is ever conscious of the One as the essence of Complete, Bliss and All-Pervading and nothing else, becomes free from death and sorrows in this world.—91

यस्यारोपापवादाभ्यां यत्र सर्वे लयं गताः।
स एको वर्त्तते नान्यत् तच्चित्तेनावधार्यते।। ९२।।

That which ordains and dissolves everything at will is but One, not many. This must be firmly held in the mind.—92

पितुरन्नमयात् कोषाज्जायते पूर्वकर्मतः।
तच्छरीरं विदुर्दुःखं स्वप्राग्भोगाय सुन्दरम्।। ९३।।

The physical body is produced out of a cell from the father's (body) which had been nourished by food. Know that beautiful body to be the inheritor of sorrows resulting from past *karma*.—93

मांसास्थिस्नायुमज्जादि निर्मितं भोगमन्दिरम्।
केवलं दुःखभोगाय नाडीसन्ततिगुम्फितम्।। ९४।।

Made of flesh, bones, nerves, marrow, etc., and veins spread all over, this body is built only for the experiencing of sorrows.—94

पारमेष्ट्यमिदं गात्रं पञ्चभूतविनिर्मितम्।
ब्रह्माण्डसंज्ञकं दुःखसुखभोगाय कल्पितम्।। ९५।।

The Creator has created this body out of the five Elements and in the concept of the Universe. It has been designed so that sorrows and pleasures may be experienced in it.—95

विन्दुः शिवो रजः शक्तिरूभयोर्मेलनात् स्वयम्।
स्वप्रभूतानि जायन्ते स्वशक्त्या जड़रूपया।। ९६।।

Inanimate physical matter becomes sentient and self-conscious as a result of combination of the seminal seed (sperm), representing Lord Śiva, and the ovum, representing Śakti (Pārvatī).—96

तत्पञ्चीकरणात् स्थूलान्यसंख्यानि समासते।
ब्रह्माण्डस्थानि वस्तूनि यत्र जीवोऽस्ति कर्मभिः।। ९७।।

The numerous gross objects in the universe are all formed in accordance with the five-fold law (of contraction, expansion, attraction, repulsion and motion). In their midst the living creature exists as ordained by its *karma.*—97

तद्भूतपञ्चकात् सर्वं भोगाख्यं जीवसंज्ञकम्।
पूर्वकर्मानुरोधेन करोमि घटनामहम्।। ९८।।

All who are designated as creatures are the product of that five-fold action, and exist for the purpose of experiencing (sorrow and pleasure). Events are caused by Me in accordance with their previous *karma.*—98

अजड़ः सर्वभूतस्थो जड़स्थित्या भुनक्ति तत्।
जड़ात् स्वकर्मभिर्बद्धो जीवाख्यो विविधो भवेत्।। ९९।।

The animate (Self) in all creatures experiences (sorrows and pleasures) by dwelling in the inanimate (physical body). Bound by its own *karma,* the inanimate assumes different forms.—99

भोगायोत्पद्यते कर्म ब्रह्माण्डाख्ये पुनः पुनः।
जीवश्च लीयते भोगावसाने च स्वकर्मभिः।। १००।।

It is due to this experiencing that fresh *karma* as produced again and again in the matrix of the universe. Hence when such experiencing (of the fruits of *karma*) are over, along with *karma* that caused them, the creature ceases to be (i.e., merges in the Supreme Being).—100

Here ends chapter I of *Śivasamhitā,* entitled
'The Path of Harmony'.

CHAPTER II

Fundamentals of Yoga

देहेस्मिन् वर्त्तते मेरुः सप्तद्वीप समन्वितः।
सरितः सागराः शैलाः क्षेत्राणि क्षेत्रपालकः।। १।।

Within this body dwells the mountain of Meru, and it is surrounded by seven islands as well as lakes, seas, hills, plains and their presiding deities.—1

ऋषयो मुनयः सर्वे नक्षत्राणि ग्रहास्तथा।
पुण्यतीर्थानि पीठानि वर्त्तन्ते पीठदेवता।। २।।

Also there dwell *ṛṣis* (conveyers of knowledge), *munis* (sages) and all the stars and planets, holy places of pilgrimage and temples, as well as the gods residing in those temples.—2

सृष्टिसंहारकर्तारौ भ्रमन्तौ शशिभास्करौ।
नभोवायुश्च वह्निश्च जलं पृथ्वी तथैव च।। ३।।

(In this body) wander the sun and the moon—the cause of creation and destruction. In the same way there are the five elements—the sky, air, fire, water, and earth.—3

त्रैलोक्यांने भूतानि तानि सर्वांनि देहतः।
मेरुं संवेष्टय सर्वत्र व्यवहारः प्रवर्त्तते।। ४।।

All creatures that exist in the three worlds (heaven, earth and hell) are also in this very body. Those are attached to the Mt. Meru (represented by the spinal column) and are ever engaged in doing their own duties.—4

जानाति यः सर्वमिदं स योगी नात्र संशयः।। ५।।

He who knows all this is undoubtedly a yogi.—5

ब्रह्माण्डसंज्ञिते देहे यथा देशे व्यवस्थितः।
मेरुशृङ्गे सुधारश्मी द्विरष्टकलायुतः।। ६।।

In this universe-patterned body, each of these objects is located in its own place. At the top of the Meru mountain (spinal column) is the moon, casting down its light of sixteen *kalās** (phases).—6

वर्त्ततेऽहर्निशं सोऽपि सुधां वर्षत्यधोमुखः।
ततोऽमृतं द्विधाभूतं याति सूक्ष्मं यथा च वै।। ७।।

This moon is constantly pouring down its ambrosian gleam which, bifurcating further down, assumes a subtle form.—7

इड़ामार्गेण पुष्ट्यर्थं याति मन्दाकिनीजलम।
पुष्णाति सकलं देहमिड़ामार्गेण निश्चितम्।। ८।।

One shaft (of the moon's ray) goes through the channel of Iḍā** like the waters of the Mandākinī, and as it goes along, it nourishes the entire structure of the body.—8

एष पीयूषरश्मिर्हि वामपार्श्वेव व्यवस्थितः।
अपरः शुद्धदुग्धाभो हर्षकर्षितमण्डलः।
मध्यमार्गेण सृष्ट्यर्थं मेरौ संयाति चन्द्रमाः।। ९।।

This ambrosian shaft is directed down the left. The other one—pure, milky and infused with bliss—enters the central passage of the spinal column (*meru*) to which the moon is attached, and it is meant for the purpose of creation.—9

मेरुमूले स्थितः सूर्यः कलाद्वादशसंयुतः।
दक्षिणे पथि रश्मिभिर्वहत्यूर्द्ध्वं प्रजापतिः।। १०।।

At the base of the spinal column is stationed the sun, with its twelve attributes.† It is the lord of creation, and its rays shoot upward through the right channel (i.e., the Piṅgalā nerve).—10

पियूषरश्मिनिर्यासं धातूंश्च ग्रसति ध्रुवम्।
समीरमण्डलैः सूर्यो भ्रमते सर्वविग्रहे।। ११।।

As the sun wanders across the space within the body, the essence of its ambrosian rays permeates the substance (*dhātus*‡) of the body.—11

*The sixteen *kalās* of the moon are from New Moon to Full Moon, both inclusive.

**Iḍā is the psychic nerve on the left side of the body. On the right is the Piṅgalā and in the centre, threading through the spinal column, is the Suṣumnā.

The upper reaches of the river Ganges, flowing over the mountain bed, is known as the Mandākinī. Its water is always crystal clear.

†The twelve *kalās* of the sun are its twelve characters as it passes through the twelve signs of the Zodiac in the course of one year.

‡*Dhātus* or constituents of the body are seven in number, viz., flesh, bone, marrow, fat, blood, lymph, and seminal fluid.

एषा सूर्यापरामूर्त्तिः निर्वाणं दक्षिणे पथि।
वर्त्तते लग्नयोगेन सृष्टिसंहारकारकः।। १२।।

This is the psychic form of the sun that sets on the right side of the body and is the means of creation and destruction. It appears in the body at the appropriate time.—12

सार्धलक्षत्रयं नाड्यः सन्ति देहान्तरे नृणाम्।
प्रधानभूता नाड्यस्तु तासु मुख्याश्चतुर्दश।। १३।।

There are three and a half lakh channels (physical and psychic nerves) within man's body. Of these fourteen are principal.—13

सुषुम्नेडा पिङ्गला च गान्धारी हस्तिजिह्विका।
कुहूः सरस्वती पूषा शङ्खिनी च पयस्विनी।। १४।।
वारुण्यलम्बुषा चैव विश्वोदरी यशस्विनी।
एतासु तिस्रो मुख्यास्युः पिंङ्गलेड़ासुषुम्निका।। १५।।

(Their names are) Suṣumnā, Iḍā, Piṅgalā, Gāndhārī, Hastijihvā, Kuhū, Saraswatī, Pūṣā, Śaṅkhinī, Payaswinī, Vāruṇi, Alambuṣā, Viśwodarī, and Yaśaswinī. Of these only three—Piṅgalā, Iḍā and Suṣumnā—are important.—14 and 15

तिसृष्वेका सुषुम्नैव मुख्या सा योगवल्लभा।
अन्यास्तदाश्रयं कृत्वा नाड्यः सन्ति हि देहिनाम्।। १६।।

Of these three, Suṣumnā is the main that is specially chosen for the purpose of yoga. The others exist in the body with its support.—16

सर्वाश्चाधोमुखा नाड्यः पद्मतन्तुनिभाः स्थिताः।
पृष्ठवंशं समाश्रित्य सोमसूर्याग्निरूपिणी।। १७।।

All these downward nerves are thin as fibres of a lotus, and hang down from the spinal column in the form of the sun, the moon and fire.—17

तासां मध्ये गता नाड़ी चित्रा सा मम वल्लभा।
ब्रह्मरन्ध्रञ्च तत्रैव सूक्ष्मात् सूक्ष्मतरं गतम्।। १८।।

Of these the middle one—Citrā* or Suṣumnā—is the most dear to Me. It is finer than fine, and through it goes the Brahma-randhra (Passage of Knowledge).—18

*Citrā or Citrinī is another name for the Suṣumnā *nāḍī*, which is also sometimes called Sāvitrī (*savitṛ*, generator, mother).

पञ्चवर्णोज्ज्वला शुद्धा सुषुम्ना मध्यचारिणी।
देहस्योपाधिरूपा सा सुषुम्नमध्यरूपिणी।। १९।।

Five-coloured, bright and pure, the Suṣumnā* takes the middle path. Holding as it does a central position, it forms the staff of life.—19

दिव्यमार्गमिदं प्रोक्तममृतानन्दकारकम्।
ध्यानमात्रेण योगीन्द्रो दुरितौघं विनाशयेत्।। २०।।

It has been described as the Divine Way and the cause of Eternal Bliss. By meditating upon it the yogis are able to destroy all sins and impiety.—20

गुदात्तु द्वयङ्गुलादूर्द्धं मेढ्रात्तुद्वयङ्गुलादधः।
चतुरङ्गुलं विस्तारमाधारं वर्त्तते समम्।। २१।।

Two finger-width above the anus and half a finger-width away from the genitals is a four-finger wide base (for the Suṣumnā).**—21

तस्मिनाधारपाथोजे कर्णिकायां सुशोभना।
त्रिकोणावर्त्तते योनिः सर्वतन्त्रेषु गोपिता।। २२।।

In the core of that Mūlādhāra lotus there is a beautiful little triangular cavity, which is the secret of all Tantras.—22

तत्र विद्युल्लताकारा कुण्डली परदेवता।
सार्धत्रिकारा कुटिला सुषुम्नामार्गसंस्थिता।। २३।।

There abides, coiled three and a half times and like a flexible electric cord, the presiding deity (Serpent Power) guarding the path of the Suṣumnā.—23

जगत्संसृष्टिरूपा सा निर्माणे सततोद्यता।
वाचामवाच्या वाग्देवी सदा देवैर्नमस्कृता।। २४।।

Representing creation of the world, she is constantly engaged in the act of creation. She is the goddess of speech, beyond words (indescribable), and is adored by the gods as such.—24

इड़ानाम्नी तु या नाड़ी वाममार्गे व्यवस्थिता।
सुषुम्नां सा समाश्लिष्य दक्षनासापुटं गता।। २५।।

*Suṣumnā, which reflects the sun, carries the five principal colours of the rainbow, viz., red, purple, blue, green, and yellow.

**Sacrum (L. = sacred bone) is a triangular-shaped bone at the tail-end of the spine. It is the root-support for Suṣumnā where is located the Mūlādhāracakra.

A finger-width is about 1.5 centimetre.

Iḍā, the *nāḍī* placed on the left, intertwines with the Suṣumnā, and then reaches the right nostril.—25

पिङ्गलानाग या नाड़ी दक्षमार्गे व्यवस्थिता।
मध्यनाड़ीं समाश्लिष्य वामनासापुटं गता।। २६।।

The *nāḍī* named Piṅgalā is placed on the right. It too intertwines the Suṣumnā and goes up to the left nostril.—26

इड़ापिङ्गलोर्मध्ये सुषुम्ना या भवेत् खलु।
षट्स्थानेषु च षट्शक्तिं षट्पद्मं योगिनो विदुः।। २७।।

Thus wedged in between Iḍā and Piṅgalā, the Suṣumnā *nāḍī* carries six lotuses, endowed with six *śaktis* (forces) at six points. These only the yogis know.—27

पञ्चस्थानसुषुम्नाया नामानि स्युर्बहूनि च।
प्रयोजनवशात्तानि ज्ञातव्यानीह शास्त्रके।। २८।।

The other five points* (excluding Mūlādhāra) have many names, which will be revealed in this *śāstra* as and when necessary.—28

अन्या यास्त्यपरा नाड़ी मूलाधारात् समुत्थिता।
रसनामेढ्रवृषनपादाङ्गुष्ठं च नासिकाम्।। २९।।
कुक्षिनेत्राङ्गुष्ठकर्णं सर्वाङ्गं पायुकुक्षिकम्।
लब्ध्वा निवर्त्तते सा वै यथादेशसमुद्भवा।। ३०।।

Apart from these, the other *nāḍīs* that originate from the Mūlādhāra reach the various parts of the body like eyes, ears, nose, tongue, fingers, stomach, intestines, genitals, thumbs and toes, and then return to the source (i.e., Mūlādhāra).—29 and 30

एताभ्य एव नाड़ीभ्यः शाखोपशाखतः क्रमात्।
सार्धलक्षत्रयं जातं यथाभागव्यवस्थितम्।। ३१।।

Branching off progressively, these *nāḍīs* become three and a half lakhs in number and occupy their respective position in the body.—31.

एता भोगवहा नाड्यो वायुसंचाररक्षकाः।
ओतप्रोताभिसंव्याप्य तिष्ठन्त्यस्मिन् कलेवरे।। ३२।।

These activated nerves sustain the respiration, and they dwell in the body as its warp and woof.—32

*The other five points or *cakras* are: Swādhiṣṭhāna, Maṇipura, Anāhata, Viśuddha and Ājñā. The seventh *cakra*, Sahasrāra, is at the brain-centre.

सूर्यमण्डलमध्यस्थ कला द्वादश संयुत:।
बस्तिदेशे ज्वलद्वह्निर्वर्त्तते चान्नपाचक:।। ३३।।
वैश्वानराग्निर्विज्ञेयो मम तेजोंशसम्भव:।
करोति विविधं पाकं प्राणिनां देहमास्थित:।। ३४।।

The food-consuming fire (heat) that dwells inside the bowels is composed of the twelve attributes of the sun. The cosmic fire is only a part of My effulgence. It is I who transmute matter within the body of all creatures.—33 and 34

आयु:प्रदायको वह्निर्वलं पुष्टिं ददाति च।
शरीरपाटवञ्चापि ध्वस्तरोगसमुद्भव:।। ३५।।

This fire is the bestower of strength, vigour and longevity. It nourishes the body and makes it possible for it to resist disease.—35

तस्माद्वैश्वानराग्निञ्च प्रज्वाल्य विधिवत् सुधी:।
तस्मिन्नन्नं हुनेत् योगी प्रत्यहं गुरुशिक्षया।। ३६।।

Hence, by igniting that cosmic fire (within the body) the wise yogi, as directed by his guru, properly consumes his food every day.—36

ब्रह्माण्डसंज्ञके देहे स्थानानि स्युर्बहूनि च।
मयोक्तानि प्रधानानि ज्ञातव्यानीह शास्त्रके।। ३७।।

(In fact) in this cosmically-constituted body there are many points (organs), but I have spoken only of the main ones necessary for the understanding of this yoga-*śāstra*.—37

नानाप्रकारनामानि स्थानानि विविधानि च।
वर्त्तन्ते विग्रहे तानि कथितुं नैव शक्यते।। ३८।।

These exist in the body under different names and are located at various spots, which I need not describe just now.—38

इत्थं प्रकल्पिते देहे जीवो वसति सर्वग:।
अनादिवासनामालाऽलंकृत: कर्मभृङ्खल:।। ३९।।

Within the body thus visualized dwells the *Ātman*, which is chained to it by *karma*, and is adorned with a necklace of endless desires.—39

नानाविधगुणोपेत: सर्वव्यापारकारक:।
पूर्वार्ज्जितानि कर्माणि भुनक्ति विविधानि च।। ४०।।

In this way a creature is invested with various qualities that cause all the events for it. It thus experiences the fruits accrued to it from its own previous *karma.*—40

यद्यत् संदृश्यते लोके सर्वं तत् कर्मसम्भवम्।
सर्वान् कर्मानुसारेण जन्तुर्भोगान् भुनक्ति वै।। ४१।।

Whatever are seen in this world as a creature's experiences are really the product of its own *karma,* experienced by it now in accordance with the law of *karma.*—41

ये ये कामादयो दोषाः सुखदुःखप्रदायकाः।
ते ते सर्वे प्रवर्त्तन्ते जीवकर्मानुसारतः।। ४२।।

Frailties such as passion etc. are the cause of all pleasures and pains. All these (pleasures and pains) prevail in accordance with the law of *karma.*—42

पुण्योपरक्तचैतन्यैः प्राणान् प्रीणाति केवलम्।
वाह्ये पुण्यमयं प्राप्य भोज्यवस्तु स्वयंभवेत्।। ४३।।

A mind endowed with virtue always causes a thing to take a virtuous shape—one that is suitable for its enjoyment and such as would please the heart.—43

ततः कर्मबलात् पुंसः सुखम्वा दुःखमेव वा।
पापोपरक्तचैतन्यं नैव तिष्ठति निश्चितम्।। ४४।।

In the same way a vice-infested mind never stays peaceful (i.e., it causes pain). Thus men experience pleasure and pain through the force of *karma.*—44

न तद्भिन्नो भवेत् सोऽपि न तद्भिन्नन्तु किञ्चन।
मायोपहितचैतन्यात् सर्ववस्तु प्रजायते।। ४५।।

It is never otherwise; nor is there anything else than that. All things grow out of a *māyā*-captivated mind.—45

यथा कालोपभोगाय जन्तूनां विविधोद्भवः।
यथा दोषवशच्छुक्तौ रजतारोपणं भवेत्।
तथा स्वकर्मदोषाद्वै ब्रह्मण्यारोप्यते जगत्।। ४६।।

Just as time is experienced by different beings in different ways, and just as, owing to illusion, a piece of white shell (mother-of-pearl) is confused with silver—in the same way, due to the fault of one's own *karma,* the Brahman gets obscured by world phenomena.—46

सवासना भ्रमोत्पन्नोन्मूलनातिसमर्थनम्।
उत्पन्नञ्चेदीदृशं स्यात् ज्ञानं मोक्षप्रसाधनम्।। ४७।।

The delusion born of one's own desires cannot be uprooted wholly. However when this sort of knowledge (i.e., the consciousness of delusion) dawns, then that becomes a means of deliverance (*mokṣa*).—47

साक्षाद्विशेषदृष्टिस्तु साक्षात्कारिणि विभ्रमे।
कारणं नान्यथा युक्त्या सत्यं सत्यं मयोदितम्।। ४८।।

The cause of delusion lies in the particular perspective of the viewer; it is not linked to anything else, I tell you truly.—48

साक्षात्कारभ्रमं साक्षात् साक्षात्कारिणि नाशयेत्।
स हि नास्तीति संसारे भ्रमो नैव विवर्त्तते।। ४९।।

The viewer's delusion can be dispelled only by recognizing the reality. There is nothing in this world that is not obscured by delusion.—49

मिथ्याज्ञाननिवृत्तिस्तु विशेष दर्शनाद्भवेत्।
अन्यथा न निवृत्तिस्याद्दृष्यते रजतभ्रमः।। ५०।।

The delusion can be dissolved only by specific observation. Otherwise, when left unresolved, the same may cause (as stated earlier) a white shell to be mistaken for silver.—50

यावन्नोत्पद्यते ज्ञानं साक्षात्कारे निरञ्जने।
तावत् सर्वाणि भूतानि दृष्यन्ते विविधानि च।। ५१।।

So long as the Reality is not seen, and knowledge is gained thereby, everything and all beings appear in their diverse forms.—51

यदा कर्मार्जितं देहं निर्वाणसाधनं भवेत्।
तदा शरीरवहनं सफलं स्यान्न चान्यथा।। ५२।।

When this body, acquired as a result of *karma*, is made a means for achieving *nirvāṇa*, then only it becomes worthwhile; not otherwise.—52

यादृशी वासनामूला वर्त्तते जीवसङ्गिनी।
तादृशं वहते जन्तुः कृत्याकृत्य विधौ भ्रमम्।। ५३।।

Whatever be the basic desire of a creature, the same becomes its life companion. It moves through life accordingly, subjected to the delusions of right and wrong.—53

संसारसागरं तर्तुं यदीच्छेद्योगसाधकः।
कृत्वा वर्णाश्रमं कर्म फलवर्जं समाचरेत्।। ५४।।

Hence a yogi desirous of crossing this ocean of *saṃsāra* (world phenomena) should perform deeds (*karma*) befitting his position in life, but without expecting their fruit.—54

विषयासक्तपुरुषा विषयेषु सुखेप्सवः।
वचोभिरुद्धनिर्वाणाद्वर्त्तन्ते पापकर्मणि।। ५५।।

People attached to worldly attractions and desiring pleasure from those, persist in their evil deeds despite the good advice given in the scriptures regarding *nirvāṇa*.—55

आत्मानमात्मना पश्यन्न किञ्चिदिह पश्यति।
तदा कर्मपरित्यागे न दोषोऽस्ति मतं मम।। ५६।।

When one sees one's own Self only and nothing else, then, in My view, there is no harm if the performance of all deeds (good as well as evil) is abandoned.—56

कामादयो विलीयन्ते ज्ञानादेव न चान्यथा।
अभावे सर्वतत्वानां समं तत्वं प्रकाशते।। ५७।।

All desires disappear only through knowledge. When the sense of plurality fades away, the light of Oneness dawns.—57

Here ends chapter II of *Śivasaṃhitā* entitled
'Fundamentals of Yoga'.

CHAPTER III

The System and its Practice

हृद्यस्ति पंकजं दिव्यं दिव्यलिङ्गेन भूषितम्।
कादिठान्ताक्षरोपेतं द्वादशार्णविभूषितम्।। १।।

Inside the heart there is a divine lotus, endowed with divine glory, that has twelve petals, each indicating the twelve letters beginning with *ka* (क) and ending with *ṭha* (ठ).*—1

प्राणो वसति तत्रैव वासनाभिरलंकृतः।
अनादिकर्मसंश्लिष्टः प्राप्याहंकारसंयुतः।। २।।

There, co-mingled with desires that accumulate as a result of innumerable past *karma,* and invested with egoism, dwells the *prāṇa* (the vital force).—2

प्राणस्य वृत्तिभेदेन नामानि विविधानि च।
वर्त्तन्ते तानि सर्वाणि कथितुं नैव शक्यते।। ३।।

This *prāṇa* assumes different names in accordance with the different propensities (prevailing in the body). It is not possible for Me to describe all of those here.—3

प्राणोऽपानः समानश्चोदानो व्यानश्च पञ्चमः।
नागः कूर्मश्च कृकरो देवदत्तो धनञ्जयः।। ४।।

Prāṇa, apāna, samāna, udāna, and *vyāna* are the five (inflowing airs). *Nāga, kūrma, kṛkara, devadatta,* and *dhanañjaya* are the other five (outflowing airs).—4

दशनामानि मुख्यानि मयोक्तानीह शास्त्रके।
कुर्वन्ति तेऽत्र कार्याणि प्रेरितानि स्वकर्मभिः।। ५।।

*The letters are mystic symbols (16 vowels and 34 consonants) used to indicate the character of each psychic centre within the body. These letters invested with sound, are also the basis of *mantras* that are recited to invoke psychic power.

These are the principal ten names mentioned by Me in this *śāstra*. Propelled by one's own *karma*, these operate here (within the body).—5

अत्रापि वायवः पञ्च मुख्या स्युर्दशतः पुनः।
तत्रापि श्रेष्ठकर्तारौ प्राणापानौ मयोदितौ।। ६।।

Of these ten airs, the first five are more important. And, out of these, *prāṇa* and *apāna* are of the utmost significance.—6

हृदि प्राणो गुदेऽपानः समानो नाभिमण्डले।
उदानो कंठदेशस्थो व्यानं सर्वशरीरगः।। ७।।

Prāṇa flows into the heart, *apāna* to the anus, *samāna* to the navel, *udāna* to the throat, while *vyāna* pervades the entire body.—7

नागादि वायवः पञ्च कुर्वन्ति ते च विग्रहे।
उद्गारोन्मीलनं क्षुत्तृद् जृम्भा हिक्का च पञ्च वै।। ८।।

The five (outflowing) *nāga* and other airs cause (the following reflex actions): belching, batting of eye-lids, craving for food and water, yawning or sneezing, and hiccoughing.—8

अनेन विधिना यो वै ब्रह्माण्डं वेत्ति विग्रहम्।
सर्वपापविनिर्मुक्तः स याति परमां गतिम्।। ९।।

He who sees the universe thus represented in his own body reaches the Ultimate, being rid of all sins.—9

अधुना कथयिष्यामि क्षिप्रं योगस्य सिद्धये।
यज्ज्ञात्वा नावसीदन्ति योगिनो योगसाधने।। १०।।

Now I shall disclose a speedy method for the mastery of yoga. By knowing this the yogi would not be ever discouraged in the practice of yoga.—10

भवेद्वीर्यवती विद्या गुरुवक्त्रसमुद्भवा।
अन्यथा फलहीना स्यान्निर्वीर्या चातिदुःखदा।। ११।।

Knowledge that flows from the mouth of a guru alone bears fruit. Others, that are weak and tiresome, prove fruitless.—11

गुरुं सन्तोष्य यत्नेन यो वै विद्यामुपासते।
अविलम्बेन विद्यायास्तस्याः फलमवाप्नुयात्।। १२।।

He who gets his knowledge after meticulously satisfying his guru receives the fruit of that knowledge before long.—12

गुरुः पिता गुरुर्माता गुरुर्देवो न संशयः।
कर्मणा मनसा वाचा तस्मात् सर्वैः प्रसेव्यते।। १३।।

Undoubtedly the guru is like father, mother and god. Hence he should be obeyed by all in word, deed and thought.—13

गुरुः प्रसादतः सर्वं लभ्यते शुभमात्मनः।
तस्मात् सेव्यो गुरुर्नित्यमन्यथा न शुभं भवेत्।। १४।।

Through the guru's favour one may obtain all the beneficial things. The guru, therefore, must always be obeyed, or else nothing shall be beneficial.—14

प्रदक्षिणं त्रयं कृत्वा स्पृष्ट्वा सव्येन पाणिना।
प्रदक्षिणं नमस्कुर्यात् गुरोः पादसरोरुहम्।। १५।।

The lotus feet of the guru should be touched with the right hand after going round him thrice. Thereafter obeisance should be paid after going round once more.—15

श्रद्धयात्मवतां पुंसां सिद्धिर्भवति निश्चिता।
अन्येषाञ्च न सिद्धिः स्यात्तस्माद्यत्नेन साधयेत्।। १६।।

Success positively comes to the person who has faith and confidence in himself; others do not succeed. Hence it is necessary always to practise with confidence.—16

न भवेत् संज्ञयुक्तानां तथाविश्वासिनामपि।
गुरुपूजाविहीनानां तथा च वहुसंज्ञिनाम्।। १७।।
मिथ्यावादरतानाञ्च तथा निष्ठुरभाषिणाम्।
गुरुसन्तोषहीनानां न सिद्धिः स्यात् कदाचन।। १८।।

Success never comes to those who are worldly-minded, who lack faith, who do not adore the guru, who have many attachments, who are involved in fruitless disputes, who speak harshly, and also those who have failed to gain the grace of the guru.—17 and 18

फलिष्यतीति विश्वासः सिद्धेः प्रथमलक्षणम्।
द्वितीयं श्रद्धयायुक्तं तृतीयं गुरुपूजनम्।। १९।।
चतुर्थं समताभावं पञ्चमेन्द्रियनिग्रहम्।
षष्ठञ्च प्रमिताहारं सप्तमं नैव विद्यते।। २०।।

Full confidence that the practice (of yoga) shall succeed, is the first sign of success. The second is stability of that faith. The third is adoration of the guru; the fourth equanimity; the fifth control over the senses, and the sixth reduction in diet. There is no seventh (other) sign.—19 and 20

योगोपदेशं संप्राप्य लब्ध्वा योगविदं गुरुम्।
गुरूपदिष्टविधिना धिया निश्चित्य साधयेत्।। २१।।

After finding a yoga-qualified guru and obtaining yoga instructions from him, one should practise according to the directions given by the guru, diligently and with faith.—21

सुशोभने मठे योगी पद्मासनसमन्वितः।
आसनोपरि संविश्य पवनाभ्यास समाचरेत्।। २२।।
समकायः प्राञ्जलिश्च प्रणम्य च गुरून् सुधीः।
दक्षे वामे च विघ्नेशक्षेत्रपालाम्बिकां पुनः।। २३।।

Seated in Padmāsana (cross-legged posture) in a congenial place, the yogi should practise (correct) breathing, holding the body erect and yet at ease, but first after bowing to the wise guru and to Gaṇeśa (Destroyer of Hindrances) on the right and Ambikā (Durgā) and the Kṣetrapāla (deity presiding over all regions, i.e., Śiva).—22 and 23

ततश्च दक्षाङ्गुष्ठेन निरुद्ध्य पिङ्गला सुधीः।
इडया पूरयेद्वायुं यथाशक्त्या तु कुम्भयेत्।। २४।।
ततस्त्यक्त्वा पिङ्गलया शनैरेव न वेगतः।
पुनः पिङ्गलयापूर्य यथाशक्त्या तु कुम्भयेत्।। २५।।

Thereafter the yogi should block the right nostril (entrance to the Piṅgalā nerve) with his right thumb, and then take in air through the left nostril (entrance to the Iḍā nerve); then holding this air inside as long as possible, release the same slowly (i.e., not too quick) through the right nostril. And again, taking in air through the right nostril, and holding it as long as possible, perform the *kumbhaka.**—24 and 25

इडया रेचयेद्वायुं न वेगेन शनैः शनैः।
एवं योगविधानेन कुर्याद्विंशति कुम्भकम्।। २६।।

When releasing the air through Iḍā it should not be quick, but gradual. In this manner the *kumbhaka* should be performed twenty times.—26

*Holding or retention of breath inside the lungs is called *kumbhaka* (potted).

सर्वद्वन्द्वविनिर्मुक्तः प्रत्यहं विगतालसः।
प्रातःकाले च मध्याह्ने सूर्यास्ते चार्धरात्रिके।
कुर्यादेवं चतुर्वारं कालेष्वेतेषु कुम्भकान्।। २७।।

Freeing the mind of all worries this type of *kumbhaka* should be practised four times every day—morning, mid-day, evening, and midnight—without fail.—27

इत्थं मासत्रयं कुर्यादनालस्यं दिने दिने।
ततो नाडी विशुद्धिः स्यादविलम्बेन निश्चितम्।। २८।।

When this has been practised diligently and regularly for three months, the *nāḍīs* will get positively purified before long.—28

यदा तु नाडी शुद्धिः स्याद्योगिनस्तत्वदर्शिनः।
तदा विध्वस्तदोषश्च भवेदारम्भकुम्भकः।। २९।।

And when the *nāḍīs* of the yoga-aspirant become pure, then it will be possible for him to start the practice of proper *kumbhaka.*—29

चिन्हानि योगिनो देहे दृश्यन्ते नाडिशुद्धितः।
कथ्यन्ते तु समस्तान्यङ्गानि संक्षेपतो मया।। ३०।।

As a result of the *nāḍīs* getting cleansed, certain signs become apparent in the body of the yogi. These I shall describe in brief.—30.

समकायः सुगन्धिश्च सुकान्तिः स्वरसाधकः।
प्रौढवह्नि सुभोगी च सुखी सर्वाङ्गसुन्दरः।। ३१।।

The body becomes supple, complexion bright, the voice resonant and breath fragrant. His appetite increases, he is cheerful and contented, and all his limbs work in good order.—31

सम्पूर्णहृदयो योगी सर्वोत्साहबलान्वितः।
जायते योगिनोऽवश्यमेते सर्वकलेवरे।। ३२।।

Due to these (improvements) the yogi is always joyful at heart, optimistic and strong in all parts of his body.—32

आरम्भश्च घटश्चैव तथा परिचयस्तदा।
निष्पत्तिः सर्वयोगेषु योगावस्था भवन्ति ताः।। ३३।।

There are four stages in the practice of yoga—the beginning, the *ghaṭa* (i.e., *kumbhaka*), its mastery, and the end.—33

आरम्भः कथितोऽस्माभिरधुना वायुसिद्धये।
अपरं कथ्यते पश्चात् सर्वदुःखौघनाशकम्।। ३४।।

I have already spoken about the beginning. The mastery of breath and others which dispel the sorrows and afflictions will be related later.—34

अथ वर्ज्यं प्रवक्ष्यामि योगविघ्नकरं परम्।
येन संसारदुःखाब्धिं तीर्त्वा यास्यन्ति योगिनः।। ३५।।

Now I shall describe those things which are obstacles in the way of yoga and which should therefore be avoided. These are the ones by crossing which the yogi goes beyond the ocean of sorrows and afflictions of the world.—35

अम्लं रुक्षं तथा तीक्ष्णं लवणं सार्षपं कटुम्।
बहूलभ्रमणं प्रातःस्नानं तैलविदाहकम्।। ३६।।
स्तेयं हिंसा जनद्वेषञ्चाहंकारमनार्जवम्।
उपवासमसत्यञ्च मोहञ्च प्राणिपीडनम्।। ३७।।
स्त्रीसंगमग्निसेवाञ्च वह्वालापं प्रियाप्रियम्।
अतीवभोजनं योगी त्यजेदेतानि निश्चितम्।। ३८।।

The yogi should positively renounce food that is sour, acrid, hot (peppery), saline, bitter, pungent or fried in oil, as well as things like fasting, early morning bath, vagrancy, stealing, violence, jealousy, pride, cheating, lying, cruelty to animals, company of women, too many acquaintances, gossip or argumentative talks, fire-tending, craving and gluttony.—36–38

उपायञ्च प्रवक्ष्यामि क्षिप्रं योगस्य सिद्धये।
गोपनीयं साधकानां येन सिद्धिर्भवेत् खलु।। ३९।।

And now I am disclosing a quick way to achieve success in yoga. But if it is to be really (fully) mastered, it must be kept a secret.—39

घृतं क्षीरञ्च मिष्टान्नं ताम्बूलं चूर्णवर्जितम्।
कर्पूरं निष्ठुरं मिष्टं सुमठं सूक्ष्मवस्त्रकम्।। ४०।।
सिद्धान्तश्रवणं नित्यं वैराग्यगृहसेवनम्।
नामसंकीर्त्तनं विष्णोः सुनादश्रवणं परम्।। ४१।।
धृतिः क्षमा तपः शौचं ह्रीमतिर्गुरुसेवनम्।
सदैतानि परं योगी नियमानि समाचरेत्।। ४२।।

He who follows these rules, viz., use of only clarified butter, milk, sweet preparations, betel-leaves without lime, camphor, water (soft and dirt-free), a congenial place of abode, frugal dress, regular study of scriptures, singing the praises of the Lord, listening to sweet music, serving the guru humbly and with contentment, and practising forgiveness, austerity and purity of mind—is the best among yogis.—40–42

अनिलेऽर्कप्रविष्टे च भोक्तव्यं योगिभिः सदा।
वायौ प्रविष्टे शशिनि शीयते साधकोत्तमैः।। ४३।।

The yogi should always take his meals when the air (breath) enters the sun (i.e., Piṅgalā). When the air enters the moon (Iḍā) the conscientious yogi goes to bed.*—43

सद्योभुक्तेऽपिक्षुदिते नाभ्यासः क्रियते बुधैः।
अभ्यासकाले प्रथमं कुर्यात् क्षीराज्यभोजनम्।। ४४।।

The wise yogi should not practise (breathing exercises) either immediately after meals or on an empty stomach. Before starting the practice some milk product may be taken.**—44

ततोभ्यासे स्थिरीभूते न तादृङ्नियमग्रहः।
अभ्यासिना विभोक्तव्यं स्तोकं स्तोकमनेकधा।
पूर्वोक्तकाले कुर्याच्च कुम्भकान् प्रतिवासरे।। ४५।।

These restrictions may be relaxed once the exercises are fully mastered. But such relaxation should be gradual, when the yogi may eat various items of food in increasing quantities. Before that (i.e., until the thing has been mastered) the practice of *kumbhaka* must continue every day as stated before.—45

ततो यथेष्टा शक्तिः स्याद्योगिनो वायुसाधने।
यथेष्टं धारणाद्वायोः कुम्भकः सिध्यति ध्रुवम्।
केवले कुम्भके सिद्धे किं न स्यादिह योगिनः।। ४६।।

Thereafter, when the yogi has acquired a good deal of strength through practice and is able to hold his breath for a considerable period, the *kumbhaka* may be deemed to have been mastered.

*As a rule food should be taken only when the breath passes through the right nostril. It helps digestion. When the air flows naturally through the left nostril it is the proper condition for sleep. This, of course, does not apply to the period when breathing exercises are being practised.

**Breathing exercise, when practised soon after a meal, may lead to some respiratory trouble. Similarly, when practised on an empty stomach, it may cause consumption because of the abnormal strain on the system during low vitality.

Then, as a result of this mastery of *kumbhaka*, what cannot the yogi do?—46

स्वेदः संजायते देहे योगिनः प्रथमोद्यमे।
यदा संजायते स्वेदो मर्दनं कारयेत् सुधीः।
अन्यथा विग्रहे धातुर्नष्टो भवति योगिनः।। ४७।।

At the first attempt (of *kumbhaka*) sweat is produced in the body of the yogi. When this sweat appears the wise yogi should rub his body, so that its vitality is not lost.—47

द्वितीये हि भवेत् कम्पो दार्दूरो मध्यमे अतः।
ततोऽधिकतराभ्यासाद् गगनेचर साधकः।। ४८।।

At the second stage there is shivering in the body. Thereafter jerks, like the hopping of frogs, is felt. A longer practice would bring to the yogi the ability to float in air.—48

योगी पद्मासनस्थोऽपि भुवनुत्सृज्य वर्त्तते।
वायुसिद्धिस्तदा ज्ञेया संसारध्वान्तनाशिनी।। ४९।।

When the yogi is able to rise above terra firma while still in his Padmāsana, know that to be the mastery of the breath. It also dispels his ignorance about world phenomena.—49

तावत्कालं प्रकुर्वीत योगोक्तनियमग्रहम्।
अल्पनिद्रा पुरीषञ्च स्तोकं मूत्रञ्च जायते।
अरोगित्वमदीनत्वं योगिनस्तत्वदर्शनम्।। ५०।।
स्वेदो लाला कृमिश्चैव सर्वथैव न जायते।
कफपित्तानिलाश्चैव साधकस्य कलेवरे।। ५१।।
तस्मिन् काले साधकस्य भोज्येष्वनियमग्रहः।
अत्यल्प बहुधा भुक्त्वा योगी न व्यथते हि सः।। ५२।।

The yogi should continue practising this until such symptoms as scanty sleep, scanty excretion and scanty urine do not appear, and the body rendered free of all diseases and pains, all kinds of sweat, saliva and germs disappear and phlegm, bile, air, etc. are fully controlled. Until then the yogi must observe the diet restrictions. After that, more or less quantity of food should not trouble the yogi.—50–52

अथाभ्यासवशाद् योगी भूचरीं सिद्धिमाप्नुयात्।
येन दुर्धषजन्तूनां गतिः स्यात् पाणिताडनात्।। ५३।।

As a result of this practice the yogi gets the power of *bhūcara*,* which enables him to beat off ferocious beasts with a mere clap of the hands.—53

सन्त्यत्र बहवो विघ्ना दारुणा दुर्निवारणाः।
तथापि साधयेद्योगी प्राणैः कण्ठगतेरपि।। ५४।।

At this stage several serious obstacles arise which are difficult to overcome. But despite these, the yogi must continue the practice even though his very life may be at stake!—54

ततो रहस्युपाविष्टः साधकः संयतेन्द्रियः।
प्रणवं प्रजपेद्दीर्घं विघ्नानां नाशहेतवे।। ५५।।

Yet the yogi should sit in a solitary place, control his senses, repeat *Aum* (the mystic name of God) for a long time in order to demolish all the obstacles.—55

पूर्वार्जितानि कर्माणि प्राणायामेन निश्चितम्।
नाशयेत् साधको धीमानिहलोकोद्भवानि च।। ५६।।

By means of *prāṇāyāma* (breath-control) the wise yogi is then able to destroy positively all his *karma* acquired in previous lives as well as those that have now accrued (in this life).—56

पूर्वार्जितानि पापानि पुण्यानि विविधानि च।
नाशयेत् षोडश प्राणायामेन योगीपुङ्गवाः।। ५७।।

Expert yogis can destroy all previously-earned virtue and vice by means of sixteen *prāṇāyāmas* only.—57

पापतूलचयानाहो प्रदहेत् प्रलयाग्निना।
ततः पापविनिर्मुक्तः पश्चात् पुण्यानि नाशयेत्।। ५८।।

Sins get burnt up even as a heap of cotton gets consumed by devastating fire. Thereafter, with sins gone, even the virtues are destroyed.—58

प्राणायामेन योगीन्द्रो लब्ध्वैश्वर्याष्टकानि वै।
पापपुण्योदधिं तीर्त्वा त्रैलोक्यचरतामियात्।। ५९।।

After gaining the eight supernormal powers** by means of

***Bhūcarī* are animals that move about on land, as opposed to *khecarī*, i.e., those that fly in the air and *jalacara*, the denizens of water.

**The eight *aiśwarya* or supernormal powers are: (1) Aṇimā (minuteness or invisibility), (2) Mahimā (expansion or infinity), (3) Laghimā (weightlessness), (4) Garimā (excessive weight or gravity), (5) Prākāmya (irresistible will), (6) Iśittva (supermacy), (7) Kāmavasāya (total control of senses), and (8) Vaśittva (fascination or instant hypnotism).

prāṇāyāma, the expert yogi is able to move about freely in all three worlds, having crossed the ocean of virtue and vice.—59

ततोऽभ्यासक्रमेणैव घटादित्रितयं भवेत्।
येन स्यात् सकला सिद्धिर्योगिनस्त्वीप्सिता ध्रुवम्।। ६०।।

By such regular practice the yogi is able to complete all three stages of *prāṇāyāma*—the beginning, the intermediate and the end. Thereafter all the desired powers are positively within his control.—60

वाक्सिद्धिः कामचारित्वं दूरदृष्टिस्तथैव च।
दूरश्रुतिः सूक्ष्मदृष्टिः परकायप्रवेशनम्।। ६१।।
विन्मूत्रलेपने स्वर्णमदृश्यकरणं तथा।
भवन्त्येतानि सर्वाणि खेचरत्वञ्च योगिनाम्।। ६२।।

Powers such as prophesying, automation (moving at will), seeing the invisible, hearing the inaudible, pre-cognition, entry into another body, transforming excretion into gold and power to vanish then become possible for the yogi.—61 and 62

यदा भवेद्घटावस्था पवनाभ्यासिनः परा।
तदा संसारचक्रेऽस्मिन् तन्नास्ति यन्न साधयेत्।। ६३।।

When the yogi reaches the highest form of breath-control, i.e., *ghaṭa* or *kumbhaka*, then there is nothing whatsoever in this world that he may not be able to master.—63

प्राणापानौ नादबिन्दु जीवात्मपरमात्मनौ।
मिलित्वा घटते यस्मात्तस्माद्वै घट उच्यते।। ६४।।

It is called *ghaṭa* (created) because the five constituents, viz., *prāṇa* (expiration), *apana* (inspiration), *nada-vindu* (sound-matter), *jīvātma* (individual self) and *Paramātma* (Universal Self) conjoin to create it.—64

याममात्रं यदा धर्त्तुं समर्थः स्यात्तदाद्भुतः।
प्रत्याहारस्तदैव सान्नान्तरो भवति ध्रुवम्।। ६५।।

When it is possible to hold on to this state (of *kumbhaka*) for at least one *yāma**, then *pratyāhāra*** results; this is positive.—65

*One *yāma* equals three hours or one-eighth of a day. It is also known as *prahara*.

***Pratyāhāra* is control of the senses, so that they do not respond to external objects.

यं यं जानाति योगीन्द्रस्तं तमात्मेति भावयेत्।
यैरिन्द्रियैर्विधानज्ञस्तदिन्द्रियजयो भवेत्।। ६६।।

Thereafter whatever object the yogi perceives the same appears to him as the *Ātman*. His senses, being well regulated, are now fully under control.—66

याममात्रं यदा पूर्णं भवेदभ्यासयोगतः।
एकवारं प्रकुर्वीत तदा योगी च कुम्भकम्।। ६७।।
दण्डाष्टकं यदा वायुर्निश्चलो योगिनो भवेत्।
स्वसामर्थ्यात्तदाङ्गुष्ठे तिष्ठेद्वा तूलवत् सुधीः।। ६८।।

As soon as proficiency has been gained in holding the breath for one *yāma*, the yogi may limit the performance of *kumbhaka* to once a day only. When the yogi is able to hold his breath for eight *daṇḍas**, he becomes as light as cotton and can hold his own weight upon his thumb!—67 and 68

ततः परिचयावस्था योगिनोऽभ्यासतो भवेत्।
यदा वायुश्चन्द्रसूर्यं त्यक्त्वा तिष्ठति निश्चलम्।। ६९।।

Thereafter, as a result of constant practice, the yogi attains the state of *paricaya* (familiarity). At this stage the breath leaves the Iḍā (moon) and Piṅgalā (sun) channels and stays steady.—69

वायुः परिचितो वायुः सुषुम्नाव्योम्नि संचरेत्।
क्रियाशक्तिं गृहीत्वैव चक्रान् भित्वा सुनिश्चितम्।। ७०।।

When the air becomes 'familiar' it enters the opening of the Suṣumnā (within the spinal column) and, getting activated there, it then pierces through the *cakras* positively.—70

यदा परिचयावस्था भवेदभ्यासयोगतः।
त्रिकूटं कर्मणां योगी तदा पश्यति निश्चितम्।। ७१।।

In this *paricaya* state, which results from regular practice, the yogi becomes conscious of the triple character (*trikūṭam***) of *karma* that has entrapped him into his body.—71

ततश्च कर्मकूटानि प्रणवेन विनाशयेत्।
स योगी कर्मभोगाय कायव्यूहं समाचरेत्।। ७२।।

Hence, while trying to demolish this transmutation of *karma* by

*One *daṇḍa* equals 24 minutes. It is the same as *ghatikā*.

** *Trikūṭam* signifies the transmutation of *karma* through the process of the three primal qualities (*guṇas*)—*sattva, rajas* and *tamas*—which binds the Self to the body.

reciting *Praṇava* (*Auṃ*), the yogi constructs within himself (a sort of) an inner fortress, so that his *karma* may get consumed within it.—72

अस्मिन् काले महायोगी पञ्चधा धारणाञ्चरेत्।
येन भूरादिसिद्धिः स्यात् तत्तद्भूतभयापहा।। ७३।।

During this period the good yogi should contemplate upon the Five Elements, so that when earth, fire, etc. are mastered there is no fear of any harm from these.—73

आधारे घटिका पञ्च लिङ्गस्थाने तथैव च।
तदूर्द्ध्वं घटिका पञ्च नाभौ हृन्मध्यके तथा।। ७४।।
भ्रूमध्योर्द्ध्वे तथा पञ्च घटिका धारयेत् सुधीः।
तथा भरादिना नष्टो योगीन्द्रो न भवेत् खलु।। ७५।।

The wise yogi should concentrate for five *ghatikās* (i.e., two hours) on each of the following *cakras* within his body: Mūlādhāra placed at the sacrum, Swādhiṣṭhāna at the base of the genitals, Maṇipura near the navel, Anāhata near the heart, Viśuddha near the throat, and Ājñāpura between the eyebrows. When this is done, the yogi becomes immune to the ravages caused by earth, water, fire, etc.—74 and 75

मेधावी पञ्चभूतानां धारणां यः समभ्यसेत्।
शतब्रह्मगतेनापि मृत्युस्तस्य न विद्यते।। ७६।।

One who diligently practises such concentration on the Five Elements becomes immortal. There is no death for him even in a hundred of Brahmā's days.*—76

ततोऽभ्यासक्रमेणैव निष्पत्तिर्योगिनो भवेत्।
अनादिकर्मबीजानि येन तीर्त्वामृतं पिवेत्।। ७७।।

In this way, and after constant practice, the yogi completes his task of ending the eternal flow of *karma* and then, by thus crossing over, he drinks the ambrosia of immortality.—77

यदा निष्पत्तिर्भवति समाधेः स्वेन कर्मणा।
जीवन्मुक्तस्य शान्तस्य भवेद्धीरस्य योगिनः।। ७८।।
यदा निष्पत्तिसम्पन्नः समाधिः स्वेच्छया भवेत्।

*One day of Brahmā the creator, also called a *kalpa*, equals 8,640,000,000 years on earth. Obviously, eternity is implied.

गृहीत्वा चेतनां वायुः क्रियाशक्तिञ्च वेगवान्।
सर्वान् चक्रान् विजित्वाशु ज्ञानशक्तौ विलीयते।। ७९।।

When he has completed the work of ending *karma*, and has reached *samādhi*, the yogi becomes free of the bondage of life and is perfectly serene and peaceful. Upon such completion, *samādhi* comes automatically when the vital air (*prāṇa*), gaining consciousness, force and speed, forges through all the *cakras* and finally merges with the force of Knowledge.—78 and 79

इदानीं क्लेशहान्यर्थं वक्तव्यं वायुसाधनम्।
येन संसारचक्रेऽस्मिन् भोगहानिर्भवेत् ध्रुवम्।। ८०।।

And now I shall relate the several methods of breath-control, by practising which all sufferings can be ended and the cycle of births and deaths snapped positively.—80

रसनां तालुमूले यः स्थापयित्वा विचक्षणः।
पिवेत् प्राणानिलं तस्य रोगाणां संक्षयो भवेत्।। ८१।।

By holding the tongue against the palate and then slowly drawing in the vital air (*prāṇa*), the expert yogi can get rid of all his ailments.—81

काकचञ्च्वा पिवेद्वायुं शीतलं वा विचक्षणः।
प्राणापानविधानज्ञः स भवेन्मुक्तिभाजनः।। ८२।।

Again, the expert yogi who knows how to draw in cool air through the lips shaped like a crow's beak, and also the way to control his inspiration and expiration, is the one who is qualified for *mukti* (deliverance).—82

सरसं यः पिवेद्वायुं प्रत्यहं विधिना सुधीः।
नश्यन्ति योगिनस्तस्य श्रमदाहजरामयाः।। ८३।।

All fatigue, restlessness, debility and diseases disappear when the yogi meticulously practises this sucking in of succulent air every day.—83

रसनामूर्ध्वगां कृत्वा यश्चान्द्रसलिलं पिवेत्।
मासत्रयेण योगीन्द्रो मृत्युं जयति निश्चितम्।। ८४।।

The good yogi who, by turning up the tongue, tastes the ambrosia dripping from the moon,* will undoubtedly conquer death within a month.—84

*Moon is the symbol of intelligence in the mind.

राजदन्तबिलं गाढं सम्पीड्य विधिना पिवेत्।
ध्यात्वा कुण्डलिनीं देवीं षण्मासेन कविर्भवेत्।। ८५।।

(Similarly) when air is taken in after firmly pressing the tip of the tongue into the gap near the front teeth, and at the same time meditating on the goddess Kuṇḍalinī,* the yogi becomes omniscient within six months.—85

काकचञ्च्वा पिवेद्वायुं सन्ध्ययोरुभयोरपि।
कुण्डलिन्या मुखे ध्यात्वा क्षयरोगस्य शान्तये।। ८६।।

To cure wasting diseases suck in every morning and evening cool air through the lips shaped like a crow's beak (i.e., as while whistling), and meditating at the same time on the image of the Kuṇḍalinī.—86

अहर्निशं पिवेद्योगी काकचञ्च्वा विचक्षणः।
दूरश्रुतिर्दूरदृष्टिस्तथा स्याद्दर्शनं खलु।। ८७।।

The expert yogi who does this constantly, soon acquires the powers of hearing the inaudible, seeing the invisible, and of becoming invisible himself.—87

दन्तैर्दन्तान् समापीड्य पिवेद्वायुं शनैः शनैः।
उर्द्ध्वजिह्वासुमेधावी मृत्युं जयति सोऽचिरात्।। ८८।।

The wise yogi who drinks in air very slowly, keeping both sets of teeth well pressed and the tongue upturned, conquers death before long.—88

षण्मासमात्रमभ्यासं यः करोति दिने दिने।
सर्वपापविनिर्मुक्तो रोगान्नाशयते हि सः।। ८९।।

He who is able to practise this evey day for six months gets rid of all his ailments and becomes free of all his ills.—89

संवत्सरकृताभ्यासात् भैरवो भवति ध्रुवम्।
अणिमादिगुणान् लब्ध्वा जितभूतगणः स्वयम्।। ९०।।

After practising this for a whole year he gets all the supernormal powers of Aṇimā, etc. and having also triumphed over all Five Elements, he becomes a Bhairava** himself.—90

*Kuṇḍalinī or Serpent Power is the psychic force that lies concentrated, like a coiled serpent, at the base of the spinal column.

**Bhairava is the mighty form of the Lord Siva and is identified by its eight humours, viz. *aśitāṅga* or dark body, *ru-ru* or stern appearance, *kupita* or frown, *krodhan* or anger, *caṇḍa* or aggressive mood, *unmatta* or furious mood, *bhīṣana* or terrible mood and *saṅghāra* or destructive mood.

रसनामूर्द्धगां कृत्वा क्षणार्द्धं यदि तिष्ठति।
क्षणेन मुच्यते योगी व्याधिमृत्युजरादिभिः।। ९१।।

If the yogi is also able, at the same time (i.e., while taking in air through lips formed like a crow's beak), to hold his tongue upturned even for half a moment, he gets immunity from disease, old age and death.—91

रसनां प्राणसंयुक्तां पीड्यमानां विचिन्तयेत्।
न तस्य जायते मृत्युः सत्यं सत्यं मयोदितम्।। ९२।।

Verily I say unto thee, the yogi who (regularly) meditates with his tongue upturned while drawing in the air at the same time never, never meets with death.—92

एवमभ्यासयोगेन कामदेवो द्वितीयकः।
न क्षुधा न तृषा निद्रा नैव मूर्च्छा प्रजायते।। ९३।।

By such practice of yoga one gets an unparalleled complexion like that of a second Kāmadeva (Cupid), and then he is no longer susceptible to hunger, thirst, sleep or swoon.—93

अनेनैव विधानेन योगीन्द्रोऽवनिमण्डले।
भवेत् स्वच्छन्दचारी च सर्वापत्परिवर्जितः।। ९४।।

As a result of these practices the expert yogi gets the power to move at will on earth, free of all hindrances.—94

न तस्य पुनरावृत्तिर्मोदते स सुरैरपि।
पुण्यपापैर्न लिप्येत ह्येतदाचरणेन सः।। ९५।।

He is then not reborn on this earth and, being no longer involved in righteous and unrighteous deeds, is happy like the gods.—95

चतुरशीत्यासनानि सन्ति नानाविधानि च।
तेभ्यश्चतुष्कमादाय मयोक्तानि ब्रवीम्यहम्।
सिद्धासनं तथा पद्मासनञ्चोग्रञ्च स्वस्तिकम्।। ९६।।

Āsanas are 84 in number and these are of many types. Of these four are principal, which I am describing. These are Siddhāsana, Padmāsana, Ugrāsana, and Swastikāsana.—96

योनिं संपीड्य यत्नेन पादमूलेन साधकः।
मेढ्रोपरि पादमूलं विन्यसेत् योगवित्सदा।। ९७।।
दृष्ट्या निरीक्ष्य भ्रूमध्यं निश्चलः संयतेन्द्रियः।

विशेषोऽवक्रकायश्च रहस्युद्वेगवर्जितः।। ९८।।
एतत् सिद्धासनं ज्ञेयं सिद्धानां सिद्धिदायकम्।
येनाभ्यासवशात् शीघ्रं योगनिष्पत्तिमाप्नुयात्।। ९९।।

The yogi should first draw up one leg over the opposite thigh, pressing the perineum firmly with the heel of that foot. Next, the other leg should be brought up, and with this heel the genitals should be covered up. Thereafter, controlling the senses and keeping the mind undistracted, he should fix his thought steadily upon a point between the eyebrows. All the while the body should be kept erect, and the place where this is practised should be lonely and undisturbed. A Siddhāsana performed in this manner easily brings to the yogi the desired occult powers and the yoga is soon completed.—97–99

सिद्धासनं सदा सेव्यं पवनाभ्यासिभिः परम्।
येन संसारमुत्सृज्य लभ्यते परमा गतिः।। १००।।

This Siddhāsana is best suited for those who wish to practise breath-control. It helps one to cross the ocean of world phenomena and reach the highest goal.—100

नातः परतरं गुह्यमासनं विद्यते भुवि।
येनानुध्यानमात्रेण योगी पापाद्विमुच्यते।। १०१।।

There is no other *āsana* than this (Siddhāsana) that is prized more in this world. Even the very thought of it saves the yogi from sins.—101

उत्तानौ चरणौ कृत्वा ऊरुसंस्थौ प्रयत्नतः।
ऊरुमध्ये तथोत्तानौ पाणी कृत्वा तु तादृशौ।। १०२।।
नासाग्रे विन्यसेद् दृष्टिं दन्तमूलञ्च जिह्वया।
उत्तभ्य चिवुकं वक्ष उत्थाप्य पवनं शनैः।। १०३।।
यथा शक्त्या समाकृष्य पूरयेदुदरं शनैः।
यथा शक्त्या ततः पश्चात् रेचयेदविरोधतः।। १०४।।
इदं पद्मासनं प्रोक्तं सर्वव्याधिविनाशनम्।
दुर्लभं येन केनापि धीमता लभ्यते परम्।। १०५।।

Draw up both legs, and place them upon opposite thighs with the sole turned up. Let the hands rest upon the thighs, with palms similarly turned up. Then, pressing the gums with the tongue, fix the gaze on the tip of the nose. Thereafter, throw out the chest, lower the chin over it and draw in air slowly, filling the lungs to the maximum capacity. Later release the same slowly but continuously. This is called Padmāsana. It cures all types of diseases. Though rather difficult for common people, the wise yogi is able to grasp all this very well.—102–5

अनुष्ठाने कृते प्राणः समश्चलति तत्क्षणात्।
भवेदभ्यासने सम्यक साधकस्य न संशयः।। १०६।।

When this (Padmāsana) is practised, the vital air promptly gets regulated, and there is no doubt that with regular practice it can be fully controlled by the yogi.—106

पद्मासने स्थितो योगी प्राणापानविधानतः।
पूरयेत् स विमुक्तः स्यात् सत्यं सत्यं वदाम्यहम्।। १०७।।

Verify I say unto thee, the yogi who practises *prāṇāyāma* while seated in Padmāsana is soon released from his bondage.—107

प्रसार्य चरणद्वन्द्वं परस्परमसंयुतम्।
स्वपाणिभ्यां दृढं धृत्वा जानूपरि शिरो न्यसेत्।। १०८।।
आसनोग्रमिदं प्रोक्तं भवेदनिलदीपनम्।
देहावसादहरणं पश्चिमोत्तानसंज्ञकम्।। १०९।।

Spread out both legs, keeping them together, then place the head upon the knees, with hands holding the feet. This is called Ugrāsana. It builds up nervous energy and removes lethargy from the body. It is also known by the name of Paścimottama.*—108 and 109

य एतदासनं श्रेष्ठं प्रत्यहं साधयेत् सुधीः।
वायुः पश्चिममार्गेण तस्य सञ्चरति ध्रुवम्।। ११०।।

The yogi who practises this excellent *āsana* every day will be definitely able to get the *prāṇa* to enter the Suṣumnā *nāḍī*.—110

एतदभ्यासशीलानां सर्वसिद्धिः प्रजायते।
तस्माद्योगी प्रयत्नेन साधयेत् सिद्धिसाधकः।। १११।।

Those who practise this (Ugrāsana) get all the supernormal powers. Hence a yogi desiring success must diligently master this.—111

गोप्तव्यं सुप्रयत्नेन न देयं यस्य कस्यचित्।
येन शीघ्रं मरुतसिद्धिर्भवेद् दुःखौघनाशिनी।। ११२।।

*Cf. *GS*, II.20.

This *āsana* should be carefully kept a secret and not divulged to all and sundry. This is an *āsana* by which the control of breath is mastered, ending the endless stream of sorrows.—112

जानूर्वोरन्तरे सम्यक् कृत्वा पादतले उभे।
समकायः सुखासीनः स्वस्तिकं तत् प्रवक्ष्यते।। ११३।।

Insert the two feet into the opposite knee-bends, and then sit erect in an easy (relaxed) pose. This is called Swastikāsana.—113

अनेन विधिना योगी मारुतं साधयेत् सुधीः।
देहे न क्रमते व्याधिस्तस्य वायुश्च सिद्ध्यति।। ११४।।

When the wise yogi practises breath-control in this manner (i.e., sitting in Swastikāsana) his body is no longer afflicted by diseases and he soon masters the breath-control.—114

सुखासनमिदं प्रोक्तं सर्वदुःखप्रणाशनम्।
स्वस्तिकं योगिभिर्गोप्यं स्वस्थीकरणमुत्तमम्।। ११५।।

Being the destroyer of all afflictions, it is also called Sukhāsana (Posture of Comfort). This Swastikāsana is unknown to most yogis. However, it is the best means of keeping oneself in a healthy state.—115

Here ends chapter III of *Śivasaṃhitā*, entitled
'The System and its Practice'.

CHAPTER IV

Postures and Preludes

आदौ पूरकयोगेन स्वाधारे पूरयेन्मनः।
गुदमेढ्रान्तरे योनिस्तमाकुञ्च्य प्रवर्त्तते।। १।।

In the beginning (i.e., after getting into the appropriate sitting posture) concentrate the mind on the Mūlādhāracakra with the help of a *pūraka,** contracting at the same time the perineum.—1

ब्रह्मयोनिगतं ध्यात्वा कामं बन्धूकसन्निभम्।
सूर्यकोटिप्रतीकाशं चन्द्रकोटिसुशीतलम्।। २।।
तस्योर्द्ध्वे तु शिखा सूक्ष्मा चिद्रूपा परमा कला।
तथापिहितमात्मानमेकीभूतं विचिन्तयेत्।। ३।।

Next, visualize the Kuṇḍalinī**: fragrant like the *bandhūka* flower and entering the Brahma-mārga, illumined with the radiance of a thousand suns and moons, at the upper end of which shines a fine taper of light symbolizing Knowledge in its brightest form. Contemplate your *Ātman* to be there, as though it were wrapped in unison with this Knowledge.—2 and 3

गच्छन्ति ब्रह्ममार्गेण लिङ्गत्रयक्रमेण वै।
अमृतं तद्विसर्गस्थं परमानन्दलक्षणम्।। ४।।

Then the three forms of one's existence[+] (physical, mental and

**Pūraka* is the filling in of breath through the left nostril while the right one is blocked with thumb. The exercise suggested here is apparently meant to rouse the Kuṇḍalinī, which lies dormant within the Mūlādhāra *cakra.*

**Here the word *kāma* has been used to indicate Kuṇḍalinī, which in fact is the esoteric symbol of seminal seed transmuted into psychic force. Brahma-mārga or Brahmarandhra is the median nerve (Suṣumnā) which threads through the spinal column and is known as the Passage of Knowledge.

[+]*Linga-traya* represents the three forms of existence—physical, mental and causal—in each of which the Self stays by turn. These are also known as *sthūla śarīra, sūkṣma śarīra* and *kāraṇa śarīra.*

causal) are experienced, as though these were moving up this Passage and seeking the ambrosia of extreme bliss that oozes from the moon on top of the brain.—4

श्वेतरक्तं तेजसाढ्यं सुधाधारा प्रवर्षिणम्।
पीत्वा कुलामृतं दिव्यं पुनरेव विशेत् कुलम्।। ५।।

This Kuṇḍalinī, in the form of a rosy, energy-filled stream of nectar, goes up to the other end (i.e., Sahasrāra), tastes the divine ambrosia there and returns back to her place.—5

पुनरेव कुलं गच्छेन्मात्रायोगेन नान्यथा।
सा च प्राणसमा ख्याता ह्यस्मिंतन्त्रे मयोदितं।। ६।।
पुनः प्रलीयते तस्यां कालाग्न्यादि शिवात्मकम्।। ७।।

Repeatedly it goes up in spurts, not otherwise. This flow has been described in this *śāstra* as the vital force. Finally the Kuṇḍalinī* merges into and is lost in the fire of Knowledge, which is the *Ātman.*— 6 and 7

योनिमुद्रा परा ह्येषा बन्धस्तस्या प्रकीर्त्तितः।
तस्यास्तु बन्धमात्रेण तन्नास्ति यन्न साधयेत्।। ८।।

This Yonimudrā (i.e., the technique of rousing the Kuṇḍalinī) is superb for the purpose of capturing her (Kuṇḍalinī). And when she is captured, what else cannot be mastered by the yogi?—8

छिन्नरूपास्तु ये मन्त्राः कीलिताः स्तम्भिताश्च ये।
दग्धमन्त्राः शिखाहीना मलिनास्तु तिरस्कृताः।। ९।।
मन्दा बालास्तथा वृद्धाः प्रौढायौवनगर्विताः।
अरिपक्षे स्थिता ये च निर्वीर्याः सत्त्ववर्जिताः।। १०।।
तथा सत्वेनहीना ये खण्डिताः शतधाकृताः।
विधानेन तु संयुक्ताः प्रभवन्ति चिरेण तु।। ११।।
सिद्धिमोक्षप्रदाः सर्वे गुरुणा विनियोजिताः।। १२।।
दीक्षयित्वा विधानेन अभिषिच्य सहस्रधा।
ततो मन्त्राधिकारार्थमेषा मुद्रा प्रकीर्त्तिताः।। १३।।

Instructions regarding the practice of this (Yonimudrā) remain either incomplete, partial, routine, defective, weak, vague, condemned, or are tardy, immature, antiquated (obsolete) and over-

*Kuṇḍalinī or the transmuted sex-energy is esoterically described as Śakti, consort of Śiva. The latter is represented by the *Ātman* dwelling in the brain-centre (Sahasrāra) where Śakti unites with Śiva.

zealous, or are harmful, fruitless, devoid of good points and scrappy (broken into innumerable bits) unless those are imparted according to rules, when they become effective. For purposes of mastery of the yoga, the instructions must be imparted by a guru only. When these are properly given with a thousand blessings from him, then only they become fruitful and then only this posture can be rightly called the Yonimudrā.—9–13

ब्रह्महत्यासहस्राणि त्रैलोक्यमपि घातयेत्।
नासौ लिप्यति पापेन योनिमुद्रानिबन्धनात्।। १४।।

With the performance of this Yonimudrā one is absolved of all sins, even though he may have killed a thousand Brahmins or harmed everybody in the three worlds.—14

गुरुहा च सुरापी च स्तेयी च गुरुतल्पगः।
एतैः पापैर्न बद्धेत योनिमुद्रानिबन्धनात्।। १५।।

Killing the guru, drinking liquor, thieving, or committing adultery with the guru's wife—all such sins are shed when the Yonimudrā has been successfully performed.—15

तस्मादभ्यासनं नित्यं कर्तव्यं मोक्षकांक्षिभिः।
अभ्यासाज्जायते सिद्धिरभ्यासान्मोक्षमाप्नुयात्।। १६।।

Hence this Yonimudrā should be regularly practised by all who desire deliverance (*mokṣa*). Its practice alone can bring supernormal powers and pave the way to *mokṣa*.—16

सम्विदं लभतेऽभ्यासात् योगोऽभ्यासात् पवर्त्तते।
मुद्राणां सिद्धिरभ्यासादभ्यासाद्वायु साधनम्।। १७।।
कालवञ्चनमभ्यासात् तथा मृत्युञ्जयो भवेत्।
वाक्सिद्धिः कामचारीत्वं भवेदभ्यासयोगतः।। १८।।

It is by practice that one gains full knowledge; practice stabilizes one in yoga; practice secures the *mudrās* and supernormal powers, and practice enables one to cheat time and conquer death. Practice also confers word-power (i.e., anything spoken becomes true) and omnipotency (i.e., anything willed becomes true).—17 and 18

योनिमुद्रा परं गोप्या न देया यस्य कस्यचित्।
सर्वथा नैव दातव्या प्राणैः कण्ठगतैरपि।। १९।।

This Yonimudrā is very secret and must not be passed on to any and every person. It must not be divulged to the undeserving even though one's very life be in danger.—19

अधुना कथयिष्यामि योगसिद्धिकरं परम्।
गोपनीयं सुसिद्धानां योगं परमदुर्लभम्।। २०।।

Now I shall relate the most potent method for achieving success in yoga. This is a secret for all yoga adepts and is rather rare.—20

सुप्ता गुरुप्रसादेन यदा जागर्ति कुण्डली।
तदा सर्वाणि पद्मानि भिद्यन्ते ग्रन्थयोऽपि च।। २१।।

When the dormant Kuṇḍalinī (Serpent Power) is roused, it goes through (pierces) all the *cakras* (lotuses placed alongside the median nerve).—21

तस्मात् सर्वप्रयत्नेन प्रबोधयितुमीश्वरीम्।
ब्रह्मरन्ध्रमुखे सुप्ता मुद्राभ्यासं समाचरेत्।। २२।।

Hence, in order to understand this goddess who lies asleep at the entrance to the Passage of Knowledge, the *mudrās* (described below) should be practised.—22

महामुद्रा महाबन्धो महावेधश्च खेचरी।
जालन्धरो मूलबन्धो विपरीतकृतिस्तथा।। २३।।
उड्डानञ्चैव वज्रोली दशमं शक्तिचालनम्।
इदं हि मुद्रादशकं मुद्राणामुत्तमोत्तमम्।। २४।।

Mahāmudrā, Mahābandha, Mahāvedha, Khecarī, Jālandhara, Mūlabandha, Viparītakaraṇa, Uddāna, Vajroli, and Śakticālana are the ten best among all the other *mudrās.*—23 and 24

महामुद्रा प्रवक्ष्यामि तन्त्रेऽस्मिन् मम वल्लभे।
यां प्राप्य सिद्धाः संसिद्धिं कपिलाद्या पुरागताः।। २५।।

Of these ten, O Pārvatī, I am now describing only the Mahāmudrā, by the regular practice of which adepts such as Kapila* have achieved success.—25

अपसव्येन सम्पीड्य पादमूलेन सादरम्।
गुरूपदेशतो योनिं गुदमेढ्रान्तरालगाम्।। २६।।
सव्यं प्रसारितं पादं धृत्वा पाणियुगेन वै।
नवद्वाराणि संयम्य चिवुकं हृदयोपरि।। २७।।
चित्तं चित्तपथे दत्वा प्रारम्भेद्वायुसाधनम्।
महामुद्रा भवेदेषा सर्वतन्त्रेषु गोपिता।। २८।।

*The sage Kapila is the celebrated author of the Sāṅkhya system of philosophy.

वामाङ्गेन समभ्यस्य दक्षाङ्गेनाभ्यसेत् पुनः।
प्राणायामं समं कृत्वा योगी नियतमानसः।। २९।।

As per directions of the guru, first draw up the left leg and press its heel against the perineum in the region between the anus and the genitals. Next, stretch out the right leg and hold it with both hands. Thereafter, place the chin upon the chest and, restraining the nine apertures of the body (i.e., two eyes, two ears, two nostrils, the mouth, genitals, and anus), propagate the *prāṇa* (vital force) along the Passage of Knowledge. Know this to be the Mahāmudrā, the most mysterious in all Tantras. Thereafter repeat this performance with the left leg outstretched and the right drawn up and pressed against the perineum. *Prāṇāyāma* (breath-control) practised in this manner brings equanimity to the yogi.—26–29

मुद्रामेतान्तु सम्प्राप्य गुरुवक्त्रात् सुशोभितम्।
अनेन विधिना योगी मन्दभाग्योपि सिद्ध्यति।। ३०।।

This Mahāmudrā, when received direct from the guru, enables even an unfortunate (i.e., not yet qualified) yogi to achieve success.—30

सर्वेषामेव नाडीनां चालनं विन्दुमारणम्।
जीवनन्तु कषायस्य पातकानां विनाशनम्।। ३१।।

As a result of this Mahāmudrā all the nerve channels get activated, the sexual urge is controlled, and all enervating acids in the body are eliminated.—31

कुण्डलीतापनं वायोर्ब्रह्मरन्ध्र-प्रवेशनम्।
सर्वरोगोपशमनं जठराग्निविवर्धनम्।। ३२।।
वपुषः कान्तिममलां जरामृत्युविनाशनम्।
वाञ्छितार्थफलं सौख्यमिन्द्रियाणाञ्च मारणम्।। ३३।।

Also, the Kuṇḍalinī is energized when, together with the vital air, it enters the Passage of Knowledge. The other benefits are: freedom from diseases, a healthy appetite, a fine complexion, and no fear of decay or death. It also produces all the desired things, and there is happiness in general and a full control over one's sense-organs.—32 and 33

एतदुक्तानि सर्वाणि योगारूढस्य योगिनः।
भवेदभ्यासतोऽवश्यं नात्र कार्या विचारणा।। ३४।।

All these that I have listed are signs of the yogi who has mastered yoga, which of course is possible only through practice; and there is no doubt about it.—34

गोपनीया प्रयत्नेन मुद्रेयं सुरपूजिते।
यान्तु प्राप्य भवाम्बोधेः पारं गच्छन्ति योगिनः।। ३५।।

O adored by the gods (Pārvatī)! this *mudrā*, by knowing which the yogis cross the ocean of world phenomena, should be carefully kept a secret.—35

मुद्रा कामदुधा ह्येषा साधकानां मयोदिता।
गुप्ताचारेण कर्त्तव्या न देया यस्य कस्यचित्।। ३६।।

This Mahāmudrā that I have just described is the Kāmadhenu* for all yogis. It should therefore be zealously protected and not passed on to all and sundry.—36

ततः प्रसारितः पादौ विन्यस्य तमूरूपरि।
गुदयोनिं समाकुञ्च्य कृत्वा चापानमूर्द्धगम्।। ३७।।
योजयित्वा समानेन कृत्वा प्राणमधोमुखम्।
बन्धयेदुदरोऽत्यर्थं प्राणापानौ च यः सुधीः।। ३८।।
कथितोऽयं महाबन्धः सिद्धिमार्गप्रदायकः।
नाडीजालाद्रसव्यूहो मूर्द्धानं याति योगिनः।। ३९।।
उभाभ्यां साधयेत् पद्भ्यामेकैकं सुप्रयत्नतः।। ४०।।

Next, stretch out one leg and fold the other and place the same upon the opposite thigh. Then, contracting the anus and the perineum, propagate the *apāna* (down-flowing air), along with *samāna* (air around the navel), upward while *prāṇa* is pushed down. He who can form such a combination of *prāna* and *apāna* within his body is indeed a wise yogi. This is called Mahābandha (Great Bondage) which moves the accumulated secretions in the network of nerves right up to the brain and gives the yogi his supernormal powers. This should be practised carefully, stretching out either leg by turn.—37–40

भवेदभ्यासतो वायुः सुषुम्नामध्यसंगतः।
अनेन वपुषः पुष्टिर्दृढबन्धोऽस्थिपञ्जरे।। ४१।।
सम्पूर्णहृदयो योगी भवन्त्येतानि योगिनः।
बन्धेनानेन योगीन्द्रः साधयेत् सर्वमीप्सितम्।। ४२।।

*Kāmadhenu is the celestial cow of Hindu mythology believed to be capable of granting anything asked of her.

As a result of this practice the vital air enters the Suṣumnā *nāḍī*, thereby nourishing the body and strengthening the bones of the ribs. This helps the yogi to expand his lungs to the maximum and then this *bandha* yields all the desired results.—41 and 42

अपानप्राणयोरैकं कृत्वा त्रिभुवनेश्वरी।
महावेधस्थितो योगी कुक्षिमापूर्य वायुना।
स्फिचौ संताडयेत् धीमान् बेधोऽयं कीर्त्तितो मया।। ४३।।

O Queen of all three worlds! only that yogi is wise who can unify his *prāṇa* and *apāna* airs within himself, go into a deep meditation and then shake himself up at the end. This Mahāvedha is commended by Me.—43

वेधेनानेन संविध्य वायुना योगिपुङ्गवः।
ग्रन्थिं सुषुम्नामार्गेण ब्रह्मग्रन्थिं भिनत्त्यसौ।। ४४।।

With the help of this Mahāvedha the yogi is able to pierce through the knot (gland) near the entrance to the Suṣumnā *nāḍī* and, finally, the supreme knot known as the Brahma-granthi.*—44

यः करोति सदाभ्यासं महावेधं सुगोपितम्।
वायुसिद्धिर्भवेत्तस्य जरामरणनाशिनी।। ४५।।

One who practises this Mahāvedhamudrā secretly every day gets full control over his internal airs and thus becomes free of diseases and death.—45

चक्रमध्ये स्थिता देवी कम्पन्ते वायुताडनात्।
कुण्डल्यपि महामाया कैलासे सा विलीयते।। ४६।।

The goddess (Kuṇḍalinī) dwells within the Mūlādhāracakra, and she is roused by the controlled airs. She is the great Śakti (Force) that goes up to Kailāsa** to get united (with Śiva).—46

महामुद्रा महाबन्धौ निष्फलौ वेधवर्जितौ।
तस्माद्योगी प्रयत्नेन करोति त्रितयं क्रमात्।। ४७।।

Without this Mahāvedha, the other two, viz., Mahāmudrā and

*Brahma-granthi lies at the upper end of the Brahmarandhra (Passage of Knowledge) leading through *medulla oblongata* to the brain-centre. The latter is represented by the thousand-petalled lotus Sahasrāra. The Brahma-granthi is sometimes identified as the pineal gland.

**Mount Kailāsa is the traditional abode of the Lord Śiva. Here, the inner sanctum of the brain is compared to Kailāsa, where the goddess Kuṇḍalinī or Śakti goes to dwell with her consort Śiva, as represented by the *Ātman* or *Puruṣa*.

Mahābandha, are useless (fruitless). Hence the yogi should perform all three in the proper order.—47

एतन्त्रयं प्रयत्नेन चतुर्वारं करोति यः।
षण्मासाभ्यन्तरे मृत्युं जयत्येव न संशयः।। ४८।।

He who practises these three regularly four times a day (i.e., morning, noon, evening, and midnight) will undoubtedly triumph over death within a period of six months.—48

एतन्त्रयस्य माहात्म्यं सिद्धो जानाति नेतरे।
यज्ज्ञात्वा साधकाः सर्वे सिद्धिं सम्यक् लभन्ति च।। ४९।।

Only the adepts know the immense value of these three, not others. Mastering these, the adepts gain all supernormal powers.—49

गोपनीया प्रयत्नेन साधकैः सिद्धिमीप्सुभिः।
अन्यथा च न सिद्धिः स्यान्मुद्राणामेष निश्चयः।। ५०।।

Hence yogis who desire to gain such mastery should keep this exercise a close secret, or else this *mudrā* will not bring them those positive powers.—50

भ्रुवोरन्तर्गतां दृष्टिं विधाय सुदृढां सुधीः।
उपविश्यासने वज्रे स्थानोपद्रववर्जितः।। ५१।।
लम्बिकोर्द्धस्थिते गर्ते रसनां विपरीतगाम्।
संयोजयेत् प्रयत्नेन सुधाकूपे विचक्षणः।। ५२।।
मुद्रैषा खेचरी प्रोक्ता भक्तानामनुरोधतः।
सिद्धीनां जननी ह्येषा मम प्राणाधिकाधिके।। ५३।।

The yogi should sit on a hard seat, in a solitary place, and then fix his gaze steadily between the eyebrows. Let the tongue, upturned, go back as far as possible to the aperture (at the back of the palate) into the "well of nectar" (i.e., the sinuses) and be held carefully there. This is Khecarīmudrā, which I have revealed at the express request of My devotees. The Khecarī, O Pārvatī, is the mother of all supernormal powers.—51–53

निरन्तरकृताभ्यासात् पीयूषं प्रत्यहं पिबेत्।
तेन विग्रहसिद्धिः स्यात् मृत्युमातङ्गकेशरी।। ५४।।

He who regularly drinks this nectar every day gets a perfect body and conquers death even as a lion overpowers the elephant.—54

अपवित्रो पवित्रो वा सर्वावस्थां गतोऽपि वा।
खेचरी यस्य शुद्धा तु स शुद्धो नात्र संशयः।। ५५।।

Anyone, whether clean or unclean, and irrespective of the environment he be in, definitely becomes pure as soon as he has mastered the Khecarīmudrā.—55

क्षणार्द्धं कुरुते यस्तु तीर्णः पापमहार्णवात्।
दिव्यभोगान् प्रभुक्त्वा च सत्कुले स प्रजायते।। ५६।।

Even though he may hold on to this *mudrā* for only half a moment, that would enable him to cross the ocean of sins, enjoy a divine life, and then be reborn in a good and devout family.—56

मुद्रैषा खेचरी यस्तु सुस्थितोऽस्यामतन्द्रितः।
शतब्रह्मागतेनापि क्षणार्द्धं मन्यते हि सः।। ५७।।

One who practises this Khecarīmudrā patiently and meticulously finds eternal time reduced to a mere moment.*—57

गुरूपदेशतो मुद्रां यो वेत्ति खेचरीमिमाम्।
नाना पापरतो धीमान् स याति परमां गतिम्।। ५८।।

The wise yogi who learns this Khecarīmudrā as per guru's guidance attains, despite his many demerits, the supreme state (i.e., emancipation).—58

स्वप्राणैः सदृशो यस्तु तस्मै चापि न दीयते।
प्रच्छाद्यते प्रयत्नेन मुद्रेयं सुरपूजिते।। ५९।।

O adored by the gods (Pārvatī)! this *mudrā* should be kept a close secret and must not be divulged even to the most beloved person (as dear as one's life).—59

बद्ध्वा गलशिराजालं हृदये चिबुकं न्यसेत्।
बन्धो जालन्धरः प्रोक्तो देवानामपि दुर्लभः।। ६०।।

Bending down the chin upon the chest, the network of veins in the neck should be blocked. This constitutes the Jālandhara-bandha.** It is rare even for the gods.—60

Śata-Brahmā literally means one hundred of Brahmā's days. Since one day of Brahmā equals 8,640,000,000 years on earth, *śata-Brahmā* would seem to indicate 'eternity'.

***Prāṇāyāma* or breath-control is an integral part of all these *mudrās* and it must be practised simultaneously with each *mudrā*.

नाभिस्थो वह्निर्जन्तूनां सहस्रकमलच्युतम्।
पिवेत् पीयूषविवरं तदर्थं बन्धयेदिमाम्।। ६१।।

This (Jālandharabandha) is so-called because it intercepts the nectar oozing from the thousand-petalled lotus (*sahasrāra*) which otherwise gets consumed in the fire found within the navel. In this (Jālandhara) way the yogi is able to drink the nectar.—61

बन्धेनानेन पीयूषं स्वयं पिवति बुद्धिमान्।
अमरत्वञ्च सम्प्राप्य मोदते भुवनत्रये।। ६२।।

By means of this (Jālandharabandha) the wise yogi himself drinks the nectar, and thus attaining immortality, moves about happily in all three worlds.—62

जालन्धरो बन्ध एषः सिद्धानां सिद्धिदायकः।
अभ्यासः क्रियते नित्यं योगिना सिद्धिमिच्छता।। ६३।।

This Jālandharabandha is the bestower of supernormal powers to all who can master it. Yogis desirous of acquiring these powers must practise it regularly.—63

पादमूलेन सम्पीड्य गुदमार्गं सुयन्त्रितः।
बलादपानमाकृष्य क्रमादूर्द्ध्वं समभ्यसेत्।। ६४।।

Block the anus carefully with the heel and then draw in the *apāna* (inhaled air) to the maximum, then practise pushing it up slowly but firmly.—64

कल्पितोऽयं मूलबन्धो जरामरणनाशिनः।
अपानप्राणयोरैक्यं प्रकरोत्यधिकल्पितम्।। ६५।।

This is Mūlabandha, devised for conquering decay and death. By this the *apāna* and *prāṇa* get more or less equalized.—65

ब्रन्धेनानेन सुतरां योनिमुद्रा प्रसिद्ध्यति।
सिद्धायां योनिमुद्रायां किं न सिद्ध्यति भूतले।। ६६।।

This *bandha,* therefore, is a distinguishing feature of the Yonimudrā. And once this Yonimudrā is mastered, what else cannot be mastered on this earth?—66

बन्धस्यास्य प्रसादेन गगने विजितानिलः।
पद्मासने स्थितो योगी भुतमुत्सृज्य वर्त्तते।। ६७।।

By the grace of this Mūlabandha the yogi conquers the air in the sky. He can then rise above the ground even while sitting in

Padmāsana.—67

सुगुप्ते निर्जने देशे बन्धमेनं समभ्यसेत्।
संसारसागरं तर्तुं यदीच्छेद् योगिपुङ्गवः।। ६८।।

This Mūlabandha should be practised in a solitary place and in secret if the yogi is really desirous of crossing the ocean of world phenomena.—68

भूतले स्वशिरो दत्वा खे नयेच्चरणद्वयम्।
विपरीतकृतिश्चैषा सर्वतन्त्रेषु गोपिता।। ६९।।

Placing the head on the ground, let both the legs go up. This is Viparītakaraṇamudrā, which is one of the secrets preserved in all Tantras.—69

एतां यः कुरुते नित्यमभ्यासं याममात्रकं।
मृत्युं जयति स योगी प्रलये नापि सीदति।। ७०।।

The yogi who practises this for one *yāma* (three hours), conquers death. He is not destroyed even at the time of the final dissolution of the universe!—70

कुरुतेऽमृतपानं स सिद्धानां समतामियात्।
स सिद्धः सर्वलोकेषु बन्धमेनं करोति यः।। ७१।।

When he drinks the nectar*, he becomes equal to all other adepts. Having mastered this *mudrā*, he becomes a master in all three worlds.—71

नाभेरूर्द्धमधश्चापि तानं पश्चिममाचरेत्।
उड्डानो बन्ध एषः स्यात् सर्वदुःखौघनाशनः।। ७२।।
उदरे पश्चिमं तानं नाभेरूर्द्धन्तु कारयेत्।
उड्डानाख्यो ह्ययं बन्धो मृत्युमातङ्गकेशरी।। ७३।।

Push the navel up and down as you contract and expand the stomach. This is the Uddānabandha, the practice of which removes all pains and diseases. *Or*, pull in the stomach to the maximum, pushing up the navel as well. This too is called Uddāna. It bestows on one the strength of a lion that overpowers the elephant.—72 and 73

*The nectar, apparently, is the psychic energy produced in the brain which gets consumed by the digestive process. Esoterically, the brain is the 'moon' and the navel, as repository of the fire of hunger, is the 'sun'. Through the practice of Viparītakaraṇamudrā—which is virtually standing upon one's head—the energy which normally gets wasted in the act of digestion, is preserved by the yogi by means of this inverse posture.

नित्यं यः कुरुते योगी चतुर्वारं दिने दिने।
तस्य नाभेस्तु शुद्धिः स्याद् येन शुद्धो भवेन्मरुत्।। ७४।।

The yogi who practises this regularly four times a day gets his intestines automatically cleansed and, because of this cleansing, the air within the body also gets purified.—74

षण्मासमभ्यसन् योगी मृत्युं जयति निश्चितम्।
तस्योदराग्निर्ज्वलति रसवृद्धिस्तु जायते।। ७५।।

When this is practised for six months the yogi is positively able to conquer death. This practice ignites the fire (appetite) in the stomach and there is an increase of (digestive) juices.—75

अनेन सुतरां सिद्धिर्विग्रहस्य प्रजायते।
रोगाणां संक्षयश्चापि योगिनो भवति ध्रुवम्।। ७६।।

In this way the body becomes perfect and the yogi is soon able to eliminate all diseases.—76

गुरोर्लब्ध्वा तु यत्नेन साधयेत्तु विचक्षणः।
निर्जने सुस्थिते देशे बन्धं परमदुर्लभम्।। ७७।।

Having obtained correct instructions from the guru, the wise yogi should proceed to practise this with care in a solitary and congenial place. This *bandha* is indeed incomparable.—77

वज्रोलीं कथयिष्यामि संसारध्वान्तनाशिनीम्।
स्वभक्तेभ्यः समासेन गुह्याद्गुह्यतमामपि।। ७८।।

Now I shall relate for the benefit of My devotees the most secret of all *mudrās*, namely, Vajroli, which is a dispeller of all worldly illusions.—78

स्वेच्छयावर्त्तमानेपि योगोक्तनियमैर्विना।
मुक्तो भवेद्गृहस्थोऽपि वज्रोल्याभ्यासयोगतः।। ७९।।

Through the practice of this Vajrolimudrā even a householder—provided he is eager for it—can become free (achieve deliverance) even though he may not have followed all of yoga instructions.—79

वज्रोल्यभ्यासयोगोऽयं भोगे युक्तोऽपि मुक्तिदः।
तस्मादतिप्रयत्नेन कर्त्तव्यो योगिभिः सदा।। ८०।।

The practice of Vajroli bestows deliverance even upon those who are bound to their worldly attractions. It is the duty of all yogis, therefore, to see that it is practised with due care.—80

आदौ रजः स्त्रियायोन्या यत्नेन विविधत् सुधीः।
आकुञ्च्य लिङ्गनालेन स्वशरीरे प्रवेशयेत्।। ८१।।
स्वकं विन्दुञ्च संवध्य लिङ्गचालनमाचरेत्।
दैवाच्चलति चेदूर्द्धे निरुद्धो योनिमुद्रया।। ८२।।
वामभागेऽपि तद्विन्दुं नीत्वा लिङ्गं निवारयेत्।
क्षणमात्रं योनितोऽयं पुमांश्चालनमाचरेत्।। ८३।।
गुरूपदेशतो योगी हुंहुंकारेण योनितः।
अपानवायुमाकुञ्च्य बलादाकृष्य तद्रजः।। ८४।।

The wise one should first absorb into his own body the ovarial fluid in the vagina by contracting the duct of his own organ, and thereafter perform coitus without ejecting the seminal fluid. Should the latter tend to issue, it must be restrained by means of the Yonimudrā (mentioned earlier). Next, the same seminal fluid should be diverted to the channel on the left (Iḍā) and the coitus stopped for a while. Thereafter, in accordance with the instructions of the guru, he should, with a long in-take of *apāna* (inspiration), extract with one triumphal effort the remaining ovarial fluid in the vagina—81–84

अनेन विधिना योगी क्षिप्रं योगस्य सिद्धये।
गव्यभुक् कुरुते योगी गुरुपादाब्जपूजकः।। ८५।।

In this manner the yogi is able to master his yoga quickly and, being a worshipper of the lotus-feet of his guru, he soon qualifies for the best of food (i.e., nectar issuing from the Sahasrāra).—85

विन्दुर्विधुमयो ज्ञेयो रजः सूर्यमयस्तथा।
उभयोर्मेलनं कार्यं स्वशरीरे प्रयत्नतः।। ८६।।

Know thee that the seminal fluid is the 'moon' and the ovarial fluid the 'sun'. It is necessary to coalesce the two within one's own body.—86

अहं विन्दु रजः शक्तिरुभयोर्मेलनं यदा।
योगिनां साधनवतां भवेद्दिव्यं वपुस्तदा।। ८७।।

In fact *I* am the seminal fluid and the ovarial fluid is Śakti. When the two are united in the body of the yogi, he attains a divine body.—87

मरणं विन्दुपातेन जीवनं विन्दुधारणात्।
तस्मादतिप्रयत्नेन कुरुते विन्दुधारणम्।। ८८।।

Death follows the wastage of this seminal fluid; its preservation is life. Hence it is necessary to preserve this fluid zealously.—88

जायते म्रियते लोको विन्दुना नात्र संशयः।
एतज्ज्ञात्वा सदा योगी विन्दुधारणमाचरेत्।। ८९।।

Undoubtedly the cause of man's birth and death is this seminal fluid. Knowing this, the yogi should practise the retention of this fluid.—89

सिद्धे विन्दौ महायत्ने किं न सिद्ध्यति भूतले।
यस्य प्रसादान्महिमा ममाप्येतादृशी भवेत्।। ९०।।

When this seminal fluid has been meticulously controlled, everything else in this world can be easily controlled. In fact, by its grace I Myself have become like this!—90

विन्दुः करोति सर्वेषां सुखं दुःखञ्च संस्थितम्।
संसारिणां विमूढानां जरामरणशालिनाम्।। ९१।।

People under delusion, and being a constant prey of decay and death in this world, can make their pleasure and pain equal by a control of the seminal fluid.—91

अयं शुभकरो योगो योगिनामुत्तमोत्तमः।
अभ्यासात् सिद्धिमाप्नोति भोगेयुक्तोऽपि मानवः।। ९२।।

It is a beneficial form of yoga, and is extremely beneficial for the yogis. Even people engaged in worldly life get success when such control is practised.—92

स काले साधितार्थोऽपि सिद्धो भवति भूतले।
भुक्त्वा भोगानशेषान् वै योगेनानेन निश्चितम्।। ९३।।

Success comes in this very life when it is practised in good time. This yoga positively ends the travails of worldly life.—93

अनेन सकला सिद्धिर्योगिनां भवति ध्रुवम्।
सुखभोगेन महता तस्मादेनं समभ्यसेत्।। ९४।।

Through it the yogi gets all the powers quickly, and he experiences immense joy. Hence it should be practised regularly.—94

सहजोल्यमरोली च वज्रोल्या भेदतो भवेत्।
येन केन प्रकारेण विन्दुं योगी प्रधारयेत्।। ९५।।

Sahajoli and Amaroli are the two other forms of Vajroli. By either of these methods the seminal fluid can be conserved – 95

दैवाच्चलति चेद्वेगे मेलनं चन्द्रसूर्ययोः।
अमरोलिरियं प्रोक्ता लिङ्गनालेन शोषयेत्।। ९६।।

Should the seminal fluid get unavoidably emitted, and there is a union of the moon (seminal fluid) and the sun (ovarial fluid), the same should be sucked back through the duct of the organ. This is called Amaroli.—96

गतं विन्दुं स्वकं योगी बन्धयेत् योगिमुद्रया।
सहजोलिरियं प्रोक्ता सर्वतन्त्रेषु गोपिता।। ९७।।

When the yogi is able to control, by means of the Yonimudrā, and stop the discharge of his seminal fluid, it is called Sahajoli. It is a secret preserved in all Tantras.—97

संज्ञाभेदाद्भवेद्भेदः कार्यं तुल्यगतिर्यदि।
तस्मात् सर्वप्रयत्नेन साध्यते योगिभिः सदा।। ९८।।

These (Sahajoli and Amaroli) are different only in name; in effect they are the same. Therefore either can be used by the yogi—but all with due care.—98

अयं योगो मया प्रोक्तो भक्तानां स्नेहतः परम्।
गोपनीयं प्रयत्नेन न देयो यस्य कस्यचित्।। ९९।।

This yoga has been described by Me because of My great affection for My devotees. Otherwise it is a secret, and is not to be divulged to all and sundry.—99

एतद्गुह्यतमं गुह्यं न भूतं न भविष्यति।
तस्मादतिप्रयत्नेन गोपनीयं सदा वुधैः।। १००।।

There never has been a more mysterious yoga than this one—either in the past or ever shall be in the future. Hence the wise one should carefully keep it a secret.—100

स्वमूत्रोत्सर्गकाले यो बलादाकृष्य वायुना।
स्तोकं स्तोकं त्यजेन्मूत्रमूर्द्धमाकृष्य तत्पुनः।। १०१।।
गुरूपदिष्टमार्गेण प्रत्यहं यः समाचरेत्।
विन्दुसिद्धिर्भवेत्तस्य महासिद्धिप्रदायिका।। १०२।।

One who, after a deep inspiration, restrains the flow of his urine—releasing it little by little and again holding it back—and practises this every day as per directions of the guru, achieves mastery over his seminal fluid also. This confers all kinds of power upon him.—101 and 102

षण्मासमभ्यासेद् यो वै प्रत्यहं गुरुशिक्षया।
शताङ्गनोपभोगेऽपि तस्य विन्दुर्न नश्यति।। १०३।।

If this is practised for six months as per directions of the guru, then the seminal fluid will not be wasted even if he were to come in contact with a hundred women!—103

सिद्धे विन्दौ महायत्ने किं न सिद्ध्यति भूतले।
ईशत्वं यत्प्रसादेन ममापि दुर्लभो भवेत्।। १०४।।

Once the key to this control of the seminal fluid is found, what else cannot be performed in this world? My own rare divinity, too, is the result of such happy control.—104

आधारकमले सुप्ता चालयेत् कुण्डलीं दृढाम्।
अपानवायुमारुह्य बलादाकृष्य बुद्धिमान्।
शक्तिचालनमुद्रेयं सर्वशक्तिप्रदायिनी।। १०५।।

With a deep *apāna* (inspiration) the wise yogi stirs up the Kuṇḍalinī lying dormant in the Mūlādhāracakra and urges it to move up. This is known as Śakticālana, a *mudrā* that bestows all kinds of power.—105

शक्तिचालनमेतद्धि प्रत्यहं यः समाचरेत्।
आयुर्वृद्धिर्भवेत्तस्य रोगाणाञ्च विनाशनम्।। १०६।।

One who practises this Śakticālanamudrā every day is able to ward off all diseases, and he thus increases his longevity.—106

विहाय निद्रां भुजगी स्वयमूर्द्ध्वे भवेत् खलु।
तस्मादभ्यासनं कार्यं योगिना सिद्धिमिच्छता।। १०७।।

Thereafter the Serpent (Kuṇḍalinī) wakes up, and then automatically moves upward. For this, however, practice is necessary by the yogi desiring success.—107

यः करोति सदाभ्यासं शक्तिचालनमुत्तमम्।
येन विग्रहसिद्धिः स्यादणिमादिगुणप्रदा।
गुरूपदेशविधिना तस्य मृत्युभयं कुतः।। १०८।।

He who practises this superb Śākticālanamudrā every day—a *mudrā* that perfects the body and brings the supernormal powers of Aṇimā, etc.—in accordance with the directions of the guru, for him there is no fear of death.—108

मुहूर्तद्वयपर्यन्तं विधिना शक्तिचालनम्।
यः करोति प्रयत्नेन तस्य सिद्धिरदूरतः।
युक्तासनेन कर्तव्यं योगिभिः शक्तिचालनम्।। १०९।।

Even if this Śakticālanamudrā is performed diligently and properly for only a couple of moments, success would not be far from that yogi. He should, however, perform this while seated in the prescribed posture (*āsana*).—109

एतत्तु मुद्रादशकं न भूतं न भविष्यति।
एकैकाभ्यासने सिद्धिः सिद्धो भवति नान्यथा।। ११०।।

These ten *mudrās* are unique—never disclosed before, nor shall be in future. With the practice of just one of these, success in yoga is assured.—110

Here ends chapter IV of *Śivasaṃhitā* entitled
'Postures and Preludes'

CHAPTER V

Rājayoga

श्रीदेव्युवाच–

ब्रूहि मे वाक्यमीशान परमार्थधियं प्रति।
ये विघ्नाः सन्ति लोकानां चेन्मयि प्रेम शंकरः।। १।।

Pārvatī then spoke thus:

O Īśāna, O Śaṅkara! do tell me what are the obstacles in the path of people who aspire for the Supreme.—1

श्रीईश्वर उवाच—

शृणु देवि प्रवक्ष्यामि यथा विघ्नाः स्थिताः सदा।
मुक्तिं प्रति नराणाञ्च भोगः परमबन्धकः।। २।।

The Lord said:

O Devī, listen! I am relating all of those obstacles that stand in the way of man's deliverance. For men, the greatest bondage is gratification of desires.—2

नारी शय्यासनं वस्त्रं धनमस्य विडम्बनम्।
ताम्बूलं भक्षयानानि राज्यैश्वर्यविभूतयः।। ३।।
हेमरूप्यं तथा ताम्रं रत्नञ्चागुरुधेनवः।
पाण्डित्यं वेदशास्त्राणि नृत्यं गीतं विभूषणम्।। ४।।
वंशी वीणा मृदङ्गश्च गजेन्द्रश्चाश्ववाहनम्।
दारापत्यानि विषया विघ्ना एते प्रकीर्तिता।। ५।।

Women, a cosy bed or seat, fine clothes, wealth—all are deceptive. Also betel-chewing, too much food, posh vehicles, large estates, extensive powers, possession of lots of gold, silver, copper, gems, perfumes, hordes of cattle, or the display of knowledge of scriptures, or skill in dancing and music, or talent for playing instruments such as the flute, the *vīṇā*, the *mṛdaṅga*, or skill in riding elephants, horses, etc., and attachment to one's wife and children—all these are considered as obstacles.—3–5.

भोगरूपा इमे विघ्ना धर्मरूपानिमान् शृणु।। ६।।

These (above) obstacles are in the form of selfish enjoyment. Now listen to those that are in the form of virtuous acts.—6

स्नानं पूजातिथिर्होमं तथा सौख्यमयी स्थितिः।
व्रतोपवास नियमो मौनमिन्द्रियनिग्रहः।। ७।।
धैयो ध्यानं तथ मन्त्रो दानं ख्यातिर्दिशासु च।
वापीकूपतडागादि प्रासादारामकल्पना।। ८।।
यज्ञं चान्द्रायणं कृच्छ्रं तीर्थानि विषयानि च।
दृश्यन्ते च इमा विघ्ना धर्मरूपेण संस्थिताः।। ९।।

Holy bath, prayers, serving the guests, performing *homa* (offerings to fire), pleasant companionship, a scrupulous observance of fasting, silence, restraint of senses, meditation and *mantras,* gifts given to earn a name, plans made for building ponds, wells, reservoirs, palaces and gardens, and things like performance of *yajna* or practice of austerities such as the Cāndrāyaṇa vow, or going on pilgrimages—all these are viewed as obstacles in the form of virtuous acts.—7–9

यत्तु विघ्नं भवेज्ज्ञानं कथयामि वरानने।
गोमुखाद्यासनं कृत्वा धौती प्रक्षालनं वसेत्।। १०।।
नाडीसञ्चारविज्ञानं प्रत्याहार निरोधनम्।
कुक्षिसञ्चालनं क्षीरप्रवेश इन्द्रियाध्वना।। ११।।

O Pārvatī, let Me now tell you about the obstacles that come in the form of ignorance. These are: performing Gomukha and other *āsanas* without the preliminary (internal and external) cleansing, restraining of senses and activating the *nāḍīs* by artificial means, and causing bowel-movements by enema.—10 and 11

नाडीकर्माणि कल्याणि भोजनं श्रूयतां मम।
नवं धातुरसं छिन्दि घण्टिकास्ताडयेत् पुनः।। १२।।

Now listen to the things that are beneficent for the health of the *nāḍīs.* Make a small incision under the palatine papilla (uvula) and massage it again and again with fresh saliva.—12

एककालं समाधिः स्याल्लिङ्गभूतमिदं शृणु।
संगमं गच्छ साधूनां संकोचं भज दुर्जनात्।
प्रवेशे निर्गमे वायोर्गुरुलक्ष्यं विलोकयेत्।। १३।।

Again listen to the way in which *samādhi* is achieved during one's lifetime. Keep the company of the pious, and renounce that of the wicked. Also, mind how you breathe (inhale and exhale); do so only as advised by the guru.—13

पिण्डस्थं रूपसंस्थञ्च रूपस्थं रूपवर्जितम्।
ब्रह्मै तस्मिन्मतावस्था हृदयञ्च प्रशाम्यति।। १४।।

That which dwells within the body in the form of beauty—which is beauty without form—is the eternal Brahman (*Ātman*). When the mind is suffused with this knowledge, it is the *samādhi.*—14

इत्येते कथिता विघ्नाज्ञानरूपे व्यवस्थिता।। १५।।

Thus far I have described the obstacles that appear in the form of ignorance.—15

मन्त्रयोगो हठश्चैव लययोगस्तृतीयतः।
चतुर्थो राजयोगः स्यात् स द्विधाभाववर्जितः।। १६।।

Now there are four types of yoga: Mantrayoga, Layayoga, Haṭhayoga and Rājayoga. The last one dispels the illusion of duality.—16

चतुर्धा साधको ज्ञेयो मृदुमध्याधिमात्रकः।
अधिमात्रतमः श्रेष्ठो भवाब्धौ लंघनक्षमः।। १७।।

Like yoga, the yogis too are of four types: ordinary, middling, good and very good. The last type is the best, being capable of crossing the ocean of world phenomena.—17

मन्दोत्साही सुसंमूढो व्याधिस्थो गुरुदूषकः।
लोभी पापमतिश्चैव वह्वाशी वनिताश्रयः।। १८।।
चपलः कातरो रोगी पराधीनोऽतिनिष्ठुरः।
मन्दाचारो मन्दवीर्यो ज्ञातव्यो मृदुसाधकः।। १९।।
द्वादशाब्दे भवेत् सिद्धिरेतस्य यत्नतः परम्।
मन्त्रयोगाधिकारी स ज्ञातव्यो गुरुणा ध्रुवम्।। २०।।

Half-hearted, steeped in ignorance, diseased, rejected by the guru, greedy, wicked-minded, a glutton, surrounded by women (a ladies' man), fickle, gloomy, weak, helpless (dependent on others), cruel, unclean (of dirty habits) and lethargic—know all these to be the signs of an ordinary yoga aspirant. These must labour for twelve years before they can achieve success. However, when duly instructed by the guru, these very persons qualify for the Mantrayoga.—18–20

समबुद्धिः क्षमायुक्तः पुण्याकांक्षी प्रियम्वदः।
मध्यस्थः सर्वकार्येषु सामान्यः स्यान्न संशयः।। २१।।
एतज्ज्ञात्वैव गुरुभिर्दीयते युक्तितो लयः।। २२।।

Even tempered, forgiving, eager to do good, soft-spoken, with equal interest in all work and without doubts—to such (middling type) as may be deserving, the guru imparts the Layayoga.—21 and 22

स्थिरबुद्धिर्लये युक्तः स्वाधीनो वीर्यवानपि।
महाशयो दयायुक्तः क्षमावान् सत्यवानपि।। २३।।
शूरो लयस्य श्रद्धावान् गुरुपादाब्जपूजकः।
योगाभ्यासरतश्चैव ज्ञातव्यश्चाधिमात्रकः।। २४।।
एतस्य सिद्धिः षड्वर्षैर्भवेदभ्यासयोगतः।
एतस्मै दीयते धीरैर्हठयोगश्च साङ्गकः।। २५।।

A balanced mind, already engaged in Layayoga, self-reliant, energetic, of liberal outlook, compassionate, forgiving, speaking only the truth, courageous, enthusiastic about Layayoga, devoted to guru and the practice of yoga—these belong to the *adhimātra* or fairly good type of yogis. To these the guru imparts the knowledge of Haṭhayoga. By practising the same, they achieve success within six years.—23–25

महावीर्यान्वितोत्साही मनोज्ञः शौर्यवानपि।
शस्त्रज्ञोऽभ्यासशीलश्च निर्मोहश्च निराकुलः।। २६।।
नवयौवनसम्पन्नो मिताहारी जितेन्द्रियः।
निर्भयश्च शुचिर्दक्षो दाता सर्वजनाश्रयः।। २७।।
अधिकारी स्थिरो धीमान् यथेच्छावस्थितः क्षमी।
सुशीलो धर्मचारी च गुप्तचेष्टः प्रियम्बदः।। २८।।
शान्तो विश्वाससम्पन्नो देवतागुरुपूजकः।
जनसङ्गविरक्तश्च महाव्याधिविवर्जितः।। २९।।
अधिमात्रतम व्रतज्ञश्च सर्वयोगस्य साधकः।
त्रिभिः संवत्सरैः सिद्धिरेतस्य स्यात् न संशयः।। ३०।।

Endowed with immense energy and enthusiasm, of imposing personality, bold, learned, studious, unattached to worldly objects, unperturbed, full of fresh vigour, frugal in diet, master of his senses, of clean habits, fearless, efficient, sheltering all, commanding respect, benevolent, steady, intelligent, confident, forgiving, noble, just, doing good by stealth, polite, peaceful, trustworthy, adoring the guru and gods, shunning crowds, free of contagious diseases, good at keeping all vows and practising yoga—for such *adhimātratama* (very good) yogis success is assured within three years.—26–30

सर्वयोगाधिकारी स नात्र कार्या विचारणा।। ३१।।

Such (very good) yogis are entitled to receive all forms of yoga, and for them there is no need for further scrutiny.—31

प्रतीकोपासना कार्या दृष्टादृष्टफलप्रदा।
पुणति दर्शनादत्र नात्र कार्या विचारणा।। ३२।।

(Next) it is necessary to practise contemplation upon one's own reflection. Such contemplation brings forth both seen and unseen results. There is no doubt that viewing one's own image is sanctifying.—32

गाढातपे स्वप्रतिविम्बमैश्वरं निरीक्ष्य निश्चलितलोचनद्वयम्।
यदा नभः पश्यति स्वप्रतीकं नभोऽङ्गने तत्क्षणमेव पश्यति।। ३३।।

If you fix your gaze upon your own shadow cast by a blazing sun, and thereafter lift the eyes to the horizon, you can at once see your own image reflected against the sky.—33

प्रत्यहं पश्यते यो वै स्वप्रतीकं नभोऽङ्गने।
आयुर्वृद्धिर्भवेत्तस्य न मृत्युः स्यात् कदाचन।। ३४।।

He who sees his own reflection in the expanse of the sky every day, prolongs his longevity and never dies.—34

यदा पश्यति सम्पूर्ण स्वप्रतीकं नभोऽङ्गने।
तदा जयः समायाति वायुं निर्जित्य सञ्चरेत्।। ३५।।

When such an image is seen in the sky clearly then there is a sense of triumph over the air, and the yogi feels that he can float in the sky.—35

यः करोति सदाभ्यासं चात्मानं विन्दते परम्।
पूर्णानन्दैकपुरुषं स्वप्रतीकप्रसादतः।। ३६।।

One who practises this, and thus sees himself at a distance, receives the grace of the all-blissful Supreme Being.—36

यात्राकाले विवाहे च शुभे कर्माणि सङ्कटे।
पापक्षये पुण्यवृद्धौ प्रतीकोपासनञ्चरेत्।। ३७।।

This discipline of image-reflection should be practised at all times—during travel, at a marriage ceremony, on all auspicious occasions as well as at times of adversity—with a view to reducing the sins and increasing the virtues.—37

निरन्तरं कृताभ्यासादन्तरे पश्यति ध्रुवम्।
तदा मुक्तिमवाप्नोति योगी नियतमानसः।। ३८।।

After a regular practice for some time the yogi begins to see this image within himself. This brings about concentration of the mind, which finally leads to emancipation.—38

अंगुष्ठाभ्यामुभे श्रोत्रे तर्जनीभ्यां द्विलोचने।
नासारन्ध्रे च मध्याभ्यां अनामाभ्यां वदने दृढम्।। ३९।।
निरुद्धयन् मरुतं योगी यदेवं कुरुते भृशम्।
तदा लक्षणमात्मानं ज्योतिरूपं प्रपश्यति।। ४०।।

When the yogi blocks his breath by first plugging the ears with the two thumbs, closing the eyes with the index fingers, the nostrils with middle fingers, and then pressing tight the mouth with the ring fingers, and holds the breath thus, he gets a glimpse of his own *Ātman* in the form of radiant light.—39 and 40

तत्तेजो दृश्यते येन क्षणमात्रं निराविलम्।
सर्वपापैर्विनिर्मुक्तः स याति परमां गतिम्।। ४१।।

He who sees this light with rapt attention even for half a moment gets rid of all his sins, and soon attains the supreme state.—41

निरन्तरकृताभ्यासात् योगी विगतकल्मषः।
सर्वदेहादि विस्मृत्य तदभिन्नः स्वयं भवेत्।। ४२।।

The yogi who practises this for a long time becomes sinless and transcends all forms of existence,* and finally merges into That (Supreme Being).—42

यः करोति [illegible]यासं गुप्ताचारेण मानवः।
स वै ब्रह्मविलीनः स्यात् पापकर्मरतो यदि।। ४३।।

The person who practises this (form of visualization of his own *Ātman*) in secret, ultimately merges into the Brahman despite his previous sins.—43

गोपनीयं प्रयत्नेन सद्यः प्रत्ययकारकः।
निर्वाणदायको लोके योगोऽयं मम वल्लभः।। ४४।।

*The four forms of existence are: physical, spiritual, divine, and causal.

When practised in secret it bears fruit instantly. O My dear Pārvatī! this yoga brings about *nirvāṇa* in this very world.—44

नादः सञ्जायते तस्य क्रमेणाभ्यासतश्च वै।
मत्तभृङ्गवेणुवीणासदृशः प्रथमो ध्वनिः।। ४५।।
एवमभ्यासतः पश्चात् संसारध्वान्तनाशनः।
घण्टानादसमः पश्चात् ध्वनिर्मेघरवोपमः।। ४६।।
ध्वनौ तस्मिन् मनो दत्वा यदा तिष्ठति निर्भयः।
तदा सञ्जायते तस्य लयस्य मम वल्लभे।। ४७।।

Its constant practice generates a number of sounds. At first the yogi hears a buzzing sound—like that made by a hornet intoxicated (by honey in flowers). Then it is like a musical note on the flute. Thereafter it is like the vibrations of a *vīṇā* (the Indian lute). Next it is like the ringing of bells—as though dispelling the illusion of world phenomena. Finally, it is like a thunderclap. If the yogi boldly remains concentrated despite even this, then, O My dear, he really gets involved in the Supreme (merges with the Supreme).—45–47

तत्र नादे यदा चित्तं रमते योगिनो भृशम्।
विस्मृत्य सकलं वाह्यं नादेन सह शाम्यति।। ४८।।

When the yogi's mind is enraptured with that sound, he becomes obvious to all external world and his mind gets harmonized with the sound.—48

एतदभ्यासयोगेन जित्वा सम्यक् गुणान् बहून्।
सर्वारम्भपरित्यागी चिदाकाशे विलीयते।। ४९।।

As a result of this the yogi conquers all three Qualities of Nature (*guṇas*) and then, released from the cycle of births and deaths, he merges into the Universal Soul.—49

नासनं सिद्धसदृशं न कुम्भसदृशं बलम्।
न खेचरीसमा मुद्रा न नादसदृशो लयः।। ५०।।

There is no *āsana* that is better than the Siddhāsana, no force equal to the one generated by *kumbhaka*, no *mudrā* more potent than the Khecarīmudrā and no *laya* more effective than the one caused by *nāda* (sound).—50

इदानीं कथयिष्यामि मुक्तस्यानुभवं प्रिये।
यज्ज्ञात्वा लभते मुक्तिं पापयुक्तोऽपि साधकः।। ५१।।

Now I shall describe, O dear, the actual method of liberation. When the yogi knows this he is able to achieve his own deliverance despite all his previous sins.—51

समभ्यर्चेश्वरं सम्यक् कृत्वा च योगमुत्तमम्।
गृह्णीयात् सुस्थितो भूत्वा गुरुं सन्तोष्य बुद्धिमान्।। ५२।।
जीवादि सकलं वस्तु दत्वा योगविदं गुरुम्।
सन्तोष्याति प्रयत्नेन योगोऽयं गृह्यते बुधैः।। ५३।।
विप्रान सन्तोष्य मेधावी नानामङ्गलसंयुतः।
ममालये शुचिर्भूत्वा प्रगृह्णीयात् शुभात्मकम्।। ५४।।
सन्यस्यानेन विधिना प्राक्तनं विग्रहादिकम्।
भूत्वा दिव्यवपुर्योगी गृह्णीयाद्वक्ष्यमाणकम्।। ५५।।

The wise yogi should start this excellent yoga after first doing obeisance to the Lord and then, after satisfying the guru and sitting down with a composed mind, accept the instructions from him. He should accept the instructions only after scrupulously satisfying the guru (in regard to his keenness) and, as an earnest, offering him goods and cattle. He should also satisfy some noble persons (Brahmins) before entering My temple and there, in auspicious surroundings, accept the instructions from the guru after duly renouncing the propensities of his senses and assuming a fresh divine (pure) body for the purpose of yoga.—52–55

पद्मानस्थितो योगी जनसङ्गविवर्जितः।
विज्ञाननाडीद्वितयमङ्गुलीभ्यां निरोधयेत्।। ५६।।

The yogi should then sit in Padmāsana in a solitary place and press his nostrils with the fingers to stop the breath.—56

सिद्धे तदा विभर्ति सुखरूपी निरञ्जनः।
तस्मिन् परिश्रमः कार्यो येन सिद्धो भवेत् खलु।। ५७।।

As the mastery of this breath-control leads to a vision of the Clear Light, it is necessary to work hard for its success.—57

यः करोति सदाभ्यासं तस्य सिद्धिर्न दूरतः।
वायुसिद्धिर्भवेत्तस्य क्रमादेव न संशयः।। ५८।।

Success is not far away for him who practises this regularly. He undoubtedly gets a command over his breath gradually.—58

सकृत् यः कुरुते योगी पापौघं नाशयेद् ध्रुवम्।
तस्य स्यान्मध्यमे वायोः प्रवेशो नात्र संशयः।। ५९।।

For the yogi who practises this well, the heap of sins vanish. He is then positively able to direct his vital air into the middle nerve (Suṣumnā).—59

एतदभ्यासशीलो यः स योगी देवपूजितः।
अणिमादिगुणं लब्ध्वा विचरेद्भुवनत्रये।। ६०।।

The yogi who practises this is adored even by the gods. Having acquired the supernormal powers of Aṇimā, etc. he can then move about in all the three worlds.—60

यो यथास्यानिलाभ्यासात्तद्भवेत्तस्य विग्रहः।
तिष्ठेदात्मनि मेधावी स पुनः क्रीडते भृशम्।। ६१।।

With whatever object in view the breath-control is practised the body gains the same quality. Having acquired that power, the yogi can then exercise it at will.—61

एतद्योगं परं गोप्यं न देयं यस्य कस्यचित्।
सप्रमाणैः समायुक्तस्तमेव कथ्यते ध्रुवम्।। ६२।।

This yoga is most secret and is not to be divulged indiscriminately to all. It should be told only to those who are positively qualified to receive it.—62

योगी पद्मासने तिष्ठेत् कण्ठकूपे यदा स्मरन्।
जिह्वां कृत्वा तालुमूले क्षुत्पिपासा निवर्त्तते।। ६३।।

When a yogi, sitting in Padmāsana, concentrates upon the hollow of his throat, keeping the tongue upturned against the palate, all his thirst and hunger disappear.—63

कण्ठकूपादधःस्थाने कूर्मनाड्यस्ति शोभना।
तस्मिन् योगी मनो दत्वा चित्तस्थैर्यं लभेद्भृशम्।। ६४।।

Just below the hollow of the throat is the Kūrma *nāḍī*. By concentrating upon it the yogi positively gets stability of the mind.—64

शिरःकपाले रुद्राक्ष्यो विधिवत् चिन्तयेद्यदि।
तदा ज्योतिः प्रकाशं स्याद्विद्युत्तेजः समप्रभम्।। ६५।।

When one concentrates upon the Rudra-eye* in the centre of the forehead, then a light like the flash of lightning issues from it.—65

***Rudrākṣi* or the Rudra-eye is the third eye of Lord Śiva which is located between the eyebrows. Esoterically, it is equated to the mental eye of man.

एतच्चिन्तनमात्रेण पापानां संक्षयो भवेत्।
दुराचारोऽपि पुरुषो लभते परमं पदम्।। ६६।।

With such concentration all the sins are shed, and even a wicked person can then attain the final goal.—66

अहर्निशं यदा चिन्तां तत् करोति विचक्षण:।
सिद्धानां दर्शनं तस्य भाषणञ्च भवेद्ध्रुवम्।। ६७।।

The wise yogi who concentrates like this day and night gets a vision of the Masters. He can actually talk with them.—67

तिष्ठन् गच्छन् स्वपन् भुञ्जन् ध्यायेच्छून्यमहर्निशम्।
तदाकाशमयो योगी चिदाकाशे विलीयते।। ६८।।

The yogi who contemplates upon the Void day and night even while sitting, walking, sleeping or eating, assumes the form of the sky and merges in the expanse of the mind.—68

एतज्ज्ञानं सदा कार्यं योगिना सिद्धिमिच्छता।
निरन्तरकृताभ्यासात् मम तुल्यो भवेद्ध्रुवम्।। ६९।।

Knowing all this, yogis who wish to master the yoga must always practise it. Through unremitting practice they can surely become like me.—69

एतज्ज्ञानबलाद्योगी सर्वेषां वल्लभो भवेत्।
सर्वान् भूतान् जयं कृत्वा निराशीरपरिग्रह:।। ७०।।

With this kind of knowledge the yogi endears himself to all. Having triumphed over all Elements he becomes detached and has a distaste for all worldly objects.—70

नासाग्रे दृश्यते येन पद्मासनगतेन वै।
मनसो मरणं तस्य खेचरत्वं प्रसिध्यति।। ७१।।

One who concentrates his gaze upon the tip of his nose while sitting in Padmāsana brings his mind (thoughts) to naught. He thus attains the state of Khecara.—71

ज्योति: पश्यति योगीन्द्र: शुद्धं शुद्धाचलोपमम्।
तत्राभ्यासबलेनैव स्वयं तद्रक्षको भवेत्।। ७२।।

That good yogi then sees the purest of pure Clear Light. After he has practised it for long he becomes his own protector.—72

उत्तानं शयने भूमौ सुप्त्वा ध्यायन्निरन्तरम्।
सद्य: श्रमविनाशाय स्वयं योगी विचक्षण:।

शिरः पश्चात्तु भागस्य ध्याने मृत्युञ्जयो भवेत्।। ७३।।

The wise yogi who lies flat (supine) on the ground and concentrates his thoughts for some time, gets rid of all his lethargy. When the thoughts are concentrated upon the back of the head, he is able to conquer death.—73

भ्रूमध्ये दृष्टिमात्रेण ह्यपरः परिकीर्तितः।। ७४।।

Another way is to concentrate upon the centre of the forehead between the eyebrows.—74

चतुर्विधस्य चान्नस्य रसस्त्रेधा विभज्यते।
तत्र सारतमो लिङ्गदेहस्य परिपोषकः।। ७५।।
सप्तधातुमयं पिण्डमेति पुष्णाति मध्यगः।
याति विन्मूत्ररूपेण तृतीयः सप्ततो वहिः।। ७६।।

Food goes into the body in four different ways.* There it is transformed into three substances. Of the latter the best extract goes to nourish the psychic field. The second best turns into the seven constituents of the physical body. The last goes out in the form of urine and excretions.—75 and 76

आद्यभागद्वयं नाड्यः प्रोक्तास्ताः सकला अपि।
पोषयन्ति वपुर्वायुमापादतलमस्तकम्।। ७७।।

The first two kinds of extracts stated above nourish all the physical and psychic channels as well as the airs circulating within the body from head to foot.—77

नाडीभिराभिः सर्वाभिर्वायुः सञ्चरते यदा।
तदैव न रसो देहे साम्येनेह प्रवर्तते।। ७८।।

When the airs flow evenly through all the *nāḍīs*, then there is no excess of juice in the body; it remains normal.—78

चतुर्दशानां तन्त्रेह व्यापारो मुख्यभागतः।
ता अनुग्राणहीनाश्च प्राणसञ्चारनाडिकाः।। ७९।।

The fourteen *nāḍīs* mentioned in this *śāstra* (II.13-15) are without any auxiliaries. These govern the operation of the senses and are the main channels of consciousness.—79

*The four ways in which food goes into the body are through (1) *cavvya* (mastication), (2) *cosya* (sucking), (3) *lehya* (lapping), and (4) *peya* (drinking).

The seven constituents of body are: (1) blood, (2) lymph, (3) marrow, (4) fat, (5) flesh or tissue, (6) bone, and (7) seminal fluid.

गुदाद्द्व्यङ्गुलश्चोर्द्धं मेढ्रैकाङ्गुलतस्त्वधः।
एवञ्चास्ति समं कन्दं समताचतुरङ्गुलम्।। ८०।।
पश्चिमाभिमुखी योनिर्गुदमेढ्रान्तरालगा।
तत्र कन्दं समाख्यातं तत्रास्ति कुण्डली सदा।। ८१।।
संवेष्टय सकला नाडी सार्द्धत्रिकुटिलाकृतिः।
मुखे निवेश्य सा पुच्छं सुषुम्नाविवरे स्थिता।। ८२।।

Now there is a compound bone which forms a four-finger wide platform (for the spinal column). It is located two-fingers above the anus and one finger below the genitals. Upon this platform, placed in the rear of the pelvic region, is to be found the Kuṇḍalinī coiled three and a half times around the root of the *nāḍīs*, lying like a serpent with its tail in its mouth, and blocking the entrance of the Suṣumnā *nāḍī*.—80-82

सुप्ता नागोपमा ह्येषा स्फुरन्ति प्रभया स्वया।
अहिवत् सन्धिसंस्थाना वाग्देवी बीजसंज्ञका।। ८३।।

Here she lies asleep, glowing with her own light; and guarding the crucial junction (of sacrum and the tail-end of the backbone) where lies the Seed of Speech.—83

तत्र बन्धूकपुष्पाभं कामबीजं प्रकीर्तितम्।
कलहेमसमं योगे प्रयुक्ताक्षररूपिणम्।। ८४।।

Here shines like a rosy *bandhūka* flower, or dull gold, the Seed of Sex. In yoga it is described as *Akṣara* or the Imperishable.—84

सुषुम्नापि च संश्लिष्टा बीजं तत्र वरं स्थितम्।
शरच्चन्द्रनिभं तेजस्त्वयमेतत् स्फुरत् स्थितम्।। ८५।।
सूर्यकोटिप्रतीकाशं चन्द्रकोटिसुशीतलम्।
एतन्त्रयं मिलित्वैव देवी त्रिपुरभैरवी।। ८६।।

This Seed, encircled by the Suṣumnā, is well-settled here. It radiates a bright light such as is seen coming from an autumn moon—as brilliant as though ten million suns and moons had got together! These three (the sun, the moon and the seed) constitute the Tripura-Bhairavī*—85 and 86

बीजसंज्ञं परं तेजस्तदेव परिकीर्तितम्।
क्रियाविज्ञानशक्तिभ्यां युतं यत् परितो भ्रमेत्।। ८७।।

*Tripura-Bhairavī is another name of Durgā, the supreme deity presiding over all three worlds. Durgā is also the goddess Śakti, consort of Śiva.

This great brilliance has been described as the Essence of the Seed. It operates in association with the forces of action (motion) and knowledge (consciousness).—87

उत्तिष्ठद्विशतन्त्वम्भः सूक्ष्मं शोणशिखायुतम्।
योनिस्थं तत् परं तेजः स्वयम्भूलिङ्गसंस्थितम्।। ८८।।

It moves up and down with the fluid in the body, in the form of an extremely fine red flame. It is very powerful while it is in the pelvic cavity close to the sex-organ, and is self-generated.—88

आधारपद्यमेतद्धि योनिर्यस्यास्ति कन्दतः।
परिस्फुरद्वादिसान्त चतुर्वर्णं चतुर्दलम्।। ८९।।

Here it is that the supporting lotus (Mūlādhāra) is found. Its core lies in the sacrum and its four petals, of four different hues indicated by the four letters beginning with *va* (व) and ending with *sa* (स), sparkle beautifully.—89

कुलाभिधं सुवर्णाभं स्वयम्भूलिङ्गसंगतम्।
द्विरण्डो यत्र सिद्धोस्ति डाकिनी यत्र देवता।। ९०।।

At one end of the golden-hued (petal) is the organ of procreation. The key-word for its mastery is Dviraṇḍa and its presiding deity is Ḍākinī.*—90

तत्पद्ममध्यगा योनिस्तत्र कुण्डलिनी स्थिता।
तस्या ऊर्द्धे स्फुरत्तेजः कामबीजं भ्रमन्मतम्।। ९१।।

In the core of this (Mūlādhāra) lotus dwells the goddess Kuṇḍalinī, endowed with the brilliance of the seminal seed radiating all over.—91

यः करोति सदा ध्यानं मूलाधारे विचक्षणः।
तस्य स्याद्दार्दुरीसिद्धिर्भूमित्याग क्रमेण वै।। ९२।।

The wise one who meditates upon this Mūlādhāra soon masters the power called Dārduri (frog-like) as a result of which he can gradually leave the ground.—92

वपुषः कान्तिरुत्कृष्टा जठराग्नि विवर्धनम्।
आरोग्यञ्च पटुत्वञ्च सर्वज्ञत्वञ्च जायते।। ९३।।

He gains as excellent glow all over his body, his appetite increases and he becomes healthy, smart and efficient.—93

*Dviraṇḍa is another name for Śiva in his aggressive mood, while Ḍākinī represents the goddess Śakti or Force.

भूतभव्यं भविष्यञ्च वेत्ति सर्वं सकारणम्।
अश्रुतान्यपि शास्त्राणि सरहस्यं वदेत् ध्रुवम्।। ९४।।

He knows all past, present and future, as well as other causes, and the mysteries of untaught *śāstras* become clear to him.—94

वक्त्रे सरस्वती देवी सदा नृत्यति निर्भरा।
मन्त्रसिद्धिर्भवेत्तस्य जपादेव न संशयः।। ९५।।

Saraswatī, the goddess of Speech, always dwells upon his lips (i.e., wise words come out of his mouth), as a result of which he is able to master the *mantras* with positive success—95

जरामरणदुःखौघान् नाशयति गुरोर्वचः।। ९६।।

This (Mūlādhāra contemplation) sweeps away decay, death and a flood of sins: such are the (infallible) words of the guru!—96

इदं ध्यानं सदा कार्यं पवनाभ्यासिना परम्।
ध्यानमात्रेण योगीन्द्रो मुच्यते सर्वकिल्विषात्।। ९७।।

This meditation should be done only after the breathing exercise. By such meditation the best among the yogis are freed from their impurities.—97

मूलपद्मं यदा ध्यायेत् स्वयम्भूलिङ्गसंज्ञकम्।
तदा तत् क्षणमात्रेण पापौघं नाशयेद् ध्रुवम्।। ९८।।

When the yogi meditates upon the image of Śiva in the Mūlādhāra lotus, all his sins vanish instantly.—98

यं यं कामयते चित्तं तं तं फलमवाप्नुयात्।
निरन्तरकृताभ्यासात् तं पश्यति विमुक्तिदम्।। ९९।।

Then whatever he thinks in his mind bears fruit definitely. By constant practice of this he finds the way to his deliverance.—99

पहिरभ्यन्तरे श्रेष्ठं पूजनीयं प्रयत्नतः।
ततः श्रेष्ठतमं ह्येतन्नान्यदस्ति मतं मम।। १००।।

Hence it is desirable to try for it with body and soul (i.e., outwardly and inwardly). In My view this is the best way, and there is none other like it.—100

आत्मसंस्थं शिवं त्यक्त्वा बहिरस्थं यः समर्चयेत्।
हस्तस्थं पिण्डमुत्सृज्य भ्रमते जीविताशया।। १०१।।

He who neglects the Śiva (*Ātman*) installed within him and seeks the one installed outside, is like a man who casts away the morsel of food in his hand and goes round looking for sustenance elsewhere.—101

आत्मलिङ्गार्चनं कुर्यादनालस्यं दिने दिने।
तस्य स्यात्सकला सिद्धिर्नात्र कार्या विचारणा।। १०२।।

He who worships his own Self (*Ātman*) assiduously, day after day, soon gets all the powers. There is no scope for any doubt about this.—102

निरन्तरकृताभ्यासात् षण्मासात् सिद्धिमाप्नुयात्।
तस्य वायुर्प्रवेशोऽपि सुषुम्नायां भवेद्ध्रुवम्।। १०३।।

Success is assured when this is practised unremittingly for six months. In this way the vital air can be made to enter the Suṣumnā *nāḍī* positively.—103

मनोजयञ्च लभते वायुविन्दुविधारणम्।
ऐहिकामुष्मिकी सिद्धिर्भवेन्नैवात्र संशयः।। १०४।।

The yogi finally masters his mind, gains control over the vital air and the seminal fluid. Undoubtedly he gets power, both in this world as well as in the other.—104

द्वितीयन्तु सरोजं यल्लिङ्गमूले व्यवस्थितम्।
तद्बादिलान्तषड्वर्णैः परिभास्वरषड्दलम्।। १०५।।
स्वाधिष्ठानाभिधं तत्तु पङ्कजं शोणरूपकम्।
बालाख्यो यत्र सिद्धोऽस्ति देवी यत्रास्ति राकिनी।। १०६।।

The second lotus is based at the root of the genitals. It has six petals, indicated by the letters *ba* (ब) to *la* (ल). It is called Swādhiṣṭhāna. This lotus is red as blood. The key to its mastery is Bāla and its presiding deity is Rākinī.*—105 and 106

यः ध्यायति सदा दिव्यं स्वाधिष्ठानारविन्दकम्।
तस्य कामाङ्गनाः सर्वे भजन्ते काममोहिताः।। १०७।।

He who always meditates upon the beautiful Swādhiṣṭhāna lotus is sought after by lovelorn damsels.—107

विविधाञ्चाश्रुतं शास्त्रं निःशंको वै भवेद्ध्रुवम्।
सर्वरोगाविनिर्मुक्तो लोके चरति निर्भयः।। १०८।।

He can propound with ease even those *śāstras* that have not been

*Bāla and Rākinī are variants of Śiva and Śakti.

learnt by him directly. Free of all ailments, he is able to move about in this world without care—108

मरणं खाद्यते तेन स केनापि न खाद्यते।
तस्य स्यात् परमा सिद्धिरणिमादिगुणान्विता।। १०९।।
वायुः सञ्चरते देहे रसवृद्धिर्भवेद्ध्रुवम्।
आकाशपङ्कजगलात्पीयूषमपि वर्द्धते।। ११०।।

Such a yogi conquers death, though he himself cannot be conquered by anybody. He acquires the great supernormal powers of Aṇimā etc., his vital air flows evenly in his body, the vitality improves and the nectar from the top lotus (Sahasrāra) overflows.—109 and 110

तृतीयं पङ्कजं नाभौ मणिपुरसंज्ञकम्।
दशारं डादिफान्तार्णैः शोभितं हेमवर्णकम्।। १११।।

The third lotus, called Maṇipura, is located near the navel. It has ten petals, all golden-hued, and are indicated by the ten letters beginning with *ḍa* (ड) and ending with *pha* (फ).—111

रुद्राख्यो यत्र सिद्धोऽस्ति सर्वमंगलदायकः।
तत्रस्था लाकिनी नाम्नी देवी परमधार्मिका।। ११२।।

The key-word for its mastery is Rudra, the bestower of benefices, and it is presided over by Lākinī,* the embodiment of highest virtue.—112

तस्मिन् ध्यानं सदा योगी करोति मणिपूरके।
तस्य पातालसिद्धिः स्यान्निरन्तरसुखावहा।। ११३।।

The yogi who meditates upon this Maṇipura lotus becomes a master of the nether world, and remains always happy.—113

ईप्सितञ्च भवेल्लोके दुःखरोगविनाशनम्।
कालस्य वञ्चनञ्चापि परदेहप्रवेशनम्।। ११४।।
जाम्बूनदादिकरणं सिद्धानां दर्शनं भवेत्।
ओषधिदर्शनञ्चापि निधीनां दर्शनं भवेत्।। ११५।।

He gets all the desired things in this world, is free from misery and disease, and can enter another body by 'cheating time.'** He can turn other metals into gold, discover rare herbs and treasures,

*Rudra and Lākinī are, again, the different names of Śiva and Śakti.

**'Cheating time'—i.e., Time, which inevitably disintegrates all composite bodies, has no effect on him.

and can meet the great adepts.—114 and 115

हृदयोऽनाहतं नाम चतुर्थं पङ्कजं भवेत्।
कादिठान्तार्णसंस्थानं द्वादशच्छदशोभितम्।
अतिशोणं वायुबीजं प्रसादस्थानमीरितम्।। ११६।।

The fourth lotus—Anāhata—is located near the heart. It has twelve petals, all intense red, which are indicated by the letters beginning with *ka* (क) and ending with *ṭha* (ठ). It contains the Seed of Air and throws up happiness all around.—116

पद्मस्थं तत्परं तेजो बाणलिङ्गं प्रकीर्तितम्।
तस्य स्मरणमात्रेण दृष्टादृष्टफलं लभेत्।
सिद्धः पिनाकी यत्रास्ते काकिनी यत्र देवता।। ११७।।

The heat that dwells within this lotus is called Bāṇaliṅga (heat). The yogi meditating upon this lotus gets the fruit of all seen and unseen things instantly. Its key-word is Pinākī and the presiding deity is Kākinī.*—117

एतस्मिन् सततं ध्यानं हृत्पाथोजे करोति यः।
क्षुभ्यन्ते तस्य कान्ता वै कामार्ता दिव्ययोषितः।। ११८।।

He who thus meditates upon the heart-lotus is sought after by lovelorn damsels even in heaven.—118

ज्ञानञ्चाप्रतिमं तस्य त्रिकालविषयं भवेत्।
दूरश्रुतिर्दूरदृष्टिः स्वेच्छया खगतां व्रजेत्।। ११९।।

He becomes an embodiment of knowledge and knows everything happening in past, present and future. He can hear inaudible sounds, see invisible things, and float in the air at his own sweet will.—119

सिद्धानां दर्शनञ्चापि योगिनां दर्शनं तथा।
भवेत् खेचरीसिद्धिश्च खेचराणां जयस्तथा।। १२०।।

Through the mastery of this Khecarī (levitation) power he commands all the creatures of the air. He also meets the great adepts and yogis of the past.—120

यो ध्यायति परं नित्यं बाणलिङ्गमद्वितीयकम्।
खेचरीभूचरीसिद्धिर्भवेत्तस्य न संशयः।। १२१।।

Anyone who meditates upon this unparalleled Bāṇaliṅga un-

*Pinākī and Kākinī are different forms of Śiva and Śakti.

doubtedly can master both the Khecarī and Bhūcarī powers.—121

एतद्ध्यानस्य माहात्म्यं कथितुं नैव शक्यते।
ब्रह्माद्योः सकला देवा गोपयन्ति परन्त्विदम्।। १२२।।

I need not extol the glories of this meditation any further. Brahmā and the other gods keep it a secret from others.—122

कण्ठस्थानस्थितं पद्मं विशुद्धं नाम पञ्चमम्।
धूम्रवर्णं स्वरोपेतं षोडशच्छदशोभितम्।। १२३।।

The fifth lotus, named Viśuddha, is located in the throat. It has sixteen petals, all smoke coloured, and are indicated by the sixteen (short and long) vowels beginning with *a* (अ) and ending with *aḥ* (अः).—123

छगलाण्डोऽस्ति सिद्धोऽत्र शाकिनी चाधिदेवता।
ध्यानं करोति यो नित्यं स योगीश्वरपण्डितः।। १२४।।

He is truly a wise and capable yogi who meditates upon this lotus. The key-word is Chagalāṇḍa and the presiding deity is Śākinī.*—124

किं तस्य योगिनोऽन्यत्र विशुद्धाख्ये सरोरुहे।
चतुर्वेदा विभासन्ते सरहस्या निधेरिव।। १२५।।

For a yogi who has mastered Viśuddha, where is the need for him to hunt for knowledge? The four Vedas and their mysteries are revealed to him just like the treasures of Kuvera.**—125

रहःस्थाने स्थितो योगी यदा क्रोधवशो भवेत्।
तदा समस्तं त्रैलोक्यं कम्पते नात्र संशयः।। १२६।।

Even if this yogi were to express displeasure at something while sitting at a remote and solitary place, all the three worlds would begin to tremble. There is no doubt about this.—126

इह स्थाने मनो यस्य दैवाद्याति लयं यदा।
तदा वाह्यं परित्यज्य स्वान्तरे रमते ध्रुवम्।। १२७।।

When his mind gets thoroughly absorbed in the (Viśuddha) lotus, he remains in an inner bliss and loses consciousness of the external world.—127

*Chagalāṇḍa (blue-throated) and Śākinī represents Śiva and Śakti. Śiva is also known as Nīlakaṇṭha (blue-throated) since he holds by his yogic feat all the poison of this world in his throat.

**Kuvera is the mythological *yakṣa* king who is believed to be entrusted with the task of guarding the wealth of the gods.

तस्य न क्षतिमायाति स्वशरीरस्य शक्तितः।
संवत्सरसहस्रोऽपि वज्रातिकठिनस्य वै।। १२८।।

His body does not decay during this time, for he can just wish and make it as hard as a thunderbolt, so that it can last a thousand years!—128

यदा त्यजति तद्ध्यानं योगीन्द्रोऽवनिमण्डले।
तदा वर्षसहस्राणि तत्क्षणं मन्यते कृती।। १२९।।

And when he finishes with that meditation the master-yogi feels as though a thousand years on this earth were only a moment!—129

आज्ञापद्मं भ्रुवोर्मध्ये हक्षोपेतं द्विपत्रकम्।
शुक्लाख्यं तन्महाकालः सिद्धो देव्यत्र हाकिनी।। १३०।।

The Ājñāpura lotus is located between the eyebrows. It has two petals, indicated by the letters *ha* (ह) and *kṣa* (क्ष). Its key-word is Śukla, representing Eternal Time, and it is presided over by the deity called Hākinī.—130

शरच्चन्द्रनिभं तत्राक्षरबीजं विजृम्भितम्।
पुमान् परमहंसोऽयं यज्ज्ञात्वा नावसीदति।। १३१।।

Here it is that the Seed of Immortality bursts forth, like an autumn moon, into the Paramahaṃsa state.* With that kind of knowledge nobody ever suffers.—131

एतदेव परं तेजः सर्वतन्त्रेषु गोपितम्।
चिन्तयित्वा परं सिद्धिं लभते नात्र संशयः।। १३२।।

This (Seed of Immortality) has been regarded in the Tantras as a super force which, when contemplated upon, undoubtedly brings the maximum success.—132

तुरीयं त्रितयं लिङ्गं तदाहं मुक्तिदायकः।
ध्यानमात्रेण योगीन्द्रो मत्समो भवति ध्रुवम्।। १३३।।

This (Ājñāpura) completes the three main divisons, i.e., it is the fourth (Turīya) stage. I call it the 'bestower of Deliverance' because the yogi can become like Me by meditating upon it.**—133

*Paramahaṃsa (Supreme Swan) is a person who, like a swan, can extract the milk of Reality from the concoction that is world phenomena.

**Turīya is the fourth stage, so called because it is here that the twisting of the three principal nerves ends; after this only the Suṣumṇā proceeds further up to the Sahasrāra. Rising from Mūlādhāra, the Iḍā and Piṅgalā intertwine with the Suṣumnā

इडा हि पिंगला ख्याता वरुणासीति होच्यते।
वाराणसी तयोर्मध्ये विश्वनाथोऽत्र भाषितः।। १३४।।

Iḍā and Piṅgalā have been described as the rivers Varuṇā and Asi* at the confluence of which is located Vārāṇasī or Kāśī, the seat of Viśwanātha (Lord of the Universe).—134

एतत् क्षेत्रस्य माहात्म्यमृषिभिस्तत्त्वदर्शिभिः।
शास्त्रेषु बहुधा प्रोक्तं परं तत्त्वं सुभाषितम्।। १३५।।

The holy significance of this place (Kāśī) has been described in the various *śāstras* as well as by the sages and philosophers.—135

सुषुम्ना मेरुणा याता ब्रह्मरन्ध्रं यतोऽस्ति वै।
ततश्चैषा परावृत्या तदाज्ञापद्मदक्षिणे।
वामनासापुटं याति गंगेति परिगीयते।। १३६।।

The Suṣumnā passes through the spinal column (*meru*) wherein is to be found the Brahmarandhra (Passage of Knowledge). There, girdling the Ājñā lotus on the right, the Gaṅgā or Iḍā joins the left nostril.**—136

ब्रह्मरन्ध्रे हि यत्पद्मं सहस्रारं व्यवस्थितम्।
तत्र कन्दे हि या योनिस्तस्यां चन्द्रो व्यवस्थितः।। १३७।।

Crowning the Brahmarandhra is enshrined the thousand-petalled Sahasrāra, at the base of which is a cavity in which is located the Moon.—137

त्रिकोणाकारतस्तस्याः सुधा क्षरति सन्ततम्।
इडायाममृतं तत्र समं स्रवति चन्द्रमाः।। १३८।।

It is triangular (crescent) in shape, and from this Moon constantly drips ambrosia which feeds the Iḍā.—138

अमृतं वहते धारा धारारूपं निरन्तरम्।
वामनासापुटं याति गंगेत्युक्ता हि योगिभिः।। १३९।।

and cross each other at three points, thus diving the trunk into three main divisions. Iḍā and Piṅgalā rise like the two serpents seen in the winged wand of the Greek god Hermes. They end at the back of the two nostrils, just below the Ājñāpuracakra stationed between the eyebrows.

*Varuṇā and Asi are two small tributaries of the river Gaṅgā which flows past the city of Benares.

**Iḍā, Piṅgalā and Suṣumnā have been here designated respectively as Gaṅgā, Yamunā and Saraswatī. Earlier, however, Iḍā and Piṅgalā were compared to the two tributaries of the Gaṅgā, viz., Varuṇā and Asi.

This ambrosia flows in a continuous stream which, passing through the left nostril, enters the Iḍā. The yogis call it the Gaṅgā.—139

आज्ञापङ्कजदक्षांसाद्वामनासापुटं गता।
उद्ग्वहेति तत्रेडा वरणासमुदाहृता।। १४०।।

It is the upper (up-flowing) part of the Iḍā, which encircles the Ājñā, lotus on the right, that has been designated as the Varuṇā.—140

ततो द्वयमिहस्थाने वाराणस्यान्तु चिन्तयेत्।। १४१।।

Hence both (Iḍā and Piṅgalā) as well as Vārāṇasī should be visualized at this point.—141

तदाकारा पिङ्गलापि तदाज्ञाकमलान्तरे।
दक्षनासापुटे याति प्रोक्तास्माभिरसीति वै।। १४२।।

In the same way Piṅgalā too encircles the Ājñā lotus on the left and then joins the right nostril. It has been designated as Asi.—142

मूलाधारे हि यत्पद्मं चतुष्पत्रं व्यवस्थितम्।
तत्र मध्ये हि या योनिस्तस्यां सूर्यो व्यवस्थितः।। १४३।।

Now, within the Mūlādhāra lotus, which has four petals, there is a small cavity in which dwells the Sun.—143

तत्सूर्यमण्डलाद्वारं विषं क्षरति सन्ततम्।
पिङ्गलायां विषं यत्र स्वयं यात्यति तापनम्।। १४४।।

From this orb constantly oozes poison (passion) and this self-generated heat infects the Piṅgalā.—144

विषं तत्र वहन्ती या धारारूपं निरन्तरम्।
दक्षनासापुटं याति कल्पितेयन्तु पूर्वकम्।। १४५।।

This poison continuously flows up and, as described earlier, comes up to the right nostril.—145

आज्ञापङ्कजवामांशाद्दक्षनासापुटं गता।
उदग्वहा पिङ्गलापि पुरासीति प्रकीर्तिता।। १४६।।

Encircling the Ājñā lotus on the left and coming round to the right nostril, this upper region of the Piṅgalā has been described earlier as the river Asi.—146

आज्ञापद्ममिदं प्रोक्तं यत्र प्रोक्तो महेश्वरः।
पीठत्रयं ततश्चोर्द्ध निरुक्तं योगचिन्तकैः।
तद्विन्दुनादशक्त्याख्यो भालपद्मे व्यवस्थितः।। १४७।।

The Ājñāpura, mentioned earlier as the seat of Eternal Time, is located in the forehead (between the eyebrows). Yoga thinkers have visualized three platforms just above it—one each for Matter, Sound and Force.—147

यः करोति सदा ध्यानमाज्ञापद्मस्य गोपितम्।
पूर्वजन्मकृतं कर्म विनश्येदविरोधतः।। १४८।।

He who regularly meditates upon this Ājñā lotus in secret liquidates his *karma* acquired in previous lives without much difficulty.—148

इह स्थितो यदा योगी ध्यानं कुर्यान्निरन्तरम्।
तदा करोति प्रतिमाप्रतिजल्पमनर्थवत्।। १४९।।

When the yogi, through constant practice, gets stabilized in such meditation, he loses the sense of duality. He has then no use either for the original or the image of it.—149

यक्षराक्षसगन्धर्वा अप्सरोगणकिन्नराः।
सेवन्ते चरणौ तस्य सर्वे तस्य वशानुगाः।। १५०।।

Then *yakṣas* (divine guards), *rākṣasas* (monsters), *gandharvas* (divine musicians), *apsarās* (divine dancers), and *kinnaras* (half-human and half-animal divine beings)—all worship at his feet and obey him.—150

करोति रसनां योगी प्रविष्टां विपरीतगाम्।
लम्बिकोर्द्धेषु गर्त्तेषु कृत्वा ध्यानं भयापहम्।। १५१।।
अस्मिन् स्थाने मनो यस्य क्षणार्धं वर्ततेऽचलम्।
तस्य सर्वाणि पापानि संक्षयं यान्ति तत्क्षणात्।। १५२।।

Above the palatine papilla (uvula) is a small aperture (sinus). When the yogi takes his upturned tongue and holds it there while meditating, even though that meditation may be but for a short duration, he gets rid of all his accumulated sins.—151 and 152

यानि यानीह प्रोक्तानि पञ्चपद्मे फलानि वै।
तानि सर्वाणि सुतरामेतज्ज्ञानाद्भवन्ति हि।। १५३।।

All the benefits spoken of by Me for the other five lotuses can be obtained quicker when this (Ājñācakra) is known —153

यः करोति सदा ध्यानमाज्ञापद्मे विचक्षणः।
वासनाया महाबन्धं तिरस्कृत्य प्रमोदते।। १५४।।

The wise yogi who regularly practises meditation on the Ājñācakra gets freed from the great snare of desires, and thereafter lives happily.—154

प्राणप्रयाणसमये तत् पद्मं यः स्मरन् सुधीः।
त्यजेत् प्राणान् स धर्मात्मा परमात्मनि लीयते।। १५५।।

The wise one who remembers this lotus at the time of relinquishing his breath (i.e., at death) gets merged into the Supreme.—155

तिष्ठन् गच्छन् स्वपन् जाग्रत् यो ध्यानं कुरुते नरः।
पापकर्माणि कुर्वाणो न हि मज्जति किल्विषे।
योगी द्वन्दविनिर्मुक्तः स्वीयया प्रभया स्वयम्।। १५६।।

The man who always meditates upon this, whether while walking, sitting, sleeping or awake, never gets tainted by unrighteous deeds. Such a yogi, through his own efforts, gets released from the illusion of dualities.—156

द्विदलध्यानमाहात्म्यं कथितुं नैव शक्यते।
ब्रह्मादिदेवताश्चैव किञ्चिन्मत्तो विदन्ति हि।। १५७।।

I am unable to extol the glories of meditation upon this two-petalled one (i.e., Ājñācakra). Even Brahmā and the other gods have learnt only a little of it from Me.—157

अत ऊर्ध्वं तालुमूले सहस्रारं सुशोभितम्।
अस्ति तत्र सुषुम्नाया मूलं सविवरं स्थितम्।। १५८।।

Higher above and over the roof of the palate is enshrined the Sahasrāra. Here ends the upper end of the Suṣumnā *nāḍī*.—158

तालुमूले सुषुम्ना सा अधोवक्त्रा प्रवर्तते।
मूलाधारयोन्यन्ता सर्वनाडीसमाश्रिताः।
ता बीजभूतास्तत्वस्य ब्रह्ममार्गप्रदायिकाः।। १५९।।

The Suṣumnā terminates over the roof of the palate and then turns downwards. Being connected with the Mūlādhāra it serves as common support (afferent and efferent) for all other nerves, thus conveying the essence (seed) of perception (to the brain) through the channel of Brahma-mārga.—159

तालुस्थाने च यत् पद्मं सहस्रारं पुरोदितम्।
तत् कन्दे योनिरेकास्ति पश्चिमाभिमुखी गता।। १६०।।

The Sahasrāra lotus located over the roof of the palate has a small cavity placed laterally in its stamen.—160

तस्यां मध्ये सुषुम्नायां मूलं सविवरं स्थितम्।
ब्रह्मरन्ध्रं तदेवोक्तमामूलाधारपङ्कजम्।। १६१।।

The Suṣumnā, which comes up from the Mūlādhāra and passes through the Brahmarandhra, opens up here into this cavity.—161

तत्र रन्ध्रे तु तच्छक्तिः सुषुम्नाकुण्डली सदा।
सुषुम्नायां सदा शक्तिश्चित्रा स्यान्मम वल्लभे।
तस्यां मम मते कार्या ब्रह्मरन्ध्रादिकल्पना।। १६२।।

In this Passage is to be found a force that is the Suṣumnā's own psychic power (Kuṇḍalinī). This force is known as Citrā. Hence in My view, O Pārvatī, it is advisable to meditate upon this Brahmarandhra itself.—162

यस्य स्मरणमात्रेण ब्रह्मज्ञत्वं प्रजायते।
पापक्षयश्च भवति न भूयः पुरुषो भवेत्।। १६३।।

Meditation upon the Brahmarandhra brings the knowledge of Brahman or the Supreme. Then all sins are wiped off and one is not reborn again.—163

प्रवेशितं चलाङ्गुष्ठं मुखे स्वस्य निवेशयेत्।
तेनात्र न वहत्येव देहचारी समीरणः।। १६४।।

If one takes his big toe into his mouth and holds it there, he can thereby stop the flow of the psychic air within his body.—164

तेन संसारचक्रेऽस्मिन् भ्रमतीत्येव सर्वदा।
तदर्थं ये प्रवर्तन्ते योगी न प्राणधारणे।। १६५।।

It is the flow of this (psychic air) that is the motive power for the cycle of births and deaths. That is why yogis try to control this vital air.—165

तत एवाखिला नाडी विरुद्धा चाष्टवेष्टनम्।
इयं कुण्डलिनी शक्ती रन्ध्रं त्यजति नान्यथा।। १६६।।

When the flow in the nerves surrounding the Suṣumnā is reversed, the Serpent Power vacates the entrance to the Brahmarandhra (at the Mūlādhāra).—166

यदा पूर्णासु सर्वासु संनिरुद्धोऽनिलस्तदा।
बन्धत्यागे कुण्डलीन्या मुखं रन्ध्राद्बहिर्भवेत्।। १६७।।

When the flow of this air is checked, and there is no escape for it through any of the (other) *nāḍīs*, then the Kuṇḍalinī is forced to abandon its position at the entrance of the Brahmarandhra.—167

सुषुम्नायां सदैवायं वहेत् प्राणसमीरणः।
मूलपद्मास्थितो योनिर्वामदक्षिणकोणतः।
इडापिङ्गलोर्मध्ये सुषुम्ना योनिमध्यगा।। १६८।।

The vital air then flows freely through the Suṣumnā *nāḍī*. (As already explained) on the either side of the Mūlādhāra are placed the Iḍā and the Piṅgalā with the Suṣumnā in the centre.—168

ब्रह्मरन्ध्रन्तु तत्रैव सुषुम्नाधारमण्डले।
यो जानाति स मुक्तः स्यात् कर्मबन्धाद्विचक्षणः।। १६९।।

The Brahmarandhra starts with Suṣumnā from the Mūlādhāra. He who knows this is indeed wise and must soon be liberated from the bondage of his *karma*.—169

ब्रह्मरन्ध्रमुखे तासां संगमं स्यादसंशयः।
यस्मिन् स्नाने स्नातकानां मुक्तिः स्यादविरोधतः।। १७०।।

At the mouth of the Brahmarandhra is to be found their confluence (i.e., of Iḍā, Piṅgalā and Suṣumnā). Those who bathe (meditate) at this confluence are positively liberated.—170

गंगायमुनयोर्मध्ये वहत्येषा सरस्वती।
तासान्तु संगमे स्नात्वा धन्यो याति परां गतिम्।। १७१।।

This is like the confluence of the Gaṅgā, Yamuṇā and Saraswatī (at Prayāg, Allahabad), bathing at which place helps the fortunate one to attain the supreme state.—171

इडा गंगा पुरा प्रोक्ता पिङ्गला चार्कपुत्रिका।
मध्या सरस्वती प्रोक्ता तासां संगोऽतिदुर्लभम्।। १७२।।

Earlier, Iḍā has been named as the Gaṅgā, Piṅgalā as the Yamunā, and in between lies the Saraswatī (daughter of Sun). The confluence of these three is unique indeed.—172

सितासिते संगमे यो मनसा स्नानमाचरेत्।
सर्वपापविनिर्मुक्तो याति ब्रह्म सनातनम्।। १७३।।

When the mind takes a dip at the junction of the bright and the dark,* it rids itself of all the impurities, and thereafter proceeds to the Eternal Brahman.—173

त्रिवेण्या संगमे यो वै पितृकर्म समाचरेत्।
तारयित्वा पितॄन् सर्वान् स याति परमां गतिम्।। १७४।।

He who performs the funeral rites of his forefathers at *triveṇī* (at the confluence of the three rivers) helps them (the forefathers) to shed their sins and attain the supreme state.—174

नित्यनैमित्तिकं काम्यं प्रत्यहं यः समाचरेत्।
मनसा चिन्तयित्वा तु सोऽक्षयं फलमाप्नुयात्।। १७५।।

He who has this (sacred confluence) in his mind while he peforms his ordinary, particular and desired deeds (*karma*) gets the eternal (divine) fruits of those *karma.*—175

सकृद्यः कुरुते स्नानं स्वर्गे सौख्यं भुनक्ति सः।
दग्धान् पापानशेषान् वै योगी शुद्धमतिः स्वयम्।। १७६।।

The yogi who thus bathes (his mind) even once enjoys the pleasures of heaven after his impurities are washed away and his mind has turned pure.—176

अपवित्रः पवित्रो वा सर्वावस्थां गतोऽपि वा।
स्नानाचरणमात्रेण पूतो भवति नान्यथा।। १७७।।

Whether one be clean or unclean, and whatever may be the condition in which he is placed, once such a bath has been performed he becomes absolutely pure.—177

मृत्युकाले प्लुतं देहं त्रिवेण्याः सलिले यदा।
विचिन्त्य यस्त्यजेत् प्राणान् स तदा मोक्षमाप्नुयात्।। १७८।।

He who breathes his last while thinking that his body is flooded with the waters of the *triveṇī*, always attains emancipation.—178

नातः परतरं गुह्यं त्रिषु लोकेषु विद्यते।
गोप्तव्यं स प्रयत्नेन न चाख्येन कदाचन।। १७९।।

Indeed nothing is more mysterious than this in all the three worlds. Hence it should be kept a secret and not disclosed to others.—179

* *Sitāsit* literally means the white and non-white. The water of the Gaṅgā appears white,against the dark (bluish) colour of the water of the Yamunā.

ब्रह्मरन्ध्रे मनोदत्त्वा क्षणार्धं यदि तिष्ठति।
सर्वपापविनिर्मुक्तः स याति परमां गतिम्।। १८०।।

For, he who can truly concentrate his mind upon the Brahmarandhra even for a while, gets rid of all his sins and attains the highest state.—180

अस्मिन् लीनं मनो यस्य स योगी लीयते मयि।
अणिमादिगुणान् भुक्त्वा स्वेच्छया पुरुषोत्तमः।। १८१।।

The yogi whose mind is thus absorbed gets merged in Me. He enjoys all the supernormal powers of Aṇimā etc. and thereafter, at his own choice, reaches the highest state.—181

एतद्रन्ध्रज्ञानमात्रेण मर्त्यः संसारेऽस्मिन् वल्लभो मे भवेत् सः।
पापं जित्वा मुक्तिमार्गाधिकारी, ज्ञानं दत्वा तारयत्यद्भुतं वै।। १८२।।

He who cognizes his Brahmarandhra in this very world becomes very dear to Me. That man triumphs over his sins and, being himself destined for deliverance, imparts knowledge to others, thus helping them to cross (the world phenomena).—182

चतुर्मुखादित्रिदशैरगम्यं योगिवल्लभम्।
प्रयत्नेन सुगोप्यं तद्ब्रह्मरन्ध्रं मयोदितम्।। १८३।।

The Four-faced One (Brahmā) and other gods are still uninitiated in the mystery of this Brahmarandhra. Hence what has been said by Me now should be kept a close secret by all good yogis.—183

पुरा मयोक्ता या योनिः सहस्रारसरोरुहे।
तदधो वर्तते चन्द्रस्तद्ध्यानं क्रियते बुधैः।। १८४।।

Now the little cavity spoken of by Me earlier, and which is found inside the *sahasrāra*, lotus, has below it the Moon. The wise yogi should meditate upon it.—184

यस्य स्मरणमात्रेण योगीन्द्रोऽवनिमण्डले।
पूज्यो भवति देवानां सिद्धानां सम्मतो भवेत्।। १८५।।

By concentrating on this, the good yogi earns the respect of the gods and becomes equal to the adepts.—185

शिरःकपालविवरे ध्यायेद्दुग्धमहोदधिम्।
तत्र स्थित्वा सहस्रारे पद्मे चन्द्रं विचिन्तयेत्।। १८६।।

(The yogi should) visualize a vast ocean of milk existing within his cranium in the midst of which has bloomed the Sahasrāra lotus with the Moon within it.—186

शिरःकपालविवरे द्विरष्टकलया युतः।
पीयूषभानुं हंसाख्यं भवेत्तं निरञ्जनम्।। १८७।।

That Moon in the cavity of the head should be visualized as the Clear Light, shaped like a swan, and shedding ambrosia enriched with the sixteen phases of the Moon.—187

निरन्तरं कृताभ्यासात्त्रिदिने पश्यति ध्रुवम्।
दृष्टिमात्रेण पापौघं दहत्येव स साधकः।। १८८।।

As a result of continuous practice one can see it (Clear Light) within three days. Seeing it the yogi's sins are burnt up in no time.—188

अनागतञ्च स्फुरति चित्तशुद्धिर्भवेत् खलु।
सद्यः कृत्वापि दहति महापातकपञ्चकम्।। १८९।।
अनुकूल्यं ग्रहा यान्ति सर्वे नश्यन्त्युपद्रवाः।
उपसर्गाः शमं यान्ति युद्धे जयमाप्नुयात्।। १९०।।

The future then becomes apparent, the mind turns pure, and even though one may have committed one of the five Great Sins (*mahāpātaka*),* the same gets obliterated. All the celestial bodies (i.e., their influence) become favourable, all hindrances vanish, all problems get solved, and success crowns all efforts.—189 and 190

खेचरीभूचरीसिद्धिर्भवेच्छिरेन्दु दर्शनात्।
ध्यानादेव भवेत् सर्वं नात्र कार्या विचारणा।। १९१।।
सतताभ्यासयोगेन सिद्धो भवति नान्यथा।
सत्यं सत्यं पुनः सत्यं मम तुल्यो भवेद्ध्रुवम्।। १९२।।
योगशास्त्रञ्च परमं योगिनां सिद्धिदायकम्।। १९३।।

When the Moon (Clear Light) within the head is seen and is meditated upon, all wishes are automatically fulfilled. In due course, and by constant practice of this yoga, one can become as adept, and not otherwise. In the *Yogaśāstra* this has been described as one of the best of yogas, a bestower of supernormal powers upon the yogi. Verily, those who practise this become just like Me.—191–93

*The five *mahāpātaka* are described as: (1) killing a Brahmin, (2) taking liquor, (3) thieving, (4) committing adultery with the guru's wife, and (5) associating with those who have committed one or more of the aforesaid four categories of crime.

अत ऊर्द्धं दिव्यरूपं सहस्रारं सरोरुहम्।
ब्रह्माण्डाख्यस्य देहस्य वाह्ये तिष्ठति मुक्तिदम्।। १९४।।
कैलासो नाम तस्यैव महेशो यत्र तिष्ठति।
अकुलाख्यो विलासी च क्षयवृद्धि विवर्जितः।। १९५।।

Further up, spreading out like a wide lake, is the divine configuration of the Sahasrāra. It is outside the cosmic universe within the body (cf. II.1–4) and it is the key to Emancipation. It has been designated Kailāsa where dwells Maheśa (Great God) and it is described as limitless, resplendent and constant (i.e., without the qualities of increase and decrease).—194 and 195

स्थानस्यास्य ज्ञानमात्रेण नृणां संसारेऽस्मिन् सम्भवो नैव भूयः।
भूतग्रामं सन्तताभ्यासयोगात् कर्तुं हर्तुं स्याच्च शक्तिः समग्राः।। १९६।।

For those men who know this place there is no return to earth (i.e., no re-birth). All creatures subject to the law (cycle) of births and deaths can develop the necessary powers and neutralize it through yoga.—196

स्थाने परे हंसनिवासभूते, कैलासनाम्नीह निविष्टचेताः।
योगी हृतव्याधिरधःकृताधिरायुश्चिरं जीवति मृत्युमुक्तः।। १९७।।

The yogi whose mind gets fixed on this place called Kailāsa where dwells the Swan (the symbol of Pure Knowledge) will be able to banish all his ailments, prolong his longevity and, being free from death, can live on eternally (i.e., become an immortal).—197

चित्तवृत्तिर्यदा लीना कुलाख्ये परमेश्वरे।
तदा समाधिसाम्येन योगी निश्चलतां व्रजेत्।। १९८।।

When all propensities of the mind break up at this point and submerge into the Supreme, the yogi becomes motionless. He attains the equability of *samādhi.*—198

निरन्तरकृतध्यानाज्जगद्विस्मरणं भवेत्।
तदा विचित्रसामर्थ्यं योगिनो भवति ध्रुवम्।। १९९।।

When he continues with this meditation he becomes oblivious of the world. The yogi then develops extraordinary powers.—199

तस्माद्गलितपीयूषं पिबेद्योगी निरन्तरम्।
मृत्योर्मृत्युं विधाय स कुलं जित्वा सरोरुहे।। २००।।

The yogi then drinks deep the nectar that flows (from the Moon) and, dealing a death-blow to Death, crosses over to that

Wide Lake (Sahasrāra).—200

अत्र कुण्डलिनीशक्तिर्लयं याति कुलाभिधा।
तदा चतुर्विधा सृष्टिर्लीयते परमात्मनि।। २०१।।

Here it is that the Kuṇḍalinī force terminates, and here it is that the cause of the four-fold births* ends in the Supreme.—201

यज्ज्ञात्वा प्राप्य विषयं चित्तवृत्तिर्विलीयते।
तस्मिन् परिश्रमं योगी करोति निरपेक्षकः।। २०२।।

Upon achieving the desired objective, modifications in the mind of the yogi subside. The wise yogi therefore always works diligently and relentlessly for this objective.—202

चित्तवृत्तिर्यदालीना तस्मिन् योगी भवेद्ध्रुवम्।
तदा विज्ञायतेऽखण्ड ज्ञानरूपी निरञ्जनः।। २०३।।

When the propensities in the yogi's mind finally quiesce, the Clear Light is revealed in full in the Knowledge-form.—203

ब्रह्माण्डवाह्ये संचिन्त्य स्वप्रतीकं यथोदितम्।
तमावेश्य महच्छून्यं चिन्तयेदविरोधतः।। २०४।।

The yogi, as stated earlier, should visualize his own image out in the universe—in the Great Space enveloped in darkness—and meditate upon it diligently.—204

आद्यमध्यान्तशून्यन्तं कोटिसूर्यसमप्रभम्।
चन्द्रकोटिप्रतीकाशमभ्यस्य सिद्धिमाप्नुयात्।। २०५।।

This Void, which is infinite and without beginning, middle or end, absorbs the light of ten million suns and ten million moons. Meditation on this will bring success to the yogi.—205

एतद्ध्यानं सदा कुर्यादनालस्यं दिने दिने।
तस्य स्यात् सकला सिद्धिर्वत्सरान्नात्र संशयः।। २०६।।

He who energetically pursues this form of meditation day after day undoubtedly gets all the supernormal powers.—206

क्षणार्द्धं निश्चलं तत्र मनो यस्य भवेद्ध्रुवम्।
स एव योगी मद्भक्तः सर्वलोकेषु पूजितः।। २०७।।
तस्य कल्मषसंघातस्तत्क्षणादेव नश्यति।। २०८।।

*The four-fold births are: (1) *svedaj* or birth caused by exudation, e.g., plants, etc., (2) *aṇḍaj* or birth out of eggs, e.g., birds, reptiles, etc., (3) *piṇḍaj* or birth out of a cell, e.g., mammals and human beings, and (4) *manaj* or birth out of the mind, e.g., spirit bodies, etc.

The yogi who gets his mind steadily fixed there (in the Void) even for half a moment is indeed a faithful devotee of Mine and will be adored in all the three worlds. His accumulated sins will get dissipated promptly.—207 and 208

यं दृष्ट्वा न प्रवर्तन्ते मृत्युसंसारवर्त्मनि।
अभ्यासेत्तं प्रयत्नेन स्वाधिष्ठानेन वर्त्मना।। २०९।।

This self-determined path which, when followed, does not bring one back to this death-dominated world, should therefore be practised earnestly.—209

एतद्ध्यानस्य माहात्म्यं मया वक्तुं न शक्यते।
यः साधयति जानाति सोऽस्माकमपि सम्मतः।। २१०।।

I need not stress the great importance of such practice, for he who practises thus knows that he can thereby become like Me.—210

ध्यानादेव विजानाति विचित्रेक्षण सम्भवम्।
अणिमादिगुणोपेतो भवत्येव न संशयः।। २११।।

Quite a number of things become instantly possible with this meditation, and there is no doubt that supernormal powers like Aṇimā etc. can then be easily enjoyed.—211

राजयोगो मयाख्यातः सर्वतन्त्रेषु गोपितः।
राजाधिराज योगोऽयं कथयामि समासतः।। २१२।।

I have thus described the Rājayoga, which is the most mysterious among all Tantras. It is the king (best) of Rājayogas that I have told you in brief.—212

स्वस्तिकऽ्यासनं कृत्वा सुमठे जन्तुवर्जिते।
गुरुं संपूज्य यत्नेन ध्यानमेतत् समाचरेत्।। २१३।।

This meditation is to be started after first doing obeisance to the guru, and thereafter seated in Swastikāsana (easy posture) at a congenial and uncrowded temple or holy place.—213

निरालम्बं भवेज्जीवं ज्ञात्वा वेदान्तयुक्तितः।
निरालम्बं मनोकृत्वा न किञ्चित् साधयेत् सुधीः।। २१४।।

The wise yogi should be completely unattached (in his mind) in accordance with the precepts of Vedānta, and he should never meditate even for a while until his mind is totally composed.—214

एतद्ध्यानान्महासिद्धिर्भवत्येव न संशयः।
वृत्तिहीनं मनः कृत्वा पूर्णरूपः स्वयं भवेत्।। २१५।।

Only such meditation will bring the maximum success, because a mind that is propensity-less automatically takes on the form of the Self (*Ātman*).—215

साधयेत् सततं यो वै स योगी विगतस्पृहः।
अहं नाम न कोऽप्यस्मिन् सर्वदात्मैव विद्यते।। २१६।।

To the yogi who regularly practises this form of non-attachment, the word 'I' has no meaning, for he sees everything around him as his own *Ātman*.—216

को बन्धः कस्य वा मोक्षः एवं पश्येत् सदा हि सः।
एतत् करोति यो नित्यं स मुक्तो नात्र संशयः।। २१७।।

What is bondage and what is freedom?—this is how he views (life) always. When he is constantly in this state he undoubtedly becomes emancipated.—217

स एव योगी सद्भक्तः सर्वलोकेषु पूजितः।
अहमस्मीति च जपन् जीवात्मपरमात्मनोः।
अहं त्वमेतदुभयं त्यक्त्वाखण्डं विचिन्तयेत्।। २१८।।

He alone is a true yogi, a good devotee and dear to all, who accepts the idea and always reminds himself that the *Ātman* and the *Paramātman* are both 'I', and thus abandons the duality of 'You' and 'I'.—218

अध्यारोपापवादाभ्यां यत्र सर्वं विलीयते।
तद्बीजमाश्रयेद्योगी सर्वसङ्गविवर्जितः।। २१९।।

Detached from all obejcts the yogi goes direct to the essence (seed), when all delusions get dissolved.—219

अपरोक्षं चिदानन्दं पूर्णं त्यक्त्वा प्रगाकुलम्।
परोक्षमपरोक्षञ्च कृत्वा मूढा भ्रमन्ति वै।। २२०।।

Abandoning the Real, the Blissful and the Whole, an ignorant person always seeks to convert the deluding unreality into a reality.—220

चराचरमिदं विश्वं परोक्षं यः करोति च।
अपरोक्षं परंब्रह्म त्यक्त्वा तस्मिन् विलीयते।। २२१।।

But he who considers all moving and unmoving world as unreal, and abandons the same, gets merged into the Real which is the Supreme Brahman.—221

ज्ञानकारणमज्ञानं यथा नोत्पद्यते भृशम्।
अभ्यासं कुरुते योगी तदा सङ्गविवर्जितः।। २२२।।

So long as the knowledge of the cause of ignorance does not develop in the yogi sufficiently enough, so long must he continue this practice of non-attachment.—222

सर्वेन्द्रियाणि संयम्य विषयेभ्यो विचक्षणः।
विषयेभ्यः सुषुप्तेव तिष्ठेत् सङ्गविवर्जितः।। २२३।।

He should thus remain detached, withdraw his senses from all objects of desire, thereby putting to sleep his craving for objects.—223

एवमभ्यासतो नित्यं स्वप्रकाशं प्रकाशते।
श्रोतुर्बुद्धिसमर्थार्थं निवर्तन्ते गुरोर्गिरः।
तदभ्यासवशादेकं स्वतो ज्ञानं प्रवर्तते।। २२४।।

With kind of regular practice, the Light within appears (glows) by itself. Then, hearing and understanding the sweet words of the guru are no longer necessary; for Knowledge prevails automatically as a result of such meditation.—224

यतो वाचो निवर्तन्ते अप्राप्य मनसा सह।
साधनादमलं ज्ञानं स्वयं स्फुरति तद्ध्रुवम्।। २२५।।

That Pure Knowledge, where words do not reach and which the mind cannot conceive, glows automatically after such meditation.—225

हठं विना राजयोगो राजयोगं विना हठः।
तस्मात् प्रवर्तते योगी हठे सद्गुरुमार्गतः।। २२६।।

Haṭhayoga without Rājayoga and Rājayoga without Haṭhayoga are equally ineffective. Hence the yogi should first practise Haṭhayoga on the lines advised by a competent guru.—226

स्थिते देहे जीवति च योगो न श्रियते भृशम्।
इन्द्रियार्थोपभोगेषु स जीवति न संशयः।। २२७।।

He who does not take advantage of yoga while still in this body and alive, undoubtedly lives only for the gratification of his senses.—227

अभ्यासपाकपर्यन्तं मितान्नं शरणं भवेत्।
अन्यथा साधनं धीमान् कर्तुं पारयतीह न।। २२८।।

Until the practice gets easy and signifies perfection, food should be taken in small quantity only. Otherwise the wise yogi will find it difficult to achieve success.—228

अतीव साधुसंलापो वदेत् संसदि बुद्धिमान्।
करोति पिण्डरक्षार्थं वह्वालापविवर्जितः।। २२९।।
त्यज्यते त्यज्यते सङ्गं सर्वथा त्यज्यते भृशम्।
अन्यथा न लभेन्मुक्तिं सत्यं सत्यं मयोदितम्।। २३०।।

The wise yogi should speak gently in an assembly, eat only to preserve the body, avoid too much talk, and positively keep away from the company of many people. Without these, I say very truly, he cannot attain Emancipation.—229 and 230

गुह्ये वै क्रियतेऽभ्यासः सङ्गं त्यक्त्वा तदन्तरे।
व्यवहाराय कर्तव्यो वाह्ये सङ्गानुरागतः।। २३१।।
स्वे स्वे कर्मणि वर्तन्ते सर्वे ते कर्मसम्भवाः।
निमित्तमात्रं करणे न दोषोऽस्ति कदाचन।। २३२।।

In between meeting people he should practise in private. For, onviously, routine duties must be performed in the company of others, and everybody has to perform these in accordance with his station in life. Therefore, there is no harm if such duties are performed.—231 and 232

एवं निश्चित्य सुधिया गृहस्थोऽपि यदाचरेत्।
तदा सिद्धिमवाप्नोति नात्र कार्या विचारणा।। २३३।।

If even a householder wisely practises while keeping this in mind, he shall positively achieve success.—233

पापपुण्य विनिर्मुक्तः परित्यक्ताङ्गसाधकः।
यो भवेत् स विमुक्तः स्यादगृहे तिष्ठन् सदागृही।। २३४।।
पापपुण्यैर्न लिप्येत योगयुक्तः सदागृही।
कुर्वन्नपि तदा पापं स्वकार्ये लोकसंग्रहे।। २३५।।

The yogi who rejects sensual pleasures and is free from both virtue and vice becomes, because of such renunciation, a recluse—even though he may be a householder. As a recluuse engaged in performance of yoga he is not besmirched by either virtue or vice. And, as a householder, he does not sin when he does his duties for the sake of other people.—235 and 235

अधुना प्रवक्ष्यामि मन्त्रसाधनमुत्तमम्।
ऐहिकामुष्मिकसुखं येन स्यादविरोधतः।। २३६।।

Now I shall speak about the great *mantra* technique, by means of which everlasting happiness can be gained here as well as hereafter.—236

अस्मिन्मन्त्रवरे ज्ञाते योगसिद्धिर्भवेत् खलु।
योगेन साधकेन्द्रस्य सर्वैश्वर्यसुखप्रदा।। २३७।।

By knowing this excellent *mantra* technique the yogi can achieve positive success. This yoga bestows all supernormal powers and happiness upon an expert yogi.—237

मूलाधारेऽस्ति यत्पद्मं चतुरदलसमन्वितम्।
तन्मध्ये वाग्भवं बीजं विस्फुरन्तं तडित्प्रभा।। २३८।।
हृदये कामबीजन्तु बन्धूककुसुमप्रभम्।
आज्ञारविन्दे शक्त्याख्यं चन्द्रकोटिसमप्रभम्।। २३९।।
बीजत्रयमिदं गोप्यं भुक्तिमुक्तिफलप्रदम्।
एतन्मन्त्रत्रयं योगी साधयेत् सिद्धिसाधकः।। २४०।।

Within the four-petalled Mūlādhāra lotus is the Seed of Speech, glowing like a spark of electricity. The Seed of Desire is in the heart (Anāhata lotus), blooming like a red *bandhūka* flower. In the Ājñā lotus (between the eyebrows) shines the Seed of Force, like ten million moons. The three Seeds are the determining causes of bondage and emancipation, and hence must be kept a secret. A yogi aspiring for success must master these three *mantras.*—238-40

एतन्मन्त्रं गुरोर्लब्ध्वा न द्रुतं न विलम्बितम्।
अक्षराक्षरसन्धानं निःसन्दिग्धमना जपेत्।। २४१।।

After obtaining these *mantras* from the guru he should carefully recite them word for word, neither too fast nor too slow, dwelling upon their meaning and significance, and with full faith.—241

तद्गतश्चैकचित्तश्च शास्त्रोक्तविधिना सुधीः।
देव्यास्तु पुरतो लक्षं हुत्वा लक्षत्रयं जपेत्।। २४२।।

With one pointedness of mind resulting therefrom, the wise yogi should next pray before the Goddess in accordance with the rites prescribed in the scriptures, and repeat the *mantras* three hundred thousand times, after performing *homa* for a hundred thousand times.—242

करवीरप्रसूनैस्तु गुडक्षीराज्यसंयुतैः।
कुण्डे योन्यान्तु ते धीमान् जपान्ते जुहुयात् सुधीः।। २४३।।

Thereafter he should offer (to the *homa* fire) fresh oleander flowers as well as some raw sugar, milk and clarified butter, putting all these into the *homa* receptacle.—243

अनुष्ठाने कृते धीमान् पूर्णसेवा कृता भवेत्।
ततो ददाति कामान् वै देवी त्रिपुरभैरवी।। २४४।।

When this has been done, the wise yogi has completed all the necessary rites. Then (propitiated by his prayers) the Goddess Tripura-Bhairavī bestows upon the yogi all that he asks for.—244

गुरुं सन्तोष्य विधिवल्लब्ध्वा मन्त्रवरोत्तमम्।
अनेन विधिना युक्तो मन्दभाग्योऽपि सिद्ध्यति।। २४५।।

In this way, i.e., after properly satisfying the guru and obtaining from him the best of *mantras*, even a not-so-lucky yogi achieves success.—245

लक्षमेकं जपेद्यस्तु साधको विजितेन्द्रियः।
दर्शनात्तस्य क्षुभ्यन्ते योषितो मदनातुराः।
पतन्ति साधकास्याग्रे निर्लज्जा भयवर्जिताः।। २४६।।

The yogi who, having controlled his senses, recites these *mantras* a hundred thousand times is sought after by lovelorn damsels, who boldly and shamelessly throw themselves before him.—246

जप्तेन चेद् द्विलक्षेण ये यस्मिन्विषये स्थिताः।
आगच्छन्ति यथा तीर्थं विमुक्त कुलविग्रहाः।
ददते तस्य सर्वस्वं तस्यैव च वशे स्थिताः।। २४७।।

Should the *mantras* be repeated two hundred thousand times, even the family deities, freed from the images (i.e., assuming human form), appear before the yogi at his yoga-sanctified place and remain at his command to fulfil his wishes.—247

त्रिभिर्लक्षैस्तथा जप्तैर्मण्डलीकं समण्डलम्।
वशमायान्ति ते सर्वे नात्र कार्या विचारणा।। २४८।।
षडभिर्लक्षैर्महीपालः स एव बलवाहनः।। २४९।।
लक्षैर्द्वादशकैज्जप्तैर्यक्षरक्षोरगेश्वराः।
वशमयान्ति ते सर्वे आज्ञां कुर्वन्ति नित्यशः।। २५०।।

After the *mantras* have been repeated three hundred thousand times all the potentates from different regions, together with their retinue, surrender to the yogi. Similarly, their recitation for six hundred thousand times earns the yogi the powers of a sovereign or emperor, and twelve hundred thousand times extends his sway to the three worlds when the kings of *yakṣas* in heaven, of *rākṣasas* on earth and of *nāgas* (serpents) in the nether world—all submit to him and carry out his commands at all times.—248–50

त्रिपञ्चलक्षजप्तैस्तु साधकेन्द्रस्य धीमतः।
सिद्धविद्याधराश्चैव गन्धर्वाप्सरसाङ्गणाः।। २५१।।
वशमायान्ति ते सर्वे नात्र कार्या विचारणा।
हठात् श्रवणविज्ञानं सर्वज्ञत्वं प्रजायते।। २५२।।
तथाष्टादशभिर्लक्षैर्देहेनानेन साधकः।
उत्तिष्ठन् मेदिनीं त्यक्त्वा दिव्यदेहस्तु जायते।
भ्रमते स्वेच्छया लोके छिद्रां पश्यति मेदिनीम्।। २५३।।

After completing the *mantras* fifteen hundred thousand times, the persevering yogi establishes an undoubted sway over learned adepts, *gandharvas* (divine singers) and *apsarās* (divine dancers), when he discerns all divine sound and becomes omniscient. Thereafter, with eight hundred thousand repetitions, the yogi is able to rise bodily from the earth and, assuming a divine form, move about in the universe watching the tiny little earth below.—251–53

अष्टाविंशतिभिर्लक्षैर्विद्याधरपतिर्भवेत्।
साधकस्तु भवेद्धीमान् कामरूपो महाबलः।। २५४।।
त्रिंशल्लक्षैस्तथा जप्ते ब्रह्मविष्णुसमो भवेत्।
रुद्रत्वं षष्टिभिर्लक्षैरमायित्वमशीतिभिः।। २५५।।
कोटचैकया महायोगी लीयते परमे पदे।
साधकस्तु भवेद्योगी त्रैलोक्ये सोऽतिदुर्लभः।। २५६।।

Twentyeight hundred thousand times makes the yogi strong and handsome like the God of Love and he becomes the chief among the divine learned. When three million times have been completed, he is like Brahmā and Viṣṇu, and with six million repetitions he gains the qualities of Śiva. Eight million times places him in Eternal Bliss, and after ten million repetitions he merges into the Supreme. Such a yogi, however, is very, very rare indeed in all three worlds.—254–56

त्रिपुरे त्रिपुरन्त्वकं शिवं परमकारणम्।
अक्षयं तत्पदं शान्तमप्रमेयमनामयम्।
लभतेऽसौ न सन्देहो धीमान् सर्वमभिप्सितम्।। २५७।।

O Pārvatī! (Mistress of Three Worlds), Śiva the Demolisher of Three Worlds is the Primordial Cause. He is eternal. Immortality, peace, abundance and well-being are to be found at His feet. In seeking Him the wise yogi no doubt achieves all of these.—257

शिवविद्या महाविद्या गुप्ताञ्चाग्रे महेश्वरी।
सद्भाषितमिदं शास्त्रं गोपनीयमतो बुधैः।। २५८।।

O Pārvatī! this knowledge of Śiva is a great knowledge. It is essentially a mystery. Hence the wise yogi should keep this knowledge, as revealed by Me, a close secret.—258

हठविद्या परं गोप्या योगिना सिद्धिमिच्छता।
भवेद्वीर्यवती गुप्ता निर्वीया च प्रकाशिता।। २५९।।

All yogis aspiring for success must keep this Haṭhayoga a zealously-guarded secret. It weakens when it becomes known to all.—259

य इदं पठते नित्यमाद्योपान्तं विचक्षणः।
योगसिद्धिर्भवेत्तस्य क्रमेणैव न संशयः।
स मोक्षं लभते धीमान् य इदं नित्यमर्चयेत्।। २६०।।

The wise one who reads this (*śāstra*) regularly from beginning to end will definitely master this yoga in due course. With continued practice, he shall attain Emancipation.—260

मोक्षार्थिभ्यश्च सर्वेभ्यः साधुभ्यः श्रावयेदपि।
क्रियायुक्तस्य सिद्धिः स्यादक्रियस्य कथम्भवेत्।
तस्मात् क्रियाविधानेन कर्तव्या योगिपुङ्गवैः।। २६१।।

It may be recited to all such pious persons as may be aspiring for Emancipation. However, only those who act upon it shall achieve success, not the inactive ones. Hence the yogis should conscientiously practise this according to the rules laid down here.—261

यदृच्छालाभसन्तुष्टः सन्त्यक्तान्तरसङ्गकः।
गृहस्थश्चाप्यनासक्तः स मुक्तो योगसाधनात्।। २६२।।

He who is contented with whatever he has got and has conquered his senses through the practice of yoga, is really free and unattached even though he may be a householder.—262

गृहस्थानां भवेत् सिद्धिरीश्वराणां जपेन वै।
योगक्रियाभियुक्तानां तस्मात् संयतते गृही।। २६३।।

A householder achieves success by repeating the name of the Supreme while engaged in the practice of yoga. Hence the householder should earnestly engage himself in this task.—263

गेहे स्थित्वा पुत्रदारादिपूर्णः सङ्गं त्यक्त्वा चान्तरे योगमार्गे।
सिद्धेश्चिह्नं वीक्ष्य पश्चात् गृहस्थः क्रीडेत् सो वै मन्मतं साधयित्वा।। २६४।।

A householder who, while residing at home amidst his wife and children, abandons all attachments and inwardly treads the path of yoga, ere long sees the signs of success, and then, having mastered the yoga, lives happily ever after.—264

Here ends chapter V of *Śivasaṃhitā* entitled 'Rājayoga'.

Book II

Gheraṇḍasaṃhitā

LESSON ONE

The Six-fold System

BENEDICTION

आदीश्वराय प्रणमामि तस्मै येनोपदिष्टा हठयोगविद्या।
विराजते प्रोन्नतराजयोगमारूढमिच्छन् विधियोग एव।।

I bow to that Primordial Supreme Being who has taught this science of Haṭhayoga, which is the best means (ladder) for climbing up to Rājayoga for all those who desire to do so.

GHAṬASTHAYOGA

एकदा चण्डकापालिर्गत्वा घेरण्ड कुट्टिमम्।
प्रणम्य विनयाद् भक्त्या घेरण्डं परिपृच्छति।। १।।

Once upon a time Caṇḍakāpāli (a yoga aspirant) went to the cottage of sage Gheraṇḍa and, humbly approaching and doing obeisance to him, spoke thus.—1

घटस्थयोगं योगेश तत्वज्ञानस्य कारणम्।
इदानीं श्रोतुमिच्छामि योगेश्वर वद प्रभो।। २।।

"O best of yogis! I am desirous of learning the secret of that yoga which concerns the physical body (*ghaṭastha*).* Be gracious enough to tell me that, O Lord of yogis!—2

Gheraṇḍa said:

साधु साधु महाबाहो यन्मां त्वं परिपृच्छति।
कथयामि हि ते वत्स सावधानवधारय।। ३।।

O ardent One! (lit. 'of mighty arms') what thou hast asked me is most excellent. I shall surely tell you, my child! Now listen to me

Ghaṭastha (within pot) is the physical body in which *prāṇa, apāna, nāda-vindu, jīvātmā,* and *Paramātmā* are conjoined.

attentively.—3

नास्ति मायासमं पाशं नास्ति योगात् परं बलम्।
नास्ति ज्ञानात् परो बन्धुर्नाहंकारात् परो रिपुः।। ४।।

There is no greater snare than Illusion, no greater friend than Knowledge and no greater enemy then Pride. (Similarly) there is no greater power than that of Yoga.—4

अभ्यासात् कादिवर्णानि यथा शास्त्राणि बोधयेत्।
तथा योगं समासाद्य तत्वज्ञानञ्च लभ्यते।। ५।।

Just as by first learning the alphabets (a, b, c, etc.) one is able (gradually) to comprehend difficult treatises, so is the Supreme Knowledge gained by first mastering yoga.—5

सुकृतैर्दुष्कृतैः कार्यैः जायते प्राणिनां घटः।
घटादुत्पद्यते कर्म घटीयन्त्रं यथा भ्रमेत्।। ६।।

The physical body of all creatures is the product of their good and evil actions. As the machine of the physical body works, yet more actions result.—6

उर्द्धाधो भ्रमते यद्वद् घटीयन्त्रं गवां वशात्।
तद्वत् कर्मवशाज्जीवो भ्रमते जन्ममृत्युभिः।। ७।।

Even as the body-machine instinctively moves up and down, so do all creatures move through life and death driven by their own actions (*karma*).—7

आमकुम्भ इवाम्भस्थो जीर्यमाणः सदा घटः।
योगानलेन संदह्य घटशुद्धिं समाचरेत्।। ८।।

A pot made of unbaked clay will always melt away when filled with water (i.e., unless it has been baked first). The human pot must similarly be purified first in the fire of yoga.—8

शोधनं दृढता चैव स्थैर्यं धैर्यञ्च लाघवम्।
प्रत्यक्षञ्च निर्लिप्तञ्च घटस्य सप्तसाधनम्।। ९।।

For the purpose of learning yoga, seven disciplines are essential: Purity, Firmness, Stability, Perseverance, Buoyancy, Knowledge, and Serenity.—9

षट्कर्मणा शोधनञ्च आसनेन भवेद्दृढम्।
मुद्रया स्थिरता चैव प्रत्याहारेण धीरता।। १०।।

प्राणायामाल्लाघवञ्च ध्यानात् प्रत्यक्षमात्मनि।
समाधिना निर्लिप्तञ्च मुक्तिरेव न संशयः।। ११।।

Purity is achieved through six-fold practices: Firmness through postures, Stability through exercises, Perseverance through abstenance, Buoyancy through breath-control, Knowledge through concentration, and Serenity through superconsciousness, which undoubtedly leads to Emancipation.—10 and 11

धौतिर्वस्तिस्तथा नेतिर्लौलिकी त्राटकं तथा।
कपालभातिश्चैतानि षट्कर्माणि समाचरेत्।। १२।।

The six-fold purifications to be practised are: Dhauti, Vasti, Neti, Lauliki, Trāṭaka, and Kapālabhāti*—12

Details of these processes are explained in the verses that follow.

I. Dhauti

अन्तर्धौतिर्दन्तधौतिर्हृद्धौतिर्मूलशोधनम्।
धौतिं चतुर्विधा कृत्वा घटं कुर्वन्तु निर्मलम्।। १३।।

Dhauti is of four kinds: *antar-dhauti* (internal cleansing), *danta-dhauti* (cleansing of teeth and face), *hṛd-dhauti* (cleansing of the oesophagus), and *śodhan-dhauti* (cleansing of the lower intestines). By these processes the physical body should be purified.—13

A. *Antar-dhauti*

वातसारं वारिसारं वह्निसारं वहिष्कृतम्।
घटस्य निर्मलार्थाय अन्तर्धौतिश्चतुर्विधा।। १४।।

Antar-dhauti, again, is sub-divided into four types: *vāta-sāra* (airy), *vāri-sāra* (watery), *vanhi-sāra* (fiery), and *vahiṣkṛta* (expulsion). All four are necessary for cleansing the physical body.—14

i. *Vāta-sāra*

काकचञ्चुवदास्येन पिबेद्वायुं शनैः शनैः।
चालयेदुदरं पश्चाद्वर्त्मना रेचयेच्छनैः।। १५।।

*Dhauti is both external and internal cleansing; Vasti is cleansing of the lower intestines (a form of self-induced enema); Neti is cleansing of the passage between nose and mouth by passing through it a thin strip of cloth or string; Lauliki is contraction and rotation of bowels; Trāṭaka is an eye-exercise involving fixation of gaze upon a point; Kapālabhāti is cleansing of the sinuses by taking in water or air through the nose and expelling the same through the mouth or, conversely, sucking in water and air through the mouth and expelling the same through the nose.

वातसारं परं गोप्यं देहनिर्मलकारणम्।
सर्वरोगक्षयकरं देहानलविवर्धकम्।। १६।।

Curl up the lips like a crow's beak (as when whistling) and draw in air slowly little by little; then rotate the same within the stomach and finally release it slowly through the nether end. This *vāta-sāra* process, which is very secret, purifies the system, increases the appetite and protects the body from all diseases.—15 and 16

ii. *Vāri-sāra*

आकण्ठं पूरयेद्वारि वक्त्रेण च पिबेच्छनैः।
चालयेदुदरेनैव चोदराद्रेचयेदधः।। १७।।
वारिसारं परं गोप्यं देहनिर्मलकारणम्।
साधयेत् तत् प्रयत्नेन देवदेहं प्रपद्यते।। १८।।
वारिसारं परां धौतिं साधयेद्यः प्रयत्नतः।
मलदेहं शोधयित्वा देवदेहं प्रपद्यते।। १९।।

Sip in water slowly through the mouth and fill yourself to the maximum; then rotate the bowels and release the same through the nether end (i.e , urinate). This *vāri-sāra* process is also secret. If practised carefully it will cleanse the system and give the body a fine complexion. It is the best form of Dhauti since, when practised carefully, it purges the body of all its impurities and makes it divine (beautiful).—17–19

iii. *Agni-sāra*

नाभिग्रन्थिं मेरुपृष्ठे शतवारञ्च कारयेत्।
अग्निसारमेषा धौतिर्योगिनां योगसिद्धिदा।
उदरामयजं त्यक्त्वा जठराग्निं विवर्धयेत्।। २०।।
एषा धौतिः परा गोप्या देवानामपि दुर्लभा।
केवलं धौतिमात्रेण देवदेहो भवेद्ध्रुवम्।। २१।।

Contract the muscles of the stomach (around the navel) as far as to touch the backbone (i.e., to the maximum extent possible) and relax the same again. This should be done a hundred times. This is *agni-sāra*, the best Dhauti for yogis desiring success in yoga. By this process all stomach troubles disappear and the appetite improves. This Dhauti, too, is secret—rare even for the best of beings. It positively gives one a beautiful and robust body.—20 and 21

iv. *Vahiṣkṛta*

काकीमुद्रां शोधयित्वा पूरयेदुदरं मरुत्।
धारयेदर्द्धयामस्तु चालयेदधोवर्त्मना।
एषा धौतिः परा गोप्या न प्रकाश्या कदाचन।। २२।।

Adopting the Kāki posture (i.e., protruding lips like a crow's beak) fill up the stomach with air to the full, and then let it pass out of the nether end. This is to be practised for an hour and a half. This Dhauti* is secret and must not be divulged to anybody.—22

नाभिमग्नो जले स्थित्वा शक्तिनाडीं विसर्जयेत्।
कराभ्यां क्षालयेन्नाडीं यावन्मलविसर्जनम्।
तावत् प्रक्षाल्य नाडीञ्च उदरे वेशयेत् पुनः।। २३।।
इदं प्रक्षालनं गोप्यं देवानामपि दुर्लभम्।
केवलं धौतिमात्रेण देवदेहो भवेद्ध्रुवम्।। २४।।

Immerse up to the waist in water (in a tub or in a stream) and let the *śakti-nāḍi*** (lower intestines) be expelled into it. Thereafter, using hands, rinse the *nāḍi* until all excretion sticking to it is thoroughly cleansed. After the washing is over, place back the intestines into the bowel. This washing process is secret and is not known even to the best of beings. Through this Dhauti alone the body can be made positively beautiful.—23 and 24

यामार्द्धं धारणाशक्तिं यावन्न साधयेन्नरः।
वहिष्कृतं महद्धौतिस्तावच्चैव न जायते।। २५।।

This *vahiṣkṛta* (expulsion of rectum), which is a great Dhauti, cannot be practised so long as one has not become proficient in holding his breath for at least three hours.—25

B. *Danta-dhauti*

दन्तमूलं जिह्वामूलं रन्ध्रञ्चकर्णयुग्मयोः।
कपालरन्ध्रं पञ्चैते दन्तधौतिर्विधीयते।। २६।।

Danta-dhauti is of five types: *danta-mūla* (root of teeth or gums), *jihvā-mūla* (root of tongue), *karṇa-randhra* (openings of ears), and *kapāla-randhra* (sinuses).—26

*This, and the *vāta-sāra* Dhauti described earlier, are apparently one and the same.

**The *śakti-nāḍi* is the descending colon, or lower section of the alimentary canal. Here, however, the last six inches of the colon, viz., the rectum, seems to be indicated. In this yogic practice the rectum alone is forced out, the faeces manually removed, and then the expelled portion drawn up into its normal place.

i. *Teeth and Gums*

खादिरेण रसेनाथ मृत्तिकया च शुद्धया।
मार्जयेद्दन्तमूलञ्च यावत् किल्विषमाहरेत्।। २७।।
दन्तमूलं परा धौतिर्योगिनां योगसाधने।
नित्यं कुर्यात् प्रभाते च दन्तरक्षणहेतवे।
दन्तमूलं धावनादि कार्येषु योगिनां मतम्।। २८।।

The teeth and gums should be massaged with the juice of catechu and pure earth* (clay) until all foul accretion is removed. This type of oral cleansing is best for those engaged in practising yoga. The best of yogis think that such washing of teeth and gums, when done every morning, is most beneficial for the preservation of teeth.—27 and 28

ii. *Tongue and Throat*

अथातः संप्रवक्ष्यामि जिह्वाशोधनकारणम्।
जरामरणरोगादीन् नाशयेद्दीर्घलम्बिका।। २९।।

Now I shall describe the way to clean the tongue.** By doing this, not only disease and decay are stemmed but the tongue also becomes longer.—29

तर्जनीमध्यमानामा अङ्गुलित्रययोगतः।
वेशयेद्गलमध्ये तु मार्जयेल्लम्बिकामूलम्।
शनैः शनैर्मार्जयित्वा कफदोषं निवारयेत्।। ३०।।
मार्जयेन्नवनीतेन दोंहयेच्च पुनः पुनः।
तदग्रं लौहयन्त्रेण कर्षयित्वा शनैः शनैः।। ३१।।
नित्यं कुर्यात् प्रयत्नेन रवेरुदयकेऽस्तके।
एवं कृते च नित्यं च लम्बिका दीर्घतां ब्रजेत्।। ३२।।

The index, middle and ring fingers—the three together—should be inserted into the throat and with these the papilla beneath the tongue (uvula) should be rubbed. With repeated massage, all phlegm will be eliminated. Thereafter, the tongue should be massaged with butter; but, before that, it should be scraped

*Pure earth, without particles of sand or stone, when made into clay and applied to the skin, is known to yield therapeutic results.

**As mentioned later in connection with the practice of *mudras*, elongation of the tongue is essential to enable it to reach the aperture at the base of the palate, through which ambrosia trickles down from the nectary of the Sahasrāra lotus on top of the brain. Such elongation is often achieved by making a small incision in the membrane under the tongue.

carefully with a metal scraper. This should be done everyday, morning and night. By doing so the papilla will be tougher and longer.—30–31

iii. *The Ears*

तर्जन्यनामिकायोगान्मार्जयेत् कर्णरन्ध्रयोः।
नित्यमभ्यासयोगेन नादान्तरं प्रकाशयेत्।। ३३।।

With the aid of the index or ring finger the aperture of the ears should be rinsed. When regularly done every day, the perception of sound becomes keener.—33

iv. *The Forehead*

वृद्धाङ्गुष्ठेन दक्षेण मार्जयेद्भालरन्ध्रकम्।
एवमभ्यासयोगेन कफदोषं निवारयेत्।। ३४।।
नाडी निर्मलतां याति दिव्यदृष्टिः प्रजायते।
निद्रान्ते भोजनान्ते च दिनान्ते च दिने दिने।। ३५।।

The soft parts (sides) of the forehead should be massaged with the right thumb. This practice prevents cough, soothens the nerves and improves the eye-sight.Everyday it should be done on rising from bed, after meals, and before retiring at night.—34 and 35

C. *The Oesophagus*

हृद्धौतिं त्रिविधां कुर्याद्दण्डवमनवाससा।। ३६।।

Hṛd-dhauti is done in three ways: (i) by inserting a *daṇḍa* (twig), (ii) by *vamana* (vomitting out water), and (iii) by inserting *vāsa* (a strip of cloth).—36

रम्भादण्डं हरिद्रादण्डं वेत्रदण्डं तथैव च।
हृन्मध्ये चालयित्वा तु पुनः प्रत्याहारेच्छनैः।। ३७।।
कफपित्तं तथा क्लेदं रेचयेदूर्द्धवर्त्मना।
दण्डधौति विधानेन हृदरोगम् नाशयेद्ध्रुवम्।। ३८।।

i. *Daṇḍa-dhauti* is practised by inserting into the oesophagus (gullet) a (short, thin and tender) stalk of the plantain-tree, or a twig of the turmeric plant, or a (tender) shoot of cane, and moving the same up and down slowly. In this way all phlegm, bile and slime sticking there comes out of the mouth and thus respiratory (heart) diseases are positively cured.—37 and 38

भोजनान्ते पिबेद्वारि चाकण्ठपूरितं सुधीः।
ऊर्द्धदृष्टिं क्षणं कृत्वा तज्जलं वमयेत् पुनः।

नित्यमभ्यासयोगेन कफपित्तं निवारयेत्।। ३९।।

ii. *Vamana-dhauti* is practised by drinking water to the maximum capacity after a meal and then lifting up the face and expelling (vomitting out) the same. A regular practice of this will protect one from attacks of cough and bile.—39

चतुरङ्गुलविस्तारं सूक्ष्मवस्त्रं शनैर्ग्रसेत्।
पुनः प्रत्याहारेदेतत् प्रोच्यते धौतिकर्मकम्।। ४०।।
गुल्मज्वरप्लीहाकुष्ठकफपित्तं विनश्यति।
आरोग्यं बलपुष्टिञ्च भवेत्तस्य दिने दिने।। ४१।।

iii. *Vāsa-dhauti* is practised by slowly swallowing up a four-finger (about 6 cm) wide strip of fine cloth (gauze), then expelling out the same. This is known as cleansing of the oesophagus. By this all types of diseases due to excess of phlegm, bile or wind and causing fevers, sores, spleen troubles, etc. disappear and one grows healthier and stronger every day.—40 and 41

D. *The Posterior*

अपानक्रूरता तावत् यावन्मूलं न शेधयेत्।
तस्मात् सर्वप्रयत्नेन मूलशोधनमाचरेत्।। ४२।।
पीतमूलस्य दण्डेन मध्यमाङ्गुलिनापि वा।
यत्नेन क्षालयेदगुह्यं वारिणा च पुनः पुनः।। ४३।।
वारयेत् कोष्ठकठिन्यमामाजीर्णं निवारयेत्।
कारणं कान्तिपुष्ट्योश्च दीपनं वह्निमण्डलम्।। ४४।।

As long as the posterior (lower orifice of the bowels) is not cleansed properly, the down-flowing air (*apāna*) remains feculent. It is necessary, therefore, to cleanse the posterior carefully. It should be washed again and again either with the aid of a piece of turmeric-root or direct with the middle finger. This practice prevents stomach troubles, such as dysentery and dyspepsia, cures constipation, improves appetite, and generally bestows an all-round robust health.—42–44

II. Vasti

जलवस्तिः शुष्कवस्तिर्वस्तिः स्याद्द्विविधा स्मृता।
जलवस्तिं जले कुर्याच्छुष्कवस्तिं सदा क्षितौ।। ४५।।

It is to be remembered that Vasti is of two kinds: wet and dry. Wet Vasti is practised with water, and the dry with air.—45

नाभिमग्नजले पायुं न्यस्तवानुत्कटासनम्।
आकुञ्चनं प्रसारञ्च जलवस्तिं समाचरेत्।। ४६।।
प्रमेहञ्च उदावर्त्तं क्रूरवायुं निवारयेत्।
भवेत् स्वच्छन्ददेहश्च कामदेवसमो भवेत्।। ४७।।
वस्तिं पश्चिमोत्तानेन चालयित्वा शनैरधः।
अश्विनीमुद्राया पायुमाकुञ्चयेत् प्रसारयेत्।। ४८।।
एवमभ्यासयोगेन कोष्ठदोषो न विद्यते।
विवर्द्धयेज्जठराग्नि आमवातं विनाशयेत्।। ४९।।

Dipping the posterior in water up to the waist (navel) and sitting on toes in the Utkaṭa* posture, the *jala* (wet) Vasti is practised by contracting and distending the rectum. The water is sucked in slowly through the rectum in accordance with the Aświnī process, and later slowly released. This practice prevents constipation, nettle-rash, diabetes, urinary troubles, and all diseases caused by an excess of fetid gas. It also promotes a good appetite and the body becomes strong and beautiful like that of Kāmadeva (god of Love)!—46–49

III. Neti

वितस्तिमानं सूक्ष्मसूत्रं नासानाले प्रवेशयेत्।
मुखान्निर्गमयेत् पश्चात् प्रोच्यते नेतिकर्म तत्।। ५०।।
साधयेन्नेतिकर्माणि खेचरीसिद्धिमाप्नुयात्।
कफदोषो विनश्यन्ति दिव्यदृष्टिः प्रजायते।। ५१।।

Take a fine thread about nine inches long (span-length) and pass it up the nose, and let it come out of the mouth. This is called the Neti method of cleansing. It cures colds, improves the eyesight and helps in gaining the Khecarī (i.e., the power of levitation).—50 and 51

IV. Lauliki

अमन्दवेगे तुन्दञ्च भ्रामयेदुभपार्श्वयोः।
सर्वरोगन्निहन्तीह देहानल विवर्धनम्।। ५२।।

Rotate the stomach rapidly from one side to another. This exer-

*The Utkaṭa posture is made by raising oneself on toes, heels up, and resting the hump upon the heels. The Aświnīmudrā comprises distention and contraction of the rectum. When practised in water it is wet Vasti; when with air, it is called dry Vasti.

cise is best for preventing all kinds of diseases and increasing energy in the body.—52

V. Trāṭaka

निमेषोन्मेषकं त्यक्त्वा सूक्ष्मलक्ष्यं निरीक्षयेत्।
यावदश्रूणि पतन्ति त्राटकं प्रोच्यते बुधैः।। ५३।।
एवमभ्यासयोगेन शाम्भवी जायते ध्रुवम्।
नेत्ररोगाः विनश्यन्ति दिव्यदृष्टिः प्रजायते।। ५४।।

Fix the gaze upon a fine object (point) and, without batting the eye, keep on gazing until the eyes begin to water. The wise men have described it as Trāṭaka. Such practice cures all eye troubles, bestows a keen eye-sight, and concentration of mind suitable for Śāmbhavi* is positively gained.—53 and 54

VI. Kapālabhāti

वातक्रमेण व्युतक्रमेण शीतक्रमेण विशेषतः।
भालभातिं त्रिधा कुर्यात, कफदोषं निवारयेत्।। ५५।।

Kapālabhāti is of three types: (i) *vāta-krama* (by deep breathing), (ii) *vyut-krama* (by short breaths), and (iii) *śīta-krama* (by slow, easy breaths). When the sinuses are cleansed in this way, all cough and cold disappear.—55

इडया पूरयेद्वायुं रेचयेत् पिङ्गला पुनः।
पिङ्गलया पूरयित्वा पुनश्चन्द्रेण रेयचेत्।। ५६।।
पूरकं रेचकं कृत्वा वेगेन न तु चालयेत्।
एवमभ्यासयोगेन कफदोषं निवारयेत्।। ५७।।

Take a deep breath through the left nostril (after closing the right nostril with the right thumb), and release the same through the right (nostril). Next fill in through the right (nostril)—i.e., after closing the left with the left thumb—and later release through the left. Neither the inspiration nor the expiration should be performed rapidly (i.e., inhaling and exhaling should be slow and uniform). This practice helps to get rid of cold and cough.—56 and 57

नासाभ्यां जलमाकृष्य पुनर्वक्त्रेण रेचयेत्।
पायं पायं व्युत्क्रमेण श्लेष्मदोषं निवारयेत्।। ५८।।

*Śāmbhavi *mudrā* is practised with thoughts concentrated and fixed on the centre of the forehead between the eyebrows.

Draw in water through the nose (both nostrils), and release the same through the mouth. Both processes should be accomplished in short spurts. This practice prevents accumulation of phlegm.—58

शीतकृत्य पीत्वा वक्त्रेण नासानालैर्विरेचयेत्।
एवमभ्यासयोगेन कामदेवसमो भवेत्।। ५९।।
न जायते वार्द्धक्यञ्च जरा नैव प्रजायते।
भवेत् स्वच्छन्ददेहश्च कफदोषं निवारयेत्।। ६०।।

Sip in water slowly through the mouth and expel the same through the nose. With this practice too cough and cold are cured and the body becomes perfectly healthy; there is then neither aging nor decay and one looks as handsome as Kāmadeva (god of Love) himself!—59 and 60

Here ends Lesson One entitled 'The Six-fold System' incorporated in *Gheraṇḍasaṃhitā*.

LESSON TWO

Āsanas or Modes of Installation

Śrī Gheraṇḍa said:

आसनानि समस्तानि यावन्तो जीवजन्तवः।
चतुरशीतिलक्षाणि शिवेन कथितं पुरा।। १।।

There are as many *āsanas* (modes of installation) as the number of living beings! Of yore, however, the Lord Śiva spoke of about 84,00,000 only.—1

तेषां मध्ये विशिष्टानि षोडशानां शतं कृतम्।
तेषां मध्ये मर्त्यलोके द्वात्रिंशदासनं शुभम्।। २।।

Of these, 1600 are important ones, but out of these again only 32 are suitable (beneficial) for this world.—2

TYPES OF ĀSANAS

सिद्धं पद्मं तथा भद्रं मुक्तं वज्रञ्च स्वस्तिकम्।
सिंहञ्च गोमुखं वीरं धनुरासनमेव च।। ३।।
मृतं गुप्तं तथा मात्स्यं मत्स्येन्द्रासनमेव च।
गोरक्षं पश्चिमोत्तानं उत्कटं संकटं तथा।। ४।।
मयूरं कुक्कुटं कूर्मं तथा चोत्तानकूर्मकम्।
उत्तानमण्डूकं वृक्षं मण्डूकं गरुडं वृषम्।। ५।।
शलभं मकरं उष्ट्रं भुजंगञ्च योगासनम्।
द्वात्रिंशदासनानि स्युर्मर्त्यलोके च सिद्धिदम्।। ६।।

The names of the 32 *āsanas* suitable for practice* in this world are: Siddha, Padma, Bhadra, Mukta, Vajra, Swastika, Siṃha, Gomukha, Vīra, Dhanuṣa, Mṛta, Gupta, Matsya, Matsyendra, Gorakṣa, Paścimottāna, Utkaṭa, Saṅkaṭa, Mayūra, Kukkuṭa, Kūrma,

*All the *āsanas* are to be practised while sitting on the floor.

Uttānakūrmaka, Maṇḍūka, Uttānamaṇḍūka, Vṛkṣa, Garuḍa, Vṛṣa, Śalabha, Makara, Uṣṭra, Bhujaṅga, and Yoga.—3–6

i. *Siddhāsana*

योनिस्थानेकमङ्घ्रिमूलघटितं सम्पीड्य गुल्फेतरे।
मेढ्रे संप्रणिधाय चिबुकमथोकृत्वा हृदिप्यायिनम्।।
स्थाणुः संयमितेन्द्रियोऽचलदृशा पश्यन् भ्रुवोरन्तरं।
एवं मोक्षो विधीयते फलकरं सिद्धासनं प्रोच्यते।। ७।।

Placing the sole of one foot against the pelvic region and firmly pressing the genitals with the ankle of the other, bend down the chin upon the chest and, after fully controlling all your senses and keeping a calm mind, fix the gaze steadfastly on the centre of the eye-brows. This is known as Siddhāsana, which is useful for purposes of attaining *mokṣa* (emancipation).—7

ii. *Padmāsana*

वामोरूपरि दक्षिणं हि चरणं संस्थाप्य वामं तथा
दक्षोरूपरि पश्चिमेन विधिना कृत्वा कराभ्यां दृढम्।
अङ्गुष्ठे हृदये निधाय चिबुकं नासाग्रमालोकयेत्
एतद्व्याधिसमूहनाशकरं पद्मासनं चोच्यते।। ८।।

Draw up the right foot and place it over the left thigh; similarly, the left one over the right thigh. Then, crossing your arms behind the back, firmly catch the respective big toes. Thereafter, let the chin rest upon the chest and fix the gaze on the tip of the nose. This is known as Padmāsana, a posture that removes all disorders of the body.—8

iii. *Bhadrāsana*

गुल्फौ च वृषणस्याधो व्युत्क्रमेण समाहितः।
पादाङ्गुष्ठे कराभ्याञ्च धृत्वा च पृष्ठदेशतः।
जालन्धरं समासाद्य नासाग्रमवलोकयत्।
भद्रासनं भवेदेतत् सर्वव्याधिविनाशनम्।। ९।।

Slowly press with both ankles the region below the scrotum, then hold the big toes with your arms crossed behind the back. Thereafter, contract the muscles of the neck in the manner of Jālandhara while fixing the gaze on the tip of the nose. This is Bhadrāsana,*

*This *āsana* involves relaxation of the shoulder muscles when arms are stretched out to their maximum length behind the back; hence it must be practised cautiously but resolutely.

which eradicates all diseases.—9

iv. *Muktāsana*

पायुमूले वामगुल्फं दक्षगुल्फं तथोपरि।
शिरोग्रीवा समं कृत्वा मुक्तासनन्तु सिद्धिदम्।। १०।।

Set the left ankle below the genitals, and over them the right one. Then sit erect, keeping the head, neck and body in one line. This is Muktāsana, useful for the success of yoga.—10

v. *Vajrāsana*

जङ्घाभ्यां वज्रवत् कृत्वा गुदपार्श्वे पदावुभौ।
वज्रासनं भवेदेतत् योगिनां सिद्धिदायकम्।। ११।।

Fold both legs and contract (muscles of) the shanks making them hard as thunderbolt. Thereafter (without crossing the shins), adjust them on either side of the anus. This is Vajrāsana,* which helps yogis to achieve success in yoga.—11

vi. *Swastikāsana*

जानूर्वोरन्तरे कृत्वा योगी पादतले उभे।
ऋजुकायः समासीनः स्वस्तिकं तत् प्रचक्षते।। १२।।

When the yogi sits up erect with the soles of his feet tucked into the folds between knee and thigh, it is called Swastikāsana.—12

vii. *Siṃhāsana*

गुल्फौ च वृषणस्याधो व्युत्क्रमेणोर्द्धतां गतः।
चिविमूलो भूमिसंस्थः कृत्वा च जान्वोरूपरि।
व्यात्तवक्त्रो जलन्धरञ्च नासाग्रमवलोकयेत्।
सिंहासनं भवेदेतत् सर्वव्याधिविनाशनम्।। १३।।

Fold back the legs and bend down so that both ankles touch the region below the scrotum, slightly moving it up. Then, placing the head between the knees and the chin resting on ground, expand the face in the Jālandhara manner while gazing at the tip of the nose at the same time. This is Siṃhāsana,** suitable for curing all ailments.—13

viii. *Gomukhāsana*

पादौ च भूमौ संस्थाप्य पृष्ठपार्श्वे निवेशयेत्।
स्थिरकायं समासाद्य गोमुखं गोमुखाकृति।। १४।।

*While squatting in this posture the two hands should rest upon the thighs, with palms up.

**This is the Lion Pose. In this the elbows should rest on the ground, with the arms stiff, fists tight, mouth opened wide and eyes full of glare.

Squat on the ground and draw up both legs over the shoulders (back of neck) one after the other and sit motionless. This cow-faced formation is known as Gomukhāsana.*—14

ix. *Vīrāsana*

एकपादमथैकस्मिन् विन्यसेदूरुसंस्थितम्।
इतरस्मिन्स्थिता पश्चाद्वीरासनमितीरितम्।। १५।।

Lift one leg and place it over the other thigh; the other leg should remain folded behind (under the seat). This has been described as Vīrāsana.—15

x. *Dhanurāsana*

प्रसार्य पादौ भुवि दण्डरूपौ करौ च पृष्ठे धृतपादयुग्मम्।
कृत्वा धनुस्तुल्य परिवर्तिताङ्गं निगड्य योगी धनुरासनं तत्।। १६।।

Spread out both legs straight as two sticks; then, crossing hands behind the back and bending forward bow-like, catch the two legs. Thus 'enshackled,' the yogi is in Dhanurāsana.—16

xi. *Mṛtāsana*

उत्तानं शववद्भूमौ शयानस्तु शवासनम्।
शवासनं श्रमहरं चित्तविश्रान्तिकारकम्।। १७।।

Lying prostrate on the ground, face upward like a dead person, fully relaxed: this is known as Śavāsana.** It relieves fatigue and brings about mental tranquillity.—17

xii. *Guptāsana*

जानूर्वोरन्तरे पादौ कृत्वा पादौ च गोपयेत्।
पादोपरि च संस्थाप्य गुदं गुप्तासनं विदुः।। १८।।

Draw in both feet and insert (hide) the toes of each into the bend of the opposite knee. Then (resting on both palms and raising the body), place the posterior over the crossed legs. Know this to be Guptasana.—18

xiii. *Matsyāsana*

मुक्तपद्मासनं कृत्वा उत्तानशयनञ्चरेत्।
कूर्पराभ्यां शिरो वेष्टय मत्स्यासनस्तु रोगहा।। १९।।

*This formation, with the knees pressing the face on either side, lends the appearance of a cow's head, i.e., broad on top and narrow below.

**Śavāsana is the same as Mṛtāsana, both words signifying "a corpselike posture."

Form a free Padmāsana (i.e., a Padmāsana without the hands behind) and lie back, face up, with the arms enfolding (pressing) the head. This is Matsyāsana,* which combats all diseases.—19

xiv. *Paścimottāsana*

प्रसार्य पादौ भुवि दण्डरूपौ संन्यस्तभालश्चितियुग्ममध्ये।
यत्नेन पादौ च धृतौ कराभ्यां योगीन्द्रपीठं पश्चिमोत्तानमाहुः।। २०।।

Stretch out both legs on the ground, straight as sticks. Then bend and place the forehead over the knees and let the hands hold the feet. One school of yogis call this Paścimottāsana.—20

xv. *Matsyendrāsana*

उदरं पश्चिमाभ्यासं कृत्वा तिष्ठति यत्नतः।
नम्राङ्गवामपादं हि दक्षजानूपरि न्यसेत्।
तत्र याम्यं कूर्परञ्च याम्यं करे च वक्त्रकम्।
भ्रुवोर्मध्ये गतां दृष्टिं पीठं मात्स्येन्द्रमुच्यते।। २१।।

Sit up straight (steady), and draw in the stomach. Then put the calf of the left leg over the right knee. Next, support the face on the right palm, resting the right elbow (on the ground), and then keep the gaze fixed on the centre of the eyebrows. The yogi school call this Matsyendrāsana.—21

xvi. *Gorakṣāsana*

जानूर्वोरन्तरे पादौ उत्तानव्यक्तसंस्थितौ।
गुल्फौ चाच्छाद्य हस्ताभ्यामुत्तानाभ्यां प्रयत्नतः।
कंठसङ्कोचनं कृत्वा नासाग्रमवलोकयेत्।
गोरक्षासनमित्याह योगिनां सिद्धिकारणम्।। २२।।

Draw up both feet and place them, soles up, between the knee and thigh, carefully covering the ankles with open palms. Then, contracting the neck muscles, concentrate on the tip of the nose. This is Gorakṣāsana, which has been described by the yogis as the secret of success in yoga.—22

xvii. *Utkaṭāsana*

अङ्गुष्ठाभ्यामवष्टभ्य धरां गुल्फौ च खे गतौ।
तत्रोपरि गुदं न्यस्य विज्ञेयमुत्कटासनम्।। २३।।

Sit on toes, with heels up, and let the rump rest upon them (heels). This is known as Utkaṭāsana.—23

*During the performance of Matsyāsana, the legs must remain interlocked as prescribed for Padmāsana.

xviii. *Saṅkaṭāsana*

वामपादं चितेर्मूलं संन्यस्य धरणीतले।
पाददण्डेन याम्येन वेष्टयेद्वामपादकम्।
जानुयुग्मे करयुग्ममेतत् संकटासनम्।। २४।।

Keep the left leg fixed, level with the ground, and then enfold it with the right one midway around the shin; thereafter place both hands upon the knees. This is Saṅkaṭāsana.—24

xix. *Mayūrāsana*

धरामवष्टभ्य करयोस्तलाभ्यां तत्कूपरे स्थापितनाभिपार्श्वम्।
उच्चासनो दण्डवदुत्थितः खे मायूरमेतत् प्रवदन्ति पीठम्।। २५।।

Lie down on the ground, face down; then with elbows pressing either side of the navel and palms resting on the ground, lift yourself up like a level rod. One school of yogis call it Mayūrāsana.—25

xx. *Kukkuṭāsana*

पद्मासनं समासाद्य जानूर्वोरन्तरे करौ।
कूर्पराभ्यां समासीनो मञ्चस्थः कुक्कुटासनम्।। २६।।

Form a Padmāsana (*sans* crossing of arms), and hold the hands between thighs and knees. Then, with the help of the elbows, lift the body up. This is Kukkuṭāsana.—26

xxi. *Kūrmāsana*

गुल्फौ च वृषणस्याधो व्युत्क्रमेण समाहितौ।
ऋजुकायशिरोग्रीवं कूर्मासनमितीरितम्।। २७।।

Squat with ankles brought together and touching the region below the scrotum; then straighten up the body, neck and head in one line. This is called Kūrmāsana.*—27

xxii. *Uttānakūrmakāsana*

कुक्कुटासनबन्धस्थं कराभ्यां धृतकन्धरम्।
पीठं कूर्मवदुत्तानमेतदुत्तानकूर्मकम्।। २८।।

Form a Kukkuṭāsana—except that the hands (instead of being placed below thighs) should grip the neck. Then raise the back into a hump, like that of a turtle. This is Uttānakūrmakāsana.—28

xxiii. *Vṛkṣāsana*

वामोरुमूलदेशे च याम्यपादं निधाय तु।
तिष्ठेत्तु वृक्षवद्भूमौवृक्षासनमिदं विदुः।। २९।।

*While performing Kūrmāsana the hands should hold the shins.

Stretch out the left leg and, under this thigh, shove in about one-fourth of the right leg, keeping the body steady like a tree planted on the ground. Know this to be Vṛkṣāsana.—29

xxiv. *Maṇḍūkāsana*

पादतलौ पृष्ठदेशे अङ्गुष्ठे द्वे च संस्पृशेत्।
जानुयुग्मं पुरस्कृत्य साधयेन्मण्डूकासनम्।। ३०।।

Sit with the legs folded back, soles up and the two big toes touching each other; the knees in front should be close together and the hands straight down. This posture is known as Maṇḍūkāsana.—30

xxv. *Uttānamaṇḍūkāsana*

मण्डूकासनमध्यस्थं कूर्पराभ्यां धृतं शिरः।
एतद्भेकवदुत्तानमेतदुत्तानमण्डूकम्।। ३१।।

Form a Maṇḍūkāsana (as above), and then clasp the head with the two elbows. This frog-like formation is known as Uttānamaṇḍū-kāsana.—31

xxvi. *Garuḍāsana*

जङ्घोरुभ्यां धरां पीड्य स्थिरकायो द्विजानुना।
जानूपरि करयुग्मं गरुडासनमुच्यते।। ३२।।

Sit with both shins touching the ground and the knees and body perfectly steady. Then place both hands over the knees. This is called Garuḍāsana.—32

xxvii. *Vṛṣāsana*

याम्यगुल्फे पायुमूलं वामभागे पदेतरम्।
विपरीतं स्पृशेद्भूमिं वृषासनमिदं भवेत्।। ३३।।

Draw up the right ankle and place it under the rump. Then the left leg (held straight) should be turned over leftward so that (the side of) the foot is level with the ground. This makes a Vṛṣāsana.—33

xxviii. *Śalabhāsana*

अधास्यः शेते करयुग्मं वक्षे भूमिमवष्टभ्य करयोस्तलाभ्याम्।
पादौ च शुन्ये च वितस्ति चोर्द्ध्वं वदन्ति पीठं शलभं मुनीन्द्राः।। ३४।।

Lie down, face downwards, with both hands under the chest and palms touching the ground. Thereafter lift the legs span-high (about 9 ins. from the ground) and hold them there. The sages have named it Śalabhāsana.—34

xxix. *Makarāsana*

अधास्यः शेते हृदयं निधाय भूमौ च पादौ प्रसार्यमाणौ।

शिरश्च धृत्वा करदण्डयुग्मे देहाग्निकारकं मकरासनं तत्।। ३५।।

Lie down, face downwards, with the chest touching the ground and both legs extended fully. Thereafter, press the head with the two arms. This makes Makarāsana, which is most invigorating for the body.—35

xxx *Uṣṭrāsana*

अधास्यः शेते पदयुग्मव्यस्तं पृष्ठे निधायापि धृतं कराभ्याम्।

आकुञ्चयेत् सम्यगुदरस्यगाढं औष्ट्रञ्च पीठं योगिनो वदन्ति।। ३६।।

Lie down flat, face downwards, and draw up the legs to touch the back. Then, holding them with both hands, contract (the muscles of) the abdomen firmly. One school of yogis call this Uṣṭrāsana.—36

xxxi. *Bhujaṅgāsana*

अङ्गुष्ठनाभिपर्यन्तमधोभूमौ विनिर्न्यसेत्।

करतलाभ्यां धरां धृत्वा ऊर्द्धशीर्षः फणीव हि।

देहाग्निर्वर्द्धते नित्यं सर्वरोगविनाशनम्।

जागर्ति भुजगीदेवी साधनात् भुजगासनम्।। ३७।।

Lie down flat, face downwards. Then raise the upper half of the body with the help of the arms, palms touching the ground; the nether half of the body should remain level with the ground. Next tilt the head back like a serpent's hood. The practice of this Bhujaṅgāsana removes all ailments, invigorates the body and awakens the serpent-goddess (Kuṇḍalinī).—37

xxxii. *Yogāsana*

उत्तानौ चरणौ कृत्वा संस्थाप्य जान्वोरुपरि।

आसनोपरि संस्थाप्य उत्तानं करयुग्मकम्।

पूरकैर्वायुमाकृष्य नासाग्रमवलोकयेत्।

योगासनं भवेदेतत् योगिनां योगसाधने।। ३८।।

Place each foot, sole up, upon the opposite knee and let the hands drop down straight, resting on the lap with open palms. Then take in a full breath and, while holding it, concentrate on the tip of the nose. This constitutes Yogāsana, said to be the best for yogis engaged in practising yoga.—38

Here ends Lesson Two entitled 'Āsanas or Modes of Installation' incorporated in *Gheraṇḍasaṃhitā*.

LESSON THREE

Mudrās or Mystic Exercises

Śrī Gheraṇḍa said:

महामुद्रा नभोमुद्रा उड्डीयानं जलन्धरम्।
मूलबन्धं महाबन्धं महावेधश्च खेचरी।। १।।
विपरीतकरी योनिर्वज्रोली शक्तिचालनी।
तडागी माण्डूकी मुद्रा शाम्भवी पञ्चधारणा।। २।।
अश्विनी पाशिनी काकी मातङ्गी च भुजङ्गिनी।
पञ्चविंशति मुद्राणि सिद्धिदानीह योगिनाम्।। ३।।

There are twenty-five types of *mudrās* that bring success to the yogi. These are: Mahāmudrā, Nabhomudrā, Uḍḍīyāna, Jālandhara, Mūlabandha, Mahābandha, Mahāvedha, Khecarī, Viparītakarī, Yoni, Vajroli, Śakticālani, Taḍāgī, Māṇḍūkī, Śāmbhavī, Pañcadhāraṇā, Aświnī, Pāśinī, Kākī, Mātaṅgī, and Bhujaṅginī.—1–3

i. *Mahāmudrā*

पायुमूलं वामगुल्फे संपीड्य दृढयत्नतः।
याम्यपाद प्रसार्याय करैर्धृतपदाङ्गुलः।। ४।।
कण्ठसंकोचनं कृत्वा भ्रुवोर्मध्ये निरीक्षयेत्।
महामुद्राभिधा मुद्रा कथ्यते चैव सूरिभिः।। ५।।
क्षयकासं गुदावर्त्तं प्लीहाजीर्णं ज्वरन्तथा।
नाशयेत् सर्वरोगांश्च महामुद्राति सेवनात्।। ६।।

Draw up the left leg and firmly set its ankle against the rump (anus). Next stretch out the right leg and hold its toes. Thereafter, contracting the muscles of the neck, fix attention on the centre of the eyebrows. This posture, the practice of which combats diseases such as consumptive cough, constipation, spleen troubles and fevers, has been described by the gods as Mahāmudrā.—4–6

ii. *Nabhomudrā*

यत्र यत्र स्थितो योगी सर्वकार्येषु सर्वदा।
ऊर्द्धजिह्वः स्थिरो भूत्वा धारयेत् पवनं सदा।
नभोमुद्रा भवेदेषा योगिनां रोगनाशिनी।। ७।।

Wherever the yogi may be stationed, and whatever may be the work in which he is engaged, he should always practise the control of his breath with the tongue unturned. This is the Nabhomudrā, by which yogis keep themselves fit.—7

iii. *Uḍḍīyāna*

उदरे पश्चिमं तानं नाभेरूर्द्धन्तु कारयेत्।
उड्डीयानं कुरुते यत्तदविश्रान्तं महाखगः।।
उड्डीयानं त्वसौ बन्धो मृत्यु मातङ्ग-केशरी।। ८।।
समग्रात् बन्धनात् ह्येतत् उड्डीयानं विशिष्यते।
उड्डीयाने समभ्यस्ते मुक्तिः स्वाभाविकी भवेत्।। ९।।

Draw in the abdomen to the utmost, pushing up the bowels above the navel, and then let these be suspended there in space as long as possible. This is the Uḍḍīyāna exercise which dominates diseases even as the lion treats an elephant. Of all the exercises the practice of Uḍḍīyāna that is most distinguished inasmuch as it smoothens the path to *mukti* (deliverance).—8 and 9

iv. *Jālandhara*

कण्ठसंकोचनं कृत्वा चिबुकं हृदये न्यसेत्।
जालन्धरे कृते बन्धे षोडशाधारबन्धनम्।
जालन्धरं महा मुद्रा मृत्योश्च क्षयकारिणी।। १०।।
सिद्धं जालन्धरं बन्धं योगिनां सिद्धिदायकम्।
षण्मासमभ्यसेत् यो हि स सिद्धो नात्रसंशयः।। ११।।

Contract the muscles of the neck and let the chin rest upon the chest. Jālandhara is a great *mudrā* which combats death and with its performance the next sixteen (i.e., main) *mudrās* may be dispensed with. Six months of practice makes one an adept and, with the mastery of this *mudrā*, yogis achieve success (i.e., get the desired psychic powers).—10 and 11

v. *Mūlabandha*

पार्ष्णिणा वामपादस्य योनिमाकुञ्चयेत्ततः।
नाभिग्रन्थि मेरुदण्डे संपीड्य यत्नतः सुधीः।। १२।।

मेढ्रं दक्षिणगुल्फे तु दृढबन्धं समाचरेत्।
जराविनाशिनी मुद्रा मूलबन्धो निगद्यते।। १३।।

The wise yogi should first press hard the pelvic region with his left heel and then with the right ankle push the genitals on to one side; thereafter the muscles of the stomach should be contracted to the extent till they touch the spinal column. This *mudrā*, described as Mūlabandha, prevents aging.—12 and 13

संसार सागरं तर्तुमभिलषति यः पुमान्।
विरले सुगुप्तो भूत्वा मुद्रमेनां समभ्यसेत्।। १४।।
अभ्यासात् बन्धनस्यास्य मरुत्सिद्धिर्भवेद् ध्रुवम्।
साधयेत् यत्नतो तर्हि मौनी तु विजितालसः।। १५।।

A person desirous of crossing the ocean of world phenomena should practise this *mudrā* secretly in a solitary place. Its practice will lead to success in mastering the airs (within the body), take away all lethargy and bring tranquillity to the mind.—14 and 15

vi. *Mahābandha*

वामपादस्य गुल्फे तु पायुमूलं निरोधयेत्।
दक्षपादेन तद्गुल्फं संपीड्य यत्नतः सुधीः।। १६।।
शनैः शनैश्चालयेत् पार्ष्णिं योनिमाकुञ्चयेच्छनैः।
जालन्धरे धारयेत् प्राणान्महाबन्धो निगद्यते।। १७।।
महाबन्धो परो बन्धो जरामरणनाशनः।
प्रसादादस्य बन्धस्य साधयेत् सर्ववाञ्छितम्।। १८।।

Block the anus with the ankle of the left leg. Then slowly keep pressing it (ankle) with the right heel while contracting the rectum at the same time and holding the breath in the Jālandhara way (i.e., by contracting the neck muscles and lowering the chin on the chest). This is described as Mahābandha, which is propitious for overcoming decay and death and which yields the desired (yoga) results.—16–18

vii. *Mahāvedha*

रूपयौवनलावण्यं नारीणां पुरुषं विना।
मूलबन्ध-महाबन्धौ महावेधं विना तथा।। १९।।
महाबन्धं समासाद्य उड्डान-कुम्भकं चरेत्।
महावेधः समाख्यातो योगिनां सिद्धिदायकः।। २०।।

The two (above-noted) Mūlabandha and Mahābandha *mudrās*

are fruitless without the Mahāvedha even as youth and beauty of women are useless without there being men to observe them! When Mahābandha is accomplished along with Uḍḍīyāna (i.e., contraction of stomach muscles) and *kumbhaka* (holding of breath), it is called Mahāvedha. It is the royal road to success for yogis.—19 and 20

महाबन्ध-मूलबन्धौ महावेध समन्वितौ।
प्रत्यहं कुरुते यस्तु स योगी योगवित्तमः।। २१।।
न च मृत्युभयं तस्य न जरा तस्य विद्यते।
गोपनीयः प्रयत्नेन वेधोऽयं योगिपुङ्गवैः।। २२।।

Mahāvedha is a combination of Mūlabandha and Mahābandha. The yogi who performs this (Mahāvedha) every day is a real adept; there is no fear of decay or death for him. Hence yogis always keep it a close secret.—21 and 22

viii. *Khecarī*

जिह्वाधो नाडीं संछिन्नां रसनां चालयेत् सदा।
दोहयेन्नवनीतेन लौहयन्त्रेण कर्षयेत्।। २३।।
एवं नित्यं समभ्यासाल्लम्बिका दीर्घतां व्रजेत्।
यावद्गच्छेद् भ्रुवोर्मध्ये तदा गच्छति खेचरी।। २४।।

Make an incision in the membrane located under the tongue and rub the place with butter. Next, after scraping the tongue with a metal scraper, keep the tongue moving in the mouth. When this is practised regularly the (main) papilla under the tongue (uvula) gets longer. When the same is able to enter (with an unturned tongue) the sinus between the eyebrows, Khecarī is accomplished.—23 and 24

रसनां तालुमध्ये तु शनैः शनैः प्रवेशयेत्।
कपालकुहरे जिह्वा प्रविष्टा विपरीतगा।
भ्रुवोर्मध्ये गता दृष्टिर्मुद्रा भवति खेचरी।। २५।।

Let the tongue move along the palate little by little till it reaches the entrance to the sinus (leading into the forehead), where it turns over. When it is felt that it has touched the cavity between the eyebrows, Khecarī is accomplished.—25

न च मूर्च्छा क्षुधा तृष्णा नैवालस्यं प्रजायते।
न च रोगो जरामृत्युर्दिव्यदेहः प्रजायते।। २६।।

नाग्निना दह्यते गात्रं न शोषयति मारुतः।
न देह क्लेदयन्त्यापो दंशयेन्न भुजङ्गमः।। २७।।
लावण्यञ्च भवेद् गात्रे समाधिर्जायते ध्रुवम्।
कपालवक्त्रसंयोगे रसना रसमाप्नुयात्।। २८।।

(When this *mudrā* is practised) there is neither lethargy, hunger nor thirst; nor do diseases, decay and death afflict the yogi. His body is not affected by fire, wind, or water, and snake-bites have no effect on him. The body is then all radiant, and fit for *samādhi*. The tongue, too, tastes the ambrosia issuing from the passage between the mouth and the forehead.—26–28

नानारससमुद्भूतमानन्दञ्च दिने दिने।
आदौ लवणक्षारञ्च ततस्तिक्तकषायकम्।। २९।।
नवनीतं घृतं क्षीरं दधि तक्र मधूनि च।
द्राक्षारसञ्च पीयूषं जायते रसनोदकम्।। ३०।।

Day after day different kinds of delectable secretions ooze (from this passage). At first it is saline, then alkaline, then bitter and acrid; later it is like butter, clarified butter, milk, curd, whey and honey. Finally, the tongue tastes a fine grape-juice and then nectar itself.—29 and 30

ix. *Viparītakarī*

नाभिमूले वसेत् सूर्यस्तालुमूले च चन्द्रमा।
अमृतं ग्रसते सूर्यस्ततो मृत्युवशो नरः।। ३१।।
ऊर्ध्वे च नीयते सूर्यश्चन्द्रश्च अध आनयेत्।
विपरीतकरी मुद्रा सर्व तन्त्रेषु गोपिता।। ३२।।
भूमो शिरश्च संस्थाप्य करयुग्मं समाहितः।
ऊर्ध्वपादः स्थिरो भूत्वा विपरीतकरी मता।। ३३।।
मुद्रेयं साधयेन्नित्यं जरामृत्युञ्च नाशयेत्।
स सिद्धः सर्वलोकेषु प्रलयेऽपि न सीदति।। ३४।।

(Normally) the psychic Sun and the psychic Moon dwell at the root of the navel and the palate respectively. This Sun absorbs the (immortal) ambrosia (flowing from the Moon), leading man on to his (inevitable) death. When, however, this Sun is taken upward and the Moon is brought down by reversing oneself—with the head touching the ground and the body and legs held straight up—it becomes a *Viparītakarī* (opposite position). This *mudrā* is a secret in all Tantras. He who regularly practises this *mudrā* cheats both decay and death, becomes master of all three worlds, and is not affected by even the Cosmic Chaos!*—31–34

x. *Yoni*

सिद्धासनं समासाद्य कर्णचक्षुर्नसोमुखम्।
अङ्गुष्ठतर्जनीमध्यानामादिभिश्च साधयेत्।। ३५।।
काकीभिः प्राणं संकृष्य अपाने योजयेत्ततः।
षट्चक्राणि क्रमाद्ध्यात्वा हुं हंस मनुना सुधीः।। ३६।।
चैतन्यमानयेद् देवीं निद्रिता या भुजङ्गिनी।
जीवने सहितां शक्तिं समुत्थाप्य कराम्बुजे।। ३७।।
शक्तिमयः स्वयं भूत्वा परः शिवेन सङ्गमम्।
नाना सुखं विहारञ्च चिन्तयेत् परमं सुखम्।। ३८।।
शिवशक्तिसमायोगादेकान्तं भूवि भावयेत्।
आनन्दञ्च स्वयं भूत्वा अहं ब्रह्मेति सम्भवेत्।। ३९।।
योनिमुद्रा परा गोप्या देवानामपि दुर्लभा।
सकृत्तु लाभसंसिद्धिः समाधिस्थ स एव हि।। ४०।।

Sit in the manner of Siddhāsana, and close the ears with the two thumbs, eyes with the index fingers, nostrils with middle fingers, and the mouth with ring fingers. Next, curl up the lips to form a "crow beak" (as while whistling) and then, drawing in to the full the vital air (*prāṇa*) let the same be yoked to *apāna* (the down-flowing air within the body). Next propagate the same through the six *cakras* (psychic centres) one after another with the sounds of *huṃ* (हु) and *haṃs* (हंस्) as prescribed by the wise. It is then that the sleeping goddess called Serpent-Power (Kuṇḍalinī) is roused which, joining with life's vital power, becomes activated in the form of Śakti and seeks union with Śiva (residing at the summit on top of the brain). The yogi then experiences bliss in many forms and feels as though he is the Brahman itself, enjoying the company of Śiva and Pārvatī! This Yonimudrā is most secret, rare even for the gods and, if practised properly, can bring about the desired success in *samādhi*.—35–40

ब्रह्महा भ्रूणहा चैव सुरापी गुरुतल्पगः।
एतैः पापैर्न लिप्येत योनिमुद्रा निबन्धनात्।। ४१।।
यानि पापानि घोराणि उपपापानि यानि च।

*The last statement, obviously, is a rhetorical exaggeration meant to emphasize the great benefits of this exercise.

तानि सर्वाणि नश्यन्ति योनिमुद्रा निबन्धनात्।
तस्मादभ्यासनं कुर्याद्यदि मुक्तिं समिच्छति।। ४२।।

The practice of Yonimudrā absolves one of all sins, major as well as minor, such as killing a child, killing a Brahmin, drunkenness, or adultery committed with the guru's wife. All these are nullified by Yonimudrā, and hence those desirous of attaining *mukti* (deliverance) should practise this *mudrā.*—41 and 42

xi. *Vajroli*

धरामवष्टभ्य करयोस्तलाभ्यां
ऊर्द्ध्वं क्षिपेत् पादयुगं शिरः खे।
शक्तिप्रबोधाय चिरजीवनाय
वज्रोली मुद्रा मुनयो वदन्ति।। ४३।।

Place the palms of the hand on the ground and lift the legs and head up. This Vajrolimudrā,* say the sages, lends vigour and longevity.—43

अयं योगो योगश्रेष्ठो योगिनां मुक्तिकारणम्।
अयं हितप्रदो योगो योगिनां सिद्धिदायकः।। ४४।।

This exercise is one of the best of yogas, and serves as a means of *mukti* to the yogis. This is also useful for mastering yoga itself.—44

एतद्योगप्रसादेन विन्दुसिद्धिर्भवेद् ध्रुवम्।
सिद्धे विन्दौ महायत्ने किं न सिद्ध्यति भूतले।। ४५।।

The practice of this *mudrā* helps to get a positive control over the seminal fluid; and once this control has been assiduously achieved, what else cannot be mastered upon this earth?—45

भोगेन महता युक्तो यदि मुद्रां समाचरेत्।
तथापि सकला सिद्धिस्तस्य भवति निश्चितम्।। ४६।।

Even if this exercise is practised by a person leading a family life, it will definitely produce for him the desired success.—46

xii. *Śakticālanī*

मूलाधारे आत्मशक्तिः कुण्डली परदेवता।
शयिता भुजगाकारा सार्द्धत्रिबलयान्विता।। ४७।।
यावत् सा निद्रिता देहे तावज्जीवः पशुर्यथा।

*Vajrolimudrā implies lying on the ground face down, and then raising only the head and legs straight, while the rest of the body remains level with the ground.
Cf. *Śivasaṃhitā*, IV.78–94.

ज्ञानं न जायते तावत् कोटियोगं समभ्यसेत्।। ४८।।
उद्घाटयेत् कवाटञ्च यथा कुञ्चिकया हठात्।
कुण्डलिन्याः प्रबोधेन ब्रह्मद्वारं प्रभेदयेत्।। ४९।।

At the Mūlādhāracakra (cf. *Śivasaṃhitā*, V.89) is installed the goddess Kuṇḍalinī, representing man's vital force. She lies dormant—like a serpent coiled three-and-a-half rounds. While she is asleep, man is but an animal; he does not get the necessary knowledge (for self-realization) despite his practice of countless yogas. But when the Kuṇḍalinī suddenly wakes up, the doors of the Brahmarandhra* are opened as though by a key, and she enters therein.—47–49

नाभिं संवेष्ट्य वस्त्रेण न च नग्नो वहिःस्थितः।
गोपनीय गृहे स्थित्वा शक्तिचालनमभ्यसेत्।। ५०।।
वितस्तिप्रमितं दीर्घं विस्तारे चतुरङ्गुलम्।
मृदुलं धवलं सूक्ष्मं वेष्टनाम्बरलक्षणम्।
एवमम्बरयुक्तञ्च कटिसूत्रेण योजयेत्।। ५१।।
भस्मना गात्र संलिप्तं सिद्धासनं समाचरेत्।
नासाभ्यां प्राणमाकृष्य अपानं योजयेत् बलात्।। ५२।।
तावदाकुञ्चयेद् गुह्यं शनैरश्विनीमुद्रया।
यावद्गच्छेत् सुषुम्नायां वायुः प्रकाशयेद् हठात्।। ५३।।
तदा वायुप्रबन्धेन कुम्भिका च भुजङ्गिनी।
बद्धश्वासस्ततो भूत्वा ऊर्द्धमार्गं प्रपद्यते।। ५४।।

The Śakticālan exercise is to be practised in a secluded place, not outside, and not while wholly naked but with a piece of cloth wrapped round the waist. It should be four-finger wide (6 cm) and about a span (22 cm) long. The cloth should be soft, white and fine, and should hang from the waist by a string tied round it. After smearing the body with ash, sit down in Siddhāsana; then draw in air from the nostrils (*prāṇa*) and yoke it to *apāna* (the down-flowing air in the body), at the same time gently contracting the rectum in the manner of Aświnīmudrā (see *infra*, p. 134). So long as the air (i.e., the combined *prāṇa* and *apāna*) does not enter the Suṣumnā (median nerve), the pressure has to be maintained. Thereupon, aided by the restricted air of *kumbhaka*, the Serpent Power, having thus been choked, takes the upward path (i.e., the Passage of Knowl-

*Brahmarandhra, or the Passage of Knowledge as it is esoterically designated, is located in the median nerve called Suṣumnā.

edge).—50-54

विनाशत्तिं चालनेन योनि मुद्रा न सिद्ध्यति।
आदौ चालनमभ्यस्य योनिमुद्रां समभ्यसेत्।। ५५।।

Since the Yonimudrā cannot be mastered without this Śakticālinī, the practice of this *mudrā* is essential in the first instance.—55

इति ते कथितं चण्डकापाले शक्तिचालनम्।
गोपनीयं प्रयत्नेन दिने दिने समभ्यसेत्।। ५६।।

O Caṇḍakāpāli! I have now told you of this Śakticālan exercise, but it has to be practised very secretly and very carefully day after day.—56

मुद्रेयं परमा गोप्या जरामरणनाशिनी।
तस्मादभ्यासनं कार्यं योगिभिः सिद्धिकाङ्क्षिभिः।। ५७।।

This *mudrā* is most secret. It is a deterrent for decay and death, and hence yogis who wish to master it must practise it assiduously.—57

नित्यं योऽभ्यसते योगी सिद्धिस्तस्य करे स्थिता।
तस्य विग्रहसिद्धिः स्याद्रोगाणां संक्षयो भवेत्।। ५८।।

The yogi who practises it every day has success in the palm of his hand. When it is mastered the body becomes perfect and all ailments disappear.—58

xiii. *Taḍāgi*

उदरं पश्चिमोत्तानं कृत्वा च तडागाकृति।
तडागी सा परामुद्रा जरामृत्युविनाशिनी।। ५९।।

Lie down and pull in the stomach to the maximum, so as to form the shape of a deep pool or pond (i.e., hollow). This is Taḍāgimudrā which is excellent for overcoming decay and death.—59

xiv. *Māṇḍūki*

मुखं समुत्थितं कृत्वा जिह्वामूलं प्रचालयेत्।
शनैर्ग्रसेदमृतस्तन्माण्डूकीमुद्रिकां विदुः।। ६०।।

Lift up the face, and then roll the tongue inside the closed mouth and slowly draw out the ambrosia from the Moon (at the root of the palate). This is known as Māṇḍūkimudrā.—60

बलितं पलितं नैव जायते नित्ययौवनम्।
न केशे जायते पाको यः कुर्यान्नित्य माण्डूकीम्।। ६१।।

He who performs this Māṇḍūki exercise regularly does not become bent and old, and his hair never turns grey. He remains ever-young.—61

xv. *Śāmbhavi*

नेत्राञ्जनं समालोक्य आत्मारामं निरीक्षयेत्।
सा भवेच्छाम्भवी मुद्रा सर्वतन्त्रेषु गोपिता।। ६२।।
सत्यं सत्यं पुनः सत्यं सत्यमुक्तं महेश्वरः।
शाम्भवीं यो विजानीयात् स च ब्रह्म न चान्यथा।। ६३।।

With eyes wide-open, concentrate upon your own image (i.e., visualize your own image out in space). This constitutes the Śāmbhavimudrā, which is not mentioned in all Tantra works. He who masters this Śāmbhavi is indeed no less than the Brahman. As stated by the Lord Śiva, this is true and thrice true.—62 and 63

xvi. *Pañca-dhāraṇā*

कथिता शाम्भवी मुद्रा शृणुष्व पञ्चधारणाम्।
धारणाणि समासाद्य किं न सिध्यति भूतले।। ६४।।
अनेन नरदेहेन स्वर्गेषु गमनागमः।
मनोगतिर्भवेत्तस्य खेचरत्वं न चान्यथा।। ६५।।

Having described the Śāmbhavimudrā, now listen to the Pañca-dhāraṇā (five-fold visualizations). It enables the mind to communicate with heaven (space) even when the body dwells on earth, and also gives the mind the quality of Khecara (i.e., power to float in air).—64 and 65

1. *Pārthivi-dhāraṇā*

यत्तत्वं हरितालदेशरचितं भौमं लकारान्वितं
बेवाग्रं कगलासने सहितं वृत्वाहृदिस्थायिनग्।
प्राणांस्तत्र विनीय पञ्चघटिकां चित्तान्वितां धारये-
देषा स्तम्भकरी क्षितिजयकरी कुर्यादधोधारणा।। ६६।।

Visualize the quintessence of Earth—yellow-hued and symbolized by the letter "L" (ल) installed upon the four-petalled lotus (Anāhata) within the heart. Next, restraining the vital air (*prāṇa*) and holding it there, concentrate (meditate) upon it for two hours. This Pārthivi-dhāraṇā tranquillizes the mind and takes it out into the wide space.—66

पार्थिवीधारणामुद्रा यः करोति हि नित्यशः।
मृत्युञ्जयः स्वयं सोऽपि स सिद्धो विचरेद् भुवि।। ६७।।

Whosoever practises this Pārthivi-dhāraṇā regularly becomes like the Lord of Death (another designation of Śiva) and so can move about freely in the universe.—67

2. *Āmbhasi-dhāraṇā*

शङ्खेन्दुप्रतिमञ्च कुन्दधवलं तत्वं कीलालं शुभं
तत्पीयूषवकारबीजसहितं युक्तं सदा विष्णुना।
प्राणांस्तत्र विनीय पञ्चघटिकां चित्तान्वितां धारये-
देषा दुःसहतापहरणी स्यादाम्भसी धारणा।। ६८।।

The quintessence of Water is to be visualized as pure nectar—white like conch, moon or the *kunda* flower—symbolized by the letter "V" (व) and ever co-mingled with fire. Drawing in the vital air (*prāṇa*) there, meditate for two hours. This is Āmbhasi-dhāraṇā, which alleviates all unbearable heat (passion).—68

आम्भसी परमा मुद्रा यो जानाति स योगवित्।
जले च गभीरे घोरे मरणं तस्य नो भवेत्।। ६९।।
इयन्तु परमा मुद्रा गोपनीया प्रयत्नतः।
प्रकाशात् सिद्धिहानिः स्यात् सत्यं वच्मि च तत्वतः।। ७०।।

The Āmbhasi is an excellent *mudrā.* He who knows it properly is never in danger of drowning in even wide and deep oceans. Hence this excellent *mudrā* should be guarded carefully, since its divulgence might lead to a positive loss of this power, I tell you truly.—69 and 70

3. *Āgneyi-dhāraṇā*

यन्नाभिस्थितमिन्द्रगोपसदृशं बीजं त्रिकोणान्वितं
तत्वं तेजोमयं प्रदीप्तमरुणं रुद्रेण यत् सिद्धिदम्।
प्राणं तत्र विनीय पञ्चघटिकां चित्तान्वितां धारये-
देषा कालगंभीरभीतिहरणी वैश्वानरी धारणा।। ७१।।

The quintessence of Fire is to be visualized as the red, velvety *indragopa* insect, triangular in shape [symbolized by the letter "R" (र)], radiant and bright as the sun dominating the dawn, and dwelling inside the navel. The vital air (*prāṇa*) is to be drawn in and held there while the mind meditates on it for two hours. This is Āgneyi-dhāraṇā, which dispels the deeply ingrained Terror of Death.—71

प्रदीप्ते ज्वलिते वह्नौ यदि पतति साधकः।
एवन्मुद्रा प्रसादेन स जीवति न मृत्युभाक्।। ७२।।

Through the grace of this *mudrā* the yogi, even if he falls into a red raging fire, continues to live and does not become a prey to death.—72

4. *Vāyavi-dhāraṇā*

यद्भिन्नाञ्जनपुञ्जसन्निभमिदं धूम्रावभासं परं
तत्वं सत्वमयं यकारसहितं यत्रेश्वरो देवता।
प्राणांस्तत्र विनीय पञ्चघटिकां चित्तान्वितां धारये-
देषा खे गमनं करोति यमिनां स्याद्वायवीधारणा।। ७३।।

The quintessence of Air is to be visualized as a glowing speck of smoky grey (variegated), symbolized by the letter "Y" (य) and the immaculate attribute of the Supreme. To this the *prāna* should be united and the mind held in concentration for two hours. This is Vāyavi-dhāraṇā, which makes it possible to float and move about in air.—73

इयन्तु परमा मुद्रा जरामृत्युविनाशिनी।
वायुना म्रियते नापि खे च गति प्रदायिनी।। ७४।।

This is an excellent *mudrā* which prevents decay and death, bestows the power to float in air, and never causes death either by or in the air.—74

शठाय भक्तिहीनाय न देया यस्य कस्यचित्।
दत्ते च सिद्धिहानिः स्यात् सत्यं वच्मि च चण्ड ते।। ७५।।

This (secret) is not to be passed on to any and every person, and certainly not to the wicked and the faithless. If so done, I tell you truly, O Caṇḍakāpāli, you shall lose the power.—75

5. *Ākāśi-dhāraṇā*

यत् सिन्धौ वरशुद्धवारिसदृशं व्योमं परं भासितं
तत्वं देव सदाशिवेन सहितं बीजं ठकारान्वितम्।
प्राणांस्तत्र विनीय पञ्चघटिकां चित्तान्वितां धारये-
देषा मोक्षकवाटभेदनकरी कुर्यान्नभोधारणा।। ७६।।

The quintessence of Space is to be visualized as a sky that is clear and bright as the pure waters of ocean, symbolized by the letter "ṭha" (ठ) and indicating Eternal Infinity. Ṭo this should be united the *prāṇa* (vital air), and the mind concentrated for two hours. This is the Ākāśi-dhāraṇā, which opens the door to *mokṣa* (emancipation).—76

आकाशीधारणामुद्रां यो वेत्ति स् च योगवित्।
न मृत्युर्जायते तस्य प्रलये नावसीदति।। ७७।।

He who knows the Ākāśi-dhāraṇā properly neither dies nor shall he be affected by the Final Dissolution (*pralaya*).—77

xvii. *Aświnī*

आकुञ्चयेद् गुदद्वारं प्रकाशयेत् पुनः पुनः।
सा भवेदश्विनी मुद्रा शक्तिप्रबोधकारिणी।। ७८।।

The Aświnīmudrā involves repeated dilation and contraction of the rectum. This exercise generates strength and confidence.—78

अश्विनी परमा मुद्रा गुह्यरोगविनाशिनी।
बलपुष्टिकरी चैव अकालमरणं हरेत्।। ७९।।

Aświnī is an excellent exercise for curing secret disorders. It also builds up vigour and prevents premature death.—79

xviii. *Pāśini*

कण्ठपृष्ठे क्षिपेत् पादौ पाशवद् दृढबन्धनम्।
सा एव पाशिनी मुद्रा शक्तिप्रबोधकारिणी।। ८०।।

Bring up the two legs over the opposite shoulders, and with the two feet hold the neck in a grip (trap). This is Pāśinimudrā, which is good for building up vigour and confidence.—80

पाशिनी महती मुद्रा बलपुष्टिविधायिनी।
साधनीया प्रयत्नेन साधकैः सिद्धिकाङ्क्षिभिः।। ८१।।

Pāśini is a great exercise for making oneself strong and vigorous. Yogis aspiring to succeed in yoga should practise it regularly.—81

xix. *Kāki*

काकचञ्चुवदास्येन पिबेद्वायुं शनैः शनैः।
काकीमुद्रा भवेदेषा सर्वरोगविनाशिनी।। ८२।।

Curl up the lips to form a "crow's beak" (as during whistling) and then draw in air through them very slowly. This is Kākimudrā, which prevents any ill-health.—82

काकीमुद्रा परा मुद्रा सर्वतन्त्रेषु गोपिता।
अस्या प्रसादमात्रेण काकवत् नीरोगी भवेत्।। ८३।।

Kākimudrā is an excellent exercise, and it has been well preserved in the works of Tantra. Its mastery makes one as healthy as a crow!*—83

xx. *Mātaṅgini*

कण्ठमग्ने जले स्थित्वा नासाभ्यां जलमाहरेत्।
मुखान्निर्गमयेत् पश्चात् पुनर्वक्त्रेण चाहरेत्।। ८४।।
नासाभ्यां रेचयेत् पश्चात् कुर्यादेवं पुनः पुनः।
मातङ्गिनी परा मुद्रा जरामृत्युविनाशिनी।। ८५।।

Sit in a tub (or in a stream) with water up to your neck. Then draw in water through the nostrils and expel the same through the mouth. Again, draw in water through the mouth and release it through the nose. This process should be repeated several times. Mātaṅginimudrā is an excellent exercise which has been devised to defeat aging and death.—84 and 85

विरले निर्जने देशे स्थित्वा चैकाग्रमानसः।
कुर्यान्मातङ्गिनीं मुद्रां मातङ्ग इव जायते।। ८६।।

The Mātaṅginimudrā should be performed when alone and in a solitary place, and also with a devoted mind. It will make one as strong as an elephant.—86

यत्र तत्र स्थितो योगी सुखमत्यन्तमश्नुते।
तस्मात् सर्वप्रयत्नेन साधयेत् मुद्रिकां पराम्।। ८७।।

Then the yogi can be happy anywhere and in whatever position he may be. Hence this good exercise should be practised with every care.—87

xxi. *Bhujaṅgini*

वक्त्रं किञ्चित् सुप्रसार्य चानिलं गलया पिबेत्।
सा भवेत् भुजंगीमुद्रा जरामृत्युविनाशिनी।। ८८।।

Keep the mouth half open and draw in air direct into the throat. This is Bhujaṅginimudrā, which prevents decay and death.—88

यावच्च उदरे रोगमजीर्णादि विशेषतः।
तत् सर्वं नाशयेदाशु यत्र मुद्रा भुजङ्गिनी।। ८९।।

All stomach complaints, especially indigestion, are quickly removed by the practice of the Bhujaṅginimudrā.—89

इदन्तु मुद्रापटलं कथितं चण्डकापाले।
वल्लभं सर्वसिद्धानां जरामरणनाशनम्।। ९०।।

O Caṇḍakāpāli! I have now described the entire series of exer-

*Traditionally, the crow is believed never to fall ill.

cises that are dear to yogis and which defeat senility and death.—90

शठाय भक्तिहीनाय न देयं यस्य कस्यचित्।
गोपनीयं प्रयत्नेन दुर्लभं मरुतामपि।। ९१।।

These must not be passed on to any and every person—particularly to the wicked and the faithless—but should be preserved carefully, since these are generally not available even to the gods.—91

ऋजवे शान्तचित्ताय गुरुभक्तिपराय च।
कुलीनाय प्रदातव्य भोगमुक्तिप्रदायकम्।। ९२।।

However, these may be communicated to those who are faithful, composed in mind, devoted to their gurus, and who come from well-bred families—for the purpose of their welfare and deliverance.—92

मुद्राणां पटलं ह्येतत् सर्वव्याधिविनाशनम्।
नित्यमभ्यासशीलस्य जठराग्निविवर्द्धनम्।। ९३।।

This series of exercises is good for overcoming all kinds of diseases, and their regular practice will surely improve the appetite.—93

तस्य न जायते मृत्युर्नास्य जरादिकं तथा।
नाग्निजलभयं तस्य वायोरपि कुतो भयम्।। ९४।।

Nor would he (i.e., the person practising these exercises) have any more fear of death by drowning, fire, wind or aging.—94

कासः श्वासः प्लीहा श्लेष्म रोगाणाञ्चैव विंशति।
मुद्राणां साधनाच्चैव विनश्यन्ति न संशयः।। ९५।।

Through the practice of these *mudrās* all respiratory diseases, as well as such diseases as are caused by an excess of bile and phlegm, are fully controlled.—95

बहुना किमिहोक्तेन सारं वच्मि च चण्ड ते।
नास्ति मुद्रासमं किञ्चित् सिद्धिदं क्षितिमण्डले।। ९६।।

O Caṇḍakāpāli! a lot more has been said about these, but I have told you only the essence in brief. Know that in the entire Universe there is naught that is worth mastering more than all these *mudras.*—96

Here ends Lesson Three entitled "Mudrās or Mystic Exercises" incorporated in *Gheraṇḍasaṃhitā.*

LESSON FOUR

Control of Senses

Śrī Gheraṇḍa said:

अथातः संप्रवक्ष्यामि प्रत्याहारमनुत्तमम्।
यस्य विज्ञानमात्रेण कामादिरिपुनाशनम्।। १।।

Now I shall tell you the best way to control the senses, the mere knowledge of which would help to overcome adverse tendencies such as passions, etc.—1

यतो यतो निश्चरति मनश्चञ्चलमस्थिरम्।
ततस्ततो नियम्यैतदात्मन्येव वशं नयेत्।। २।।

In whichever direction the fickle and unstable mind goes, bring it back resolutely under your own control.—2

पुरस्कारं तिरस्कारं सुश्राव्यं भावमायिकम्।
मनस्तस्मान्नियम्यैतदात्मन्येव वशं नयेत्।। ३।।

Reward, rebuke or flattery (sweet words), all should be regarded as delusive. Systematically withdraw the thoughts from those and bring the mind under your own control.—3

सुगन्धो वापि दुर्गन्धो घ्राणेषु जायते मनः।
तस्मात् प्रत्याहरेदेतदात्मन्येव वशं नयेत्।। ४।।

If the mind is attracted by a sweet smell (fragrance) or a bad smell (stink), withdraw the thought from those and bring the mind systematically under your own control.—4

मधुराम्लकतिक्तादिरसगादि यदा मनः।
तस्मात् प्रत्याहरेदेतदात्मन्येव वशं नयेत्।। ५।।

If the mind is attracted by things sweet, sour or bitter, withdraw all thoughts from these and bring the mind under your own control.—5

शब्दादिष्वनुरक्तानि निगृह्याक्षाणि योगवित्।
कुर्यात् चित्तानुचारीणि प्रत्याहारपरायणः।। ६।।

A yogi devoted to *pratyāhāra* systematically controls all his faculties of sound, sight, etc. and makes those follow his mind.—6

वश्यता परमा तेन जायतेऽतिचलात्मनाम्।
इन्द्रियाणामवश्यैस्तैर्न योगी योगसाधकः।। ७।।

Through supreme subjugation of the overactive (sensitive) senses, the yogi controls and is not controlled by those senses.—7

प्राणायामैर्दहेद्दोषान् धारणाभिश्च किल्विषम्।
प्रत्याहारेण विषयान् ध्यानेनानीश्वरान् गुणान्।। ८।।

Infirmities of the body are countered by *prāṇāyāma* (breath-control), sins (mental infirmities) by *dhāraṇā* (concentration), attachments (infirmities of heart) by *pratyāhāra* (withdrawals), and agnosticism (non-belief) by *dhyāna* (meditation).—8

यथा पर्वतधातूनां दोषा दह्यन्ति धाम्यताम्।
तथेन्द्रियकृता दोषा दह्यन्ते प्राणनिग्रहात्।। ९।।

Just as the blast of heat burns up a heap of impurities in a metal, similarly impurities produced by the senses are burnt up by breath-control.—9

समः समासनो भूत्वा संहृत्य चरणावुभौ।
संवृतास्यस्तथैवोरू सम्यग्विष्टभ्य चाग्रतः।। १०।।
पार्ष्णिभ्यां लिङ्गवृषणावस्पृशन् प्रयतः स्थितः।
किञ्चिदुन्नमितशिरा दन्तैर्दन्तान् न संस्पृशेत्।। ११।।
संपश्यन् नासिकाग्रं स्वं दिशश्चानवलोकयन्।
रजसा तमसो वृत्तिं सत्वेन रजसस्तथा।। १२।।
सञ्छाद्य निर्मले तत्वे स्थितो युञ्जीत योगवित्।
इन्द्रियाणीन्द्रियार्थेभ्यः प्राणादीन् मन एव च।। १३।।

Sit on a level ground and draw up both legs and hide them under the thighs. But, before that, let the sides of the feet firmly enfold the genitals. Next, lift up the face slightly and, without letting the two sets of teeth touch each other, fix the gaze at the tip of the nose and do not observe anything else in any direction. Thereafter, overpower the inertia (*tamas*) prevailing in the mind with passion (*rajas*), and again the latter with purity (*sattva*). Thus covered with immaculateness and turned into perfect equanimity, the mind will be united to *prāṇa* after the senses are separated from their objects (of desire).—10–13

निगृह्य समवायेन प्रत्याहारमुपक्रमेत्।
यसतु प्रत्याहरेत् कामान् सर्वाङ्गानीव कच्छपः।। १४।।
सदात्मरतिरेकस्थः पश्यत्यात्मानमात्मनि।
स वाह्याभ्यन्तरं शौचं निष्पाद्याकण्ठनाभितः।। १५।।
पूरयित्वा बुधो देहं प्रत्याहारमुपक्रमेत्।
तथा वै योगमुक्तस्य योगिनो नियतात्मनः।। १६।।

He who thus totally withdraws all his desires by *pratyāhāra*—even as the turtle withdraws all its limbs under the shell—becomes self-composed, sees his Self in himself and, being full and pure externally and internally owing to *pratyāhāra* and thus freed from further practice of yoga, is then his own immortal Self.—14–16

Here ends Lesson Four entitled "Control of Senses"
incorporated in *Gheraṇḍasaṃhitā*.

LESSON FIVE

Breath-Control

Śrī Gheraṇḍa said:

अथातः संप्रवक्ष्यामि प्राणायामस्य यद्विधिम्।
यस्य साधनमात्रेण देवतुल्यो भवेन्नरः।। १।।

Now I shall tell you about the method of breath-control, by mastering which man can become equal to a god.—1

आदौ स्थानं तथा कालं मिताहारं तथापरम्।
नाडीशुद्धिञ्च तत्पश्चात् प्रणायामञ्च साधयेत्।। २।।

Four things are necessary before one can practise *prāṇāyāma* (breath-control); right place, right time, right diet, and purification of nerves (*nāḍī-śuddhi*).*—2

THE PLACE

दूरदेशे तथारण्ये राजधान्यां जनान्तिके।
योगारम्भं न कुर्वीत कृते च सिद्धिहा भवेत्।। ३।।

Yoga should not be started either in a far-off place, a forest, a metropolis or a too populous place. If so done, this will be detrimental to its success.—3

अविश्वासं दूरदेशे अरण्ये रक्षिवर्जितम्।
लोकारण्ये प्रकाशश्च तस्मान्त्रीणि विवर्जयेत्।। ४।।

Being alone in a far-off place creates lack of confidence; in a forest there is a sense of insecurity, and in a populous place it is excess of publicity (lack of privacy). Therefore all three should be avoided.—4

*The word *nāḍī* stands for both physical as well as psychic channels inside the body.

सुदेशे धार्मिके राज्ये सुभक्ष्ये निरुपद्रवे।
तत्रैकं कुटीरं कृत्वा प्राचीरैः परिवेष्टितम्।। ५।।
वापीकूपतडागञ्च प्राचीरमध्यवर्त्ति च।
नात्युच्चं नातिनिम्नञ्च कुटीरं कीटवर्जितम्।। ६।।
सम्यग्गोमयलिप्तञ्च कुटीरन्तत्र निर्मितम्।
एवं स्थानेषु गुप्तेषु प्राणायामं समभ्यसेत्।। ७।।

Let there be a small hut in a good, peaceful, well-provided, undisturbed and a well-administered (lit. 'under a noble king') place, fenced round with walls, and within the compound let there be a well or pond (i.e., provision for water). The hut should be neither too high nor too low, free of insects (i.e., clean) and neat (lit. 'scoured with cow-dung'). In such a secluded place the *prāṇāyāma* should be practised all alone.—5–7

THE TIME

हेमन्ते शिशिरे ग्रीष्मे वर्षायाञ्च ऋतौ तथा।
योगारम्भं न कुर्वीत कृते योगी हि रोगदः।। ८।।

Yoga should not be commenced in the following seasons: In frosty weather, winter, summer and during the rains. If so done, the yogi will fall ill.—8

वसन्ते शरदे प्रोक्तं योगारम्भं समाचरेत्।
तथा योगी भवेत् सिद्धो रोगान्मुक्तो भवेद् ध्रुवम्।। ९।।

It is advisable that yoga should be commenced only on spring time or in autumn. When so done, the yogi will be positively successful and free of all ailments.—9

चैत्रादि फाल्गुनान्ते च माघादि फाल्गुनान्तिके।
द्वौ द्वौ मासौ ऋतुर्भागौ अनुभावश्चचतुश्चतुः।। १०।।

Beginning with the month of Caitra and ending with Phālguna, the year is divided into six bi-monthly periods, such as from beginning of Māgha (i.e., fifteenth of January) to end of Phālguna (i.e., fourteenth of March). The three seasons (i.e., summer, rains and winter) are actually experienced over four-monthly periods.*—10

*The solar year, however, starts with the Hindu month of Vaiśākha (commencing about the middle of April) and ends with Caitra (covering the period mid-March to mid-April).

वसन्तश्चैत्रवैशाखौ जैष्ठाषाढ़ौ च ग्रीष्मकौ।
वर्षा श्रावणभाद्राभ्यां शरदाश्विनकार्तिकौ।
मार्गपौषौ च हेमन्तः शिशरौ माघफाल्गुनौ।। ११।।

Vasanta (springtime) ranges over the two months of Caitra and Vaiśākha; Summer over Jaiṣṭha and Āṣāḍha; Rains over Śrāvaṇa and Bhādra: Autumn over Āświn and Kārtika, Frost over Mārga (or Agrahāyaṇa) and Pauṣa, and Winter over Māgha and Phālguna.—11

अनुभावं प्रवक्ष्यामि ऋतुणाञ्च यथोदितम्।
माघादि माघवान्तेषु वसन्तानुभवश्चतुः।। १२।।

Now I shall relate the actual experiencing of the seasons as mentioned by me. Vasanta (springtime) is experienced during the four months beginning Māgha and ending with Vaiśākha (both inclusive).—12

चैत्रादि चाषाढान्तञ्च निदाघानुभवश्चतुः।
आषाढादि चाश्विनान्तं प्रावृषानुभवश्चतुः।। १३।।

The four months beginning Caitra and ending with Āṣāḍha (both inclusive) are spring and summertime, and the four months beginning Āṣāḍha and ending Āświn (both inclusive) are rainy.—13

भाद्रादिमार्गशीर्षान्तं शरदोऽनुभवश्चतुः।
कार्तिकादि माघमासान्तं हेमन्तानुभवश्चतुः।
मार्गादि चतुरो मासान् शिशिरानुभवं विदुः।। १४।।

Autumn is experienced during Bhādra to Mārga (both inclusive). Frost during Kārtika to Māgha (both inclusive) and Winter during Mārga to Phālguna.*—14

वसन्ते वापि शरदे योगारम्भं समाचरेत्।
तदा योगो भवेत् सिद्धो विनायासेन कथ्यते।। १५।।

Begin the yoga either during Vasanta (springtime), or in Śarad (autumntime). Then the yoga becomes successful without much difficulty.—15

*It will be observed that the four principal seasons—summer, rains, autumn and winter—overlap each other and are experienced in six spells of weather designated as Vasanta, Grīṣma, Varṣā, Śarad, Hemanta, and Śiśira. For obvious reasons, these are not experienced uniformly at all latitudes.

THE DIET

मिताहारं विना यस्तु योगारम्भन्तु कारयेत्।
नाना रोगो भवेत्तस्य किञ्चिद्योगो न सिद्ध्यति।। १६।।

He who commences the practice of yoga without first controlling his diet becomes a victim of many diseases. His yoga also does not succeed.—16

शाल्यान्नं यवपिण्डं वा गोधूमपिण्डकं तथा।
मुद्गंमाषचणकादि शुभ्रञ्च तुषवर्जितम्।। १७।।
पटोलं पनसं मानं कक्कोलञ्च शुकाशकम्।
द्राढिकां कर्कटीं रम्भां डुम्बरीं कण्टकण्टकम्।। १८।।
आमरम्भां वालरम्भां रम्भादण्डञ्च मूलकम्।
वार्त्ताकीं मूलकं ऋद्धिं योगी भक्षणमाचरेत्।। १९।।

The yogi may freely take all these: *śali* (a kind of fine rice), wheat and barley flour, pulses such as *mūṃga, māṣa* and gram—clean and without husk; *patol* (gourd), *panasa* (jack-fruit), *māna* (gherkin), and *kakkol* (mulberry)—without the skin; *drāḍhika* (ginger), *karkaṭi* (cucumber), *rambhā* (banana), and *ḍumbari* (figs)—prickleless; raw and green plantains as well as their tender stem and root; brinjals and radishes.—17–19

बालशाकं कालशाकं तथा पटोलपत्रकम्।
पञ्चशाकं प्रशंसीयाद्वास्तूकं हिलमोचिकाम्।। २०।।

Five kinds of leafy vegetables are advised, viz., *bālaśāka, kāla-śāka, patol-patra, vāstūka,* and *hilāmocikā.*—20

शुद्धं सुमधुरं स्निग्धं उदरार्द्धं विवर्जितम्।
भुज्यते सुरसं प्रीत्या मिताहारमिमं विदुः।। २१।।

Take only pure, tasty and nutritious food, and soft drinks, keeping half the stomach unfilled. This, when eaten with satisfaction, is known as *mitāhāra* (balanced diet).—21

अन्नेन पूरयेदर्द्धं तोयेन तु तृतीयकम्।
उदरस्य तुरीयांशं संरक्षेद्वायुचारणे।। २२।।

Half of the stomach should be filled with food, the third-quarter with water, and the fourth part should be left free for the movement of air.—22

कट्वम्लं लवणं तिक्तं भृष्टञ्च दधितक्रकम्।
शाकोत्कटं तथा मद्यं तालञ्च पनसन्तथा।। २३।।
कुलत्थं मसूरं पाण्डुकुष्माण्डं शाकदण्डकम्।
तुम्बी कोल कपित्थञ्च कण्टविल्वं पलाशकम्।। २४।।
कदम्बं जम्बीरं बिम्बं लकुचं लशुनं विषम्।
कामरङ्गं पियालञ्च हिङ्गुशाल्मलीकेमूकम्।
योगारम्भे वर्जयेच्च पथस्त्रीवह्निसेवनम्।। २५।।

When commencing yoga, avoid things that are hot, sour, salty, bitter or fried; also curd, whey, any strong-smelling vegetable (e.g., spring onions), liquor made from palm and jackfruit juice (toddy), pulses like *kulattha* and *masūra* (lentil), ripe (yellow) pumpkins, stalks of leafy vegetables, *tumbi* (bitter gourd), *kol* (sour berries), *kapittha* (sour wood-apple), *kaṇṭa-vilva* (wild castor) and fruits of *palāśa, kadamba, jambīra* (citron), *bimba* (red cherry), *lakuca* (bread-fruit), *laśuna* (garlic), *kāmaraṅga* (pummelo), *piyāla* (hazel-nut), *hiṅgu* (asafoetida), *śālmali* and *kemūka.* These are harmful. Avoid also going out in the streets, the company of women and nearness to fire.—23–25

नवनीतं घृतं क्षीरं गुडं शर्करादि चैक्षवम्।
पक्वरम्भां नारिकेलं दाडिम्बमशिवासवम्।
द्राक्षास्तु नवनीं धात्रीं रसमम्लं विवर्जितम्।। २६।।

Not harmful are fresh butter,clarified butter, milk, jaggery, cane-sugar, sugarcane, ripe bananas, cocoanuts, pomegranates, fresh grapes and *dhātri* (myrobalan)—provided it is not sour.—26

एलाजातिलवङ्गञ्च पौरुषं जम्भूजाम्बूलम्।
हरीतकीं खर्जुरञ्च योगी भक्षणमाचरेत्।। २७।।

But the yogi may take such stimulating stuff as cardamoms, *jāti-phal* (nutmeg), cloves, *jambhu* (lime), *jāmbula* (rose apple), *harītaki* (yellow myrobalan), and dates.—27

लघुपाकं प्रियं स्निग्धं यथा धातुप्रपोषणम्।
मनोऽभिलषितं योग्यं योगी भोजनमाचरेत्।। २८।।

Whatever is easily digestible, pleasing and nutritious and builds up energy—such suitable food may be taken by the yogi according to his liking.—28

काठिन्यं दुरितं पूतिमुष्णं पर्य्युषितं तथा।
अतिशीतञ्चातिचोग्रं भक्ष्यं योगी विवर्जयेत्।। २९।।

But the yogi must not take anything that is hard (i.e., not well cooked), spoiled, stale, smelly, hot and fermented, nor such stuff as may be too hot or too cold.—29

प्रातःस्नानोपवासादि कायक्लेशविधिं विना।
एकाहारं निराहारं यामान्ते च न कारयेत्।। ३०।।

Very early morning bath or total fasting may be undertaken if these do not cause distress to the body. One meal a day, or no food for more than three hours, should be avoided.—30

एवं विधि विधानेन प्राणायामं समाचरेत्।
आरम्भे प्रथमे कुर्य्यात् क्षीराज्यं नित्यभोजनम्।
मध्याह्ने चैव सायाह्ने भोजनद्वयमाचरेत्।। ३१।।

In this manner and procedure the *prāṇāyāma* should be practised. Before commencing the course, however, let fresh butter and clarified butter be taken daily (for some days) and meals restricted to two times—at mid-way and in the evening.—31

PURIFICATION OF NĀḌĪS

कुशासने मृगाजिने व्याघ्राजिने च कम्बले।
स्थलासने समासीनः प्राङ्मुखो वाप्युदङ्मुखो।
नाडीशुद्धिं समासाद्य प्राणायामं समभ्यसेत्।। ३२।।

Sit upon a straw carpet, a deer skin, a tiger skin, a blanket or even on plain ground, facing the east and with the head erect, and then perform *prāṇāyāma* after purifying the *nāḍīs*.—32

Caṇḍakāpāli said:

नाडीशुद्धिं कथं कुर्य्यान्नाडीशुद्धिस्तु कीदृशी।
तत्सर्वं श्रोतुमिच्छामि तद्वदस्व दयानिधे।। ३३।।

O Ocean of Compassion! What is "purification" of *nāḍīs*? And how is the purification of *nāḍīs* done? Do tell me that, as I am desirous of knowing all these.—33

Śrī Gheraṇḍa said:

मलाकुलासु नाडीषु मारुतो नैव गच्छति।
प्राणायामः कथं सिद्धिस्तत्वज्ञानं कथं भवेत्।
तस्मादादौ नाडीशुद्धिं प्राणायामं ततोऽभ्यसेत्।। ३४।।

When the channels (*nāḍīs*) are cloyed with fetid matter, pure air does not circulate in them freely. How would then *prāṇāyāma* be possible, and how could the essence of knowledge be gained? Hence, cleansing of these channels is essential before *prāṇāyāma* is started.—34

नाडीशुद्धिर्द्विधा प्रोक्ता समनुनिर्मनुस्तथा।
बीजेन समनुं कुर्य्यान्निर्मनुं धौतिकर्मणा।। ३५।।

There are two ways of cleansing the *nāḍīs*—Samanu and Nirmanu.* Samanu is performed with the aid of key-*mantras* and Nirmanu through the Dhauti-process.—35

धौतिकर्म पुरा प्रोक्तं षट्कर्मसाधने यथा।
शृणुष्व समनुं चण्ड नाडीशुद्धिर्यथा भवेत्।। ३६।।

I have told you earlier about Dhauti—the Six-fold System. Listen now, O Caṇḍakāpāli, to Samanu, which leads to the purification of the *nāḍīs*.—36

उपविश्यासने योगी पद्मासनं समाचरेत्।
गुर्वादिन्यासनं कुर्याद्यथैव गुरुभाषितम्।
नाडीशुद्धिं प्रकुर्वीत प्राणायामविशुद्धये।। ३७।।

The yogi should sit in the Padmāsana posture and then, after performing *nyāsa*** before the guru and obtaining his directions in regard to the correct method of *prāṇāyāma*, practise the purification of the *nāḍīs*.—37

वायुबीजं ततो ध्यात्वा धूम्रवर्णं सतेजसम्।
चन्द्रेण पूरयेद्वायुं बीजं षोडशकैः सुधीः।। ३८।।
चतुःषष्ट्या मात्रया च कुम्भकेनैव धारयेत्।
द्वात्रिंशन्मात्रया वायुं सूर्यनाड्या च रेचयेत्।। ३९।।

First, visualize the quintessence of Air in the form of a dark, furious Force (cf. III.73) symbolised by the key-*mantra* "Yaṅg" (यं). Next, the yogi should breathe in through the Moon (i.e., Iḍā or left nostril) counting up to sixteen; retain the air in the pot (*kumbhaka*) for sixty-four measures, and finally release it through the Sun (i.e.,

*Samanu is mental; Nirmanu is physical.

***Nyāsa* is a ritual of dedication, performed in front of the guru or deity as an earnest of one's singlemindedness and devotion prior to invoking the guru's or the deity's blessings. Not unoften, it takes the form of the first *prāṇāyāma* performed by the yogi.

Piṅgalā or right nostril).*—38 and 39

नाभिमूलाद्वह्निमुत्थाप्य ध्यायेत्तेजोऽवनीयुतम्।
वह्निबीजषोडशेन सूर्यनाड्या च पूरयेत्।। ४०।।
चतुःषष्ट्या च मात्रया कुम्भकेनैव धारयेत्।
द्वात्रिंशमात्रया वायुं शशिनाड्या च रेचयेत्।। ४१।।

Visualize the fire that dwells inside the navel as the quintessence of Fire (र), co-mingled with Earth (ल), and repeat the *mantra* "Raṅg" (रं) as you breathe in through the right nostril (Sun) in sixteen measures. Then, holding the breath in *kumbhaka* for sixty-four measures, expel the same over a period of thirty-two measures through the left (Moon).—40 and 41

नासाग्रे शशधृग्बिम्बं ध्यात्वा ज्योत्स्नासमन्वितम्।
ठं बीजषोडशेनैव इडया पूरयेन्मरुत्।। ४२।।
चतुःषष्ट्या मात्रया च वंबीजेनैव धारयेत्।
अमृतप्लावितं ध्यात्वा नाडीधौतं विभावयेत्।
लकारेण द्वात्रिंशेन दृढं भाव्यं विरेचयेत्।। ४३।।

Next, visualize a bright moon at the tip of the nose and repeat the key-*mantra* "Ṭhaṅg" (ठं) sixteen times as you fill in the air through the left (Iḍā) nostril; then repeat the key-*mantra* "Vaṅg" (वं) sixty-four times while the breath is held in *kumbhaka*, suffusing with ambrosia and cleansing all the *nāḍīs*; Thereafter steadily release it (through the right) while repeating "Laṅg" (लं) for thirty-two times.**—42 and 43

एवं विधां नाडी शुद्धिं कृत्वा नाडी विशोधयेत्।
दृढोभूत्वासनं कृत्वा प्राणायामं समाचरेत्।। ४४।।

In this way the *nāḍīs* should be cleansed through the process of *nāḍī*-purification. One should sit up firmly in an *āsana* posture and then only start practising *prāṇāyāma*.—44

*For purposes of *prāṇāyāma* the ratio of inspiration, retention and expiration of breath is always the same, viz., 1.4.2. The measure or unit of time is regulated in accordance with an individual's capacity and may range from one-quarter of a second, rising gradually to one second, then one minute—and even one hour in the case of adepts.

**These *mantras*, it will be observed, relate to the Five Elements—earth, water, fire, air and sky. As described in Lesson Third (66–77), these have been symbolized by the letters "L" (ल), "V" (व), "R" (र), "Y" (य), and "Ṭh" (ठ) respectively. The sounds of "Aṅg" (अं) and "Aḥ" (अः) represent the functions of inspiration and expiration. "Aṅg" is added to all key-*mantras* to indicate the strength of air taken in, held in the lungs and thrown out—all under proper control. It also lends vibratory power to the sound; that is, when the *mantra* is properly intonated.

KUMBHAKA

सहितः सूर्यभेदश्च उज्जायी शीतली तथा।
भस्त्रिका भ्रामरी मूर्च्छा केवली चाष्ट कुम्भिकाः।।

There are eight kinds of *kumbhaka*—Sahita, Sūrya-bheda, Ujjāyī, Śītalī, Bhrastrikā, Bhrāmari, Mūrchā, and Kevalī.—45

i. *Sahita*

सहितो द्विविधः प्रोक्तः प्राणायामं समाचरेत्।
सगर्भो बीज़मुच्चार्य निर्गर्भो बीजवर्जितः।। ४६।।

For the purpose of *prāṇāyāma*, Sahita is of two kinds: Sagarbha and Nirgarbha. Sagarbha is practised with key-*mantras* and Nirgarbha without.—46

प्राणायामं सगर्भञ्च प्रथमं कथयामि ते।
सुखासने चोपविश्य प्राङ्मुखो वाप्युदङ्मुखः।
ध्यायेद्विधिं रजोगुणं रक्तवर्णमवर्णकम्।। ४७।।

First I shall tell you of Sahita *prāṇāyāma* of the Sagarbha type. Sit in Sukhāsana (Swastikāsana) posture, facing either east or north, and meditate upon the Creator, symbolized by the letter "A" (अ) and endowed with the quality of the bright red Force (*rajas*).—47

इडया पूरयेद्वायुं मात्रया षोडशैः सुधीः।
पूरकान्ते कुम्भकाद्ये कर्तव्यस्तूड्डीयानकः।। ४८।।

Breathe in through the Iḍā (left nostril) counting up to sixteen. But the *kumbhaka* (retention of air) should be preceded and followed by the Uḍḍīyānamudrā (cf. III.10).—48

सत्वमयं हरिं ध्यात्वा उकारं कृष्णवर्णकम्।
चतुःषष्ट्या मात्रया च कुम्भकेनैव धारयेत्।। ४९।।

Next, meditate upon Viṣṇu the Preserver, symbolized by the letter "U" (उ) and endowed with the quality of Purity (*satva*) in a dark blue shade.—49

तमोमयं शिवं ध्यात्वा मकारं शुक्लवर्णकम्।
द्वात्रिंशन्मात्रया चैव रेचयेद्विधिना पुनः।। ५०।।

Thereafter meditate upon Śiva the Destroyer, symbolized by the letter "M" (ग) and endowed with the quality of Inertia (*tamas*) in snow-white hue. (*Kumbhaka* being thus completed) release the breath over a measure of thirty-two.—50

पुनः पिङ्गलयापूर्य कुम्भकेनैव धारयेत्।
इडया रेचयेत् पश्चात् तद्बीजेन क्रमेण तु।। ५१।।

Repeat this by filling in air through the Piṅgalā (right nostril), retaining it in *kumbhaka* and later releasing the same gradually, keeping all the while the key-letters* in mind.—51

अनुलोमविलोमेन वारंवारञ्च साधयेत्।
पूरकान्ते कुम्भकान्तं धृतनासापुटद्वयम्।
कनिष्ठानामिकाङ्गुष्ठैस्तर्जनीमध्यमा विना।। ५२।।

In this way practise the inspiration and expiration again and again. Block both nostrils during *kumbhaka,* i.e., between the end of inspiration and the end of retention, with the aid of the thumb (on one side) and the ring and small fingers (on the other), leaving the index and middle fingers free.—52

प्राणायामं निर्गर्भन्तु विना बीजेन जायते।
एकादि शतपर्यन्तं पूरकुम्भकरेचनम्।। ५३।।

The Nirgarbha *prāṇāyāma* is practised without the key-*mantras.* Its unit of time ranges from one to one hundred in respect of inspiration, retention and expiration (i.e., it can be practised up to a maximum of 100 measures per *kumbhaka*).—53

उत्तमा विंशतिमात्रा षोडशीमात्रा मध्यमा।
अधमा द्वादशीमात्रा प्राणायामास्त्रिधा स्मृताः।। ५४।।

It should be remembered that *prāṇāyāma* is of three categories. Twenty measures and over belong to first category, sixteen to nineteen are the second, and one to twelve are the third.—54

अधमाज्जायते घर्मो मेरुकम्पश्च मध्यमात्।
उत्तमाच्च भूमित्यागस्त्रिविधं सिद्धिलक्षणम्।। ५५।।

Signs of success of each are: for the third category, sweating: for the second, shivering along the spine, while the first category bestows the power of levitation (or ability to leave the ground).—55

प्राणायामात् खेचरत्वं प्राणायामात् रोगनाशनम्।
प्राणायामाद्बोधयेच्छक्तिं प्राणायामान्मनोन्मनी।
आनन्दो जायते चित्ते प्राणायामी सुखी भवेत्।। ५६।।

Prāṇāyāma leads to Khecarī (levitation), *prāṇāyāma* overcomes

*The three key-letters *Aum* constitute the verbal symbol of the Supreme (cf. *Pātañjala Yogasūtra,* I.27–28).

all diseases, *prāṇāyāma* generates the mystic power and *prāṇāyāma* uncovers the light of the mind. The yogi who practises *prāṇāyāma* enjoys divine bliss.—56

ii. *Sūrya-bheda*

कथितं सहितं कुम्भं सूर्यभेदनकं शृणु।
पूरयेत् सूर्यनाड्या च यथाशक्ति बहिर्मरुत्।। ५७।।
धारयेद्बहुयत्नेन कुम्भकेन जलन्धरैः।
यावत् स्वेदं नखकेशाभ्यां तावत्कुर्वन्तु कुम्भकम्।। ५८।।

I have described the Sahita *kumbhaka*; now listen to the Sūrya-bheda one. In this you breathe in to the fullest capacity through the Piṅgalā (right nostril) while forming the Jālandharamudrā (cf. III.10) and retain the breath as long as possible. This *kumbhaka* is to be continued so long as sweat does not appear from head to foot.—57 and 58

प्राणोऽपानः समानश्चोदानव्यानौ तथैव च।
नागः कूर्मश्च कृकरो देवदत्तो धनञ्जयः।। ५९।।

Prāṇa, apāna, samāna, udāna, and *vyāna*: these are the five internal airs. *Nāga, kūrma, kṛkara, devadatta,* and *dhanañjaya* are the five external airs.—59

हृदि प्राणो वहेन्नित्यं अपानो गुदमण्डले।
समानो नाभिदेशे तु उदानः कण्ठमध्यगः।। ६०।।
व्यानो व्याप्य शरीरे तु प्रधानाः पञ्च वायवः।
प्राणाद्याः पञ्च विख्याता नागाद्या पञ्च वायवः।। ६१।।

Prāṇa always dwells in the heart; *apāna* in the perineum; *samāna* in the naval region; *udāna* in the throat; and *vyāna* pervades the whole body. These are the five principal airs. The first five (*prāṇa,* etc.) flow inward, the other five (*nāga,* etc.) outward.—60 and 61

तेषामपि च पञ्चानां स्थानानि च वदाम्यहम्।
उद्गारे नाग आख्यातः कूर्मस्तून्मीलने स्मृतः।। ६२।।
कृकरः क्षुत्कृते ज्ञेयो देवदत्तो विजृम्भणे।
न जहाति मृते क्वापि सर्वव्यापी धनञ्जयः।। ६३।।

I shall now tell you of the roles played by these five (i.e., external airs). *Nāga* manifests itself through hiccups and belching; *kūrma* through the batting of eyes; *kṛkara* through sneezing; and *devadatta* through yawning. As for *dhanañjaya,* it hovers over body even after death (i.e., it remains with the corpse until cremation or disintegration of the body—long after the other nine airs have departed.)—62 and 63

नागो गृह्णति चैतन्यं कूर्मश्चैव निमेषणम्।
क्षुत्तृषं कृकरश्चैव जृम्भणं चतुर्थेन तु।
भवेद्धनञ्जयाच्छब्दं क्षणमात्रं न निःसरेत्।। ६४।।

Nāga controls the consciousness; *kūrma* the timing of eyelids (batting); *kṛkara* hunger and thirst, and the fourth (i.e., *devadatta*) yawning. *Dhanañjaya* converts into sound, and does not leave (the body) even for a moment.—64

सर्वे तु सूर्यसंभिन्ना नाभिमूलात् समुद्धरेत्।
इडया रेचयेत् पश्चात् धैर्येणाखण्डवेगतः।। ६५।।
पुनः सूर्येण चाकृष्य कुम्भयित्वा यथाविधि।
रेचयित्वा साधयेत्तु क्रमेण न च पुनः पुनः।। ६६।।

All these airs, together with the heat (Sun) concentrated in the core of the navel, should be collected and later expelled through Iḍā (left nostril) gently but in a continuous flow. Again, filling in through the Piṅgalā (right nostril), hold the breath in *kumbhaka* as prescribed, and later expel it in the same way. This should be done in short spells (i.e., not continuously) and it is not to be repeated again and again.—65 and 66

कुम्भकः सूर्यभेदस्तु जरामृत्युविनाशनः।
बोधयेत् कुण्डलीं शक्तिं देहानलं विवर्द्धयेत्।
इति ते कथितश्चण्ड सूर्यभेवनमुत्तमम्।। ६७।।

This Sūrya-bheda *kumbhaka* counters decay and death, controls the Kuṇḍalinī power and increases bodily heat. Thus, O Caṇḍakāpāli, I have now told you of the excellent *kumbhaka* called Sūrya-bheda.—67

iii. *Ujjāyī*

नासाभ्यां वायुमाकृष्य वायुं वक्त्रेण धारयेत्।
हृद्गलाभ्यां समाकृष्य मुखमध्ये च धारयेत्।। ६८।।
मुखं प्रक्षाल्य संवन्द्य कुर्याज्जालन्धरं ततः।
आशक्ति कुम्भकं कृत्वा धारयेदविरोधतः।। ६९।।
उज्जायीकुम्भकं कृत्वा सर्वकार्याणि साधयेत्।
न भवेत् कफरोगश्च क्रूरवायुरजीर्णकम्।। ७०।।

आमपातः क्षयः कासो ज्वरप्लीहा न विद्यते।
जरामृत्यु विनाशाय चोज्जायीं साधयेन्नरः।। ७१।।

Stop the nostrils and draw into the (closed) mouth the air subsisting therein. Similarly draw up the air from the lungs and throat and hold the same in the mouth. Then let this air rotate within the mouth as you perform the Jālandharamudrā, retaining the air in *kumbhaka* as long as possible. This Ujjāyī *kumbhaka* enables the yogi to perform all tasks successfully and he is never a victim of respiratory or abdominal diseases like cold, cough, consumption, fever, jaundice or rashes, being above decay and death.—68–71

iv. *Śītalī*

जिह्वया वायुमाकृष्य उदरे पूरयेच्छनैः।
क्षणं च कुम्भकं कृत्वा नासाभ्यां रेचयेत् पुनः।। ७२।।
सर्वदा साधयेद्योगी शीतली कुम्भकं शुभम्।
अजीर्णं कफपित्तञ्च नैव देहे प्रजायते।। ७३।।

Draw in air through the mouth (not nose) and let it pass over the tongue and go and fill the stomach. Then, holding it in the form of a short *kumbhaka*, release it through the nostrils. The yogi who practises this useful Śītalī *kumbhaka* shall never have his body afflicted by troubles of phlegm, bile or indigestion.—72 and 73

v. *Bhastrikā*

भस्त्रैव लौहकाराणां यथाक्रमेण संभ्रमेत्।
ततो वायुञ्च नासाभ्यामुभाभ्यां चालयेच्छनैः।। ७४।।
एवं विंशतिवारञ्च कृत्वा कुर्याञ्च कुम्भकम्।
तदन्ते चालयेद्वायुं पूर्वोक्तञ्च यथाविधि।। ७५।।
त्रिवारं साधयेदेनं भस्त्रिकाकुम्भकं सुधीः।
न च रोगं न च क्लेशमारोग्यञ्च दिने दिने।। ७६।।

Draw in and throw out air through the nostrils like the bellows of a blacksmith. After doing so for twenty times, take a deep one and perform a *kumbhaka*, at the end of which repeat the bellow-like action (twenty times). The wise one who practises this only thrice, gets rid of all pains and diseases and remains hale and hearty everyday —74–76

vi. *Bhrāmari*

अर्द्धरात्रिगते योगी जन्तूनां शब्दवर्जिते।
कर्णौपिधाय हस्ताभ्यां कुर्यात् पूरककुम्भकम्।। ७७।।

श्रृणुयाद्दक्षिणे कर्णे नादमन्तर्गतं शुभम्।
प्रथमं झिञ्झीनादञ्च वंशीनादं ततः परम्।। ७८।।
मेघझर्झरभ्रमरी घण्टाकांस्यन्ततः परम्।
तूरीभेरीमृदङ्गादि निनादानेकदुन्दुभिः।। ७९।।

After midnight, and at a (solitary) place far from populous habitation and noise, the yogi should perform a complete *kumbhaka* with ears covered with his palms. He would then hear in his right ear many (strange) sounds (coming from) within his body. At first a sound would seem like one made by crickets, then a sound as of a flute, then others like that of a thunder, a stream, a buzz, a bell, a cymbal, a horn, a trumpet, a drum and, finally, like many drums together.—77–79

एवं नानाविधो नादो जायते नित्यमभ्यसात्।
अनाहतस्य शब्दस्य तस्य शब्दस्य यो ध्वनिः।। ८०।।

In this manner many kinds of sound—sounds not actually made by anybody or any thing—are heard by one who regularly practises (this Bhrāmari *kumbhaka*).—80

ध्वनेरन्तर्गतं ज्योतिर्ज्योतिरन्तर्गतं मनः।
तन्मनो विलयं याति तद्विष्णोः परमं पदम्।
एवं भ्रामरीसंसिद्धिः समाधिसिद्धिमाप्नुयात्।। ८१।।

(The yogi then finds that) within that sound dwells fire (light) and within that fire (light) is his mind. His mind then gets merged in the Cosmic Fire*—the Supreme. In this manner the practice of Bhrāmari *kumbhaka* leads to mastery of *samādhi.*—81

vii. *Mūrchā*

सुखेन कुम्भकं कृत्वा मनश्च भ्रवोरन्तरम्।
सन्त्यज्य विषयान् सर्वान् मनोमूर्च्छा सुखप्रदा।
आत्मनि मनसो योगादानन्दो जायते ध्रुवम्।। ८२।।

Perform a *kumbhaka* at ease (i.e., without straining in any way) and then fix the thought between the eyebrows, withdrawing the mind from all other objects. This brings about a blissful mental swoon. The union of the mind and the Self positively produces a state of ecstasy.—82

*Traditionally, Viṣṇu is identified as the Preserver, one of the Holy Trinity—Brahmā, Viṣṇu and Śiva, or Creator, Preserver and Demolisher. Here, however, the word "Viṣṇu" would seem to symbolize the Cosmic Fire within (cf. *SS*, II.3 and 33–36; also *GS*, III.71). Incidentally, heat (fire) is the preserver of the body.

viii. *Kevali*

हंकारेण वहिर्याति सःकारेण विशेत् पुनः।
षट्शतानि दिवारात्रौ सहस्राण्येकविंशतिः।
अजपां नाम गायत्रीं जीवो जपति सर्वदा।। ८३।।

In the course of a day a living being recites the Ajapā, also called the Gāyatrī, 21,600 times. The breath goes out of the body with the sound of "Haṅg" (हं) and enters it with the sound of "Saḥ" (सः).*—83

मूलाधारे यथा हंसस्तथा हि हृदिपङ्कजे।
तथा नासापुटद्वन्द्वे त्रिविधं संगमागमम्।। ८४।।

Haṅgsaḥ (Haṅg + Saḥ) as a compound sound indicating the Ajapā, forms a conflux at the Mūlādhāra (in the perineum), at Anāhata (in the heart), and also within the two nostrils—thus making a triple conflux.—84

षण्णवत्यङ्गुलीमानं शरीरं कर्मरूपकम्।
देहाद्बहिर्गतो वायुः स्वभावो द्वादशाङ्गुलिः।। ८५।।

Actions of the body are limited to a range of 96 *aṅgulis* (finger-width). Normally the breath going out of the body is limited to a range of 12 *aṅgulis* only.**—85

गायने षोडशाङ्गुल्यां भोजने विंशातिस्तथा।
चतुर्विंशाङ्गुलिः पान्थो निद्रायां त्रिंशदङ्गुलिः।
मैथुने षट्त्रिंशदुक्तं व्यायामे च ततोऽधिकम्।। ८६।।

It has been said that the range (of breath) during singing extends to 16 *aṅgulis* (12 ins. approx.), during eating to 20 *aṅgulis* (15 ins. approx.), while walking to 24 *aṅgulis* (18 ins. approx.), during sleep to 30 *aṅgulis* (22½ ins. approx.), during coitus to 36 *aṅgulis* (27 ins. approx.), and more than that during athletic exer-

*Man breathes 21,600 times in 24 hours, or 15 times per minute. It works out to 4 seconds per breath, i.e., inspiration and expiration. This process is called Ajapā, i.e., that which is "not repeated consciously." Hence it has been named the natural Gāyatrī. The other Gāyatrī, which is a Vedic *mantra*, is so named because its recitation thrice a day (*gāya* = sung; *tri* = thrice)—morning, noon and evening—is incumbent, specially upon a Brahmin. Another interpretation of Gāyatrī is that it is so called because originally it was made up of three lines only: the *Rgveda* does not mention the first line now generally recited, viz., *Aum bhūḥ bhuvaḥ swaḥ*.

**The unit of measure is described in terms of *aṅgulis* or finger-width. Twelve finger-widths equal 9 ins. approx. and 96 finger-widths 6 ft. approx. Man's actions, while in one position, are limited to a range of 6 feet, i.e., 3 ft. on either side. Six feet approx. is also the average height of man.

cises.—86

स्वभावेऽस्य गतेर्न्यूने परमायुः प्रवर्द्धते।
आयुःक्षयोऽधिके प्रोक्तो मारुते चान्तराद्गते।। ८७।।

When the range is *below* normal (i.e., 12 *aṅgulis*), it promotes longevity, but when the air that goes out crosses this limit it shortens longevity.*—87

तस्मात् प्राणे स्थिते देहे मरणं नैव जायते।
वायुना घटसंबद्धो भवेत् केवलकुम्भकः।। ८८।।

Hence as long as *prāṇa* (vital air) stays within the body, death does not take place. With the Kevalī *kumbhaka* it is possible to control all airs within the body.—88

यावज्जीवो जपेन्मन्त्रमजपासंख्यकेवलम्।
अद्यावधि धृतं संख्याविभ्रमं केवलीकृते।। ८९।।

So long as a creature lives, it "recites" the Ajapā for an unspecified (unknown) number of times. But when this number is controlled by Kevalī the prescribed figure for life is upset.—89

अतएव हि कर्तव्यः केवलीकुम्भको नरैः।
केवली चाजपा संख्या द्विगुणा च मनोन्मनी।। ९०।।

Hence it is necessary for men to perform the Kevalī *kumbhaka.* The Kevalī doubles the number of Ajapās (allotted to a life) and also sublimates the mind.—90

नासाभ्यां वायुमाकृष्य केवलं कुम्भकञ्चरेत्।
एकादिकचतुःषष्टिं धारयेत् प्रथमे दिने।। ९१।।

On the first day draw in breath through both nostrils and perform only a *kumbhaka*, retaining the breath from one to sixty-four measures.**—91

केवलीमष्टधां कुर्याद्यामे यामे दिने दिने।
अथवा पञ्चधा कुर्याद्यथा तत् कथयामि ते।। ९२।।

*Longevity is pre-determined (cf. *Pātañjala Yogasūtra*, II.13 and III.23). As such the number of breaths (inspiration and expiration) in a life-time is fixed. The aim of *prāṇāyāma* is to reduce this number as much as possible and thus proportionately increase the longevity.

**Here the "measure" is fixed only for *kumbhaka* (retention of breath); the time for *pūraka* and *recaka* is apparently not so important in this exercise.

Perform the Kevalī either eight times a day (i.e., every quarter, or at intervals of three hours), or five times as I am telling you presently.—92

प्रातर्मध्याह्नसायाह्ने मध्येरात्रिचतुर्थके।
त्रिसन्ध्यमथवा कुर्यात् सममाने दिने दिने।। ९३।।

At sunrise, at midday, at sunset, at midnight and at fourth quarter of the night (i.e., three hours before sunrise). Or, (at least) do it regularly everyday at the three cardinal times, viz. at sunrise, midday and sunset.—93

पञ्चवारं दिने वृद्धिर्वारैकञ्च दिने तथा।
अजपा परिमाणञ्च यावत्सिद्धिः प्रजायते।। ९४।।

As long as full mastery is not gained the duration of the Ajapā should be increased gradually by one "measure" at a time, five times a day.*—94

प्राणायामं केवलीञ्च तदा वदति योगवित्।
कुम्भके केवली सिद्धौ किं न सिद्ध्यति भूतले।। ९५।।

Only then would the yogi properly learn both *prāṇāyāma* and the Kevalī *kumbhaka*. And, lo! when Kevalī has been mastered, what else cannot be mastered upon this earth?—95

Here ends Lesson Five entitled 'Breath-control'
incorporated in *Gheraṇḍasaṃhitā*

*If the duration of normal inspiration and expiration is prolonged, the *number* of breaths taken in and thrown out will be proportionately reduced. Since fewer number of breaths will last longer during the same (allotted) span of life, it would mean prolonged longevity.

LESSON SIX

Meditation

Śrī Gheraṇḍa said:

स्थूलं ज्योतिस्तथा सूक्ष्मं ध्यानस्य त्रिविधं विदुः।
स्थूलं मूर्त्तिमयं प्रोक्तं ज्योतिस्तेजोमयं तथा।
सूक्ष्मं विन्दुमयं ब्रह्म कुण्डली परदेवता।। १।।

Meditation has three forms: Concrete, Effulgent and Subtle. Concrete is defined as the image-form; Effulgent as the light (brilliance) form, and Subtle as the Supreme (Brahman) in micro form manifested in man as the Goddess Kuṇḍalinī.—1

i. *The Concrete*

सहस्रारे महापद्मे कर्णिकायां विचिन्तयेत्।
विलग्नसहितं पद्मं द्वादशैर्दलसंयुतम्।। २।।
शुक्लवर्णं महातेजो द्वादशैर्बीजभाषितम्।
हसक्षमलवरयूंहसखफ्रें यथाक्रमम्।। ३।।

Visualize the exalted (thousand-petalled) Sahasrāra lotus (at the top of the brain) and another lotus (Anāhata) twelve-petalled—white, brilliant and attached to its axis (*thalamus*) with each petal symbolized by the letters H, S, Kṣ, M, L, V, R, Yuṅg, H, S, Kh, and Freṅg—in this order—(ह, स, क्ष, म, ल, व, र, यूं, ह, स, ख, फ्रें) representing the twelve seeds (quintessence) of perceptions.*—2 and 3

तन्मध्ये कर्णिकायान्तु अकथादिरेखात्रयम्।
हलक्षकोण संयुक्तं प्रणवं तत्र वर्त्तते।। ४।।

Within the axis (of Anāhata) are three lines, represented by the letters A (अ), K (क) and Th (थ), forming a triangle, three angles of

*The twelve perceptions are: seeing, hearing, smelling, tasting, touch, consciousness (awareness of awareness), desire, sorrow, gratification, thinking, intelligence, reasoning, and bliss (ecstasy).

which are H (ह), L (ल) and Kṣ (क्ष)* and which holds within it the symbol of the Supreme—*Aum.*—4

नादविन्दुमयं पीठं ध्यायेत्तत्र मनोहरम्।
तत्रोपरि हंसयुग्मं पादुका तत्र वर्त्तते।। ५।।

Visualize in it a beautiful pedestal formed by *nāda-bindu* (i.e., Subtle sound indicated by the mystic Symbol) and two swans installed over them, representing a pair of (the guru's) sandals.—5

ध्यायेत्तत्र गुरुं देवं द्विभुजञ्च त्रिलोचनम्।
श्वेताम्बरधरं देवं शुक्लगन्धानुलेपनम्।। ६।।
शुक्लपुष्पमयं माल्यं रक्तशक्तिसमन्वितम्।
एवंविधगुरुध्यानं स्थूलध्यानं प्रसिध्यति।। ७।।

Next, visualize the venerable guru himself seated there—two arms, three eyes, robed in white, anointed with white sandalpaste, bedecked with a garland of white flowers and endowed with red energy. When the guru** is thus visualized it is known as Concrete Meditation.—6 and 7

ii. *The Effulgent*

कथितं स्थूलध्यानन्तु, तेजो ध्यानं शृणुष्व मे।
यद्ध्यानेन योगसिद्धिरात्मप्रत्यक्षमेव च।। ८।।

*A (अ), K (क) and Th (थ) represent respectively *ākāśa* (Space), *kāla* (Time) and *sthiti* (Stability). H (ह), L (ल) and Kṣ (क्ष) symbolize Water, Earth and Fire respectively.

**Here the guru has been equated with the Lord of yogis, Śiva Himself, who is normally visualized as described in the two verses above. The 'red energy' is the psychic force—Śakti—personified by Pārvatī, consort of Śiva.

Similar descriptions of the guru are found in some other Tantras as well. In *Nīla Tantra*, for example, the same visualization is expressed as follows:

The guru is to be visualized as Haṃsa (another name of Śiva or the Supreme) seated upon the thousand-petalled (Sahasrāra) lotus on top of head, embodiment of soothing light, bedecked with pleasing fragrance and flowers, one hand raised in token of assurance (promising protection) and the other holding a lotus, looking down graciously—a synthesis of all the gods!

In *Kaṅkālamālinī Tantra* it is described in these words: Your own guru, installed upon a glorious throne placed within the thousand-petalled lotus and enveloped in *nāda-bindu*, eternal in the midst of silvery mountains, seated in the Vīrāsana posture, decorated in a white robe and with white garlands, one hand raised in token of assurance (i.e., shielding from evil), and the Śakti-incarnate (Pārvatī) sitting on the left lap with Her right hand encircling His beautiful body and left holding a lotus, She bedecked in brilliant red apparel, and He looking on compassionately—full of Eternal Knowledge and Bliss. Thus shall the guru be visualized.

I have told you of the Concrete Meditation; now listen to the Effulgent one, the meditation of which leads to mastery of yoga and Self-realization.—8

मूलाधारे कुण्डलिनी भुजगाकाररूपिणी।
जीवात्मा तिष्ठति तत्र प्रदीपकलिकाकृतिः।
ध्यायेत्तेजोमयं ब्रह्म तेजोध्यानं परात्परम्।। ९।।

In the Mūlādhāracakra dwells the Kuṇḍalinī, serpent-like, and there is to be found also the Life Force glowing like a taper of light. Visualize there the radiant form of the Supreme (Brahman). This is the excellent Effulgent Meditation.—9

भ्रुवोमध्ये मनोर्द्धे च यत्तेजः प्रणवात्मकम्।
ध्यायेज्ज्वालावतीयुक्तं तेजोध्यानं तदेव हि।। १०।।

The bright force that dwells between the eyebrows in the brain should be visualized as *Aum* (symbol of the Supreme), enveloped in a flood of radiance. This, too, is Effulgent Meditation.—10

iii. *The Subtle*

तेजोध्यानं श्रुतं चण्ड सूक्ष्मध्यानं वदाम्यहम्।
बहुभाग्यवशाद् यस्य कुण्डली जाग्रती भवेत्।। ११।।
आत्मना सहयोगेन नेत्ररन्ध्राद्विनिर्गता।
विहरेद्राजमार्गे च चञ्चलत्वान्न दृश्यते।। १२।।
शाम्भवीमुद्रया योगी ध्यानयोगेन सिद्ध्यति।
सूक्ष्मध्यानमिदं गोप्यं देवानामपि दुर्लभम्।। १३।।

You have heard about the Effulgent Meditation, O Caṇḍakāpāli; now I shall tell you about the Subtle. In this the Kuṇḍalinī, when it is aroused at last due to great good luck, unites with the Self (*Ātman*) and emerges from the sinuses to tread the royal path (higher plane) where, due to extreme vibrations, it cannot be seen. The yogi is able to master this (subtle form of meditation) by first practising the Śāmbhavimudrā (cf. III.62–63). This Subtle Meditation, however, should be kept a secret, since it is rare even for the gods.—11–13

स्थूलध्यानाच्छतगुणं तेजोध्यानं प्रचक्षते।
तेजोध्यानाल्लक्षगुणं सूक्ष्मध्यानं विशिष्यते।। १४।।

Effulgent Meditation, no doubt, is a hundred times better than the Concrete one, but Subtle Meditation is a hundred thousand times better than the Effulgent one!—14

इति ते कथितं चण्ड ध्यानयोगः सुदुर्लभः।
आत्मसाक्षाद्भवेत् यस्मात्तस्माद्ध्यानं विशिष्यते।। १५।।

Now I have told you, O Caṇḍakāpāli, the incomparable technique of meditations. However, only that meditation is best by which Self-realization becomes possible.—15

Here ends Lesson Six entitled 'Meditation' incorporated in *Gheraṇḍasaṃhitā*

LESSON SEVEN

Superconsciousness

Śrī Gheraṇḍa said:

समाधिश्च परो योगो बहुभाग्येन लभ्यते।
गुरोः कृपाप्रसादेन प्राप्यते गुरुभक्तितः।। १।।

Samādhi (superconsciousness) is a superb yoga that is reached by great good luck, through devotion to guru and by the grace of guru.—1

विद्याप्रतीतिः स्वगुरुप्रतीतिरात्मप्रतीतिर्मनसः प्रबोधः।
दिने दिने यस्य भवेत् स योगी सुशोभनाभ्यासमुपैति सद्यः।। २।।

The yogi who, day by day, develops faith in the knowledge (of yoga), in his own guru and in himself, gains confidence in his mind and is soon able to reach this wonderful state of *samādhi*.—2

घटाद्भिन्नं मनः कृत्वा ऐक्यं कुर्यात् परात्मनि।
समाधिं तं विजानीयात् मुक्तसङ्गोदशादिभिः।। ३।।

Separating the mind from the body and uniting it with the Supreme—know this to be the state of *samādhi* when one is freed from the ten *daśās** (conditions).—3

अहं ब्रह्म न चान्योऽस्मि ब्रह्मैवाहं न शोकभाक्।
सच्चिदानन्दरूपोऽहं नित्यमुक्तः स्वभाववान्।। ४।।

(One then feels) "I am Brahman, I am no other than the Supreme; I am not subject to sorrows or grief: I am *Saccidānanda*;** I am eternal: I am free; I am my own natural Self."—4

*The ten *daśās* (conditions) of man are: (1) propensity to see, (2) propensity to hear, (3) propensity to smell, (4) propensity to taste, (5) propensity to touch, (6) feeling of sorrow, (7) feeling of anger, (8) feeling of envy, (9) feeling of hatred, and (10) sexual urge.

***Saccidānanda* (*sat* + *cit* + *ānanda*) stands for "The Supreme"—the immanence of Truth, Knowledge and Bliss.

शाम्भव्या चैव खेचर्या भ्रमर्या योनिमुद्रया।
ध्यानं नादं रसानन्दं लयसिद्धिश्चतुर्विधा।। ५।।
पञ्चधा भक्तियोगेन मनोमूर्च्छा च षड्विधा।
षड्विधोऽयं राजयोगः प्रत्येकमवधारयेत्।। ६।।

The way to *samādhi* is six-fold; Meditation, Merging with Sound, Tasting Ambrosia and Bliss—these are the four methods by which one can get lost in ecstasy with the help of Śāmbhavi, Khecarī, Bhrāmari and Yoni *mudrās.* The fifth is through *bhakti* (intense devotion) and the sixth through "Mental Swoon" (cf. V.82). This is the six-fold Rājayoga (king of yogas). Now try and identify each.—5 and 6

LAYAYOGA

i. *The Void*

शाम्भवीं मुद्रिकां कृत्वा आत्मप्रत्यक्षमानयेत्।
विन्दुब्रह्म सकृद्दृष्ट्वा मनस्तत्र नियोजयेत्।। ७।।
खमध्ये कुरु चात्मानं आत्ममध्ये च खं कुरु।
आत्मानं खमयं दृष्ट्वा न किञ्चिदपि बाध्यते।। ८।।

After performing a Śāmbhavimudrā, cognize directly your own Self. Then, visualizing the Supreme (Brahman) in a micro form, let your mind unite with it while fully concentrating upon this. Thereafter, let your Self (together with the Supreme) go out into the Void, visualizing the Void also within you. In this manner the Self should be merged with the Void without any limits whatsoever.—7 and 8

ii *The Ambrosia*

सानात् खेचरीमुद्रा रसनोर्द्ध्वगता सदा।
तदा समाधिसिद्धिः स्याद्धित्वा साधारणक्रियाम्।। ९।।

After performing a Khecarīmudrā, keep the tongue unturned all the while and follow the usual procedure (i.e., suck in the ambrosia). In this way also *samādhi* is attained.—9

iii. *Sounds*

अनिलं मन्दवेगेन भ्रामरी कुम्भकं चरेत्।
मन्दं मन्दं रेचयेद्वायुं भृङ्गनादस्ततो भवेत्।। १०।।
अन्तःस्थं भ्रामरीनादं श्रुत्वा तत्र मनो नयेत्।
समाधिर्जायते तत्र आनन्दः सोऽहमित्यतः।। ११।।

After performing a Bhrāmarīmudrā, hold a *kumbhaka* and then release the air very slowly. This would produce sounds as though made by hornets. When you hear this buzzing noise within yourself, let the mind be merged with that. It would lead to *samādhi*—a state of bliss and oneness (I am That).—10 and 11

iv. *Bliss*

योनिमुद्रां समासाद्य स्वयं शक्तिमयो भवेत्।
सुश्रृंगाररसेनैव विहरेत् परमात्मनि।। १२।।
आनन्दमयः सम्भूत्वा ऐक्यं ब्रह्मणि सम्भवेत्।
अहं ब्रह्मेति वाद्वैतं समाधिस्तेन जायते।। १३।।

After performing a Yonimudrā, visualize yourself as Śakti (consort of Lord Śiva) and with all Her bewitching charm, you too woo and play with the Supreme (Śiva). When you are in complete bliss, then only would it be possible to unite with the Supreme and realize: "I am One (*Brahman*), not two." This leads to *samādhi*.—12 and 13

BHAKTIYOGA

स्वकीयहृदये ध्यायेदिष्टदेवस्वरूपकम्।
चिन्तयेद्भक्तियोगेन परमाह्लादपूर्वकम्।। १४।।
आनन्दाश्रु पुलकेन दशाभावः प्रजायते।
समाधिं सम्भवेत्तेन सम्भवेच्च मनोन्मनीः।। १५।।

Bhaktiyoga, or the yoga of intense devotion, is practised by visualizing, with a cheerful state of mind, the image of one's own chosen deity inside one's own heart. When this produces tears of joy, thrills, and later, an insensate physical condition, it would lead to sublimation of the mind and then *samādhi*.—14 and 15

MENTAL SWOON

मनोमूर्च्छां समासाद्य मनः आत्मनि योजयेत्।
परमात्मनः समायोगात् समाधिं समवाप्नुयात्।। १६।।

Getting into a "mental swoon" (cf. V.82), let the mind be united with the Self (*Ātman*). When both (mind and Self) merge into the Supreme Soul (*Paramātman*), *samādhi* ensues.—16

इति ते कथितं चण्ड समाधिं मुक्तिलक्षणम्।
राजयोगः समाधिः स्यादेकात्मन्येव साधनम्।

उन्मनी सहजावस्था सर्वे चैकात्मवाचका।। १७।।

Thus I have described to you, O Caṇḍakāpāli, the *samādhi* that is a sign of Emancipation. *Samādhi* is attained by practising this Rāja-yoga with onepointedness. Then the mind is sublimated and brought to its own natural form, indicating oneness all round.—17

जले विष्णुः स्थले विष्णुर्विष्णुः पर्वतमस्तके।
ज्वालामालाकुले विष्णुः सर्वं विष्णुमयं जगत्।। १८।।

Then the entire universe seems full of the Supreme (Viṣṇu)—Viṣṇu in water, Viṣṇu on land, Viṣṇu on top of the mountain, Viṣṇu in fire and Viṣṇu in all beings.—18

भूचराः खेचराश्चामी यावन्तो जीवजन्तवः।
वृक्षगुल्मलतावल्लीतृणाद्या वारिपर्वताः।
सर्वं ब्रह्म विजानीयात् सर्वं पश्यति चात्मनि।। १९।।

All living creatures on land and in the sky, all trees, bushes, creepers, plants, grass, all rivers and mountains—*all* are seen as the one Supreme Brahman, and one's own Self is seen in *all*.—19

आत्मा घटस्थचैतन्यमद्वैतं शाश्वतं परम्।
घटाद्विभिन्नतो ज्ञात्वा वीतरागो विवासनः।। २०।।

Then the consciousness of duality between the Self and the Eternal Supreme is lost, and so knowing (realizing) that the Self is different from the body, one becomes unattached to objects and is devoid of desires.—20

एवंविधः समाधिः स्यात् सर्वसंकल्पवर्जितः।
स्वदेहे पुत्रदारादिबान्धवेषु धनादिषु।
सर्वेषु निर्ममो भूत्वा समाधिं समवाप्नुयात्।। २१।।

By this kind of *samādhi* all desires are abandoned. Complete *samādhi* is attained when one becomes totally indifferent to one's own body, son, wife, relations, wealth—everything.—21

तत्वं लयामृतं गोप्यं शिवोक्तं विविधानि च।
तासां संक्षेपमादाय कथितं मुक्तिलक्षणम्।। २२।।

The secret of this immortal Science of Harmony has been described in detail by the Lord Śiva Himself, and I have only summarized and told you some of the main methods of Emancipation.—22

इति ते कथितं चण्ड समाधिर्दुर्लभः परः।
यज्ज्ञात्वा न पुनर्जन्म जायते भुविमण्डले।। २३।।

O Caṇḍakāpāli, I have told you here an extremely rare *samādhi* yoga, by knowing which one is never born again on this earth.—23

Here ends Lesson Seven entitled 'Superconsciousness' incorporated in *Gheraṇḍasaṃhitā*

Book III

Pātañjala Yogasūtra

CHAPTER I

Types of Yoga

अथ योगानुशासनम्।।१।।

Now (is explained) the discipline of yoga.—1

This aphorism define the scope and purpose of the science of yoga. The word *atha* (now) signifies both an auspicious beginning as well as the scope of the work.

Discipline (*anuśāsana*) implies effort. Thus the discipline of yoga involves conscientious effort that is necessary in order to achieve the goal. The goal is *samādhi*, or superconsciousness. For this purpose all thoughts arising in the mind have to be controlled; in other words, the mind is to be trained to behave in a disciplined manner, as directed and as desired. When, finally, all irrelevant thoughts quiesce, all passions subside and all "impurities" are purged, the mind assumes the form of Pure Knowledge, which is also the natural form of the Self. The two then unite, or are "yoked." This union is called *Kaivalya* or Oneness. It is also Asamprajñāta *samādhi*, or superconsciousness.

योगश्चित्तवृत्तिनिरोधः।।२।।

Yoga is control of modifications of the mind.—2

Now yoga is defined. Yoga is the regulation and suppression of the modifications or changes that constantly take place in the mind. The mind is never at rest. As soon as one thought subsides another arises. It is active all the time—even during sleep or when one appears to be unconscious. Further, when a thought arises it tends to proliferate. This tendency is called *vṛtti* (inclination), which yoga seeks to control. Since all propensities possess the quality of fickleness, or an extravert tendency, the same have to be restrained. This is the task of yoga. Yoga not only restrains but actually reverses these tendencies to their source. In other words, the effect is pushed back to its cause. However, although such total control of the mind is beneficial for everybody, the same is rarely practised by all.

The different states of the mind are: Kṣipta or agitated, Mūḍha or ignorant, Vikṣipta or distracted, Ekāgra or concentrated, and Niruddha or controlled.

Of the above, the Kṣipta state, being born of the quality of *rajas* (passion or force), is the most unsteady and of an extravert character. It always darts towards some object or another, whether it be pleasurable or painful, and is riddled with doubts. Thus driven by the force of *rajas*, the mind is ever demon-like.

The Mūḍha (ignorant) state is the result of *tamas*, the quality of dormancy or inertia. It is puzzled by the alternatives of do-able and not do-able, and, when finally unable to decide, it does the wrong thing and succumbs to anger. Then it becomes savage and is almost like an evil spirit.

The Vikṣipta (distracted) state of mind results from entry into this field (of *rajas* and *tamas*) of the quality of *sattva* (purity). The nature of this quality is immaculateness, and it scatters both pleasure and sorrow-causing thoughts. As a result the mind is unable to concentrate. At this stage music or prayers bring comparative peace to the mind; the state is then designated 'godly'.

All three states, however, are unsuitable for the purpose of *samādhi.* Although the quality of *rajas* engenders fierce propensities, that of *tamas* the tendency to harm others and of *sattva* a contented mind, normally none of these exists in the mind exclusively; there is always a mixture of the three in unequal proportions. Only in Ekāgra and Niruddha states, the *sattva* predominates. However, the last one alone is recommended as the most suitable state of mind for purposes of *samādhi.*

Here the mention of *rajas* and *tamas,* both inferior and undesirable qualities, in supersession of *sattva* may seem somewhat irregular. Yet the two have been placed first advisedly. The reason is that it is these two that always activate a *pravṛtti* (propensity) and, obviously, unless there is a *pravṛtti* its *nivṛtti* (restraint) is out of question. The subsequent appearance of *sattva* in this field prepares the ground for the practice of yoga. And, when this ground has been thoroughly cleansed of the impurities of *rajas* and *tamas* by means of *ekāgratā* (concentration), then only a complete control of the mind (Niruddha) results. This ground is then suitable for *samādhi.*

तदा द्रष्टुः स्वरूपेऽवस्थानम्।।३।।

Then it stays in the form of the Seer (Self).—3

The mind, in fact, is only a reflector. Innumerable objects are reflected in it, and this keeps the mind perpetually busy analyzing, accepting or rejecting those impressions. All the while the mind suffers from a sense of false self-consciousness—viz. that it is the one that is "seeing" those objects—whereas, in actual fact, it is merely reflecting them. The real "seer" always is the Self which, although it witnesses the drama staged inside the mind, does not react in the least to the things seen. However, the real cause of the mind's activities is propensities, which are automatically generated within it. These have to be controlled by the practice of yoga. When these are stilled, and the mind calms down to its natural pure state, the mind becomes like a crystal that is no longer obliged to reflect shadows. It is this shadowless state of the mind which has the form of Pure Knowledge, a form that is exactly like the form in which the Self or *Ātman* dwells within the body.

वृत्तिसारूप्यमितरत्र।।४।।

Otherwise it is in the form of propensities.—4

What is the form of propensities? Propensities appear in varied forms—sometimes in the form of sorrow, sometimes as happiness, sometimes as desire, and so on. These appear, too, in different degrees. When afflicted by any of these, the mind takes on the form of that particular propensity, and again the form of the next one that comes its way. In this manner, one after another, the mind continuously keeps changing its own form in accordance with the form of the propensity that predominates it. During this process the mind never gets a chance to be its own real self. This quick-changing process also causes the reflections to appear somewhat distorted—something like the reflection of the moon seen in waves of water.

वृत्तयः पञ्चतय्यः क्लिष्टा अक्लिष्टाः।।५।।

Propensities are five-fold: painful and non-painful.—5

Here the character of the propensities is further explained. Some of these, it is observed, are painful, i.e., they lead to direct suffering, while the others are not so. All five are enumerated in the aphorism that follows.

प्रमाणविपर्ययविकल्पनिद्रास्मृतयः ।।६।।

(These are) Proof, Indeterminacy, Delusion, Dormancy, and Memory.—6

The above five types of propensities are further explained in the succeeding *sūtras.*

प्रत्यक्षानुमानागमाः प्रमाणानि।।७।।

Proofs are obtained by Direct Knowledge, by Inference, and from the Scriptures.—7

The characteristics of a propensity demanding proof are now explained. Ordinarily the proof of a thing is established by *pratyakṣa* or Direct Knowledge. When a thing is either seen or heard directly, it becomes obvious and no further proof of its existence is required. This is Instant Proof. Here the shadow of an external object is captured by the sense-organ concerned and transmitted direct to the mind, which promptly accepts the same without any hesitation. But when this same shadow has to linger for a while, and await verification by the other sense-organs, it is called *anumāna* or Inference. However, after due verification, this too is accepted as a proof. The third category of proof is *āgamas,* or the Scriptures. This is also proof, since scriptures are the already-verified and recorded truths.

विपर्य्ययो मिथ्याज्ञानमतद्रूपप्रतिष्ठितम्।।८।।

Indeterminacy is getting stuck in a state of false notion.—8

When an object is either blurred or veiled in a false cloak it is not possible to have a correct knowledge of it. This results in indeterminacy. For example, a mother-of-pearl, when seen at a distance, may well appear to be a piece of silver which, of course, it is not. A mind thus placed, is always in doubt, having formed a wrong idea of the object seen with own eyes; and this doubt persists until the real thing becomes apparent. For instance, when it is not clear in the dark whether the object seen is a pillar or a man, doubt persists. This is Indeterminacy.

शब्दज्ञानानुपाती वस्तुशून्यो विकल्पः।।९।।

Going by the sound of words only, without the reality, is Delusion.—9

Accepting a verbal statement that is not rooted in fact usually leads to mistaken conclusions. This is *vikalpa*, or Delusion. The reality must always be verifiable, since the mere description of it can never convey a full and correct idea of the thing described. For example, when we say: "The consciousness of man is his own Śelf" and again: "The blanket of Devadatta"—the difference between the two statements is that, while in the first case verification is lacking, in the second, the object, though not seen, is yet verifiable. Actually, however, "consciousness" is the "man".

अभावप्रत्ययालम्बना वृत्तिर्निद्रा।।१०।।

The propensity of Dormancy harbours a sense of deficiency—10

Dormancy (*nidrā*) is a propensity that is born of the quality of inertia (*tamas*) in an excessive measure. During dormancy the mind temporarily withdraws and dissociates itself from external objects of interest. This creates a vacuum and a sense of nothingness. It is due to this propensity that one recalls: "I slept happily" despite the absence (deficiency) of that particular "happy" experience in his mind at the moment when the statement is made.

अनुभूतविषया सम्प्रमोषः स्मृतिः।।११।।

The collection of impressions of perceived objects is Memory.—11

All objects perceived by the senses leave their impressions upon the mind. These, after they have duly furnished the "proof" of their existence, are collected and stored there for future use. When the mind *re*-cognizes them and *re*-collects them, they *re*-appear from the storehouse called Memory. Of the five types of propensities the first three, viz. Proof, Indeterminacy and Delusion, lie inhibited or dormant in the mind during the waking state. In other words, they remain stored in memory—in the unconscious part of it—during the period of Dormancy.

अभयासवैराग्याभ्यां तन्निरोधः।।१२।।

They are to be controlled through Practice and Non-attachment.—12

Now the way to control these propensities. As stated earlier the most remarkable characteristic of a propensity is its extravert tendency. A propensity always seeks action and urges action. This tendency of the propensity has to be curbed, and it is possible to do so only by means of Practice and Non-attachment. However, when a propensity's extravert tendency is restrained in this manner, it turns (being a force that is self-generated) inward and enters deep into the mind. But here again, finding itself in the wrong place and blocked, it takes another turn and darts back outward. Only repeated exercise of control would stop this inward-outward flow, whereafter the propensity finally quiesces. The exercise prescribed is: diligent practice of control and scrupulous non-attachment, i.e., taking the mind off from the propensity concerned.

तत्र स्थितौ यत्नोऽभ्यासः।।१३।।

Effort made to stabilize these (propensities) is Practice.—13

Here Practice is further explained. The kind of practice necessary to stabilize the propensities must be assiduous, involving repeated application of the mind to the essence of the object to be gained. In other words, it is the persistence of this process of constant control, exerted with determination, that constitutes real practice.

स तु दीर्घकालादरनैरन्तर्यसत्कारसेवितो दृढभूमिः।।१४।।

That, dutifully peformed over a long period, confirms the ground.—14

The special features of such practice are emphasized here. These are—long period, regularly (without break) and diligent performance. Any practice that has these features would help to stabilize the propensities and make the mind's ground firm. Thereafter the mind cannot get unsettled by the pranks of those propensities.

दृष्टानुश्रविकविषयवितृष्णस्य वशीकारसंज्ञा वैराग्यम्।।१५।।

Distaste for the seen and heard of objects, and their allurements, is Non-attachment.—15

Next, the nature of non-attachment that is required for this purpose. Here objects have been divided into two categories: objects that are seen around one's self in this world, and objects that are heard of only and which are said to be available in the Hereafter. The latter are the promised ones—heard or learnt from others, e.g., the guru or the Vedas. However, both the "seen" as well as the "heard of" objects leave their impressions upon the mind. Since these impressions come in the way of effective concentration essential for a *samādhi* they have to be restrained, indeed countered, with such thoughts as "I am the real master, not these!" In this manner their power of attraction or "allurement" can be neutralized. This is called Non-attachment.

तत्परं पुरुषख्यातेर्गुणवैतृष्ण्यम्।।१६।।

That (Non-attachment) is supreme which sheds the qualities and realizes the Self.—16

Non-attachment is of two kinds. One comprises distaste *of* and *about* objects; the other is distaste *for* their qualities. The latter kind is recommended as the best form of non-attachment since it generates *viveka* or discriminative knowledge which is essential for realizing the Self. Hence this type of non-attachment is useful for *samādhi.*

वितर्कविचारानन्दास्मितानुगमात् सम्प्रज्ञातः।।१७।।

Samprajñāta *samādhi* follows reasoning, discrimination, bliss and self-awareness.—17

Now the two forms of *samādhi*, namely, Samprajñāta and Asamprajñāta, or *with* consciousness and *without* consciousness.

Contemplation upon a single visualized object for a length of time is *samādhi.* A *samādhi*, at the end of which the object meditated upon is truly and fully known and all doubts in regard to it are dispelled, is called Samprajñāta *samādhi*, or *samādhi* with consciousness. This *samādhi* is of four kinds: (1) Savitarka (with questions or reasoning), (2) Sa-vicāra (with judgment or discrimination), (3) Sa-ānanda (with bliss), and (4) Sa-asmitā (with self-awareness). Meditation (*bhāvana*) is the repeated application of the mind to the object meditated upon. This takes two forms: one, when the mind is concentrated upon the Absolute in abstract form, and two, when the subject of concentration is Elements in concrete form. The Elements, again, are divided into Matter and Non-Matter. While Non-Matter is but one, viz., the soul within (called *Puruṣa* or *Ātman*), Matter covers 24 varieties.'*

*According to the Sāṅkhya school of philosophy, Matter has twenty-four *tattvas* or true principles, viz., five *tanmātras* or subtle forms of the elements of Fire, Water, Air, Earth, and Sky; five *bhūtas* or gross forms of the elements of Fire, Water, Air,

Of the four kinds of Samprajñāta *samādhi*, the first—Sa-vitarka (with questions) relates to meditation upon the principal elements of Matter, viz., Earth, Water, Fire, Air, and Sky (quintessence). Objects constituted of these elements, and perceived by the sense-organs, are analyzed by means of *vitarka* (reasoning) in respect of their sound and meaning, making a clear distinction between the two. When there is no such analysis and no clear appreciation of the significance and meaning of each, this same *samādhi* becomes Nir-vitarka or without reasoning.

The next, Sa-vicāra (with discrimination) is that kind of meditation in which the intrinsic character of each element is identified and then reduced to its subtle form in terms of time, space and quality. When such discrimination is not made and yet the yogi is conscious, it is called Nir-vicāra or without discrimination.

In Sa-ānanda (with bliss) *samādhi* the yogi suppresses the *rajas* and *tamas* qualities and encourages the *sattva* to pervade his mind. This form of *samādhi*, i.e., with an excess of immaculateness in the mind, is known as *videha* (non-physical). However, in this *samādhi* the mind does not cognize the Self, this being only a transitory phase of excessive *sattva* which produces bliss or ecstasy in the mind. Further, being *videha*, there is no consciousness of the physical body.

Sa-asmitā literally means "with ego". In this form of *samādhi* the yogi is aware of his consciousness and yet is unconscious about the existence of his body. Such faint awareness of one's existence, even though in a subtle form, is not considered conducive for purposes of attaining the supreme goal of Emancipation; hence this *samādhi* is known as *Prakṛti-laya* or dissolution into Nature (as opposed to dissolution into the Universal Soul or *Paramātman*). However, Sa-asmitā is a *samādhi* in which *sattva* subsists till the very end and, as such, it is regarded as a "complete *samādhi*," being the last of the four stages of Samprajñāta *samādhi*.

विरामप्रत्ययाभ्यासपूर्वकः संस्कारशेषोऽन्यः ।।१८।।

The other is by total obliteration of past impressions residual in the Unconscious.—18.

Earth, and Sky; five sense-organs or faculties of sight, hearing, smell, taste, and touch; five organs of action, viz., tongue (speech), hands, legs, genitals, and anus; and Mind; Ego; Intelligence and *mahat* (Infinity).

"The other" here refers to A-samprajñāta *samādhi.*

Virām means a halt. Modification of thoughts is halted with the aid of *viveka* (discriminative knowledge). The resolute practice of this halting process (slowing down to a halt) is *virām-pratyaya* or positive halt. In other words, it is a process of applying the brake again and again on the mind's natural tendency to modify. No sooner a propensity-endowed thought arises than it is to be countered and rejected with the firm admonition: "No! Not this!" This is *virām-pratyaya.* When, in this manner, the last vestige of thought-consciousness is curbed and eliminated, it is A-samprajñāta *samādhi* or super-consciousness. The stage immediately before this is Samprajñāta.

The A-samprajñāta *samādhi* is also known as the "seedless" *samādhi* because in this *samādhi* the very seed of normal consciousness is burnt up and destroyed. There are four stages in this form of *samādhi.* The first is when the mind is stabilized and there is no fresh proliferation of thoughts. Then begins the *samādhi* proper. With the aid of concentration, more and more of *sattva* is infused into the field formerly dominated by *rajas* and *tamas.* Concentration brings about one-pointedness, which helps to control the lingering propensities, including those resting on past impressions (*saṃskāra*). Ultimately, even the residual impressions in the Unconscious mind are totally obliterated. It is just like the smelting of gold: the ore, though mixed with zinc and other impurities, comes out as pure gold from the fire in which the zinc and other impurities are all burnt up. In the same way, in A-samprajñāta *samādhi* all past impressions, as well as the current consciousness resulting from efforts made during concentration and control, are all lost in the heights of superconsciousness.

भवप्रत्ययो विदेहप्रकृतिलयानाम्।।१९।।

For those who are world-conscious (the way is) non-physical and dissolution into Nature.—19

For those yogis who happen to be *bhava-pratyaya* (*bhava,* world; *pratyaya,* direct awareness)—that is those who are still conscious of their worldly environment—the way recommended is *videha* or renouncing of physical consciousness and *Prakṛti-laya* (merging into Nature). In fact, this is all that they may expect in *their* form of Samprajñāta *samādhi.* The other form of Emancipation, viz., merging into the Universal Soul or the Supreme Being is reserved for those who can rise to the heights of the "seedless" A-samprajñāta *samādhi.*

श्रद्धावीर्यस्मृतिसमाधिप्रज्ञापूर्वक इतरेषाम्॥२०॥

For others, Faith, Zeal, Introspection, Contemplation, and Highest Wisdom (are necessary).—20

Here "others" refers to the select few who aspire for A-samprajñāta *samādhi.*

"Faith" denotes confidence in reaching the goal that is indicated when one's thoughts constantly veer to the object sought. It is, in fact, a fundamental condition for success in any kind of *samādhi.* "Zeal" follows faith since it represents preparedness and effort to be put in for the completion of the job. "Introspection" is re-examining one's own thoughts. "Contemplation" is continued concentration on the object to be gained, while "Highest Wisdom" is the fruit of all discriminated knowledge that enables the mind to attain the desired goal.

"Faith" leads to "Zeal" which leads to "Introspection" during which all past impressions in the memory are reviewed and analyzed by means of "Contemplation" until the "Highest Wisdom" is reached. A mind thus endowed knows everything: it is then in a state of Samprajñāta *samādhi,* or *samādhi* with consciousness. But when the yogi rises even above this state—leaving behind faith, zeal, wisdom, etc.—he attains superconsciousness (A-samprajñāta *samādhi*).

तीव्रसंवेगानामासन्नः॥२१॥

With energetic effort this is quickly accomplished.—21

Again the advice is "for others".

The way to achieve success, it is emphasized, is to maintain a uniform tempo of vigorous effort. *Tīvra-saṃvega* (energetic effort) implies both speed and energy; both are needed for subduing the propensities and wiping out their traces from memory. This is the only way in which the desired result, namely A-samprajñāta *samādhi,* can be quickly achieved.

मृदुमध्याधिमात्रत्वात्ततोऽपि विशेषः॥२२॥

Their special characteristics are mild, medium and intense.—22

The degree of energy and speed necessary for this purpose is further elucidated. Each of these is divided into three categories, viz. mild, medium and intense, that is, mild energy, medium energy and intense energy; and similarly in respect of speed. Again, to clarify what is exactly meant, each of these mild, medium and intense forms is further discriminated into *excessively* mild, *moderately* mild and *simply* mild. In the same way, "medium" and "intense" can be subdivided to indicate their precise strength. Thus, in all, they make nine types of speed and energy. The classifications obviously are to help the yogi choose the correct strength of speed and energy for quickly accomplishing his *samādhi.*

ईश्वरप्रणिधानाद्वा।।२३।।

Or, by great devotion to the Supreme Being.—23

Apart from the methods described above, the author now mentions an easier one, viz. great devotion towards God. Devotion (*praṇidhāna*) is respectful loyalty and dedication, such as are indicated in all forms of worship. Sustained devotion of this type can also lead to *samādhi.*

क्लेशकर्मविपाकाशयैरपरामृष्टः पुरुषविशेष ईश्वरः।।२४।।

The Supreme Being is a Distinct Personality who is beyond the pale of afflictions, *karma*-born desires and fruits of actions.—24

Now, about the nature of that Distinct Personality (*Viśeṣa Puruṣa*) who is so very different from all other *Puruṣas.* He is different because, unlike all others, He is not touched by afflictions, desires (*āśaya* = expectations) and *karma* or their fruit. He is supreme and His powers are infinite. He is the Creator and Demolisher of the entire universe. At His will *Prakṛti* (Nature) and *Puruṣa* (Individual Soul) combine and disintegrate. He is the prime promulgator of the law of attraction and repulsion. At His behest *Prakṛti* and *Puruṣa* unite nad disunite. All His creatures are the product of such combination of *Prakṛti* and *Puruṣa.* After the combination, the changing qualities of *Prakṛti* (Nature) continue to operate and appear in the form of pleasures, pains, attachments, etc. in all beings, while the *Puruṣa* remains a silent witness of the drama. These qualities of Nature appear at first in the mind and, if left uncontrolled, breed more of their kind in an endless sequence, thereby continuously distracting the mind. As a result even the more evolved *Puruṣas* (*Mahān Ātman*) are affected by these afflictions, albeit only indirectly. (This is like the humiliation suffered by a king when the actual defeat in battle was that of his soldiers.) The *Viśeṣa Puruṣa*, however, is never touched by such afflictions even in an indirect way. That is the distinguishing characteristic of the Supreme Being. Lastly, He is the repository of Total Purity (*sattva*) and the Highest Wisdom (*Prajñā*). Being the source of His own knowledge, He is never dependent upon any other knowledge. He has no desires and generates no *karma*.

तत्र निरतिशयं सर्वज्ञत्वबीजम्।।२५।।

There (in Him) lies the seed of His infinite omniscience.—25

Having described the nature of this Supreme Being, the author now seeks to furnish the proof of His existence.

Infinite omniscience is the apparent proof of His existence. He is omniscient because He is the seed (cause) of seed—the very essence of minuteness and immensity. Both Past and Future are condensed in Him. He is thus subtler than the subtlest—almost inconceivable. The nucleus of an atom, when viewed against the immensity of Space, although conceivable through intelligence characteristic of the mind, is seldom fully and finally grasped because of the extreme limits either way. In the case of the Supreme Being no such limits exist. His infinite and omniscient character is known only through the scriptures coming down from very ancient times. Indeed Time and Space are His children; and these too are withdrawable by Him at the time of the Great Dissolution (*Mahāpralaya*).

स पूर्वेषामपि गुरुः कालेनावच्छेदात्।।२६।।

Not being bound by Time, He is the earliest and the greatest of all Teachers.—26

Being the repository of Primordial Knowledge, all knowledge flows from Him. As such He is the Teacher of Teachers. He is the Creator of the Creator (Bramhā) and other gods; the latter anyhow are all bound by Time although the extent of that Time is very, very vast indeed. The Supreme Being, being Himself the creator of Time, existed before Time came into existence.

तस्य वाचकः प्रणवः।।२७।।

His verbal symbol is *Aum*.—27

Normally a symbol is a visual expression of the thing, and hence silent. But when it is audible, the sound becomes the means of its expression. Thus the symbol establishes a link between the expressor and the expressed to; this is the characteristic of all symbols. In this case *Aum* (*Praṇava* = Prime-Knowledge-like) is the verbal symbol that establishes the necessary link between the reciter of this symbolic word and the One to whom it is directed. It is also expressive of the natural relation between the creator and the created—like that between a father and his son.

तज्जपस्तदर्थभावम्।।२८।।

It is to be repeated, and its meaning reflected upon.—28

In order to establish that link with the Supreme, the regular use of this three-and-a-half syllabled word—*Aum*—is recommended. The word *Aum* is not only to be recited but its significance must also be reflected upon at the same time. As stated above, the meaning of *Aum* or *Praṇava* is Prime Knowledge-like. This is how the Supreme One should be visualized while *Aum* is recited.

ततः प्रत्यक्चेतनाधिगमोऽप्यन्तरायाभावश्च।।२९।।

There follows introspection, and then the obstacles are removed.—29

The benefit derived from such repetition of the word *Aum* is now stated. The recitation of *Aum*, and contemplation upon its meaning and significance, result in introspection when the mind, getting indifferent to external objects, turns inward (*pratyak-cetanā* = backward thought) to examine what it has got there. It then identifies—with the aid of knowledge gained from the review—the obstacle or obstacles lying in the way, and so proceeds to remove them one by one.

व्याधिस्त्यानसंशयप्रमादालस्याविरतिभ्रान्तिदर्शनालब्ध-
भूमिकत्वानवस्थितत्वानि चित्तविक्षेपास्तेऽन्तरायाः।।३०।।

Disease, mental fatigue, doubt, carelessness, lethargy, sensual attraction, delusion and frustration caused by failure to hold the ground—are the obstacles that distract the mind.—30

The several obstacles that come in the way of *samādhi* are now listed. Basically, their cause in each case is the prevalence of *rajas* and *tamas* in the mind in an excessive measure. The mind thus becomes *vikṣipta* (distracted) and then the obstacles appear as symptoms of a disturbed mind.

Vyādhi (disease) like fever, cold, etc. is indicated by a certain disorganization of the bodily humours. *Styāna* (mental fatigue) is inability, despite effort, to concentrate. *Saṃśaya* (doubt) arises when the mind is inclined to give up the effort. *Pramāda* (carelessness) is characterized by unwillingness caused by doubt—a state of indifference. *Ālasya* (lethargy) is disposition to postpone (following the indifference) and is signified by physical and mental heaviness. *Avirati* (sensual attraction) is continuous attachment to objects desired. *Bhrānti* (delusion) is false knowledge like (as explained before) mistaking a mother-of-pearl for silver. *Darśanālabdha-bhūmi avasthiti* is frustration caused by a feeling that the ground gained has been lost.

Each of these constitutes an obstacle in the way of *samādhi*, since each hinders effective concentration necessary for the performance of *samādhi.*

दुःखदौर्मनस्याङ्गमेजयत्वश्वासप्रश्वासाविक्षेपसहभुवः ।।३१।।

With these come sorrow, a troubled mind, tremors in body, and irregular breathing.—31

The visible results of obstacles mentioned above are: sorrow, dejection and nervousness. Sorrow (*duḥkha*) distracts the mind, producing a feeling of frustration. When it is in an excessive measure, and is not controlled, it drives a person to commit suicide. *Dourmana* (troubled mind) is the effect of a multiplicity of distractions crowding the mind at the same time—a product both of external and internal influences. *Aṅga-mejaya* (tremors in body) is the apparent sign of nervousness, and so is irregular breathing (*śwasa-praśwāsa vikṣepa*). The remedy for each of these infirmities, of course, is Practice and Non-attachment as advised earlier.

तत्प्रतिषेधार्थमेकतत्त्वाभ्यासः ।।३२।।

To counter those, practise holding on to one thought.—32

The technique is now being explained, i.e., the practical way in which these obstacles can be tackled. To begin with, some form of concentration is necessary. But that is easier said than done. However, the way to start is to hold on to *some* thought for *some* time. The subject of this thought may be anything—in fact any subject or object of one's own choice. This idea is to hold on to it in the first instance and later, gradually, to prolong the period of this "holding on" while the attention remains fixed on this one subject to the exclusion of everything else. Through constant practice, this kind of "holding on" becomes easier and then there emerges the power of concentration which may be used to counter the above-stated obstacles.

मैत्रीकरुणामुदितोपेक्षाणां सुखदुःखपुण्यापुण्यविषयाणां भावनातश्चित्तप्रसादम्।।३३।।

Thoughts favouring friendliness, compassion and cheer, and disfavouring subjects of pleasure, pain, virtue and vice, bring about a peaceful mind.—33

Here another way to ward off the obstacles is given. It is the deliberate intrusion into the mind of cheerfulness, friendliness and kindly thoughts and using the same to drive away the sorrowful, unfriendly and unkind thoughts which, as we know, produce passion (*rajas*) in one form or another culminating in sorrow.

The attitude of *maitrī* (friendliness) counters the feelings of dislike or aversion for another person which normally triggers off hatred in the mind. *Karuṇā* (compassion) is the manifested form of friendliness expressed either in word or action, such as verbal sympathy or a helpful deed. *Mudita* (cheerfulness) results when the mind's attitude towards all is both friendly and compassionate. *Upekṣā* (indifference) is the forgiving attitude of the mind when the shortcomings of others are deliberately ignored, i.e., when the lapses are neither disapproved nor approved.

All four attitudes strengthen the mind's power to tackle obstacles that come in the shape of pleasure, pain and other reactions of virtue and vice. They generate confidence in the mind, and it then turns peaceful. All these concientiously cultivated attitudes have only one common purpose, viz. to prepare the ground for effective concentration. To that extent they may be regarded as an expedient with an ulterior motive—somewhat like formulas used in mathematics for the purpose of calculating and arriving at the correct answer.

प्रच्छर्दनविधारणाभ्यां वा प्राणस्य।।३४।।

Or, by regulated expulsion and induction of the breath.—34

Another method is stated: This is control of the function of breathing, or rather its regulation in a manner that could help in bringing about concentration.

Prachārdana is the act of throwing out air held in the lungs and *vidhāraṇa* is its in-take. In a general sense *prāṇa* denotes the air that is breathed out and *apāna* the air that is breathed in. But *prāṇa* also represents the vital life-force that pervades in all living beings. Although regarded only as one of the several "airs" that operate within the body (cf. *SS*, III.3–8) it is in fact the vital force that links each individual consciousness to the Universal Consciousness and is drawn from it at birth and surrendered to it at death.

The control of this *prāṇa* within the body is *prāṇāyāma.* When this subtle *prāṇa* is taken in, in the form of inhaled air (*apāna*) it is called *pūraka*; when it is released, it is *recaka* and when it is held (i.e., retained inside the lungs for some length of time) it is called *kumbhaka* (potted).

Since *prāṇa* is a force, its inherent character like all forces is motion. Hence, when restrained and held within a limited field, it reacts by driving the propensities in the mind and herding them into a concentrated shape. In other words, *prāṇāyāma* helps to concentrate the psychic power within the mind, activating and invigorating the same. This interrelation of the mind and the breathing process is convincingly demonstrated when it is noted that the breath is automatically held whenever there is any task calling for instant concentrated attention.

विषयवती वा प्रवृत्तिरुत्पन्नास्थितिनिबन्धिनी।।३५।।

Or, by fixing the thought on the particular nature of perception born of a propensity.—35

Now several other methods are shown by which the yogi may attain the much-needed concentration. One of these is by fixing the thought on the quality of a particular perception engaging his mind at the moment. Since the process of perception involves a certain amount of (limited) concentration, even this brief spell can be utilized by him to develop a longer and a more sustained concentration of the mind.

Viṣayavatī (object-bound) propensities are those which, after arising in the mind, seek their respective objects through the faculties of sight, sound, smell, taste and touch. Each such propensity selects its own "means" to inform the mind of the particular object perceived, so that the mind's attention gets restricted, for the time being, to that one perception only to the exclusion of all others. In this way the quality of one particular perception is temporarily highlighted in the mind. Thus, if a thought is restricted to one particular part of the body, say, the tip of the nose, the sense-organ feeding that part tends to produce, after some time, a concentrated perception of smell only in the form of sweet fragrance and of nothing else. Similarly, the perceptions of taste, touch, sound and sight appear in a concentrated form whenever attention is fixed for any length of time upon the tip of the tongue, the flat (middle) of the tongue, the root (end) of the tongue and the tip of the palate, respectively. This kind of individualized perception helps the mind to concentrate.

विशोका वा ज्योतिष्मती।।३६।।

Or (by visualizing oneself) as sorrowless and effulgent.—36

Another method of achieving concentration is by visualizing oneself as a picture of cheerfulness and bright light. *Jyotiṣmati* (effulgent) signifies a sparkling mind in which the intelligence shines brightly; it is then *viśoka* (sorrowless), i.e., without a trace of sorrow. This state of mind normally results from an excess of *sattva* prevailing in the mind. By means of visualization (auto-suggestion) this quality is infused into the mind and after some time the mind becomes pure and resplendent.

वीतरागविषयाद्वा चित्तम्।।३७।।

Or (by visualizing) the mind as unattached to objects.—37

Another device to gain concentration is to visualize (again through auto-suggestion) one's mind as though it were totally cut off from all objects of interest. *Vīta-rāga* (without attachments) is the state of desirelessness. A mind thus conditioned naturally turns peaceful, and so becomes favourable for concentration.

स्वप्ननिद्राज्ञानालम्बनं वा।।३८।।

Or, by recourse to knowledge gained in a dream or sleep.—38

Yet another method is to utilize the experience gained during sleep or in dreams. As explained earlier (I.10), *nidrā* (sleep) is the natural withdrawal of the mind from all external objects of interest. This is the time when the mind is alone with its past impressions, all littered around in the unconscious memory. During dream some of these impressions become more vivid, often revealing knowledge that otherwise remains unknown in the waking state. If one's thought can be consciously fixed upon one of these vivid visions, the mind would tend to concentrate.

यथाभिमतध्यानाद्वा ।।३९।।

Or, by meditation on any chosen subject.—39

Since different people have different likings, the yogi is here given the option to meditate on whatever object he prefers or finds it easy to fix his attention upon. He may, for instance, like to limit his thoughts to one of his sense-organs, or to one of the *nāḍi cakras* or, should he prefer, to any pleasing image outside. Even such contemplation would make the mind stable, and consequently fit for prolonged concentration.

परमाणु-परममहत्त्वान्तोऽस्य वशीकारः ।।४०।।

Then anything—from an atom to the vastness of infinity—can be brought under control.—40

Having shown the various methods for achieving concentration, now the benefit that is to be derived from such concentration is stated.

By using one or other of these methods the mind positively gets stabilized, and the yogi is then able to concentrate effectually. He can then conceive of the minutest of matter—such as the nucleus of an atom—and also of the greatest possible expanse indicated by infinity. Further, the gross and the fine are then equally clear to him and so he experiences no difficulty whatsoever in thinking of, or concentrating his thoughts upon, the subtlest of subtle subjects.

क्षीणवृत्तेरभिजातस्येव मणेर्ग्रहीतृग्रहणग्राह्येषु तत्स्थतदञ्जनता समापत्तिः ।।४१।।

With propensities thus destroyed, the mind attains perfect clarity—like a pure crystal that reflects the reflectable.—41

The net result of practising such control of the mind is that all propensities originating or subsisting in it get weakened and become inoperative, leaving the mind perfectly clear and without any impurity in it. The mind is then like a crystal that truly reflects the objects placed before it. Like the crystal, again, it is merely the acceptor (reflector) of all that is acceptable (reflectable) through the process of accepting (reflecting). In other words, the seer, the seen and the seeing—all come within the compass of the mind's newly-acquired power. The mind thus becomes aware of its true nature, viz. its double role of "seeing" the "seen" (objects) on the one hand, and the real "seer" (Self) on the other. All this is possible, however, only after the propensities have quiesced and the light of intelligence bursts forth in its brightest form.

शब्दार्थज्ञानविकल्पैः सङ्कीर्णा सवितर्का।।४२।।

Sa-vitarka *samādhi* is one that is achieved by analyzing the mixture of words and their meaning.—42

Now the four types of Samprajñāta *samādhi* mentioned earlier (I.17) are discussed in further detail.

Śabda (sound) and *artha* (meaning) are inherent in every word that is uttered or thought of. *Jñāna* (knowledge) is the means by which those are discriminated and their correct significance is determined, i.e., even when those are presented in a mixed-up or confused condition. The three, viz. the sound, its meaning, and the knowledge required for discrimination between the two, are thus complementary. But by analysis of parts, the whole is sought to be comprehended. During a Sa-vitarka *samādhi*, the mind is still engaged in analyzing (through reason) the sounds, their meaning, their form and their significance. In other words, the mind is then still actively conscious. It is a distinct feature of this form of *samādhi*.

स्मृतिपरिशुद्धौ स्वरूपशून्येवार्थमात्रनिर्भासा निर्वितर्का।।४३।।

Nir-vitarka *samādhi* begins when the form and its impression upon the memory fade away and only the meaning remains.—43

The nature of Nir-vitarka (without questions) *samādhi* is different from that of the previous one. Here the form suggested by the sound, as well as its impression upon the memory, fade away. In other words, the doubt in respect of the sound disappears and in its place the meaning of it alone remains. Even knowledge (i.e., reasons employed to dispel the doubt) gives way to what appears as a sure and unquestionable meaning of the sound. Thus, the very essence is known without a recourse to any analysis.

एतयैव सविचारा निर्विचारा च सूक्ष्मविषया व्याख्याता।।४४।।

In the same way are described the Sa-vicāra, the Nir-vicāra and other subtle matters.—44

All this, no doubt, is subtle matter. But the subtle, it may be explained, is only an earlier form of the gross and vice versa. As a matter of fact, both gross and fine are transient states, and are interchangeable. Thus when a sound is not heard, it still exists in its subtle form (which is its meaning). The *tanmātras* or extra-fine particles of the various Elements always exist in the form of Space, Time and Nature. The yogi who discriminates these, i.e., is conscious of these in their separate forms, is said to be in a Sa-vicāra (with discrimination) *samādhi.* He who is above such discrimination is in a state of Nir-vicāra *samādhi.*

सूक्ष्मविषयञ्चालिंगपर्यवसानम्।।४५।।

"Subtle matter" is matter that dwells in a non-physical state.—45

Now what is a "subtle" matter? A "subtle" matter is matter that exists but has no physical form. It may also be defined as non-physical matter. When physical matter disintegrates and dissolves into its very essence, it only changes its form. The gross transmutes into fine, then finer, and then still more fine—until the whole thing ends in *Pradhāna* or the primordial. This is how, in yoga, all physical matter is conceived of as non-physical or subtle.

Matter is classified into four categories: (1) *viśiṣṭa-liṅga* (specific matter), (2) *a-viśiṣṭa-liṅga* (non-specific matter), (3) *liṅga-mātra* (pseudo-physical matter), and (4) *a-liṅga* (non-physical matter). "Specific matter" comprises the physical Elements and the senses, "non-specific matter" forms the core of *tanmātras* (fine particles of Elements), "pseudo-physical" is the intelligence, and "non-physical" (subtle)—in its extreme form—is the primordial or *Pradhāna.* There is nothing subtler than that.

ता एव सबीजः समाधिः।।४६।।

All these are *samādhis* with seed.—46

So far six types of *samādhis* have been described, viz. Sa-vitarka (with questions), Nir-vitarka (without questions), Sa-vicāra (with discrimination), Nir-vicāra (without discrimination), Sa-ānanda (with bliss) and Sa-asmitā (with self-awareness). The common factor in all these *samādhis* is consciousness, which constitutes the root-support or seed (*bīja*) of each. Hence all these different forms of Samprajñāta (with consciousness) *samādhi* are known as *sa-bīja* (with seed) *samādhis.*

निर्विचारवैशारद्ये अध्यात्मप्रसादः।।४७।।

Competency is Nir-vicāra *samādhi* brings supreme bliss.—47

Of the various types of Samprajñāta mentioned above, the Nir-vicāra *samādhi* is considered the best. Why? . . .

Because Nir-vicāra *samādhi* is characterized by non-discrimination, both of gross as well as fine. In other words, it is a form of *samādhi* in which there is never any doubt in respect of either gross or fine, nor even of a mixture of the two. It is also the prelude to total purity of the mind and indicates its competency for the higher (superconscious) experience which brings on supreme bliss.

ऋतम्भरा तत्र प्रज्ञा।।४८।।

There the Highest Wisdom is filled with manifested Truth.—48

Truth is stable (static). When it is moved (expressed) it becomes *ṛta* (kinetic).

Ṛta (Truth as expressed) is always full; it is never in an incomplete state. Indeed partial truth cannot be designated as truth since a qualified truth would always lack the absolute quality that the word Truth stands for. Only Nir-vicāra *samādhi* leads to the Highest Wisdom, i.e., wisdom that is impregnated with Total Truth. The benefit of having such Highest Wisdom is stated in the *sūtra* that follows.

श्रौतानुमानप्रज्ञाभ्यां सामान्यविषयाविशेषार्थत्वात्।।४९।।

With that Highest Wisdom the common things heard of or inferred appear with special significance.—49

Wisdom is the sum total of knowledge gained over a period of time and preserved in a distilled form. Ordinarily knowledge flows into the mind through the sensual channels and collects there to form wisdom. In this way, things heard of (including the testimony of scriptures) and inferred (i.e., those that have been already verified by the other sense-organs and accepted as proof), have to go through a process of discrimination which naturally keeps the mind busy. Not so, however, for the non-discriminating Nir-vicāra state in which the Highest Wisdom impregnated with Truth enables the yogi to comprehend the special significance of all things instantly, i.e., without recourse to any form of discrimination. In short, the subtle character of all perceivable objects then becomes crystal clear to him directly.

तज्जसंस्कारोऽन्यसंस्कारविरोधी।।५०।।

Impressions resulting from that thwart all other impressions.—50

As stated earlier, the mind carries innumerable impressions (*saṃskāras*), both inherited (past) as well as the freshly acquired ones. Unless these impressions are obliterated the mind cannot assume that crystal clear state which is necessary for it to reflect the total purity of the Self.

Various methods have been suggested for checking the formation of fresh impressions, and a few also for the purpose of erazing past ones lurking in the Unconscious which tend to come up as obstacles. Now a further method is revealed which would totally obliterate all these impressions. This is the overstamping of all impressions with the Highest Wisdom acquired through practice of Nir-vicāra *samādhi.* In this way, all impressions, past as well as present, are totally wiped out.

तस्यापि निरोधे सर्वनिरोधान्निर्वीजः समाधिः।।५१।।

With this too controlled, everything has been controlled, and the seedless *samādhi* ensues.—51

Appreciating that this form of overstamping, even though it is by the Highest Wisdom itself, may again leave some sort of an impression in the mind, the author here advises that any such residual impression should also be removed. The control or elimination of this last vestige of impressions is accomplished by repeated thoughts of "Not this! Not this!" When that is finally achieved, the "seedless" or A-samprajñāta *samādhi*—when the Self or *Puruṣa* is seen in its pristine Knowledge form (I.3)—is experienced. This is superconsciousness.

Here ends chapter I of *Pātañjala Yogasūtra,*
entitled 'Types of Yoga'.

CHAPTER II

Practice of Yoga

तपःस्वाध्यायेश्वरप्रणिधानानि क्रियायोगः ।।१।।

Austerity, self-study and deep devotion to God constitute Kriyā-yoga.—1

Having described the different types of yoga and the merits of each, now the way to practise those are being explained. Kriyā-yoga (practical yoga) deals with the steps to be taken for mastering the methods prescribed for attaining *samādhi*, e.g. rules and regulations to be observed, physical postures and exercises to be practised, and the technique of inducing the mind to stabilize, concentrate and reform itself into Pure Knowledge.

Towards this end the basic requirements in a yogi are: observance of austerity, a habit of study and an attitude of devotion towards God.

Tapas (austerity) covers a whole range of self-denials designed to restrain the natural physical and mental urges—such as hunger, thirst, greed, anger, sex, etc. It envisages a severely simple living, a planned renunciation of comforts, and often a deliberate acceptance of discomforts with a view to disciplining the mind and body. Physical urges are thus controlled by undertaking periodic fasts for short or long periods as necessary. The form and length of such fasts are stipulated in advance, and are observed scrupulously.

For example, the vow called Cāndrāyaṇa involves almost total fasting for a whole month when next to nothing is taken in the shape of food. It begins on a New Moon day with total abstention of food, later increasing, according to waxing phases of the moon, by one piece of clove or pepper per day. After the Full Moon day, this in-take is gradually reduced in the same way. Sometimes the clove or pepper is substituted by a morsel of food when it is recognized that the condition of health may not permit of a more extreme form of fasting.

There are several other recognized forms of fasting—such as Prajāpatya and Sāntapanam—in which the in-take is restricted to food received (or not received) in a small begging bowl in the course of one morning, or to just one drop of water (as much as a blade of grass would hold!) for a whole week. However, such extreme mortification of the flesh, including such practices as lying on a bed of nails or standing on one leg in blazing midday sun, is very rare indeed. In fact, continued mortification of the flesh over a very long period may sometimes indicate the yogi's slow progress on the path of yoga. Normally, therefore, only a hard life—such as may be involved in sleeping on the floor, bathing in frigid water, taking a minimum quantity of simple food and baring the body to the rigours of weather—is found sufficient for the purpose of subduing the distracting urges of body and mind.

In the same way, a life of studious learning and regular devotion to God helps to tranquillize the mind and make it fit for concentration.

समाधिभावनार्थः क्लेशतनूकरणार्थश्च।।२।।

These help to attain *samādhi* and lessen the afflictions.—2

As stated above, the whole purpose of subjecting oneself to this kind of strict physical and mental discipline is to train the mind for the ultimate object of achieving the state of *samādhi.* The discipline helps to rid the mind of its afflictions, i.e., the distractions that come in the way of performing *samādhi.* In other words, the strict discipline that has been prescribed is for a specific purpose, and the same is not to be observed as a matter of course only.

Kleśa (afflictions) is the disturbing factor in the mind, and so this must be controlled first. To begin with, its strength must be weakened so that a reasonably stable atmosphere, fit for concentration and meditation, is created. This is the first step in Kriyā-yoga.

अविद्यास्मितारागद्वेषाभिनिवेशाः क्लेशाः।।३।।

The afflictions are: Ignorance, Egoism, Fondness, Aversion, and Fear of Death.—3

Now what is *kleśa?* The word *kleśa* represents all the aberrations (deviations from normal) in the mind, collectively. *Kleśa* appears in the mind in various forms: as ignorance, as egoism, as desire, as aversion and as a constant fear of death. *Avidyā* (ignorance) is nescience or absence of knowledge; *asmitā* (egoism) is systematic sefishness; *rāga* (attachment) is the craving to meet objects and persons; *dveṣa* (aversion) is hatred, and *abhiniveśa* is the natural terror of death (conversely, an yearning for continued life). All these are disturbing factors in the mind, and prevent effective concentration necessary for a *samādhi*.

अविद्या क्षेत्रमुत्तरेषां प्रसुप्ततनुविच्छिन्नोदाराणाम्।।४।।

Ignorance is the ground; the others dwell upon it either in dormant, limited, scattered or profuse condition.—4

The main culprit is *avidyā* (ignorance). It breeds the other four, viz. egoism, fondness, aversion and craving for life. The latter exist in varying strength. Some are in a dormant state (*prasupta*); others are found in a small measure (*tanu*); a few are scattered and disorganized (*vicchinna*), while the rest are profuse (*udāra*) or in sufficient strength. Thus the amount of trouble that each may create depends largely upon their individual strength. A dormant desire, for instance, would appear innocent until it is roused—like a child's desire to grasp a toy immediately it is seen by him but about which he was oblivious as long as it was out of his sight. The child's crying for the toy expresses his dormant sorrow (*kleśa*).

Tanu, vicchinna and *udāra,* however, are the more recognizable forms of afflictions. *Tanu,* being small and limited in strength, are able to generate only vague stirrings of afflictions; the resulting disturbance is but mild. The *vicchinna,* being scattered and disorganized, are unable to gather their full strength. But *udāra* (liberal), being abundant, are always in full strength and as such are the greatest obstacles in the path of yoga.

Ignorance, however, remains the mother of all these various forms of *klcśa.*

अनित्याशुचिदुःखानात्मसु नित्यशुचिसुखात्मख्यातिरविद्या।।५।।

Ignorance causes the perishable, the impure, the painfuland the non-Self to appear as imperishable, pure, pleasing and reality.—5

Now the characteristics of *avidyā* (ignorance) are stated. Ignorance produces illusion; that is, it makes one accept a substitute for the reality. "This is *like* that"—is a common form of ignorance. It is ignorance again that makes us forget, when we see a nice new article, that its form and beauty would one day perish and be unrecognizable. In the same ignorant way we judge the purity of a body mostly by its outward cleanliness, seldom realizing that internally it is full of impurities. Again, when we seek pleasure, we always ignore the pain that lurks behind it in the shape of regret or remorse that invariably follows all pleasures. Similarly, it is ignorance that keeps us in the dark about the real character of the Self.

Thus, ignorance is the root-cause of all our misconceptions. It is ignorance that always deceives us into forming a wrong idea of everything in this world.

दृग्दर्शनशक्त्योरेकात्मतैवास्मिता ।।६।।

Egoism is identification of the seen with the act of seeing.—6

Asmitā (egoism) is the "I"-consciousness—the notion that it is *my* mind that is seeing, feeling, thinking and directing all actions. This notion is false, since the mind is not the real seer and enjoyer of things seen, these being the functions of the Self only. This baseless self-importance of the mind is known as *asmitā* or egoism. The egotistic tendency merely leads up to a mix-up of the seer, the seen and the act of seeing. It is born of ignorance.

सुखानुशयी रागः ।।७।।

Attachment dwells upon pleasure.—7

Sukhānuśayī literally means 'a seeker of pleasure'. *Rāga* (attachment) is the craving for pleasure. When attachment dwells upon pleasure, it actually thrives on it and asks for more and more of it. This pleasure-seeking then becomes a matter of habit, so that the mind does not stop to discriminate between the real pleasure and *false* pleasures. Since worldly objects offer only false pleasure, which all end in sorrow or regret—attachment to such pleasures is mere ignorance.

दुःखानुशयी द्वेषः ।।८।।

Aversion dwells upon pain.—8

Dveṣa (aversion) is dislike or hatred for a person or thing. It is always rooted in sorrow, caused by some painful experience gone through earlier. It is in fact born of a desire (instinct) to escape similar pain once again, and so creates in the mind a kind of revulsion against the person or thing suspected as a potential inflector of similar pain once again. A feeling of reproachful anger then overwhelms the mind and it results in active hatred or aversion. Thus, aversion too is a product of ignorance.

स्वरसवाही विदुषोऽपि तथारूढोऽभिनिवेशः ।।९।।

The fear of death is natural to everybody, and it affects even the learned.—9

All living creatures—from the smallest insect to the most evolved, to wit, the human being—are tormented by the fear of death. All the time they move about with this "unaccountable" fear. Yet this fear is not really unaccountable. For the terror or fright of facing death is, in fact, a residuum in the Unconscious that has been brought forward from a previous birth or births. The earlier painful experience of death subsists in the unconscious mind, and it is this that creates a terror in the present life of all creatures. There is thus an instinctive revulsion against death in any form in all living creatures. Even learned people, who should know better, entertain some such thoughts as: "Let me not be parted from this body," knowing fully well that death and dissolution of the body are inevitable.

ते प्रतिप्रसवहेयाः सूक्ष्माः ।।१०।।

They should be rejected and thrown back to their finer forms.—10

All the aforementioned propensities in the mind are *kleśa*, and all these afflictions are rooted in ignorance. Hence it is ignorance that must be tackled first. However to do so it is necessary first of all to identify the culprit.

Ignorance, it is observed, exists in a fine or subtle state, although its progeny, viz. egoism, fondness, aversion and yearning for life, appear in gross forms. The remedy, therefore, would seem to lie in tackling the products first. These should all be rejected. In other words the effects should be pushed back to their common cause. How this can be done is explained in the *sūtra* that follows.

ध्यानहेयास्तद्वृत्तयः ।।११।।

Those propensities should be rejected by means of meditation.—11

The way to tackle those gross by-products of ignorance is now told. Their gross form, it is advised, should be demolished and reduced to their fine form by means of meditation. The fine form, of course, is ignorance itself,which exists in a subtle form. So the first step is to restrict this ignorance to its own confines and in its pristine form. The idea is that once it is thus restricted it would be unable to yield its by-products of egoism, aversion, desires, etc. which, after all, are its excretions and need to be cleansed.

The next step is to remove the subsisting impurities with the detergent of intense concentration. Just as dirt in a soiled piece of cloth is washed away with a detergent, or just as impurities in a metal are burnt up when treated in fire, in a similar way, the gross forms of ignorance disappear when those are exposed to the intense concentration of the mind.

क्लेशमूलः कर्माशयो दृष्टादृष्टजन्मवेदनीयः ।।१२।।

The reservoir of actions performed, whether in this (seen) or another (unseen) life, is the source of afflictions.—12

Karma (actions) is a continued process. It collects in the *karmāśaya* (storehouse of *karma*) where all actions, physical as well as mental, and whether performed in this or in a previous life or lives, find a place. In due course these actions (cause) are transmuted into afflictions (effect), and then the latter are experienced in life by the creature to whom the *karmāśaya* belongs. In other words, afflictions are the fruit of a creature's self-performed actions.

This *karmāśaya* or storehouse of *karma* is always full. Because, as some of the *karma* in it get transmuted and expended in one life, others are added on to the collection when fresh *karma* are performed in the course of the same life. This goes on from life to life, and the collection remains almost constant. For, the span of each life being limited, the fund of *karma* is never totally spent up in one life. The balance is carried over to the next life, and thence to the next, and so on. In this way, *karma*, and the fruits of *karma* in the shape of afflictions, become a part of each living creature.

This continuity, however, can be terminated by practising yoga in the prescribed manner.

सति मूले तद्विपाको जात्यायुर्भोगाः ।।१३।।

So long as the root of *karma* is there, it is bound to sprout (and transmute) into different kinds of life, lengths of life and types of experience.—13

It is now clear that *karmāśaya* or the Karma Pool is the source of all afflictions. But how is it that these afflictions are not uniform for all? In all creatures they seem to differ not only in respect of quality and quantity but also in respect of the length of time during which they subsist. The reason for such variations is now being explained.

Jāti (species), *āyu* (longevity) and *bhoga* (quanta of experience) are determined by the nature of contents in each individual's *karmāśaya.* Thus the quality of the predominating *karma* in a *karmāśaya* decides the *nature* of the next birth, including the genus of life, *environment* in which that birth shall take place and the *period* needed to consume a certain quantum of acquired *karma.* For, the environment must provide necessary opportunity to consume one's own *karma* through suitable experience of pleasure and pain. In this way, each insect, reptile, bird, fish, animal or human being is the product of its own self-acquired *karma* and experiences exactly the sort of life it deserves. In other words, each life is pre-determined by its own past actions.

ते ह्लादपरितापफलाः पुण्यापुण्यहेतुत्वात्।।१४।।

They bear fruit as pleasure and pain, caused by virtue and vice.—14

As we have seen, *karma* gets transmuted into afflictions, which then begin to bear fruit in the shape of pleasures and pains. *Hlāda* (happiness), however, is always transient, for invariably it is followed by *paritāpa* (regret)—and pain is inherent in all forms of regret. Hence both pleasure and pain have common parentage in *kleśa*, which remains the primal cause of all types of pain, including those which come in the guise of pleasure. This dual (pleasure pain) nature is due to the dual character of *karma* in the *karmasaya* where both virtue and vice are collected.

परिणामतापसंस्कारदुःखैर्गुणवृत्तिविरोधाच्च दुःखमेव सर्वं विवेकिनः।।१५।।

To the wise, these transmuted afflictions are but sorrows born of past impressions (of *karma*) and the conflict of Qualities.—15

A *vivekinaḥ* is one who can discriminate between the unreal and the real and arrive at the correct conclusion. Such a person ultimately finds out the real character of *kleśa* which, of course, is all sorrow. To him *kleśa*, irrespective of the form in which it may appear, becomes instantly apparent in its true form, and he looks upon it as the real cause of his distractions. He knows that, what at first sight seems a pleasure, has really pain behind it. For all pleasures are either preceded or followed by pain in the form of unhappiness and regret—unhappiness when the pleasure does not come as desired, and regret when it has passed over. The consequence of experiencing pleasure, too, is often painful—such as the reaction known as "hangover" which is followed by fresh cravings for pleasure.

All this is perfectly clear to the discriminating one, and he therefore abhors afflictions in every form. To him the slightest sorrow is a source of distraction even as a minute bit of silk thread getting into the eye causes a lot of irritation! A sorrow causes annoyance, which is a form of anger, and anger inevitably results in regret, which again is a form of sorrow. Thus there is a chain of pleasure-regret-annoyance-sorrow-craving-pleasure, etc.

Again, pleasure is an indeterminable quality. What is pleasure at one time may not prove to be so on another occasion, and what is pleasure to one is not so to another. This is proved by the saying: "one man's meat is another man's poison." Thus a thing becomes pleasurable only when it is *liked* and the same thing, when not liked, is painful.

Pain is experienced in different ways. Some pains are directly felt, as when we touch a piece of hot iron. Others are indirectly felt, as when a dear one suffers and we are sorry. Still others come in the form of painful memories, emanating from past impressions in the mind. A fourth type is felt, first as pleasure and then as pain; it is in fact pain sugarcoated with pleasure!

The wise one can discriminate all four types. He can not only trace each to its source in the *karmāśaya,* but also master the process of their transmutation caused by interaction of the three primal Qualities of Nature—*sattva, rajas* and *tamas.* Painful sorrow, to him, is thus the product of the natural conflict of Qualities as seen, for instance, between the controller and the controlled.

हेयं दुःखमनागतम्।।१६।।

Sorrows that are yet to come should be rejected.—16

Anāgatam (unarrived) refers to sorrows that have not yet manifested themselves, i.e., not yet transmuted from *karma* into *kleśa.* Their transmutation, it is advised, should be prevented, so that there is no further accretion of affliction in the mind. The past ones, anyhow, are past. Without fresh arrivals adding to the collection, the existing ones would be more manageable and can be tackled more effectively by the process of intense concentration.

Rejection of the "unarrived," therefore, is essential even as a matter of tactics.

द्रष्टृदृश्ययोः संयोगो हेयहेतुः ।।१७।।

The cause (of such sorrows) is the link between the seer and the seen, and this should be broken.—17

Here the technique is further explained. It consists of snapping the link between the seer and the seen, thus separating the two. When the seer (mind) is separated from the seen (afflictions), the link that causes the perception would not be there and hence there would be no more perception of afflictions by the mind. The natural flow of *kleśa,* i.e., its transmutation from fine into the gross state, would then cease because there would be no more contact between the cause and its effect. The source of supply is thus dammed.

प्रकाशक्रियास्थितिशीलं भूतेन्द्रियात्मकं भोगापवर्गार्थं दृश्यम् ।।१८।।

The seen is composed of fine Elements of Nature, endowed with the qualities of brilliance, motion and fixity, and transmuted into gross forms for purposes of perception by the senses.—18

"The seen" covers the entire gross world, including the senses which help to perceive it. Nature, as we have seen, has two phases: fine and gross. In its fine form it exists, but is not perceived because of the extra-fine particles of Elements (*tanmātras*) which are beyond the range of our sensual organs. In the gross form, however, these very Elements appear as earth, water, fire, air and sky (quintessence). They then become perceivable, and are duly cognized by the senses in their various gross form as "the seen" universe.

All gross matter carry in them the three basic Qualities of Nature, viz. brilliance, motion and inertia, designated respectively as *sattva, rajas* and *tamas.* In the ideal staste, *rajas* (force) and *tamas* (inertia) are held in equilibrium by *sattva* (immaculateness). However, constant intermixture and coalition of the three Qualities leads to the production of fresh gross matter of varied size and shape suitable for perception by the senses. In other words, it is only when matter turns gross that it is "accepted" by the senses: it is then passed on to the mind for its "enjoyment" and "consumption" (*bhogā-pavarga*).

विशेषाविशेषलिङ्गमात्रालिङ्गानि गुणपर्वाणि ।।१९।।

Phases of the Qualities are specific, non-specific, pseudo-physical and non-physical.—19

As has been stated earlier (I.45) Matter exists in four different forms: specific, non-specific, pseudo-physical and non-physical. The specific is the manifested gross form, non-specific is gross but unmanifested, pseudo-physical is fine but manifested and non-physical is fine and wholly unmanifested. When it is gross, the qualities constituting Matter are clearly defined and can be easily differentiated. When it is fine, these very qualities cannot be differentiated and so they remain undefined. When it is fine but manifest (such as intelligence), it is called pseudo-physical. And when Matter exists as extra-fine particles of Elements, and therefore totally unmanifested, it is then in its ultimate non-physical, non-manifested subtle state.

द्रष्टा दृशिमात्रः शुद्धोऽपि प्रत्ययानुपश्यः।।२०।।

The seer's work is to be see only; it remains unaffected by the seen.—20

Now the attributes of "the seer" are explained. The ultimate seer is not the mind—as appears falsely—but the Self. The Self is the real seer, and its job is to see only—that is, to be a witness to all that is presented before it by the mind. The latter is only a reflector that reflects the "seen" (sensed) world. However, the Self sees all without reacting in any way to whatever is seen by it and without getting involved in the good and bad character of the "seen" presented before it. It remains impeccable (*śuddha* = pure); that is, not liable to sin. The objects cognized by the mind are all coloured (biased) in the sense that those are indiscriminately selected by the mind; the Self is not affected by that colouring.

तदर्थ एव दृश्यस्यात्मा।।२१।।

The Self exists for that purpose of seeing alone (and for nothing else).—21

Mind and Matter combine in a creature. Actually it is the Self (soul) and Nature (physical body) that come together to form aliving being. The author here explains the cause of this combination—or rather the purpose for which the soul—itself a part of the Universal Soul—gets associated with Matter to form a living creature.

This purpose is stated to be "to see". But to see what? To see, it is explained, that the constituted Matter duly experiences the products of its own *karma.* This Matter, as we have seen, exists in the form of intelligence as well as a combination of the five Elements. Each such constituted creature is thus destined to "enjoy" the fruits of its own *karma* transmuted into various forms of *kleśa.* The Self merely witnesses the "enjoyment" which, as it happens, continues over a series of lives, punctuated with deaths and births. The common bondage of soul and body continues for an indefinite period until the Karma Pool is exhausted, or until this Pool is isolated and neutralized by means of yoga. Then only the Self is released from its duty "to see", and hence is emancipated.

कृतार्थं प्रति नष्टमप्यनष्टं तदन्यसाधारणत्वात्॥२२॥

When that is finished (completed), it (world phenomena) is over and not yet over, being necessary for others.—22

It has been said above that the Self is here for the sole purpose of seeing to the fulfilment of a creature's *karma* which appear in the form of world phenomena. The question may be asked, what happens to world phenomena when the Self's purpose is over and it gets emancipated? Normally, when the Self is no longer here, the world phenomena too should disappear. But this does not happen.

The paradox is explained by the words: "It is over and not yet over" (*naṣṭam-api-anaṣṭam*). World phenomena in fact exist to help *all* souls to "enjoy" the fruits of their respective *karmāśaya* so that, when one particular soul is liberated, the *karmāśaya* of several others remain to be "exhausted". Moreover, emancipation does not come to all at one and the same time. The world phenomena, therefore, must continue for the sake of other souls yet to be emancipated.

स्वस्वामिशक्त्योः स्वरूपोपलब्धिहेतुः संयोगः॥२३॥

Contact of two forces—that of the seer (master) and the seen—causes an object to assume its own form.—23

There is an intrinsic force in both the seer as well as the seen. While the seen (object) has its own force, the controlling or master force is that of the seer. The union of these two forces produces cognition, thereby enabling the seer to enjoy (experience) the seen (object). Thus the cause of enjoyment (experience) is this union or contact, which alone makes it possible for the seer to see the seen (object) in the desired form. In this manner all worldly objects pander to the wishes of the seeing mind.

तस्य हेतुरविद्या।।२४।।

Ignorance is its cause.—24

Now, the cause of this contact is nothing else but ignorance. Ignorance (*avidyā*), as has been explained earlier, is characterized by its lack of discriminative knowledge. This creates a sense of illusion in the mind. The illusion then lends a false shape to the seen (object), which appears in a form totally different from its real form. In other words, ignorance misguides the mind and keeps it bound to the wrong thing. However, its own strength rests wholly on the "contact".

तदभावात् संयोगाभावो हानं तद्दृशेः कैवल्यम्।।२५।।

Its absence means the absence of contact; then, when the seeing is eliminated, there is oneness.—25

The logic is clear. As long as the seer (mind) is in touch (contact) with the seen (world phenomena) it remains involved in the act of seeing. But when that contact ceases, the seeing too comes to an end. And since the cause of this contact is ignorance, the elimination of this cause ends the contact between the seer and the seen. Thereafter (owing to the snapping of the contact) the seeing mind, which is otherwise attracted to and lulled by the false world phenomena, gets isolated. It then takes on its true form—the form of the Self—and merges with the latter. Thus there is *Kaivalya* or Oneness.

विवेकख्यातिरविप्लवा हानोपायः।।२६।।

Incessant discrimination is the way to destroy that ignorance.—26

Here the way is told how that ignorance may be ended. *Viveka-khyāti* is the discriminative knowledge that enables one to distinguish the Real from the Unreal. When such discrimination is *a-viplava* (abiding), that is, not merely temporary but enduring—it grows and gathers strength and then dislodges the ignorance dwelling in the mind. Then, in the face of incessant discrimination, the Unreal gradually fades away, leaving behind the Real.

The emphasis, however, is on *a-viplava* because a short spell of discrimination may only temporarily dispel ignorance which, when first dislodged, has a tendency to recoil with redoubled force. Hence continuous discrimination is advised. Abiding discrimination leaves no room for the ignorance to return.

तस्य सप्तधा प्रान्तभूमिः प्रज्ञा ।।२७।।

The approach to that Highest Wisdom is seven-fold.—27

That state of everlasting discrimination is no doubt the highest form of Knowledge. However, this state is reached only by stages.

Thus the approach (*prānta-bhūmi*—foreground) to it passes through seven identifiable phases. The *first* phase comprises the yogi's clear awareness of what is to be done; there is no more wavering as to whether the *samādhi* is to be begun or not. The *second* phase begins with discrimination—trying to distinguish between the Real and the Unreal. The *third* is devoted to separating the two, i.e., removing the cause (ignorance) from the effect (*kleśa*). The *fourth* brings in satisfaction and confidence produced by the successful efforts made so far.

All four phases above are in the nature of preparation; the next three yield the fruit of the work accomplished up to this stage. Thus, in the *fifth* phase the yogi's mind is completely rid of all erstwhile obstacles, leaving behind no trace of *kleśa* whatsoever, In the *sixth* phase the mind becomes competent to dispense with even the qualities that constitute pseudo-physical Matter, such as intelligence. Finally, in the *seventh* phase, the mind is firmly installed in its true form, i.e., it becomes Self-like. This is the highest form of Knowledge—a state when the duality of mind and Self disappears and the two merge into one. This oneness is *Kaivalya* or Emancipation.

योगाङ्गानुष्ठानादशुद्धिक्षये ज्ञानदीप्तिराविवेकख्यातेः ।।२८।।

Through the practice of yoga disciplines—and thereby cleansing of the impurities—comes the Light of Discriminative Knowledge.—28

Yogāṅga (limbs of yoga) are the various disciplines that are prescribed to help combat ignorance and develop the discriminative power. Discriminative Knowledge in fact is the key to that Highest Wisdom called *Prajñā*.

A-viveka is non-discrimination or lack of discrimination resulting from the clouding of the mind by ignorance. The light of Knowledge dispels the darkness caused by ignorance, and the mind then gets its discriminative knowledge. In this process the various disciplines of yoga are useful and are recommended for cleansing the impurities left in the mind by ignorance and which normally act as obstacles in the way of attaining discriminative knowledge. The practice of yoga disciplines helps to wipe out all impurities in the mind by kindling in it the Light of Discrimination.

यमनियमासनप्राणायामप्रत्याहारधारणाध्यानसमाधयोऽष्टावङ्गानि।।२९।।

Yama, niyama, āsana, prāṇāyāma, pratyāhāra, dhāraṇā, dhyāna, and *samādhi* are the eight limbs of yoga.—29

The prescribed disciplines are eight in number. Of these the first seven are in the nature of camps to be established on the way to the summit, viz. *samādhi* or superconsciousness.

Yama are the restrictions, *niyama* the rules to be observed, *āsana* are the physical postures that help, *prāṇāyāma* is breath-control, *pratyāhāra* is control of the senses, *dhāraṇā* is limited concentration such as fixing the mind to any one object, *dhyāna* is continued concentration for a length of time, and *samādhi* is the state of superconsciousness. The first five help *samādhi* indirectly and the next two directly. When practised conscientiously and in due order they lead to superconsciousness.

अहिंसासत्यास्तेयब्रह्मचर्यापरिग्रहा यमा:।।३०।।

The restrictions (*yama*) are: Non-violence, Truthfulness, Non-stealing, Continence, and Non-receiving.—30

The different restrictive rules are now listed. First is the observance of Non-violence (*ahiṃsā*) in thought, word and deed; that is, violence in any form is to be abjured. Next is Truth (*satya*). A correct, uncoloured and well-weighed thought, when expressed faithfully in word or deed, means a restraint on the mind's tendency to bypass accuracy. Non-stealing (*a-steya*) is a curb on covetousness which prompts one to grab, covertly or overtly, what belongs to others. *Brahmacarya* (continence) is control of the sexual propensity. Non-receiving (*a-parigraha*) is a discipline of self-denial when gifts and services of others are not accepted. The idea is that the yogi should never place himself under an obligation to others.

All these rules are obviously intended to keep the yogi restricted to the straight and narrow path. Like all disciplines, restriction forms a basic feature of yoga.

एते तु जातिदेशकालसमयानवच्छिन्ना: सार्वभौमा महाव्रतम्।।३१।।

These constitute the Universal Code of Conduct (to be observed) irrespective of kind, place, time or occasion.—31

The restrictive rules enumerated in the previous *sūtra* are to be observed at all times and on all occasions irrespective of the location or class of the being concerned. These have been designated as the Great Vows (*mahāvratam*) and must not be violated on any pretext or by twisting their meaning in any manner, or practised with a mental reservation.

For example, it will not be perfect non-violence if the yogi were to decide that he would not kill only godly persons, and/or certainly not in a place of pilgrimage; or on a festival day; and/or never, never on the 14th day of the moon!

The same kind of conditional observance of the rules regarding Truth, Continence, etc. would no doubt make a mockery of the Universal Code of Conduct, which is meant to be observed both in letter and spirit.

शौचसन्तोषतपःस्वाध्यायेश्वरप्रणिधानानि नियमाः।।३२।।

Purity, Contentment, Austerity, Study, and Devotion to God are the regulations (*niyama*).—32

The restrictive rules (*yama*) stated earlier were in the nature of "Don'ts". The regulations now being prescribed are the "Do's"

Purity (*śauca*) is of two kinds: internal and external. The external is accomplished by washing the body with clay (in the absence of soap) and water. Internal purity is achieved when the impure thoughts that defile the mind are replaced with clean thoughts of friendliness, joy, contentment, etc.

The other "Do's" are: practice of austerity, practice of study and devotion to God—already mentioned as basic qualifications of a yogi in the opening *sūtra* of this chapter.

वितर्कबाधने प्रतिपक्षभावनम्।।३३।।

Obstructive thoughts are to be countered with their opposites.—33

Another suggestion is that wrong thoughts should be fought with right ones.

Vitarka (doubt) is the nagging, obstructive thought that pesters the mind in season and out of season. Such obstructive thoughts should be countered with thoughts of exactly the opposite quality.

For example, hatred and anger against another person can be controlled by generating thoughts of friendliness and peace towards him. Similarly, the impulse to tell a lie, or to grab what is known to be another's, can be checked by firmly reminding oneself of the vows of Truth and Non-stealing. This is the way to regulate all unseemly thoughts.

वितर्का हिंसादयः कृतकारितानुमोदिता लोभक्रोधमोहपूर्विका
मृदुमध्याधिमात्रा दुःखाज्ञानानन्तफला इति प्रतिपक्षभावनम्।।३४।।

Obstructive thoughts are those that imply doubt, violence, etc. provoked by avarice, anger or delusion. No matter whether these result in acts actually done, got done or only endorsed, and irrespective of the measure—mild, substantial or excessive—in which those exist, they always bring endless sorrow and ignorance. These are to be countered with their opposites.—34

Obstructive thoughts appear in different forms and in different measure. Initially they are all found in the mind in the form of either *vitarka* (doubt) or *hiṃsā* (hostility). These two carry in them the qualities of *tamas* and *rajas*—fixity and motion—which, as we know, are in eternal conflict. Since modification is the charater of mind, ultimately Doubt and Hostility change into Avarice, Anger and Delusion. The last three find expression in action at some suitable moment.

This action, however, appears in different forms. Some are *kṛta* (personally done), others are *kārita* (got done by another) and yet others are *anumodita* (endorsed or approved actions of others). To illustrate: a man may be killed direct in a fit of passion; *or* he may be got killed by directing another person to do so for him; *or* the killing of that person by another (without one's direct or indirect involvement) is merely approved and secretly gloated over. Each such action is a form of *hiṃsā* and hence reprehensible: in the mind they generate obstructive thoughts that bear the elements of Sorrow and Ignorance along with their disturbing properties of *rajas* and *tamas* respectively.

Similarly, Doubt (*vitarka*)—a perplexing matter by itself—is made worse by Delusion which thrives on confusion created in the mind when it is unable to choose between "do-ables" and "not do-ables". This stage is known as *moha-pūrvikā* (Delusion-filled). It generates anger or avarice, which ultimately finds expression in some kind of action as described above. The three—Anger, Avarice and Delusion—however have common moorings in Egoism.

As for the strength of each such action, the same varies and is normally related to the quantum of Avarice, Anger or Delusion that may have already got generated in the mind. Thus, these may be found in either a mild, substantial or excessive measure in direct proportion to the extent of avarice, anger or delusion then prevailing in the mind. As explained in the previous chapter (I.22) these strengths are further divisible into their sub-strengths, thus making a total of 27 types and degrees of Avarice, Anger and Delusion that the yogi must identify for himself.

अहिंसाप्रतिष्ठायां तत्सन्निधौ वैरत्यागः।।३५।।

When Non-violence is established, hostility recoils in its presence.—35

Now are explained the methods by which these obstructive thoughts may be countered. First of all *yama*, i.e., the restrictive rules that constitute the *mahāvratam*, have to be practised. Out of these, Non-violence (*ahiṃsā*) is the most potent for countering hostile thoughts in the mind. Non-violence is the opposite of Violence (*hiṃsā*) and as such, when this is infused into the mind and is firmly established there, Violence recedes in its presence. The mood of hostility then changes automatically into one of peace and neutrality.

सत्यप्रतिष्ठायां क्रियाफलाश्रयित्वम्।।३६।।

When Truth is established, the means of action are unnecessary.—36

Truth is strictly correct and impartial. It does not depend upon any device for its manifestation. It is self-evident. Hence, when this Truth is firmly installed in the mind, it dispenses with the 'means' of action and manifests itself directly and automatically. In other words, a really and wholly true thought turns into a true deed without that deed having been consciously performed. Moreover, wrong (obstructive) thoughts have no place where Truth prevails wholly.

अस्तेयप्रतिष्ठायां सर्वरत्नोपस्थानम्।।३७।।

When Non-stealing is established, all treasures present themselves.—37

Non-stealing pre-supposes non-desire. When there is no desire and no craving for any object whatsoever, then all objects lose their respective worth, or rather they become worthless. Then there is no question of a pick and choose, because all are readily available, awaiting to be beckoned by some desire or other in the mind. But when those desires are held back, the yogi is left alone in the midst of unsought treasures. All kinds of pleasurable objects present themselves before him, but they lie around uncared for.

ब्रह्मचर्यप्रतिष्ठायां वीर्यलाभ:।।३८।।

When Continence is established, virility is gained.—38

When true continence is practised, the capacity to retain the sexual fluid increases and, with that sort of control, the vital energy pervades the entire body and mind. The yogi's mental and physical efficiency are then at their best.

अपरिग्रहस्थैर्ये जन्मकथन्तासंबोध:।।३९।।

When Non-receiving is established, there is awareness of the past life's events.—39

Aparigraha (non-receiving) has been described earlier (II.30) as non-acceptance of gifts and services from others. In an extreme form, however, this non-receiving is also the non-receiving of one's own body, i.e., a reluctance to have a re-birth. The yogi works to this end as he mentally rejects the idea of a reconstituted body and tries to make the most of his present birth to get emancipated once for all. This underlying consciousness helps him to re-double his efforts, fight back the obstructive thoughts with discriminative knowledge and attain *Prajñā* (Highest Wisdom). The last one confers omniscience upon him, when he becomes aware of all past, present and future simultaneously.

शौचात् स्वाङ्गे जुगुप्सा परैरसंसर्ग:।।४०।।

With Purity established, there is then aversion for one's own body as well as for other bodies.—40

Now the regulations (*niyama*) are explained.

As stated earlier, the five *niyama* are: Purity, Contentment, Austerity, Self-study and Devotion to God. Purity of one's own self naturally comes first. It includes both physical and mental purity. When the yogi ponders upon the real nature of his physical body, he recognizes it as a mere accretion to his real Self and so develops an aversion for it. The body, anyhow, is always internally impure: this knowledge also brings on a feeling of disgust.

In the same way the purity of mind, when it is established after a course of diligent mind-control, makes the yogi conscious of the impurities existing in other minds and bodies. Then there is a disgust for those other minds and bodies, and there is no desire at all for contact with those, however attractive they may appear outwardly.

सत्वशुद्धि सौमनस्यैकाग्रतेन्द्रियजयात्मदर्शनयोग्यत्वानि च।।४१।।

Purity of mind means cheerfulness, one-pointedness, control of senses, and a capacity to see the self.—41

Sattva-śuddhi (complete purity) is achieved when the *sattva* (immaculateness) is exclusive, i.e., absolutely pure (*śuddha*). The symptoms of this state of mind are: cheerfulness, capacity to concentrate, capacity to control the senses and capacity to understand the Self. All these indicate the mind's clarity at its best.

Soumanasya (cheerfulness) is the mind's joy at not experiencing any regret. It is a feeling both of satisfaction and happiness. *Ekāgrata* (one-pointedness) is the mind's capacity to remain fixed on one object unwaveringly. *Indriya-jaya* (conquest of senses) is the mind's unquestioned supremacy over the senses, and *ātma-darśana-yogyatva* is the mind's competency to see the Self.

Total purity thus is the result of, first, *sattva* suffusing the mind, then making it cheerful and hence capable of concentration, then subduing the senses and, finally, knowing the Self.

सन्तोषादनुत्तमसुखलाभ:।।४२।।

With Contentment comes supreme joy.—42

Santoṣa (contentment) is the state of mind when it is fully satisfied with the achievement it had set out to achieve. The joy then experienced is extreme in its nature, so that this felicity is in no way comparable to the kind of happiness experienced by the enjoyment of any external object or objects.

कायेन्द्रियसिद्धिरशुद्धिक्षयात्तपस:।।४३।।

Austerity purges the impurities and helps mastery over body and senses.—43

The different forms of *tapas* (austerity) have already been explained (II.1). The practice of such austerity rids the mind of its impurities, i.e., wrong thoughts, and helps to control the senses, thereby making both body and mind fit for further efforts necessary for the purpose of *samādhi.*

स्वाध्यायादिष्टदेवतासम्प्रयोगः।।४४।।

Study of scriptures leads to direct contact with the cherished deity.—44

Swādhyāya literally means 'self-study.' The word is used here, however, to denote the sort of devoted study and recitation of Vedic *mantras* which result in concentration and, ultimately, visualization by the yogi of his own cherished form of deity.

समाधिसिद्धिरीश्वरप्रणिधानात्।।४५।।

Great devotion to God leads to *samādhi.*—45

Praṇidhāna (great devotion) implies sustained effort with an element of concentration in it (I.23). The word, in fact, is an alternative for deep meditation. This sort of great devotion to God naturally leads to *samādhi,* when the yogi is face to face with his God.

स्थिरसुखमासनम्।।४६।।

That which is a steady and comfortable posture is *āsana.*—46

Having stated the rules and regulations (*yama* and *niyama*) the author now gives the necessary directions for starting the practice of yoga.

First, *āsana* or positioning of the body. A correct position for the body during performance of yoga is the one that keeps the body steady and comfortable. There is a large variety of *āsanas*—such as Padmāsana, Siddhāsana, Swastikāsana, etc.—which are described in Book II (*G.S.,* II.1-38). The yogi, however, is advised here to select the one that is most suitable for him, bearing in mind that it should keep him steady and comfortable throughout the period he performs yoga.

प्रयत्नशैथिल्यानन्त्यसमापत्तिभ्याम्।।४७।।

. . . that sort which is effortless and lasts until the completion of the *samādhi.*—47

The "suitable" *āsana* is further explained.

The ideal *āsana* is one that can be maintained effortlessly for a long period. It should not cause stiffness in the limbs or any other kind of physical discomfort that might distract the mind. In other words, there should be no body-consciousness and the mind should be left free to project itself, if necessary, to endless space. A perfect *āsana* is indicated only when the yogi becomes confident that it needs no effort on his part either to get into that posture or to maintain it over an indefinite period without being conscious of the fact.

ततो द्वन्द्वानभिघातः ।।४८।।

Then all dualities are destroyed.—48

Dvandva (duality) is the conflict of opposites—such as heat and cold, pleasure and pain, praise and blame, amity and hostility, knowledge and ignorance, and so on. This eternal conflict of opposite forces, to which all living beings are constantly exposed, is the cause of their distractions.

In a perfect *āsana*—which is steady and comfortable and yet makes one oblivious of the physical environment—the yogi goes beyond the pale of such dualities. These then cease to exist for him.

तस्मिन् सति श्वासप्रश्वासयोर्गतिविच्छेदः प्राणायामः ।।४९।।

With that achieved, comes *prāṇāyāma* or control of the rate of inspiration and expiration.—49

The next step in yoga is the practice of *prāṇāyāma*.

Prāṇāyāma (control of *prāṇa*) is the regulation of the vital (subtle) air—as distinct from *apāna* (gross air)—that is breathed in and that brings with it the essence of life into the body. The measure and rate of its ingress and egress, and the period for which it may stay within the body each time, are carefully determined to obtain the maximum benefit of the fine particles of Elements (*tanmātras*) that nourish the body and mind of every living creature.

It has been observed that, normally, the rate of breathing (inspiration and expiration) varies according to the amount of physical and mental effort required for an occasion. Thus the "stress" in the mind at a particular moment determines how much, or how quickly, the outside air is to be taken in, how long it is to be retained inside, and then how quickly it is to be released. The control of this erratic behaviour of the breath is effected by means of *prāṇāyāma*.

बाह्याभ्यन्तरस्तम्भवृत्तिः देशकालसंख्याभिः परिदृष्टो दीर्घसूक्ष्मः ।।५०।।

That outward, inward and stationary propensity (of the breath) is determined short or long in respect of place, time and number.—50

Prāṇāyāma is further explained here.

Normal breathing is a *vṛtti* (propensity) according to which the breath automatically goes in, stays awhile inside, and then goes out again. This process varies, as stated above, according to circumstance. *Prāṇāyāma* seeks to regulate this process by specifying the place, time and number of each breath constituting the inspiration, expiration and retention of the air. In yogic language these are known as *pūraka* (filling in), *recaka* (throwing out) and *kumbhaka* (filled pitcher). With the help of *prāṇāyāma* the time, place and number of these three functions are controlled.

"Place" here signifies the distance from the nostrils, say, about twenty centimetres, to which the breath is restricted. Thus the air thrown out and the air filled in should not exceed this range.

"Time" is the time that is taken (a) in filling in this quantity of air, (b) the duration for which it is to be retained in the lungs, and (c) the time over which its release from the lungs should be spread out. Thus if the filling-in time is, say, five seconds, the retention time must be twenty seconds, and the throwing-out time should be spread over ten seconds. This ratio of 1: 4: 2 must be maintained whatever may be the unit that is adopted for the in-take. For purposes of practice, the maximum period of retention (*kumbhaka*) should not exceed 36 seconds, i.e., 9 for *pūraka*, 36 for *kumbhaka* and 18 for *recaka*.

"Number" relates to the number of times that this exercise may be performed at one sitting. A *kumbhaka* should be abandoned as soon as an *udghata* (jerk)—coming up from the navel and hitting the brain—is felt. This is the warning signal that the respiratory system would stand no further strain.

बाह्याभ्यन्तरविषयाक्षेपी चतुर्थः ।।५१।।

Reflection upon external and internal objects is the fourth.—51

Place, time and number are the three aspects of *prāṇāyāma* that have been mentioned above. There is yet a fourth one which the author is now revealing. This is linking of the breathing action to the action of the mind. In other words, it is *kumbhaka* practised simultaneously with concentration of the mind.

It is observed that whenever the mind is suddenly called upon to concentrate, the breath is automatically held up. It would appear that all serious thinking calls for a short halt in the act of breathing, proving thereby that the two acts of breathing and thinking are in a way interlinked. It follows, therefore, that if the mind is consciously concentrated for any length of time it would certainly assist in the retention of breath for the same period.

This interdependence of thought and breath is exploited in the fourth phase of *prāṇāyāma*, when the mind is deliberately fixed on some external or internal object with a view to prolonging the period of the *kumbhaka*. The net result, therefore, is twofold: concentration helps to prolong the *kumbhaka*, and *kumbhaka* helps to prolong the concentration.

The "internal" objects are the various *cakras* (psychic centres) within the body described in detail in Books I and II.

ततः क्षीयते प्रकाशावरणम्।।५२।।
With that is lifted the veil over the Light.—52

The benefit of practising this fourth form of *prāṇāyāma* is now stated.

This kind of *kumbhaka*, which combines the forces of body and mind, helps to clear up the foggy atmosphere in the mind and brushes up its pristine intelligence, which then shines forth like a strong light from which its shade has been removed.

धारणासु च योग्यता मनसः।।५३।।
And the mind then gains the ability to hold on.—53

Dhāraṇā (adherence) is the mind's capacity to hold on to one object or idea for some length of time. When the mind is scattered (*vikṣipta*) with all manner of contrary thoughts, it becomes necessary for these thoughts to be collected into one heap so that the mind may easily concentrate upon one rather than the many. Sticking to this one "object," and not allowing the same to be strewn about again, is the task of *dhāraṇa*. It is the prelude to sustained concentration.

स्वविषयासम्प्रयोगे चित्तस्वरूपानुकारे इन्द्रियाणां प्रत्याहारः।।५४।।
When the senses get detached from their own objects of perception and assume the form of mind—it is *pratyāhāra*.—54

Next comes the control of the senses.

Pratyāhāra (retreat) is renunciation by the senses of their own respective objcets of interest and their return to their master, viz. the mind. While seeing, hearing, smelling, touching or tasting, the various senses move forward to grasp their chosen objects. But when the mind asserts its superiority and firmly commands them to retreat, they follow the mind meekly—"even as bees follow the queen-bee!" This reversing process is *pratyāhāra.*

ततः परमा वश्यतेन्द्रियाणाम्।।५५।।

Then the senses are fully subjugated.—55

The practice of *pratyāhāra,* which means assertion of the mind of its superiority over the senses, ultimately leads to complete taming of the senses, so that in future they are never tempted by even the most alluring of objects and never again dart out to meet them. The control is full and final.

Here ends Chapter II of the *Pātañjala Yogasūtra*
entitled 'Practice of Yoga'.

CHAPTER III

Powers of Yoga

देशबन्धश्चित्तस्य धारणा।।१।।

Limiting the field of the mind is *dhāraṇā*.—1

The previous chapter dealt with yoga practices designed largely to discipline the body and the senses. The remaining three limbs of yoga, viz. *dhāraṇā, dhyāna* and *samādhi* deal exclusively with the mind.

Dhāraṇā (adherence) is defined here as the mind's ability to hold on to a limited field. The mind's field, as we know, is unlimited: it ranges over all manner of subjects and objects—concrete, abstract and imaginary. The first step, therefore, is to limit this wide range.

External objects, of course, are barred when the senses are withdrawn (*pratyāhāra*). The mind is then left with internal objects only. These latter are mostly structural features within the body, such as the various *cakras* alongside the spinal column, specially those which lie between the navel and the nostrils. When, therefore, the mind is confined to this area, it tends to stick to one or other of these internal "objects" found within the limited field. Moreover, owing to the earlier practice of *prāṇāyāma* and *pratyāhāra* this field, although limited, soon becomes familiar ground for the mind to work in.

तत्र प्रत्ययैकतानता ध्यानम्।।२।।

Unwavering knowledge of one object there is *dhyāna*.—2

In *dhyāna* (contemplation) the field is further constricted. The mind's range and force are restricted to one object to the exclusion of all other internal objects. All other objects then become, so to say, out of bounds for the mind, so that *visadṛśa* (dissimilar) objects do not attract attention and detract the mind. This unwavering attention to one, to the exclusion of everything else, when applied with the full force of knowledge is—*dhyāna.*

तदेवार्थमात्रनिर्भासं स्वरूपशून्यमिव समाधिः।।३।।

By that it (the object) loses its own form and only a glow of its meaning remains. This is *samādhi.*—3

Nirbhāsa (faint glow) is the essence of the object without its form; or, meaning without the sound. As a result of intense concentration upon a single object the form of that object gradually fades away and only its essence or significance remains in a formless guise. The yogi is then aware of the object without the form of object being actually present. This is the *samādhi* state of the mind.

त्रयमेकत्र संयमः।।४।।

The three together is *saṃyama.*—4

Saṃyama (control) is a Tāntric term that denotes all three aforementioned forms of mind-control, viz. *dhāraṇā, dhyāna* and *samādhi* in a collective sense, i.e., when all three operate simultaneously. Henceforward this term has been used throughout whenever such triple-control is indicated.

तज्जयात् प्रज्ञालोकः।।५।।

When that is mastered, there emerges the Light of Highest Wisdom.—5

When that kind of *saṃyama* (control) is practised, and is mastered, the mind's intelligence begins to shine.

This intelligence, however, is only a faint glow of the Highest Wisdom (*Prajñā*). For knowledge in all beings exists in various degrees, such as *samvedanā, buddhi, vitarka, viveka, vijñāna,* and *prajñā.* While in other creatures it is found in a mixed form of *samvedanā* (cognition) and *buddhi* (intelligence), which often take the form of instinct rather than intelligence, in human beings cognition and intelligence have separate identity. The latter enables the mind to reason (*vitarka*) and discriminate (*viveka*), leading up to knowledge (*jñāna*) and finally to its peak, which is *Prajñā* or Highest Wisdom. The aim of yoga is to take the mind up to that summit.

तस्य भूमिषु विनियोगः।।६।।

Its territory is divided.—6

Tasya bhūmi (its territory) refers to the area in which *saṃyama* operates.

This field is made up of both gross as well as fine matter.

The mind's range in fact extends from gross consciousness to the finest subtlety of knowledge. Normally, this field remains littered with all kinds of obstacles in the form of gross consciousness. These are to be removed one by one through the practice of *saṃyama.* Let only subtle knowledge remain.

त्रयमन्तरङ्गं पूर्वेभ्यः ।।७।।

These three are internal, as opposed to the earlier ones.—7

The "earlier ones" refers to *yama, niyama, āsana, prāṇāyāma,* and *pratyāhāra.* As compared to those, the ones now mentioned, viz., *dhāraṇā, dhyāna* and *samādhi* are internal inasmuch as these relate to the mind only.

तदपि बहिरङ्गं निर्बीजस्य।।८।।

Yet these are but external for purposes of the "seedless" (*samādhi*).—8

The "seedless" *samādhi,* as has been explained earlier, is the highest form of *samādhi.* It is also known as A-samprajñāta *samādhi* or *samādhi* without consciousness.

For reaching that highest state of superconsciousness the means of *dhāraṇā, dhyāna* and *samādhi,* although initially used, are no longer necessary when the state has been actually reached. To that extent these three are but "external". In other words, these three become superfluous in the superconscious state.

As distinct from the *sa-bīja* or with consciousness *samādhi*—where the mind is still aware of the triple-control (*saṃyama*) which brings about that state—in the *nir-bīja* (seedless) *samādhi* even the consciousness disappears. That, then, becomes superconsciousness.

व्युत्थाननिरोधसंस्कारयोरभिभव-प्रादुर्भावौ निरोधलक्षणचित्तान्वयो निरोधपरिणामः ।।९।।

Curbing the modifications (appearance and disappearance) of thoughts, as well as the impressions of such curb, is the end-product of Control.—9

Normally, the mind is in one of three states—*kṣipta* (agitated), *mūḍha* (ignorant) and *vikṣipta* (distracted). In all these states *rajas* (passion) and *tamas* (ignorance) predominate and the quality of *sattva* (purity) exists only in a weak measure. The process of control starts when, by entertaining pure thoughts, more of *sattva* is infused into the mind, thereby pushing back both *rajas* and *tamas.* The latter then take a back seat—in other words, are inhibited. Now, since every thought must leave its impression upon the mind, the controlled thoughts too register their own imprints. These however are comparatively innocuous. But when these impressions too are identified and controlled, the result is known as *nirodha-pariṇāma* or the end-product of Control.

Here the *act* of control and the *product* of control are discriminated. The act results in gradual lessening of distractions and the product indicates proportionate increase or gain in strength. The final end-product is Full Control.

तस्य प्रशान्तवाहिता संस्कारात्।।१०।।

With that purification, there is an even flow.—10

Saṃskāra here means purging or purification. This purification becomes evident when the mind assumes a tranquil state and is no more disturbed by distractions.

सर्वार्थतैकाग्रतयोः क्षयोदयौ चित्तस्य समाधि-परिणामः।।११।।

Th end-product of *samādhi* comprises concentration of all essence (meaning) and subvertion of the mind's tendency to modify.—11

Control holds the mind in equipoise. *Samādhi* dispenses with that control. The control, exercised through concentration, tends to bind the thoughts together, while modification tends to proliferate the same. The two are contradictory tendencies, and as a rule operate alternately, i.e., the modification asserts when concentration is relaxed and vice versa.

Samādhi-pariṇāma (end-product of *samādhi*) is that state of mind when this alternating process has ceased and the modifications having been finally and effectively curbed, only concentration subsists. The effort of control is then no longer necessary.

शान्तोदितौ तुल्यप्रत्ययौ चित्तस्यैकाग्रतापरिणामः।।१२।।

The end-product of Concentration is evident when emergence and subsidence (of thoughts) in the mind seem similar.—12

The inherent character of the mind is placidity or evenness, i.e., when there is no modification in it. However, modification is a tendency that is forced upon it by the senses, which keep it constantly engaged in the task of reflecting a horde of internal and external objects which the senses present before it. The mind jumps up to catch each, and the next moment subsides when it prepares for the next jump. When this up and down action is controlled, the inherent balance of the mind is restored and it becomes stable. This is the end-product of Concentration.

एतेन भूतेन्द्रियेषु धर्मलक्षणावस्थापरिणामा व्याख्याता:।।१३।।

In this manner are explained the character, symptom and product of modification of all Elements and the senses.—13

The modifications described so far related to Control, *samādhi* and Concentration. In a similar manner the modification of all Matter, both gross and fine, as well as the senses takes place. The latter belong to three categories: purely physical (*karmendriya*), cognitive (*jñānendriya*) and psychic (*buddhi* or intelligence).

The three-fold modification of Matter in respect of its form, character and condition is its "special character" (*dharmī*).

For example, an earthen pot: it first changes its past form of clay into its solid state of a particular form of pot, and then in course of time breaks and melts away into an indistinguishable fine form. Its character too changes—from particles of dust into moist clay and thence into a hard bowl or pot, and back again into the fine element of earth. The condition changes from fine to gross and again from gross to fine.

Similar modifications take place in the physical, cognitive and psychic field of the senses.

शान्तोदिताव्यपदेश्यधर्मानुपाती धर्मी।।१४।।

The "special character" is the character of emergence, subsidence and obscurity.—14

So what is this "special character"? The "special character," it is explained, is marked by its characteristics of emergence, subsidence and obscurity.

"Emergence" implies the presence of what was not there before but has manifested itself now. It has become the *present.* "Subsidence" presupposes its earlier existence, an existence that is no longer there. It is *past.* "Obscurity," on the other hand, indicates something that we know as existing but which is indistinguishable at the moment, though it may be known later. It is the *future.*

Like *rajas, tamas* and *sattva,* the three (emergence, subsidence and obscurity) are linked in a common bond and are subject to the Law of Cause and Effect. This common bondage is the "special character" called *dharmī.*

The omnigenous character of Matter may perhaps be illustrated by the changes we see in the form and character of water. Water, before it emerges as such, is in the form of condensed moisture or ice. Later, when heated, it turns into liquid and again changes into vapour and eventually is lost in thin air. It is then obscure.

क्रमान्यत्वं परिणामान्यत्वे हेतुः ।।१५।।

Continuity is maintained due to (an unbroken) series of modifications.—15

How is it possible for a single "special character" to have so many different characteristics?

To resolve the doubt it is explained that these various characteristics are in fact linked, and so form one single character. Their unbroken continuity makes the linkage possible. Since modifications continue endlessly, there is never any gap between these characteristics which flow in one continuous stream.

Once again, the earthen pot should exemplify the point. The fine particles of earth, changing into gross dust and then, with moisture, turning into clay to take the shape of a bowl or pot, is an example of the continuity process of modifications that goes on in nature. This continuity may be observed also in the process of disintegration, which reduces the pot back to its original fine form.

In the case of the mind, however, the phases of continuity in modifications are seldom cognized. The emergence, duration and subsidence of a feeling of happiness, for example, are noticed *as a whole* and are not experienced in their separate phases.

परिणामत्रयसंयमादतीतानागतज्ञानम् ।।१६।।

Saṃyama on the three phases of modifications leads to knowledge of Past and Future.—16

Now the benefits of Control, i.e., the triple-control of *dharaṇā, dhyāna* and *samādhi* that the word *saṃyama* signifies.

This kind of triple-control, when it is exercised on the modification of thoughts in the mind, brings certain powers to the mind.

One such power is the knowledge of all past and future events. This knowledge is the outcome of *saṃyama*, which neutralizes the "special character" of modifications stated above.

Thus, when the very cause of modifications, viz. continuity, is destroyed through Absolute Control, the normal flow of Past-Present-Future comes to a halt. Then both Past and Future coalesce with the Present, so that the yogi cognizes all in the present state.

शब्दार्थप्रत्ययानामितरेतराध्यासात् सङ्करस्तत् प्रविभागसंयमात् सर्वभूतरुतज्ञानम्।।१७।।

Knowledge of sounds of all creatures is gained through *saṃyama* when their meaning and significance are known by rearranging and mixing those sounds.—17

Sound is a continuity of syllables, which are its units. A particular order or sequence of these units produces a particular sound. The meaning and significance of a sound, thus, are dependent upon the way the units are arranged. Once the correct sequence of these sound-units are known, the real meaning and significance of the complete sound can also be known.

Saṃyama enables the yogi to analyze *any* sound whatsoever, after breaking it down to its units and re-arranging those if necessary. In this way he gets a full and correct knowledge of the implications of that particular sound.

संस्कारसाक्षात्करणात् पूर्वजातिज्ञानम्।।१८।।

Knowledge of previous life is gained by re-collecting past impressions and bringing those into the present.—18

Saṃskāra (past impressions) is the residuum of all impressions, both past and present, left upon the mind by thoughts that have passed through the mind. *Saṃskāra* thus may be compared to a micro-film that is kept hidden away for future use. It lies deep in the Unconscious but, like the micro-film, it can be taken out, developed and seen whenever necessary.

By means of *saṃyama*, the yogi re-collects his past impressions, re-vitalizes them, and then he has before him the full record of his own previous life or lives.

प्रत्ययस्य परचित्तज्ञानम्।।१९।।

Knowledge of another's mind is gained by concentrating on the apparent.—19

Pratyaya (direct cognition) is the experiencing of an object face to face. The object thus cognized appears always in a concrete physical form.

Such direct and close study (involving application of the method of *saṃyama*) of the physical form of another person—i.e., the physical features of that body—enables the yogi to know the contents of that person's mind.

न तत् सालम्बनं तस्याविषयीभूतत्वात्।।२०।।

That is without means (of senses), being unrelated to objects.—20

Knowledge is normally gained *through* (by means of) the senses. The senses perceive the objects and then carry their individual message for the information of the mind.

But when one mind tries to probe into another mind, the former lacks this "means" of the senses which had actually produced the knowledge in the latter. This deficiency persists even when the yogi has been able, with the aid of his *saṃyama*, to get at the contents of another's mind. As a result he sees only the *effect* prevailing in the other mind without knowing its *cause.* For example, he may correctly identify the blue colour prevailing in another mind without in any way knowing what object it is (or was) that cast that blue shade.

In other words, all reflections in another mind may be clearly distinguished by means of the practice of *saṃyama* except that the *cause* of those reflections shall always remain unidentified.

कायस्य रूपसंयमात् तत्ग्राह्यशक्तिस्तम्भे चक्षु·प्रकाशासंयोगेऽन्तर्धानम्।।२१।।

The body is rendered invisible when *saṃyama* is practised on the ray of light issuing from another's eyes and the same is cut off, neutralizing the power of seeing.—21

The beam of light issuing from one's eyes defines the form of the object seen by him. But the object is not seen when this beam is cut off.

By practising *saṃyama* on this beam, the yogi neutralizes its operation. Then nobody is able to see him. He becomes invisible to all.

एतेन शब्दाद्यन्तर्धानमुक्तम्।।२२।।

The disappearance of sound, etc. is effected in the same way.—22

All other faculties, such as hearing, smelling, tasting and touching, can be restricted and neutralized in the same way through the application of *saṃyama.*

सोपक्रमं निरुपक्रमञ्च कर्म तत्संयमादपरान्तज्ञानमप्यरिष्टेभ्यो वा ज्ञानम्॥२३॥

Knowledge of one's death or the portents thereof is gained by *saṃyama* on one's active and passive deeds (*karma*).—23

It has been stated earlier (II.13) that one's longevity is determined by the nature of one's collected *karma.* This longevity is predetermined, though ordinarily this is not known to all. The yogi, however, knows that his longevity is linked to his *karmāśaya.* He therefore practises *saṃyama* on his *karmāśaya,* and thereby comes to know in advance the exact time, place and cause of his death.

Karma collected in the *karmāśaya* fall into two categories: those that are actively performed and those that result from passive actions. These may also be termed as "premeditated" and "not premeditated".

For example, a man performs a positive action when he hangs out a damp garment in a dry and airy place. On the other hand, the same garment, if casually left in a shady corner, would take an unconscionably long time to yield the desired result.

These two types of *karma* are discriminated by the yogi who, as a result of his *saṃyama,* knows which of the two would bear fruit quicker and which at a later time. In the same way he identifies the particular *karma* that regulates his longevity and also when the same would fructify. In other words, the time and manner of his own death (*aparānta* = other end) are known to him in advance.

Ariṣṭa (portents) are signs of coming events. These are of three types: physical, psychic and providential. The *physical* are those signs which are normally seen in the body preceding its death, such as a faint pulse, cold hands and feet, or a sinking heart. *Psychic* ones come in the form of premonition, often received in a dream, or a hallucination seen while awake. The *providential* come suddenly in the form of natural calamity when it is realized that death is imminent.

Although non-yogis too are often aware of these portents, it is the yogi who, by means of his *saṃyama*, knows these positively and much in advance, and so prepares himself accordingly.

मैत्र्यादिषु बलानि।।२४।।

Strength is gained through amity, etc.—24

Mental strength is gained when certain positive thoughts are constantly entertained in the mind. It has been explained earlier (I.33) that thoughts of friendliness, cheer and compassion make the mind peaceful.

The yogi practises *saṃyama* on these qualities, and then his mind gains extra strength which enables it to overcome all kinds of hostility, jealousy and pain and, finally, to get rooted in positive and virtuous thoughts only.

बलेषु हस्तिबलादीनि।।२५।।

With that strength comes (physical) strength like that of an elephaant, etc.—25

Having developed mental strength the yogi, if he wishes, can develop physical strength also in a similar manner. As we know, a strong evil thought, when it is concentrated in the mind (in a rage, for example) produces extraordinary physical power even in a weak person. The yogi can produce similar physical reactions in a positive way through *saṃyama*, and thereby gain either the strength of an elephant, the virility of a lion or the force and speed of wind.

प्रवृत्त्यालोकन्यायात् सूक्ष्मव्यवहितविप्रकृष्टाश्र्व ज्ञानम्।।२६।।

Knowledge of the fine, the hidden and the remote is gained (by *saṃyama*) instinctively.—26

It has been stated earlier (I.35-36) that propensities are of two types: *viṣayavati* (object-bound) and *jyotismati* (effulgent). The former drag the mind toward objects, while the latter (being effulgent) merely illuminate without moving from their place. These latter are of the nature of Instinct.

When, therefore, the yogi concentrates upon his effulgent propensities, he instinctively understands the fine and the subtle. Then, even hidden treasures and remote objects become apparent to him.

भुवनज्ञानं सूर्यसंयमात्।।२७।।

Knowledge of the Universe is gained by *saṃyama* on the sun.—27

The sun is concentrated light. When the yogi practises intense concentration on this source of light, all seven phases of light—the seven "worlds" or planes of the universe—are revealed to him. The seven "worlds" are: *bhūḥ, bhuvaḥ, svaḥ, mahaḥ, janaḥ, tapaḥ,* and *satya.* These constitute the entire universe of knowledge. However, the gross universe is limited to five only, viz. Earth, Water, Fire, Air, and Sky.

चन्द्रे ताराव्यूहज्ञानम्।।२८।।

Knowledge of constellations by (*saṃyama* on) the moon.—28

Of all the heavenly bodies the moon's (apparent) motion is the fastest. It is seen in the proximity of different clusters of stars in quick succession. Hence, when the yogi practises his *saṃyama* on the moon, he gets a full knowledge about those stars also. *Saṃyama* on the sun alone would not produce this result since the stars are not visible during daytime.

ध्रुवे तद्गतिज्ञानम्।। २९।।

Knowledge of their motion by (*saṃyama* on) the firmament.—29

Motion is determined by the relative positions of two fixed or moving objects. The firmament is fixed (or is apparently so), while all the heavenly bodies—planets and stars—move at varying speeds. By exercising *saṃyama* the yogi can accurately tell the speed and character of motion of each object seen against the firmament.

Dhruva (fixed) is also the designation of the Pole-star.

नाभिचक्रे कायव्यूहज्ञानम्।। ३०।।

Knowledge of the body's structure is gained by (*saṃyama* on) the navel.—30

Having stated how to master the external world, now the mastery of the internal world, i.e., the body, is being explained.

At the centre of the body is located a sixteen-cornered congeries called the *nābhi-cakra* (navel-lotus). It is the meeting place of all nerves within the body. Hence, when the yogi practises *saṃyama* upon this organ, he obtains full knowledge of the entire structure of his body, i.e., the nature and composition of blood, bones, fluids as well as their excretions, together with the position and character of each nerve within the body.

कण्ठकूपे क्षुत्पिपासानिवृत्तिः।। ३१।।

(*Saṃyama*) on the hollow of the throat curbs hunger and thirst.—31

The body's demand for food and water—the two principal requirements for its maintenance—is normally signalled in the well of the throat—the region between the base of the tongue and the upper end of the oesophagus. So when the yogi practises *saṃyama* on this part of the body his craving for food and water is curbed and he is then able to continue his yoga as long as he desires.

To get the full effect, however, the *saṃyama* must last for at least one *ghatikā* or 24 minutes.

कूर्मनाड्यां स्थैर्यम्।। ३२।।

(*Saṃyama*) on the *kūrma-nāḍi** brings steadiness.—32

When *saṃyama* is practised on this nerve, the entire body is toned up. There is no movement or discomfort of any sort in the body, and the yogi can then continue his *āsana* undisturbed for an indefinite period.

मूर्धज्योतिषि सिद्धदर्शनम्।। ३३।।

(*Saṃyama*) on Light on the top of head brings the Masters into view.—33

Brahmarandhra (Passage of Knowledge), esoterically so called, is a psychic channel that goes through the median nerve and opens out via *medulla oblongata* into the centre of the brain, where dwells the scintillating Sahasrāracakra, the thousand-petalled lotus. It is ever illuminated with the Light of Knowledge.

When the yogi practises *saṃyama* on this part of the brain, he clearly sees all the past adepts, who seem to parade before him and talk to him.

प्रतिभाद्वा सर्वम्।। ३४।।

Or, all is known by (*saṃyama* on) radiated intelligence.—34

The author here distinguishes between the different degrees of knowledge. As stated earlier (III.5), knowledge ranges from simple cognition to the Highest Wisdom.

*The psychic nerve located below the throat is known as *kūrma-nāḍi* (cf. *S.S.*, II.13–15; *G.S.*, IV.59–64).

Pratibhā (exceptional intelligence) is the gift of inborn knowledge normally found in men of genius. When a yogi, who has brushed up his intelligence to that degree of brightness, practises *saṃyama* on the same, he sees and knows everything. (This, obviously, is an alternate method to the one mentioned in the preceding *sūtra.*)

हृदये चित्तसंवित्।। ३५।।

(*Saṃyama*) on the heart brings knowledge of all minds.—35

Hṛdaya (heart) refers here to conscience, which is supposed to dwell within the heart. It is man's moral mentor. It has the quality of absolute purity (*sattva*) and is ever available as the Inner Voice that must speak the truth despite man's intellectual conviction to the contrary. Esoterically described as *antaḥkaraṇa* (in-dwelling) its location within the body is indicated by the Anāhatacakra, the twelve-petalled lotus that lies at the lower end of the heart.

When the yogi practises *saṃyama* on this conscience (heart), everything in his own as well as in that of another mind becomes crystal clear to him.

सत्वपुरुषयोरत्यन्तासंकीर्णयो: प्रत्ययाविशेषाद् भोग: परार्थन्यस्वार्थसंयमात् पुरुष ज्ञानम्।।३६।।

Sattva and *Puruṣa* are extremely close and yet separate. They are identified by "special cognition" when it is realised that while the one exists for the other, the other abides by itself. Knowledge of the Supreme Self is gained through *saṃyama.*—36

Puruṣa, literally, is the primordial—the Supreme Self. The Self in man is a replica of this Supreme Self.

Here the author makes a fine distinction between the Supreme Self and its quality. Quality is a stuff that is "enjoyed" by the possessor of that quality. Being immaculate, the Supreme Self's quality is purity; it is thus the "enjoyer" of that quality.

This subtle distinction becomes apparent by "special cognition" when the yogi is able to discriminate between the two. That done, the yogi practises *saṃyama* on the true character of the Supreme Self and then knows all that is to be known about it. Then nothing further remains to be known.

तत: प्रातिभश्रावणवेदनादर्शास्वादवार्त्ता जायन्ते।। ३७।।

Then comes abnormal perception of sound, touch, sight, taste, and smell.—37

As stated above (III.34), *pratibhā* signifies exceptional intelligence. It is the mind's capacity to grasp what escapes ordinary intelligence. Such extraordinary intelligence is gained by the yogi as a result of his *saṃyama* on the Supreme Self, and he can thereafter hear, see, touch, taste, and smell things beyond the range of normal faculties of his senses. In other words, he acquires an abnormal power of perception.

ते समाध्युपसर्गा व्युत्थाने सिद्धयः।। ३८।।

Such supernormal powers as are obstacles for *samādhi* should be restrained.—38

This is a note of caution.

These supernormal powers are not to be exercised indiscriminately, or otherwise demonstrated in public. Such demonstrations would lead to egoism, ignorance and desire in the yogi which, undoubtedly, are obstacles for *samādhi* of the highest order.

बन्धकारणशैथिल्यात् प्रचारसंवेदनाच्च चित्तस्य परशरीरप्रवेशः।। ३९।।

By de-linking the cause of its bondage (from the effect) and by extending the mind's range of cognition, another body can be entered.—39

The individual Self and the mind are both bound to the body. The *cause* of this bondage, as we have learnt, is *karma* in the *karmāśaya.* The *purpose* of this bondage is to enable the mind (and body) to experience and expend the collected *karma.* This expending of *karma* is witnessed by the Self, while the mind only experiences and "expends" those *karma* in a varied form of *kleśa.* Because of the eternal nature of *karma,* the mind must continue to perform its task of experiencing and expending. But once its link with the cause (*karma*) is snapped, the mind would have no further work left for it to do in this body; it would then be free to do similar work in another body if that could be found for it.

The yogi achieves this kind of de-linking by practising *saṃyama* on this "cause". Then, being familiar with the psychic channels through which his mind has operated so far in his own body, he seeks similar channels in another (dead) body and projects his mind through those channels to revive the dead body and so operate all its sense-organs. This, in effect, is thought-transmission in its most powerful form.

The Ādi Śaṅkarācārya is known to have demonstrated this power when he entered a dead king's body in order to experience a non-ascetic's life. As a rule yogis develop this power in order to expend the balance of their unconsumed *karma* through another body in one and the same life. After the job is done the migrant mind naturally returns to its former body, carefully preserved by other adepts.

उदानजयाज्जलपङ्ककण्टकादिष्वसङ्ग उत्क्रान्तिश्च।। ४०।।

By mastering *udāna*, immunity is gained from deaths caused by drowning, swamps, thorns, etc.—40

Udāna is the up-flowing air in the body. It is one of the ten airs that operate within the body as part of consciousness which, in fact, is the synthesis of a number of perceptions. Consciousness or "life" may be compared to a flame that is fed by several faggots. In the case of the body the faggots are the ten airs, the principal among them being *prāṇa, apāna, udāna, samāna,* and *vyāna.* Of these, *prāṇa* is the most important. It is the vital air that is breathed in; its force is held in the heart and the rest released through the mouth or nose. *Apāna* is that part of the breath which moves down from the navel right up to the toes; *samāna* encompasses the navel, *udāna* rises from the nape and flows up to the brain, while *vyāna* is the air that pervades the entire body evenly.

When *Udāna* (which feeds the brain) is controlled through *saṃyama,* the other airs in the body get automatically restricted, thereby dulling the weight-consciousness of the body. As a result the yogi becomes excessively light, and he is then able to float in water like a straw. There is no danger for him then, even if he were to be cast in a swamp or thrown in the midst of thorns.

समानजयात् प्रज्वलनम्।। ४१।।

Mastering of *samāna* brings effulgence.—41

Samāna, the air around the navel, controls the source of heat within the body. The body's heat is actually produced in that region and later distributed all over.

But when this heat is restricted by means of *saṃyama,* it gets concentrated to an extent where it turns into light. The body of the yogi then appears effulgent. In other words, there is a glow all over him.

श्रोत्राकाशयोः सम्बन्धसंयमाद्दिव्यं श्रोत्रम्।। ४२।।

Saṃyama on the interrelation of the ear and the sky produces supernormal hearing.—42

The ear is an egocentric organ of the body inasmuch as it only accepts but neither holds nor returns. The sky, on the other hand, is the repository of all sounds. In fact, sound exists in the sky in the form of fine, unmanifested particles of the element of sound. Normally only manifested sound is heard, and that too within the limits of the ear's capacity to grasp.

But when the yogi practises *saṃyama* on the mutual relation of manifested and unmanifested sound, he develops an extra fine perception which enables him to catch seemingly inaudible sounds. In other words, sounds of even higher frequencies become audible to him. This supernormal power has been described as *divya-śrotram* or divine hearing.

कायाकाशयोः सम्बन्धसंयमाल्लघुतूलसमापत्तेश्चाकाशगमनम्।। ४३।।

Saṃyama on the interrelation of body and sky, and thereby rendering the body light as cotton wool, results in ability to float in the air.—43

The sky is one of the five constituent elements of the body. When the interrelation between this internal sky and the greater sky outside is contemplated upon through *saṃyama*, the yogi's body becomes as light as air, and then it is able to float in the air like a ball of cotton wool.

(This power is similar to the one described above in *sūtra* 40.)

बहिरकल्पितावृत्तिर्महाविदेहा ततः प्रकाशावरणक्षयः।। ४४।।

The propensity to view own body from outside is *mahāvideha*; (*saṃyama* on) this lifts the veil over the Light.—44

Mahāvideha (Great Disembodiment) is the objective view of body and mind. This is a state in which the mind, no longer fed by the senses, ceases to modify, so that obstructive thoughts—the products of *kleśa*—that normally cloud the mind and cover the light of intelligence are all swept aside. It is also a state of complete non-ego.

Hence, when *saṃyama* is practised on this *mahāvideha* the yogi's pristine intelligence is restored.

स्थूलस्वरूपसूक्ष्मान्वयार्थवत्त्वसंयमाद्भूतजयः ।। ४५ ।।

Elements are mastered by *saṃyama* on the nature of their gross and fine forms.—45

As has been explained earlier (I.44–45) all Matter in the universe exists in either gross or fine form. The two in fact are convertible—the gross into fine and vice versa.

For instance, the element of fire changes and is seen as light (a gross form) and again is felt as heat (a fine form). Similarly water, earth, air and sky (gross forms of the elements) are experienced in fine forms as moisture, smell, motion (force) and voidness (space) respectively. However, even the fine have their grades. Heat, for example, might well appear as mere warmth, an uncomfortable hotness, or scorching heat. In the same way moisture, smell, motion and voidness each have their degrees of intensity.

When these are duly discriminated by the yogi through *saṃyama*, all elements, both in their gross as well as fine forms, become amenable to him. He can then manipulate those for the purpose of yoga.

ततोऽणिमादिप्रादुर्भावः कायसम्पत्तद्धर्मानभिघातश्च ।। ४६ ।।

Then appear supernormal powers of Aṇimā, etc. whereby the properties of the body are dissolved and destroyed.—46

There are eight recognized supernormal powers that go under the common designation of *aiśwarya* (divine). These are Aṇimā, Mahimā, Laghimā, Garimā, Prākāmya, Iśittva, Kāmāvasāya, and Vaśittva.

Aṇu (atom) is the smallest part of a material substance and Aṇimā is the quality of this smallness. When the yogi gains the power of contracting himself into the minutest size, he becomes invisible.

Mahimā is the opposite of Aṇimā, i.e., the quality of expansion. It is also called Vyāpti (pervasion). With this power the yogi's body disintegrates and pervades the space. This, too, results in invisibility.

Laghimā is weightlessness, i.e., having the minimum possible weight. This power results in levitation, or ability to float in air.

Garimā is opposite of Laghimā. It is excessive gravity, when nothing can displace the yogi physically.

Prākāmya is irresistible will.

Iśittva is supremacy over all.

Kāmāvasāya is total control of senses, when neither pleasure nor pain would move the yogi.

Vaśittva is fascination, or instant hypnotism with a mere look.

All these supernormal powers come to the yogi only after he has mastered the Elements through a course of *saṃyama* as laid down in the preceding *sūtra.*

रूपलावण्यबलवज्रसंहननत्वानि कायसम्पत्।। ४७।।

The properties of the body are its form, complexion, strength and endurance.—47

The "properties of the body" mentioned in the preceding *sūtra* are listed here. These "properties" in fact are the product of coalition of the five Elements that constitute the physical body.

ग्रहणस्वरूपास्मितान्वयार्थवत्त्वसंयमादिन्द्रियजयः।। ४८।।

Mastery of senses comes from *saṃyama* on the character of their accepting forms, owning them and analyzing them.—48

Once again the nature of the senses is being explained (cf. II.18).

The act of perception comprises the spotting of an object, photographing it (so to say), possessing it and presenting it to the mind in an arranged order. The whole process, viz., "accepting" a form, owning it and later explaining it to the mind, constitutes the type of cognition that is called Perception.

When this process in all its details is controlled through *saṃyama,* the yogi achieves full mastery over his senses.

ततो मनोजवित्वं विकरणभावः प्रधानजयश्च।। ४९।।

Thereby (is produced in them) a mind-like quality, with their extravert tendency curbed and a command over their very nature.—49

Manojavittvam (mental attribute) is the mind's quality of grasping instantly the significance of anything that is presented to it.

A similar quality is bestowed upon the senses when the yogi practises *saṃyama* and fully masters them. The extravert tendency, i.e., the natural propensity of the senses to dart toward objects, is then effectively checked. In other words, the very essence (*Pradhāna* = primordial) of their character is mastered.

Such omnigenous control over the senses has been designated *madhu-pratīka* (honey-like), or distilled sweetness.

सत्वपुरुषान्यताख्यातिमात्रस्य सर्वभावाधिष्ठातृत्वं सर्वज्ञातृत्वञ्च।। ५०।।

Omnipotence and omniscience come when the distinction between the Self and *sattva* has been established.—50

Annyatā (aloofness) is the awareness of a separate existence. When such a distinction or discrimination between the Self and *sattva* or the mind's immaculate quality is firmly established, the mind becomes all-powerful. The mind's own ego gloats, as it were, that it is after all as pure as the Self! *Sattva*, on the other hand, is the quality of benign neutrality strictly maintained between *rajas* (passion) and *tamas* (ignorance); it is self-sufficient and is always in a state of equipoise. As such it is all-potent, all-knowing.

When the yogi practises *saṃyama* on this *annyatā*, i.e., on the separate and distinct character of *sattva*, the latter asserts itself, grows, and gathers strength till it becomes omnipotent and omniscient.

Such a "purged" mind is known as the state of *viśoka* (affliction-less). Some yoga books also refer to it as *vaśikāra* (subjugator of tamer).

तद्वैराग्यादपि दोषबीजक्षये कैवल्यम्।। ५१।।

When that (state) is discarded, the seed of trouble is destroyed and there is *Kaivalya*.—51

When the mind reaches that *viśoka* (affliction-less) state it revels in its achievement. A sense of false pride descends upon it, wherein of course lies the seed of ignorance. This is a serious drawback no doubt, as it might well undo all that has been gained by the yogi through his practice of *saṃyama*. Hence this state of mind must be discarded and the "seed" destroyed once for all. Then alone shall it be free of all its encumbrances and be in its natural pure state, and thus qualified for *Kaivalya* or Oneness with the Self.

स्थान्युपनिमन्त्रणे सङ्गस्मयाकरणं पुनरनिष्टप्रसङ्गात्।। ५२।।

It leads to harm (if the mind), tempted by betters, again associates with (worldly objects).—52

This is again a note of warning. At this stage the mind should not be allowed to slide back but must hold on with resoluteness to the gains of *saṃyama.*

It is a delicate stage when the mind sometimes feels tempted to try out its newly-acquired strength by yielding to some temptation or other (attachment, for example), in the hope that it would easily regain its present position now that it knows the way. But this would be a fatal mistake. For, in that case, the mind may get permanently impaired and be no more fit for *samādhi* of the highest order.

Swāmin (lord or master) here refers to one's own overriding decision, not necessarily "better".

क्षण तत्क्रमयो संयमाद्विवेकजं ज्ञानम्।। ५३।।

Saṃyama on the sequence of Time brings discriminative knowledge.—53

At this stage discrimination is most necessary, so that temptation, are recognized as such and duly rejected. Hence the way to get that discriminative knowledge is now being told.

Extreme discrimination is involved when one is able to identify the units of Time. *Kṣaṇa* (moment) is the briefest division of Time. It is the continuity of this "moment" that constitutes Time. There is only a notional interval between one "moment" and another, and yet when a 'moment" is conceived of as a unit its separate identity has to be recognized.

By practising *saṃyama* on this sequence of "moments" the yogi develops an acute sense of discrimination in himself.

जातिलक्षणदेशैरन्यतानवच्छेदात्तुल्ययोस्ततः प्रतिपत्तिः।। ५४।।

It (discrimination) is complete when the distinctions caused by the variety of kinds, signs and locations are in equilibrium.—54

Pratipatti (completion) is the successful end of a job. The standard of success in the case of discrimination is laid down here, and the completion or successful discrimination is to be measured only by this standard.

Jāti (kind), *lakṣaṇa* (sign) and *deśa* (place) are the three factors involved in any discrimination. For example, in the case of a cow and a buffalo, discrimination is to be made first in respect of kind, although both belong to the same species; next in respect of signs, e.g., the differences in colour, formation of horns, etc., and finally about the place where they are found or originally belonged to.

The same process will apply in respect of two trees, or even two fruits of the same tree.

Deep discrimination enables the yogi to determine all the factors, down to the character of the last atom, in the constitution of an object, and when all those have been properly discriminated with equal intensity, the discrimination is complete.

तारकं सर्वविषयं सर्वथा विषयक्रमञ्चेति विवेकजं ज्ञानम्।। ५५।।

Discriminative knowledge of all objects, at all times and in all respects of their sequence is *tāraka*.—55

Tāraka (means of crossing) is so called because it is this type of discriminative knowledge that helps a yogi to cross the ocean of world phenomena. It is the highest form of discriminative knowledge. It enables the yogi to know any matter, gross or fine, along with all its constituent elements and the manner of their transmutation from time to time.

This is the prelude to A-samprajñāta *samādhi* or superconsciousness.

सत्वपुरुषयो: शुद्धिसाम्ये कैवल्यमिति।। ५६।।

When *sattva* and *Puruṣa* are equally pure, there is Oneness.—56

What follows when *tāraka*, the highest form of discriminative knowledge, is gained?

Tāraka purifies the mind, whose *sattva* content is now full and unqualified. The last vestiges of *rajas* and *tamas* have departed and *sattva* is now in complete possession of the field.

Since *sattva* is total purity, which is also the quality of the Supreme Self, the two now merge and become one. This is *Kaivalya* or Oneness.

Here ends chapter III of the *Pātañjala Yogasūtra* entitled 'Powers of Yoga'.

CHAPTER IV

Towards Emancipation

जन्मौषधिमन्त्रतपःसमाधिजाः सिद्धयः ।। १ ।।

Supernormal powers come from birth, physic, *mantra*, austerity and *samādhi*.—1

The genesis of supernormal powers is now explained.

Supernormal powers result from various causes. Some apparently exist right from birth; others are acquired. The bird's power to fly in the air and the fish's to swim in water are supernormal in the sense that these defy the natural laws of gravitation and dynamics. These powers however exist in them right from birth, i.e., naturally.

On the other hand, some human beings are known to "acquire" supernormal power(s), although a few—indeed very few—also have these in them from birth, again naturally. But those who wish to acquire have to use various "means" to stimulate the inherent power within them and turn the same into a supernormal power. Their "means" often include the use of rare herbs or chemical preparations (such as some compound of mercury), the incantation of *mantras*, restrictions (austerity) exercised on their normal physical and mental urges, and a strict discipline of the mind.

The point worth nothing, however, is that all powers, whether normal or supernormal, are really inherent in the creature when it is born. Thus we find precocious children, or men of genius, with an abnormal "gift" which apparently was never acquired and yet was there right from birth, although the same became manifest only after some time. Since nothing can be *had* unless it is acquired, the presumption is that this "gift" too was acquired through some efforts made on an earlier occasion. Thus what now appears as "gift" is, in fact, a hard earned acquisition made in a previous life.

In this way a *samādhi*, when easily achieved, is really the fruit of several similar efforts made in previous lives.

जात्यन्तरपरिणामः प्रकृत्यापूरात्।। २।।

Nature completes the transformation from one kind to another.—2

Evolution is the law of Nature. During evolution some mutations take place, both in physical as well as in the mental field. In this manner one kind of species is physically changed into another; the latter then is quite different from the former. Similar transformation in the mental field results in a change of character often involving a moral change.

This kind of change is seen in the life of Viśwāmitra *muni* (who changed from a ruling Kṣatriya prince to a venerable Brahmin sage) and, more recently, in King Aśoka (who underwent a complete moral change when he abandoned wars and took to preaching and practising non-violence, compassion and *dharma*). Such mental and physical changes are completed, i.e., brought about in the desired form, by the process of mutations in their respective fields.

Howeveʳ, the motivation behind such transmutations is explained in the next *sūtra*.

निमित्तमप्रयोजकं प्रकृतीनां वरणभेदस्तु ततः क्षेत्रिकवत्।। ३।।

Nature determines the motivation, means and manner, even as the cultivator (does for his field).—3

The process of evolution is a series of mutations that take place in a manner that is determined by the actual needs of the situation—in other words, by way of natural selection. Nature provides the inner directive force which causes the mutations to take place in the way in which they would be most useful.

Thus once the mind has decided that a particular action is called for, the means and manner of its execution follow automatically. It is like the farmer who, as soon as his mind has decided that a particular part of his field needs, or does not need, water, opens or closes the appropriate channel that feeds that part. The job is done mechanically—almost instinctively—and he does not then pause even for a moment to think "how" or "when".

Similarly, all transmutations in the physical and mental fields take place naturally.

निर्माणचित्तान्यस्मितामात्रात्।। ४।।

Created minds are merely a form of Egoism.—4

What are "created minds"?

Created minds are the yogi's own positive thoughts, created within his mind to fight the negative thoughts.

When the yogi realizes that his newly-acquired powers are but a form of egoism, their motive being to possess something extra for himself—he wants to get rid of this evil of egoism which, any how, is reprehensible. He then creates new "minds" (quanta of positive thoughts) in himself which would consume the fruits of his new *karma*.

These "created minds" are of the nature of sparks that issue from one fire and that exist only temporarily before dying out. In other words, "created minds" are for a limited purpose and for a limited time.

प्रवृत्तिभेदे प्रयोजकं चित्तमेकमनेकेषाम्।। ५।।

Despite diversity of propensities, the motivator of one and many minds remains the same.—5

A number of "created minds" is bound to result in a diversity of propensities. Besides, how could all of them manage to work for one single purpose? This is explained.

The "created minds" of the yogi no doubt possess their own individual propensity. There is thus a diversity of propensities. But the motive power behind all these propensities remain the same, viz., the motivation provided by the original mind. Hence the motivation of the original mind becomes the motivator of all the freshly created minds. In other words, the original mind directs the "created minds".

It is like different organs of the body being centrally controlled. "Created minds" too are centrally controlled.

तत्र ध्यानजमनाशयम्।। ६।।

Of these, the contemplation-born ones are desireless.—6

The "creation" of diverse minds is also a supernormal power. If the yogi is not gifted with this power by birth, he has only four ways open to him to acquire the same, viz., Physics, *mantra*, Austerity, and *samādhi*.

But out of all the minds thus "created", only the one that is the product of *samādhi* is desireless (*anāśaya* = without expectations). The other three types are tinged with desire, i.e., those are *with* expectations.

कर्माशुक्लाकृष्णं योगिनस्त्रिविधमितरेषाम्।। ७।।

For yogis, *karma* is neither black nor white; for others it is of three kinds.—7

Here the adjectives used for Virtue and Vice are carefully chosen.

A-śukla (non-white) and *a-kṛṣṇa* (non-black) are the character of all *karma* performed by a yogi. His deeds cannot be called either black or white because all *karma* performed by the yogi are desireless (*anāśaya*) and hence those are not "fruitful".

For other people, however, all *karma*, being performed *with* expectations, fall into three categories, viz. black, white and grey (mixed).

ततस्तद्विपाकानुगुणानामेवाभिव्यक्तिर्वासनानाम्।। ८।।

Desires appear through transmutation of qualities of those (*karma*).—8

Now, how do, these *karma* bear fruit?

The fruit, of course, are the desires that are born of *karma*. These then take the form of *kleśa* of various types experienced in the body and mind. The "tasting" of this fruit (desire) results in more *karma*, so that fresh *karma* is added to the pool called *karmāśaya*, from which some *karma* is again drawn out for consumption. In this way the cycle continues. The same *karma* first appears as the Cause and later as its own Effect, making a rotating chain of Cause and Effect.

As stated above, all *karma* get collected in the Karma Pool called *karmāśaya*, where they exist as the essence of all previous desires born of *karma* or caused by *karma*. Through transmutation of qualities of this "essence," the Cause-*karma* changes into Effect-*karma*. It is like the seed growing into a tree and bearing fruit, which again carries the seed. The growing process, or transmutation of the qualities, is determined by Nature in accordance with the law of evolution and natural selection.

Again, it is natural selection that makes some *karma* get expended sooner than the others. Thus the time and place of their "expenditure" depend upon the "means" available for the *karma* to fructify—in other words, suitable environment and suitable opportunity.

For example, if one particular *karma* needs the experience of drowning while others, i.e., the majority have already resulted in a life to be spent in the desert, then that particular *karma* cannot obviously fructify for the simple reason that it shall have no opportunity to fructify. Hence it must await a more suitable time in future—i.e., a future birth in which to bear its fruit.

जातिदेशकालव्यवहितानामप्यान्तर्यं स्मृतिसंस्कारयोरेकरूपत्वात्।। ९।।

Despite gaps (separation and intervals) of kind, place and time, Memory and Past Impressions remain unaffected (similar).—9

This is in explanation of the previously stated theory of Cause and Effect.

First, the difference between Memory and Past Impressions (*saṃskāra*). Past Impressions lie mostly in the Unconscious. Memory carries the present impressions, which are recallable as against past impressions which cannot be consciously recalled. The latter lie hidden in the depths of the Unconscious and manifest themselves either in dreams or in the shape of instinctive acts, or as proclivities, i.e., unaccountable tendencies. Both past and present impressions, however, are similar: both represent the Effect-aspect of *karma*, viz., desires, and as such both generate fresh *karma* representing its Cause-aspect.

The law of Cause and Effect operate irrespective of the factors of kind, place and time. *Jāti* (kind) is the species of life or the form of existence; *deśa* (place) is the location—the site assigned for that existence, and *kāla* (time) is the interval between one existence (life) and another. These three factors do not influence *karma*, whereas *karma* does influence them.

As stated earlier (II.13) it is *karma* that determines the kind of life (species), its longevity and the nature of experience that it shall have. *Karma* thus ordains the conditions of life and brings to it such experiences as may help *karma* to exhaust itself. Until this task is complete, *karma* awaits a suitable opportunity for it to fructify. This opportunity, however, may not come for a long time—not even in course of a thousand births! But ultimately, it *does* come in some birth, when this particular *karma* gets the opportunity to fructify and expend itself through some appropriate experience.

In this way, the gaps of kind, place and time do not bar the ultimate and inevitable fructification of *karma*.

तासामनादित्वं चाशिषो नित्यत्वात्।। १०।।

Their beginningless and endless character is due to Continuity.—10

The Law of Continuity ("nothing is abrupt in Nature") presupposes the absence of a beginning and an end. This law also applies to *karma*, which is already subject to the law of Cause and Effect.

But what about Desire which *karma* produces?—it may be asked. When did *karma* produce the first Desire?

In answer it is explained that the essence of Thought (*bhāvastattvam*) has no beginning; it just exists, and is inherent in Thought. This "essence" has the attribute of force or motion which creates and causes new thoughts which become subject to the Law of Continuity. The continuity of *karma*, therefore, has neither a beginning nor an end.

हेतुफलाश्रयालम्बनैः संग्रहीतत्वादेषामभावे तदभावः।। ११।।

When Cause, Effect—and their support and means—combine, there is Continuity; when not, it ceases.—11

The way to end that endlessness (continuity) is now stated.

Endless experience of *karma* is due to Ignorance prevailing in the mind which does not allow the light of Knowledge to emerge and break through the continuity. Ignorance itself is the product of Desire—the propensity of attachment or craving for objects. The craving, again, is a by-product of *karma*. Hence this Wheel of *Karma*—Desire—Ignorance—Desire—*karma* which operates in accordance with the law of Cause and Effect.

The mind is the means (hub) which supports (help operation of) this wheel, so that when all four—cause, effect, means and support—cooperate, the Wheel of *Karma* rotates continuously.

This rotation can be halted, however, if any of the links—rather spokes of the wheel—is removed, thereby making continuous rotation impossible. Such cessation of the continuous rotation is achieved by the yogi when he consciously withdraws his mind—the "means" and "support"—thereby bringing the Wheel of *Karma* to a halt. The continuity then ceases.

अतीतानागतं स्वरूपतोऽस्त्यध्वभेदाद्धर्माणाम्।। १२।।

Past and Future exist in their own form, and are identified by their characters of subsidence and emergence.—12

Both Past and Future cannot be seen. Yet they exist, and their existence is as true as that of the Present which is seen. The difference between the two types of existence lies in the fact of their fine and gross characters respectively. The Present changes its gross character into fine, and becomes Past. The Future changes its fine character into gross, and becomes Present. The one disappears and the other appears. In this way Past and Future are identified by their characters of subsidence and emergence.

The fact that both Past and Future can be conceived of, also proves their existence. Normally, nothing can be conceived of unless the same has existed or exists in some form, either gross or fine.

For instance, we never conceive of horns on a rabbit for the simple reason that horny rodents do not exist and have never existed. However, if the possibility of such horns on rodents is accepted, the idea then becomes conceivable.

On the other hand, the existence of Past and Future is always conceivable.

ते व्यक्तसूक्ष्मगुणात्मानः ।। १३ ।।

They are endowed with the qualities of grossness and fineness.—13

It has been stated above that both Past and Future exist in a fine state, and that they change into gross form when they appear as Present.

The emphasis there was on the character of changing from gross to fine and from fine to gross, i.e., perpetual subsidence of Present into Past and perpetual emergence of Future into Present. It is this character of subsidence and emergence that possesses the qualities of grossness and fineness which keep interchanging.

Again, gross and fine carry in them the three primal qualities of Nature—*sattva, rajas* and *tamas.* These qualities (*guṇas*), coalescing in varied proportion, actually determine the character of grossness and fineness.

परिणामैकत्वाद्वस्तुतत्त्वम् ।।१४।।

Uniformity of an object is the result of uniformity in the process of transmutation.—14

Two uniform objects are created when the process of mutation that leads to their production is also uniform, i.e., when the quality and quantity of basic ingredients, as also the process of their mixture, are equally specific. In other words, uniformity in transmutation results in a uniform product.

This, however, is only a theory. In actual practice the products of all transmutation vary, however minutely, in respect of their form, size, weight, colour, etc. *Absolute* uniformity is a mere notion and is not seen or found anywhere in the universe—whether in man, beast, insect, plants (and their leaves), or objects meticulously constructed by man.

As we know, measurements made by the finest dial comparator or optimeter can attain accuracy only up to a point: there is always an irreducible margin of 0.000010 or so of an inch! Even the so-called "precision" parts demand lubricants of appropriate viscosity to get accurately adjusted: viscosity too leaves an indeterminable gap between *near-accuracy* and *accuracy*.

Indeed, *absolute* accuracy is beyond man's capacity when it is recognized that the judging of that accuracy is done by a being who is himself an inaccurate creature of Nature!

In principle, however, Nature *can* produce two objects precisely identical in every respect—provided of course its process of transmutation is also precisely identical in every respect.

वस्तुसाम्ये चित्तभेदात्तयोर्विविक्त: पन्था:।। १५।।

Despite the object being one and same, its reflection is diverse in different minds.—15

The cause of diversity of objects observed is now explained.

Objects appear diverse because of the diverse manner in which the mind cognizes them. Sometimes the same object appears different to different people.

For instance, an attractive woman produces three different reactions in three separate minds. One mind experiences pleasurable feelings at her sight, another—perhaps her rival's—has feelings of jealousy or regret, while a third (an ascetic's) views her with total indifference or contempt. In this way three different minds have cognized the same object in three different forms.

Again, one mind cognizes one object in different ways at different times. Thus feelings of joy, pain, disgust and indifference appear intermittently in the same one mind about the same one object. Such diversity is caused by the diverse character of shadows cast upon the mind by one and the same object on different occasions, and these shadows are then perceived by the mind in diverse manner.

Hence an object, though it may be the product of a uniform process of transmutation, appears diverse under different circumstances.

न चैकचित्ततन्त्रं वस्तु तदप्रमाणकं तदा किं स्यात्।। १६।।

If existence of an object were to depend upon one mind only, where would be the proof of its existence?—16

This is in further explanation of the character of diversity of all objects.

An object is an object so long as it is cognized as such. It is the cognition by mind that proves the existence of an object. Once the mind ceases to cognize an object its (object's) existence ceases and it is no more there. Hence the proof of existence of an object is, that it is still cognizable.

For this purpose cognition by one mind alone is not sufficient. For one mind may suspend its cognition (during *samādhi,* for instance), or refuse to cognize an object indefinitely, in which event the object would cease to exist for that mind. But in fact it does not cease to exist because several other minds are still there to cognize it; and hence its existence subsists.

The proof of an object's existence is that it is cognizable by diverse minds at the same time.

तदुपरागापेक्षित्वाच्चित्तस्य वस्तुज्ञाताज्ञातम्।। १७।।

Cognition or non-cognition of an object depends on whether or not the screen in-between is removed.—17

In order that an object may be cognized by the mind, that object must first reveal itself. However, the character of the object is to hide even as that of the mind is to seek.

This hiding character is the "screen" in-between. So long as this "screen" exists, the object remains obscure and the mind is unable to cognize it directly. The "screen" acts as a kind of filter through which knowledge of the object must seep in. In actual fact, however, this process is very rapid indeed.

Thus, when a red rose is seen, the knowledge about it passes through this "screen" in, say, the following order: first, the colour of the flower, then its fragrance, then its form (size), its exact shade, the location of the plant to which it belongs, its possible use or uses—and so on and so forth. All this knowledge about the rose the mind accepts in quick succession—but only after the mind has *re*-cognized the object's similarity with similar impressions already registered and stored in the Memory. These earlier impressions help the mind to cognize quickly.

If, somehow, this "screen" could be removed, cognition by mind would not only be instantaneous but also simultaneous for all objects. But that is not possible until and unless the mind attains the stage of *samādhi.*

सदाज्ञाताश्चित्तवृत्तयस्तत्प्रभोः पुरुषस्यापरिणामित्वात्।। १८।।

The lord of that tendency of constant cognition by mind is the Self, itself unchangeable.—18

Now the character of the Self is explained.

The character of the Self is its constancy or unchangeability—as against the character of the mind which is one of constant changing or modifications.

The Self remains unchanged because it is there to witness the changes. Since a change implies the presence of a witness to that change, a change in the Self would need another Self to witness that change, and a third Self to witness the change of the second—and so on *ad infinitum.* That, indeed, would be an absurd proposition.

Hence *Puruṣa* is the ultimate witness of all changes. It witnesses the changes as a lord—the sole onlooker of the drama that goes on within the mind, viz. the mind's constant cognition of various objects.

न तत् स्वाभासं दृश्यत्वात्।। १९।।

That (mind) has no light of its own, being a reflector of light.—19

The mind no doubt cognizes, but its cognitive power is not its own. Cognition, or the glow of Knowledge, really belongs to the Self. It is the light of the Self that finds a mirror in the mind and is reflected there, giving the latter the power to cognize. (The mind is like the moon, which has no light of its own but reflects back on earth the light it receives from the sun.)

The light of Knowledge in the mind, therefore, is actually the light that emanates from the source of all Knowledge—the Self. Hence the Self has been designated as the Seer and the mind as the Seen—the light and the thing enlightened. The seer sees the seen, whereas the seen does not see the seer.

एकसमये चोभयानवधारणात्।। २०।।

Also, because it is not possible to cognize (hold on to) both at the same time.—20

The mind, as we know, is constantly engaged in the work of cognizing various objects. It has no time left to cognize itself which, if it *had* to be cognized, would need another mind and then that second mind a third one, and so on. It would again be an endless process, an absurd proposition.

Hence, it is not possible for the mind to cognize various objects and at the same time cognize itself also.

चिन्तान्तरदृश्यबुद्धेरतिप्रसङ्गः स्मृतिसङ्करश्च।। २१।।

Assumption of other cognizing minds would be an endless process and (lead to) confusion of memory.—21

The preceding *sūtra* is further explained here.

A multiplicity of minds, if assumed, would not only be an endless process but also create a complete confusion in memory. Since each mind would be carrying its own impressions, the overcrowding and mixture of these impressions would make one compact storehouse like Memory well nigh impossible.

And even if such an omnigenous Memory were possible, recollection from that Memory of the exact form and quality of each cognized object would be a hopeless task—like looking for a small needle in a huge stack of hay!

चितेरप्रतिसंक्रामायास्तदाकारापत्तौ बुद्धिसंवेदनम्।। २२।।

When the mind reflects the light of Knowledge of the Self, it gets its own power of cognition.—22

The ultimate source of Knowledge is the Self. In fact the Self is Knowledge Personified, from which flows knowledge of all types and degrees (cf. III.5). The mind's cognitive power, too, is derived from this very source of Knowledge. Cognition, in other words, is the knowledge that is reflected upon the mind from the Self and which generates the power of cognition in the mind.

The knowledge radiated from the Self permeates the mind in the same way as the three primal Qualities—*sattva, rajas* and *tamas*—intermingle and overspread all Matter, or just as atoms constitute and permeate an object. This permeated knowledge gives the mind its power to cognize. Obviously the nearer the mind is to the Self the more is the permeation and, when the mind has absorbed this knowledge wholly, it is as pure and as immaculate as the Self's own knowledge.

द्रष्टृदृश्योपरक्तं चित्तं सर्वार्थम्।। २३।।

Coloured by both the Seer and the Seen, the mind becomes all-purposive.—23

The mind is like a mirror: it reflects whatever is close to it. When the Self is near it, it reflects the pure Knowledge of the Self. When any other object or objects are near it, it reflects the shadows of those objects. Thus the mind becomes all-purposive (*sarvārtha*).

However, reflection in the mirror is clear only when the mirror is perfectly clean. Unfortunately the average mind is mostly busy reflecting all kinds of objects. In the process it gets soiled by the by-products of *rajas* and *tamas* which prevent a clear reflection of anything—least of all of the Self which is purity itself. But when the mind's cognitive power—itself a gift of the Self—asserts (grows into *viveka* or discriminative knowledge) and brings up the inherent *sattva* in the mind, the surface of the mirror improves and there is then a better reflection of the Self in it. Thereby the mind is able to get closer to the Self—indeed it is attracted to it even as a piece of iron, when brought closer, is attracted to the magnet!

Here two types of forces have been mentioned: one, the manifested and the other, unmanifested. The unmanifested power of Knowledge is the Self itself. The manifested is the cognitive power of the mind derived from the Self. The latter the mind utilizes to stir up its inherent *sattva*; and when *that* predominates, after brushing aside both *rajas* and *tamas*, the mirror of the mind is fit to reflect the immaculateness of the Self. In this way when the purity of the Self is fully and truly reflected in the mind, proving thereby that the purity of the mind is in no way different from that of the Self, the two, being exactly the same, merge and become one.

तदसंख्येयवासनाभिश्चित्तमपि परार्थं संहत्यकारित्वात्।। २४।।

Those collected desires in the mind, having coalesced, are for "another."—24

Now the question naturally arises: what happens to the impurities (desires) "brushed aside" with the aid of *sattva* in order to render the mind more perfect for reflection? Surely all those desires could not have got expended so quickly?

It is true that all desires must await their turn, and a suitable opportunity, before they can expend themselves. But when the mind has wholly turned to the Self, and is nearer it and away from sensual objects that enable (cause) the desires to expend themselves, then the balance of those unexpended desires stay in the mind in a compounded, coalesced form. Those are then merely *seen* by "another," viz., the *Puruṣa* or Self. In other words, the residual desires in that case are no longer required to be exhausted through *bhoga*, or normal experiences of pleasure and pain.

But how is the existence of that "another" being assumed?

This assumption of "another" is somewhat like smoke on top of a hill seen from a distance. We know that there can be no smoke without fire; also that no fire can result unless there is some combustible substance below it. Now wood is a possible combustible substance, and so its existence below the fire and smoke is first assumed. Thereafter the form in which that wood could exist is determined and, finally, the conclusion is reached that the hill-top actually is covered with forest!

Similar indirect knowledge leads the mind to assume "another".

विशेषदर्शिन: आत्मभावभावनानिवृत्ति:।। २५।।

The mind's awareness of its own existence ends with "special seeing"—25

Viśeṣa-darśinaḥ (special seeing) is the power of acute discrimination. When the mind develops this sort of discriminative power it becomes aware of its true role—that of a mere medium or an instrument of communication. It then gets out of its false notion that it is the real seer of all things. Thereupon its egoism departs, and it ceases to be self-conscious.

तदा विवेकनिम्नं कैवल्यप्राग्भावं चित्तम्।। २६।।

With that deep discrimination, the mind reaches the pre-*Kaivalya* state.—26

As a sequel to this non-self-consciousness, the mind loses interest in its own work, viz. modifications. Thoughts in the mind cease to modify which, of course, comes as a blessing in disguise since it is exactly this state of mind that is suitable for the highest *samādhi.* It is the prelude to *Kaivalya.*

तच्छिद्रेषु प्रत्ययान्तराणि संस्कारेभ्यः।। २७।।

That (special discrimination) comes after piercing through the obstacles of past impressions.—27

True discrimination is hard to come by. There are always hindrances in the way, right up to the very last moment. Even at the final stage some past impression or other may crop up and stand in the way of full discrimination.

For example, the mind may be suddenly reminded of its erstwhile role when it happened to be so active modifying thoughts and thus be made self-conscious once again. Hindrances may also appear in the form of some doubt, lethargy, illusion, etc.

But, at this stage, there should be no slipping back, it is advised; these should be "pierced through."

हानमेषां क्लेशवदुक्तम्।। २८।।

These are to be rejected—like Sorrow, etc. mentioned earlier.—28

The way to get over these obstacles is now stated.

All these obstacles, it is advised, should be tackled in the same manner as Sorrow, Ignorance, Egoism, etc. mentioned earlier (II.10–11).

In other words, the only way to counter such obstacles is to push them back to their fine form by means of intense meditation.

प्रसंख्यानेऽप्यकुसीदस्य सर्वथा विवेकख्यातेर्धर्ममेघः समाधिः।।२९।।

When the collection (of obstacles) has exhausted, and discrimination is constant, there comes the *samādhi* called Dharmamegha.—29

This is the penultimate stage. When every possible obstacle has been overcome, and the discriminative power has got stabilized, the mind gets into a trance which, in Tāntric parlance, is known as *Dharmamegha,* or the Cloud of Virtue.

This Cloud descends upon the yogi, washing away whatever residual impurities that might have still stuck to his mind, thus rendering it crystal clear so that the full brightness of Knowledge may be found reflected in it.

ततः क्लेशकर्मनिवृत्तिः।। ३०।।

There ends all *kleśa* and *karma.*—30

As a result of the bursting of *Dharmamegha*, all *kleśa* (afflictions), as well as the cause of those afflictions, viz. desires born of *karma*, disappear from the mind. The mind, then, is no longer a helpless victim of the two.

तदा सर्वावरणमलापेतस्य ज्ञानस्यानन्त्यात् ज्ञेयमल्पम्।। ३१।।

Then the veil over Knowledge is lifted, and this Knowledge, being free and unlimited, makes all the Knowable shrink into insignificane.—31

When the cause of afflictions (*kleśa*) is thus removed, the ignorance that clouded the mind so far also vanishes. This releases the mind's intelligence (knowledge) from its "bondage," enabling it to grow to its maximum limit.

Since there is no limit to which knowledge may not grow, this knowledge, when it is in its infinite form, makes all knowable things seem so insignificantly small. For, largeness and smallness are but relative; so that *infinite* knowledge, when compared to the *limited* knowledge normally available to the mind, is very vast indeed!

ततः कृतार्थानां परिणामक्रमसमाप्तिर्गुणानाम्।।३२।।

With that is accomplished the termination of constant transmutation of the *guṇas.*—32

It is the job of the *guṇas* (the three primal Qualities) to transmute, and this they do through the natural process of intermingling and coalescing. The process results in the production of various objects, species and senses that enable living being to perceive their pleasures and pains.

But when no *karma*—or its product *kleśa*—is left in the mind, the work of the Qualities cannot proceed. For the *guṇas* operate only because there is something to operate on. In other words, the manufacturing process ceases when the raw material is not available. In the same way the Self is now without *guṇas,* i.e., *Nirguṇa.*

Kṛtārtha (satisfaction) is the happy end (termination) of a continuous toil.

क्षणप्रतियोगी परिणामापरान्तनिर्ग्राह्यः क्रमः।। ३३।।

A racing "moment," uncaptured till the end, is the continuity of Time.—33

A moment is the briefest division of Time. (cf. III.53). It races at a speed that prevents its "capture" and identification as a separate unit of Time. The units (moments) overlap one another so quickly and move forward at such tremendous speed that they leave behind only a continuity that is loosely termed as Time.

For purposes of identification, however, this Time (or rather the continuity of Time) is divided into seconds, minutes, hours, days, months, years and ages. In actual fact the entire Time, viz. all Past, Present and Future, is but one unit, and hence the yogi compresses all this into one—i.e., the Present. In other words, by terminating the continuity he brings Time to a halt.

पुरुषार्थशून्यानां गुणानां प्रतिप्रसवः कैवल्यं-
स्वरूपप्रतिष्ठा वा चितिशक्तिरिति।। ३४।।

Kaivalya is neutralization of the three *guṇas*, thereby depriving the Self of the products of their transmutation; or, it is the installation of the Power of Knowledge in its own true form.—34

And so to *Kaivalya.*

Like the continuity of Time, there is a continuity in the process of mutations caused by the interaction of the three *guṇas.*

Mutations take place because there is always something in Nature that is amenable to mutation. That "something" again naturally possesses the three primal qualities of *tamas*, *rajas* and *sattva*, which automatically start their work of transmutation. Normally, the continuity of this transmuting process cannot be broken.

Yet the yogi has found a way to break this continuity. Through the process of yogic disciplines and deep discrimination he has, at last, been able to eliminate from his mind both *tamas* and *rajas*, and thereby isolated the *sattva.* He has thus not only spring-cleaned his mind but gone forth to cut off the route through which his *karma* (in the form of ignorance, sorrow, etc.) have been flowing in from his *karmāśaya* after being transmuted in the natural way. He has transcended Time, and now he has transcended Nature itself!

As a result, the yogi's mind is now Purity itself—the form in which his Self abides. There is no distinction now between his Self and his Mind. In the bargain his Self is now released from its duty of witnessing whatever his Mind so far did in order to experience the transmuted fruits of his *karma*.

Since he has now successfully stalled the process of transmutation itself, there is nothing else left for the Self to witness any more. Its job of witnessing is over, and the Self is now free—unbonded—unlimited. It is now beyond Time, Space and Causation. It is Emancipated!

Here ends chapter IV of *Pātañjala Yogasūtra*
entitled 'Towards Emancipation'.

Glossary

(Botanical names of Indian plants, flowers and fruits mentioned in yoga books)

Āmlakī: (myrobalan) Emblica officinalis
Bāla-ṣāka: (leafy vegetable) Pisum arvence
Bandhūka: (a bright red flower, also called *oṣṭha-puṣpa* or lip flower) Pentaptera tomentosa
Bilva: (wood-apple) Aegle marmelos
Bimba: (Indian cherry) Coccinia indica
Caṇaka: (gram) Cicer arietinum
Daḍimba: (pomegranate) Punica gratanum
Dhātṛ: (same as *āmlakī*)
Drākṣā: (grape) Vitis vinifera
Drāṛhikā: (ginger) Zedoarium
Dumbari: (fig) Ficus hispida
Haritaki: (yellow myrobalan) Terminalia chebula
Haritāli: (Indian corn) Zea Mays
Hilmocikā: (leafy vegetable) Enhydra fluctuans
Hingu: (asafoetida) Ferula foetida
Jambira: (citron) Citrus medica
Jambhu: (citron) Citrus grandis
Jambulā: (rose-apple) Syzygium fruticosa
Jāti-phal: (nutmeg) Beleric myrobalans
Kadamba: (a flowering tree which blossoms with the roaring of thunder-clouds) Anthocephauls indicus
Kakkula: (mulberry) Morus indica
Kāla-śāka: (leafy vegetable) Cassia sophera
Kāmrañga: (citron) Averrhoa carambola
Kaṇṭa-phala: (castor) Datura metel Linn
Kapittha: (sour wood-apple) Forenia limonia
Karabi: (oleander or rose-bay) Nerium oleander
Karkaṭi: (cucumber) Cucumis sativus

Kemuka: (leafy vegetable) Costus speciosus
Khadira: (catechu) Acacia catechu
Kharjura: (date-palm) Phoenix dactylifera
Kol: (berry) Zizyphus jujuba
Kulattha: (a kind of pulse) Phaseolus multiflorus
Kunda: (a kind of jasmine) Jasminum grandiflorum
Kuṣmāṇḍa: (pumpkin) Benincasa hispida
Lakuca: (bread-fruit) Artocarpus altilis
Laśuna: (garlic) Allium sativum
Māna: (gherkin) Alocasia indica
Māśa: (a pulse) Lens esculenta
Masūra: (lentil) Lens culinaris
Mūlaka: (radish) Raphanus sativus
Palāśa: (parrot tree) Butea frondosa
Panasa: (jackfruit) Artocarpus heterophylla
Paṭol-patra: (leafy vegetable) Trichosanthes dioica
Piyāla: (hazel-nut) Corylus ferox
Rambhā: (banana) Musa sapientum
Śālmali: (silk-cotton tree) Salmalia malabaricum
Tāmbūla: (betel-leaf) Piper betel Linn
Tumbi: (gourd) Langenaria vulgaris
Vārtāki: (egg-plant, brinjal) Solanum melongena
Vastuka: (leafy vegetable) Chenopodium album

Index

EVEREST

1863

KÜRŞAT BAŞAR

1963 yılında İstanbul'da doğdu. İ.Ü. Felsefe Bölümü'nü bitirdi. Birçok dergi ve gazetede yöneticilik yaptı. *Cumhuriyet*, *Yeni Yüzyıl*, *Star*, *Akşam* gibi birçok gazetede köşe yazıları yazdı. 90'lı yıllarda başladığı televizyon programlarına halen devam ediyor.

1989 yılında yayınlanan ilk kitabı *Kış İkindisinin Evinde*'yle *Haldun Taner Öykü Ödülü*'nü aldı. 2011 yılında kurduğu "Kürşat Başar Orkestrası"yla *Keşke Burada Olsaydın* ve *Kaldığımız Yerden* adlı iki albüm yayınladı.

KİTAPLARI:

1989 *Kış İkindisinin Evinde* (öykü) (Haldun Taner Öykü Ödülü)
1990 *Konuştuğumuz Gibi Uzaklara* (roman)
1992 *Sen Olsaydın Yapmazdın, Biliyorum* (roman)
1996 *Aşkı Bulmanın ve Korumanın Yolları* (roman)
2000 *İğreti Yaşamlar* (yazılar/denemeler)
2003 *Başucumda Müzik* (roman)
2006 *Çok Güldük Ağlamayalım* (yazılar/denemeler)
2006 *Sanki Bir Roman Kahramanı/Doğan Hızlan* (biyografi)
2014 *Yaz* (roman)
2018 *Bazen Unutmak İstersin* (deneme)
2019 *Aklımda Hep Sen* (roman)

KÜRŞAT BAŞAR

Aklımda Hep Sen

§

Yayın No: **1863**
Türkçe Edebiyat: **753**

Aklımda Hep Sen
Kürşat Başar

Kapak tasarımı: Füsun Turcan Elmasoğlu
Sayfa tasarımı: M. Aslıhan Özçelik

1. Basım: Haziran 2019 (100.000 adet)

ISBN: 978 - 605 - 185 - 405 - 2
Sertifika No: 43949

Baskı ve cilt: Melisa Matbaacılık
Matbaa sertifika no: 12088
Çiftehavuzlar Yolu Acar Sanayi Sitesi, No: 8
Bayrampaşa/İstanbul
Tel: (0212) 674 97 23 Faks: (0212) 674 97 29

EVEREST YAYINLARI
Alemdar Mahallesi Ticarethane Sokak No: 15 34110
Cağaloğlu-İstanbul
Tel: (212) 513 34 20-21 Faks: (212) 512 33 76
e-posta: info@everestyayinlari.com
www. everestyayinlari.com
www. twitter. com/everestkitap
facebook.com/everestyayinlari

Everest, Alfa Yayınları'nın tescilli markasıdır.

Aklımda Hep Sen

Tren uçsuz bucaksız ormanların arasından geçiyor. Beni, bu bilmediğim ülkenin sonbaharından, kırmızı, sarı yaprakların, düzenli bir hayatı simgeleyen küçük evlerin, kasabaların arasından gitmem gereken yere, son istasyona taşıyor.

Belki benim için de son istasyona…

Görüntüler hızla geçiyor yanımdan. Burada, olduğum yerde duruyorum aslında ama tam da hayat gibi, nelerle karşılaşacağımı bilmediğim bir geleceğe doğru gidiyorum.

Bir yandan da geçmişi izliyorum ve anlar hızla gelecekten geçmişe doğru yanımdan akıp gidiyor.

İşte şimdi burada, sanki elimdeki dürbünle uzaklara bakıyormuş gibi biraz puslu, biraz titrek görüntüleri izliyorum ve kendimi oralarda, geçmişte bir yerlerde görüyorum.

Uzak geçmişi bugüne getiren bir dürbünle…

Olup biten ne varsa anlatmak istiyorum, anneannem derdi hep, hayat fırtınadaki bulutlar gibi geçip gidiyor ve siz değişen görüntülere, ışığa bakarken birdenbire kendinizi bambaşka bir yerde buluyorsunuz.

Nerede mi?

Nerede olacak?

Hayatın sonunda tabii...

Üstelik hayatın sonunda olsanız da olmasanız da, bir gün gelip geçmişe bakmak, en azından zaman zaman bir yerlerden çıkıp gelen ve birbirine bağlanmayan anıları, oraya buraya, karmakarışık çekmecelere, dolaplara tıkıştırılmış dosyaları, belgeleri toplar gibi yeniden yaşamanızı sağlar.

Belki benim için biraz erken ama bu garip yolculuğun sonunda ne olacağını ben dahil hiç kimse bilmediği için en azından unutmak istemediğim şeyleri yeniden biraraya getirmek istiyorum.

Kimbilir belki de tutunabileceğim tek şey bu olduğu için...

Ne olursa olsun, iyi ya da kötü, içlerinden bazıları kaybolup gitse de anılar aşinadır bize...

O yüzden onların yanında rahatım, çünkü dediğim gibi bir sonraki durakta ne olacağını bile bilmiyorum.

Karşı koltukta oturan yaşlıca şişman yabancı uyukluyor. Parmaklarını birbirine kenetleyip göbeğinin üstüne koymuş, arasıra başparmağını çeviriyor, dışarı bakıyor, yeniden gözlerini kapıyor. Ara ara dalıyor, iç geçiriyor. Giyimine, haline, tavrına bakılırsa (eski moda ama kaliteli yün takım, klasik çizgili kravat, yakasında, benim bilmediğim ama herhalde bir aidiyete işaret eden rozet) hayatını iyi geçirmiş birine benziyor. Uzun bir evlilik, çocuklar hatta torunlar, pazar günleri ailecek toplandıkları güzel, bahçeli bir ev…

Öyle mi?

Kimbilir. Hiç kimse aslında göründüğü gibi değil. Belki de aklıma bile gelmeyecek garip bir hayatı oldu ve gözlerini kapadığında herkesten gizlediği hayatının ayrıntılarını düşünüyor. Belki yaşamın bir yerinde geri alınamayacak yanlış bir karar verdiğini…

Yeniden dışarı bakıyorum, trenin ritmine göre sallanıyoruz yerimizde, kimi zaman tekdüzeleşen, kimi zaman değişen o sesle birlikte görüntüleri eşleştirmeye çalışıyorum. Kendimce bir oyun işte…

Evimden çok uzaktayım.

Zaten benim evim var mıydı, gerçekte hiç oldu mu ondan da emin değilim. Tek bildiğim, herhalde tam da bu yüzden, kendi içimde bir ev kurduğum.

Evet evim var, içimde, benimle her yere gelen bir ev.

Zaten asıl önemli olan da budur belki.

Annem evine çok düşkündü. Bütün hayatını o evin içine eşyalar, anmalıklar, biblolar, süsler doldurmakla geçirdi. Gittiği her yerden ne bulduysa alıp o eve koydu. Neredeyse artık bize yer kalmayacak kadar çok eşyanın içinde, orada sonsuza dek yaşayabileceği bir ev yaptığını sanmış olmalı.

Eski kralların yalnızca bir odada yaşasalar da kendilerine devasa saraylar hatta öldükten sonra da korunacakları muhteşem mezarlar yapmaları gibi…

Ama onlar nasıl bir hayat yaşayacaklarına ve nasıl öleceklerine karar verdikleri halklarını ve düşmanlarını korkutmak için yapmışlardı bunları.

Anneminki yalnızca başa çıkamadığı ya da asla sevemediği dünyadan kaçma ve kendisine ait mükemmel bir hayat kurma çabasıydı herhalde.

Şöyle dönüp bakınca insanın hayatında belirli günler, anlar, resimler ötekilerin önüne geçiyor. Yaşarken aklınıza gelmeyecek rastlantılarla, yalnızca birkaç saniyelik bir gecikmeyle değişen geleceğin dönüm noktaları aslında sayılı resimle anlatılabiliyor.

Evet evet tam da eski filmlerdeki dış sesin tonlamasıyla, 'kader denilen örümceğin ağlarını ördüğü' anlardan bahsediyorum.

Benim çocukluğumda habire 'iç gösteren gözlük' diye birşey çıkartırlardı. Gazetelerde bile böyle haberler çıkar, buna inanan da çok olurdu.

Keşke kaderin ağlarını gören bir gözlük bulsalardı.

İyi olmaz mıydı?

Evet çok uzaklarda, bilmediğim bir yerde, bilinmeyen bir yolculuktayım ama keyfim yerinde ya da en azından ben hala öyle sanmak istiyorum.

Tren sallandıkça gözlerim kapanıyor, yarı uyur yarı uyanık bir haldeyim.

Her zaman olduğu gibi gerçekle düşün arasında...

Ben...Ebru...

Dediğim gibi benim evim içimde.

Onu ne zaman yaptığımı çok iyi hatırlıyorum.

İşte o, zaman içinde kafamda değiştirip farklılaştırsam da unutulmaz resimlerden biri, belki de en önemlisi, okuldan eve geldiğim o sıradan günlerden biri.

Okul evimize çok yakındı. Her gün Seda'yla birlikte yürüyerek gider çıkışta da yine yürüyerek eve gelirdik.

Seda bir sokak ötemizde otururdu.

Uzun, sıkıcı bir yaz daha bitmişti. En azından artık ortaokula gideceğimiz için mutluyduk. Büyümüştük işte sonunda.

Seda, eteklerinin altına çıt çıt dikip okuldan çıkınca eteklerini katlayan ablaları anlatıyordu. Biz de yapar mıydık? Yapardık tabii annem farketmezse...

"Annem mi etmeyecek," dedim, "delirdin herhalde, ne çıt çıtı, düğme yerinden iplik çıksa farkeder o..."

"Ben yaparım," dedi Seda. Ne garip o konuşmayı hala hatırlamam...

Çünkü ilk kez, annesi olmadığı için mutluymuş gibi söylemişti bunu...

Eve geldim. Annem her zamanki gibi okulda neler olduğunu sordu, ben de her zamanki gibi geçiştirdim. Neden çocuklara okulda olanları sorarlar bilmem. Çocuklar, iş yerinde bugün ne oldu diye sorar mı büyüklere?

Kurabiyeyle meyve suyu getirdi annem. Elimi yüzümü yıkadım, üstümü değiştirdim, çünkü beş dakika bile formayla otursam laf edeceğini bilirdim.

Annem saçını topuz yapmıştı, anlaşılan yine kuaföre gitmişti benden sonra. Mutfakta yemekle uğraşırken ödev var mı, Seda nasılmış gibi sorular sormaya devam ediyordu.

"Matematikse baban gelmeden birazını yap istersen sonra televizyona dalacaksın yine..."

Henüz oniki yaşındaydım ve kaç yıldır artık bu konuşmalara alışmıştım. Annelerin işi bu gibi görünüyordu, söylenmek... Ama annem başkalarından biraz daha fazla söyleniyordu galiba, bana, babama, herkese...

Her nedense hiç birimiz bir türlü onun istediği mükemmellikte olamıyorduk.

Yine de artık öğrenmiştim, özellikle eve girdiğim zaman onunla biraz konuşmazsam, kendi dünyama çekilirsem işi iyice abartır, bütün gece bunu mesele ederdi.

O yüzden laf olsun diye, bildiğim halde, "Fatma nerede anne?" diye sordum.

Elinde bez mutfaktan çıktı, anlaşılan tam yerinden yakalamıştım.

"Nerede olacak yine bugün erken izne çıkacağım diye tutturdu, sürekli bir hastalık, bir gün annesi, bir gün dedesi, bir gün bilmemnesi... Derdi bitmiyor bunun..."

Aklım tabii ki başka yerdeydi ama dinliyor gibi göründüm çünkü anlaşılan bugün de Fatma'ya takmıştı.

"Yok göndereceğim ben bunu da, kadın bulmak kolay değil, gelen gideni aratıyor..." Yanıma gelip saçlarımı okşadı sonra da kokladı eğilip.

"E, sen terlemişssin, ne yapıyorsunuz okulda anlamıyorum ki, teneffüste yine koşturdunuz değil mi?"

"Yok anne sıcaktı işte ben ne yapayım?"

"Neyse neyse baban gelmeden bir duşa gir bari... Dur şu böreği fırına koyayım da... Seversin sen bak ıspanaklı börek var..."

"Yaşasın..."

İşte böyle bir gündü. Ötekilerden pek farkı olmayan...

Ben okuldan gelirim, bu konuşma benzer şekilde her gün tekrarlanır, akşama doğru babam gelir, o fazla konuşmaz, benim kafamı okşar öper, üstünü değişir, ajansı açar, annem yine ona da olan biteni anlatır, belki nadiren birileri gelecekse hazırlık yapılır yoksa akşam ben odama gider ders çalışırım, onlar içerde oturur, televizyon izler, sonra da yatma saati...

Özellikle maç varsa babam onu kaçırmaz, annem her ne kadar söylense de maç sonrası tartışmalarını bile kendi kendine sanki duyacaklarmış gibi onlara cevap yetiştirerek izlerdi.

Nasıl anneme göre kimse tam istediği gibi değilse babama göre de hemen herkes aptaldı, salaktı, budalaydı hatta çok kızdığı zaman söylediği şekliyle 'habenneka'ydı.

Politikacılar, gazeteciler, sporcular, artık akla kim geliyorsa hepsine sinirlenirdi.

Ama onun siniri bile fazla üst perdeden değildi.

Bazen annem, "Canım sen niye sinirleniyorsun ilgisiz adamlara, sana ne?" dediği zaman, "Doğru doğru bunlara sinirlenmeye bile değmez, sen bana çay koy," diye iki dakika önceki sözlerinden vazgeçerdi.

Ayda birkaç kez de babamın iş seyahatleri vardı. O zamanlar ya annemin bir arkadaşı gelir ya ikimiz yalnız kalırdık. O zaman hiç adeti olmasa da ya benimle yatar ya da geç yatmama izin verirdi.

Eğer yatmak istemezsem ve ısrar ediyorsa tam yatacakken ona olmadık bir soru sorardım. Ölümden sonra hayat var mı gibilerinden... O zaman kuşkuya kapılır, bana cevap vermesi gerektiğini düşünürdü ve en az bir yarım saati daha uyumadan geçirebilirdim.

Babamın seyahatleri her günkü hayatımı biraz değiştirdiği için ve tabii bana mutlaka kimsede olmayan hediyeler getireceği için iyiydi.

Şikayetçi miydim bu hayattan? Bilmem... Pek farkında değildim. Bizimkisi de böyle bir hayattı işte. Ama sanki şu salondaki kahverengi koltuklar bile yıllardır suren bu duzenden yorgun hatta üzgün gibi gelirdi bana.

Banyoda biraz oyalandım. Hayatta en sevdiğim şey bugün bile sıcak sudur. Su üstüme aksın öyle saatlerce oturabilirim.

Banyodan çıktım, annem saçlarımı kuruttu, fırçaladı, topladı, masa kuruldu, kapı çaldı.

Babam geldi.

Uzun boylu, yapılı bir adamdı babam. Şişman değildi ama iri yarıydı. Saçları erkenden beyazlaşmış ama dökülmemişti. Onları kısa kestirir, kendi gençliğindeki Cary Grant gibi oyuncuların tarzını beğenirdi. Pek fazla konuşup gülmezdi. Aslında yüzünden ne düşündüğünü tam anlayamadığınız insanlardandı. Kızdı mı, sevindi mi, nadiren belli ederdi. Genel olarak suratı asıktı.

Tok, kısık bir sesle konuşurdu. Sesi öyle anneminki gibi inip çıkmazdı. Yine annem gibi eliyle koluyla da konuşmazdı. Sakin bir adamdı kısacası.

Sanki her zaman çok derin konular düşünürmüş de günün birinde bütün bunları birdenbire anlatacakmış gibi bir hali vardı.

Gerçi hiç anlatmadı, ayrı...

Zaten annem öyle bir düzen kurmuştu ki, babamın belki başka türlü davranma şansı da kalmamıştı. Başkalarıyla konuşurken bile ondan üçüncü şahıs olarak, Kemal Bey diye sözederdi.

Manavdan birşey alırken bile "Kemal bey onu sevmez, sen şunlardan ver," diye konuşurdu.

Sanki babamın kendi istekleri yoktu, onun yerine hepsini annem bilirdi.

Ben de babamla siz diye konuşurdum. Bu annem için asalet göstergesi miydi, bir tür disiplin miydi bilmiyorum. Başka çocuklarla babalarını görüp aklım erdiğinde sormuştum. O zaman da bunun saygıyla ilgili olduğuna dair uzun bir nutuk dinlemiştim.

Babam küçükken benimle oynardı. Haftasonları gezmeye giderdik. Beni at gibi sırtına alıp dolaştırır, ellerimden tutup çevirerek uçak oynatır, tatillerde denizde omuzuna bindirip gezdirirdi.

Galiba o zamanlar daha çok gülerdi.

Gece yanlarında uyumak istesem annemin tüm karşı çıkmalarına rağmen babam izin verirdi.

Sonra buna kesin bir yasak koydu annem.

Ben büyümeye başladım ve babamla oyunlar da giderek azaldı. Sonra artık bazen keyfi yerindeyse yanına çağırır, kendince hoşuma gideceğini veya birşeyler öğreneceğimi düşünerek aldığı kutu oyunlarını oynamak isterdi. Ben bazılarından çok sıkılsam da onunla oynamak için sesimi çıkartmazdım. Bana soru sorduğunda aslında ona neler anlatmak isterdim ama yapamazdım.

Babam geldi beni öptü, annemi öptü, içeri geçti. Biraz sonra annem de yanına gitti.

Yemeğe oturmadıkları için merak edip içeri gittim, odalarının kapısı aralıktı, benim odamın hemen yanındaydı.

"Seyahate mi gidiyorsun, birden mi çıktı bu, söylemedin," dedi annem.

"Evet," dedi babam.

"Nereye peki?"

Ses gelmedi.

"Ne oldu Kemal bey bir terslik mi var?" dedi annem.

Bir terslik vardı, evet. Çocuklar konuşmaları bazen anlamaz ama belki seslerden olup biteni sezerler.

Annemin sesinde bir gariplik vardı.

Babamsa konuşmuyordu.

"Birşey olmadı," dedi sonunda, "gidiyorum, kendinize iyi bakın, sonra konuşuruz."

Ben odama geçtim, babam elinde bavulla dışarı çıktı, kapıdan beni gördü, gelip öptü ama aceleyle, başımı okşadı her zamanki gibi... Sanki bana söyleyecekleri varmış da bir an düşünüp vazgeçmiş gibi geldi bana.

Kapıdan çıktı gitti.

Her zamanki gibi seyahate mi gidiyordu? Öyleyse annem niye onu uğurlamamıştı?

Annemin yanına gittim.

Yatağın yanındaki koltuğa oturmuştu.

Loş odada öylece oturuyordu.

"Anne," dedim, "nereye gidiyor babam? Seyahate mi?"

O zaman bana baktı. Titreyen bir sesle,

"Evet kızım," dedi, "seyahate..."

İnsanın babası ölür.

İnsanın babası, annesi boşanır.

İnsanın anne, babası kavga eder, sonra biri öfkeyle çıkar gider.

İnsanın babası seyahate gidiyorum diye bir gün ansızın çıkıp gider mi?

Benimki gitti.

Hiçbir şey söylemeden.

O an'ı, onun kapıdan çıkıp gitme anını şimdi hayal meyal hatırlıyorum, nedense bazen bir an dönüp bana bakmış gibi geliyor, bazense bunu sonradan uydurduğumu düşünüyorum.

Ama insan öyle bir bakışı kendi kendine uyduramaz...

Annem yemekte konuşmadı. Gözü bir yere takılmış gibi televizyona baktı ve sessizce yemeğini yedi. Ben bir terslik olduğunu biliyordum ama anlamamış gibi yaptım.

Belki de böyle düşünmek o an işime geldi. Yani babamın her zamanki gibi iş gezisine gittiğini ve tabii ki bir iki gün sonra geri geleceğini düşünmek...

Belki de sorsam annemin duymak istemeyeceğim şeyler söyleyeceğinden korktum.

Hep korkarım kötü şey duymaktan.

O yüzden sormam.

Hala bugün de öyle...

Annem ki her zaman, en kötü olayda bile istifini bozmayıp kendi gibi davranmayı bilirdi, şimdi konuşamıyordu. Benim bildiğim annem ne olursa olsun benimle her zamanki gibi konuşup sorun yokmuş, herşey yolundaymış gibi yapardı. Ama yapamıyordu.

Kimseyi aramadı.

Kimseyle konuşmadı.

Sonunda, "Yemeğim bitti, ödevimi yapayım," diyince, "Tamam," dedi sadece.

Allahın cezası matematik ödevinin kafama girmesi pek mümkün değildi o akşam ama uyduruktan çalıştım işte. Sonra biraz kitap okudum...

Bilmediğim bir ülkede, bilmediğim bir zamanda, mahallenin çocukları karşı çeteler kurmuş birbiriyle savaşıyordu. Anlamsız yere acıklı bir kitaptı.

Annemin kuralları: Her akşam en az on sayfa...

İçeri gitsem? Onunla konuşsam? Neler olup bittiğini sorsam?

Keşke anneannem olsaydı, o herşeyi çözerdi.

Bilemedim ne yapacağımı...

Biraz daha oyalandım. Annem içerde sevdiği diziyi izliyordu.

Sonra gelip, "Ödevler bitti," dedim. Kontrol etmek istemedi bu kez.

Giyinirken yanıma geldi, çantamı topladım, ödevleri, kitapları koydum. Yatarken yanımdaki küçük lambayı açtı, lambanın için den şelale akardı, onu izleyerek uyurdum ben. Beni öptü, okşadı, biraz yanımda kaldı, ben de ona sarıldım çünkü üzgündü. O söylemese de ben biliyordum. Sonra dönüp kıvrıldım ve uykuya dalmış gibi yaptım ki, gitsin.

Çünkü ağlamak istiyordum. Nedenini bilmiyordum ama ağlamak istiyordum ve onun görmesini istemiyordum.

Biraz sonra üstümü örtüp alnımdan öptü ve gitti. Şelaleyi kapadım, yorganı kafama çektim ve ağlamaya başladım.

Kimsenin bana açıklama yapmasına gerek yoktu.

Ben karanlıkta ağlayıp uyurken annem bütün gece salonda oturmuş.

On yedi yılda yarattığı bu mükemmel düzene bakarak... İstanbul'un en güzel manzaralarından birine bakan, ünlü tasarımcıların imzasını taşıyan mobilyalar, en pahalı ağaçlardan lambriler, dünyanın dört bir yanından tek tek toplanmış biblolar, objeler, resimler, heykellerle doldurulmuş bir ev...

Yıllarla kurulmuş bir hayat.

Mumlara, sürekli yenilenen renkli çiçeklerle dolu kristal vazolara, gümüş ve kristal şekerliklere, tablalara, geçmiş hep bizimle kalsın diye zamandan kesilmiş fotoğrafların konulduğu çerçevelere, en küçük ayrıntılara kadar tıka basa doldurulmuş bu evde öylece oturmuştu karanlıkta.

Belki bütün bu yılları düşünerek... Belki bundan sonrasını düşünerek... Belki de düşünemeden...

Bazen annem o bayat konulu, dokunaklı eski filmleri izlerken ağlardı. Ben de o komik filmlere ağlamasına gülerdim. O zaman bana, "Günün birinde sen de bunları anlayacaksın," derdi.

Gerçekten de insan bazı şeyleri ancak "günün birinde" anlayabiliyormuş.

Kendi başına gelince, hayatı biraz daha öğrenince, en beklenmedik şeylerin olabileceğini görünce, yaşananların hiç de öyle gülüp geçilecek gibi olmayabileceğini farkedince herhalde...

Ve bir gün gelip, onlar ne kadar basit, ne kadar sıradan, ne kadar uydurma anlatılırsa anlatılsın, hatta bir reklam filmine sığdırılmış ya da uydurma bir şarkının sözleri haline getirilmiş olursa olsun artık gülemiyormuşsunuz...

Ben de anladım ama çok sonra...

Babam o akşam öylesine çıkıp gitti ve bir daha da hiç gelmedi.

Birkaç gün geçti. Sonra birkaç gün daha geçti. Yavaş yavaş neler olduğu ortaya çıkmaya başlayıncaya kadar bekledik.

Annem onun belki birşeye kızdığını, belki işle ilgili sorun olduğunu, hatta belki bize söyleyemediği bir hastalığa yakalandığını düşündü.

Ama çok geçmeden gerçekleri öğrenecektik.

Çoğumuz zaman zaman yaşadığımız hayatı tümüyle değiştirebilmeyi, yeniden başlasak nasıl olacağını hayal etmişizdir.

Büyük ikramiye kazananların ortadan kaybolduğuna dair hikayeler bana hep bunu hatırlatır.

Ama babama ikramiye çıkmamıştı. Amcamla ortak şirketlerinin hesabını zaman içinde gizlice yurtdışına aktarmış, orada kimsenin bilmediği bir hayat kurmuş, ev almış, evlenmiş, belki yeni bir kimlik bile edinmişti.

Amcam onun peşine düşmedi. Her nedense kendisinden çalınan parayla da ilgilenmedi. Galiba kardeşinin bu yaptığından o denli utandı ki bu konuda hiç konuşmadı.

Zaten bizimle de görüşmedi.

Yengem öldükten sonra yaşlı bakıcısıyla oturduğu evinde birkaç yıl sonra hayatını kaybetti. Cenazesine sadece üç beş kişinin geldiğini duyduk.

Anneme bir tanıdığımızın, onun son yıllarını sürekli içerek ve uyuyarak geçirdiğini söylediğini hayal meyal hatırlıyorum.

İnsan hayatını değiştirmek isteyebilir değil mi?

Benim anlayamadığım, bunu neden anneme söylemediğiydi. Ne olursa olsun boşanmak isteyen birini yanınızda zorla tutamazsınız. Birkaç kez bunu anneme sormak istedim ama soramadım. Bu konuyu açmanın onu her zaman fazlasıyla inciteceğini düşündüm.

Yıllarca güvendiğiniz, hep yanınızda olan birinin, çocuğunuzun babasının hem yalancı hem de sahtekar çıkması o kadar utanılacak birşeydi ki amcamın da annemin de bu konuda hiç konuşmaması belki en doğrusuydu.

Sanırım her ikisi de bu durumu açıkça söyleyip konuşmanın asıl kendilerine hakaret, hayat boyu inandıklarını boşa çıkaran inanılmaz bir felaket olduğunu düşünüyorlardı.

Ben uzun zaman bunları bir biçimde bize açıklayacağını düşündüm. Parayla mı ilgiliydi? İşlediği suçun ortaya çıkacağını düşündüğü için mi kaçmıştı yalnızca? Yoksa orada aşık olduğu bir kadının ona artık son bir şans vermesi, onu zorlaması yüzünden mi böyle yapmıştı?

İnsan en azından mektup yazıp bunları anlatamaz mıydı?

Ama bilmiyordum ki, özellikle duyguların, insan davranışının çılgınca savrulmalarının aslında böyle basit açıklaması yoktur. Deli gibi sevdiğiniz birine onun sizi neden öyle sevmediğini sorduğunuzda vereceği cevap neyi açıklayabilir ki?

Ve açıklasa bile sahiden sizi rahatlatır mı?

Annem yine de uzun süre bunlara inanmadı.

Herkese hatta Seda'ya bile babamın uzun bir iş seyahatine gittiğini söyleyerek oyalandık.

Ama sonunda anneannem geldi ve duruma el koydu.

Doğrusu o günlerde tam olarak ne düşündüğümü, ne hissettiğimi hatırlamıyorum. Şaşkındım galiba. Çok üzülmüş müydüm? Bilmiyorum. O ilk geceden sonra ağladığımı da sanmıyorum.

Sürekli gelen gidenlerle bu konu konuşuluyor, herkes ben gelince fısıldamaya başlıyor, kimileri babamın bir maceraya kalkıştığını, zamanla hatasını anlayıp döneceğini, kimileri namussuz bir kadına kapıldığı için yakında zaten kapıya konulacağını, paraları bitince kadının onu bırakacağını, kimileri de beni özleyip nasıl olsa yakında arayacağını söylüyordu.

Büyüdükçe, yıllar geçtikçe bunları unuttum. Ya da galiba unuttuğumu sandım. Öylesine derin, sonsuz bir uçuruma gömdüm ki tüm bunların üstesinden rahatlıkla geldiğimi sandım. Öyle ki artık babamın yüzünü bile doğru dürüst hatırlamıyordum. Bir keresinde Seda, "Peki ben ne yapayım, benim annem de babam da yok ve onları hiç görmedim," demişti. Öyle ya, babam da kazada ölmüş olabilirdi. Bunu böylece kabullenmek çok mu zor?

Evet zormuş.
Bunu ancak yıllar yıllar sonra anlayabildim.

Yine de bu sorular, nasıl bunca yıl herkesten gizli bir hayat daha sürdürdüğü, nasıl en sevdiklerinin hayatını ve parasını çalıp yine de herşey yolundaymış gibi davranabildiği, nasıl böylesine bir parçalanmışlıkla yaşayabildiği soruları aklımdan hiç çıkmadı.

Ta ki, Ferhat'ın sergisine gidip o resmi görene kadar.

Dev tuvalde sayısız insan figürü... İşçiler, köylüler, kadınlar, erkekler, sanatçılar, ünlüler, çıplak kadınlar, çarşaflı kadınlar, sporcular, zenginler, yoksullar, sarışınlar, esmerler, güzeller, çirkinler... Her türden insan vardı bu resimde...

Ama hepsinin yüzleri farklıydı. Bir taraftan bakınca başka, biraz eğilince başka bir yüzünü görebiliyordunuz insanların.

Aslında korkunç bir resimdi. Çünkü bir yüzüyle gülerken bir yüzüyle ağlayan, hem sevimli hem ürkütücü yüzlerdi bunlar.

Bana önce çok komik birşey hatırlattı. Tuvalete girdiğimde çocukluğumdan beri yer döşemesine bakarım ve çizgilerde, kendiliğinden oluşmuş damarlarda yüzler, desenler bulmaya çalışırım.

Ama bu dev resmin başka bir özelliği vardı. Yüzleri değişmeyen yalnızca aralarda görünen küçük çocuklar ve hayvanlardı.

O zaman Ferhat'ın burada ne anlatmak istediğini düşünmeye başladım. Bu resim bizim dışarıya verdiğimiz fotoğrafla gerçek kimliğimizi, belki farklı kimliklerimizi, gizlenmiş yüzlerimizi anlatıyordu.

Çocuklar ve hayvanlar başka kimliklere gizlenemez.

Onlar bizi bir başkası olarak kandırmazlar.

Yanıma geldi ve şaşkın şaşkın bakakaldığım resmin önünde benimle birlikte eserine baktı. O sırada sergiyi gezenler, bir kadınla bir erkeğin konuşmasını dinliyorlardı. Banttan verilen bu konuşma oldukça garipti. Çünkü söylenen sözler farklı anlamlara çekilebilirdi. Aynı konuşmayı herkes farklı biçimde yorumlayabilirdi.

"Ne o," dedi, "bütün figürleri tek tek inceliyorsun galiba?"

Ona baktım ve ağlamamak için kendimi zor tuttum.

Resmin altında bir yazı vardı. Bu resmi artık yaşamayan bir arkadaşına ithaf etmişti.

Ve ben o arkadaşının kim olduğunu biliyordum.

Onu ihbar eden ve ülkesinden kaçmasına neden olan kişiydi o.

"Bu herkesin bir başkası olduğu bir dünyanın resmi mi?" diye sordum.

"Bir başkası mı?" dedi, gülerek, "Hayır, birçok başkası olduğu bir resim.."

Ama bu çok sonraydı...

Şimdi düşünüyorum da gerçekten çok garip geliyor bütün bunlar.

Hani insanın filmlerde gördüğü, gazetelerde okuduğu ama benim başıma gelmez dediği türden...

Ama gelmişti işte.

Hayatı boyunca işiyle evi arasında yaşayan, iş gezileri dışında pek bir yere gitmeyen, fazla arkadaşı olmayan hatta hiç arkadaşı olmayan silik bir adamın yıllar sonra birdenbire çıkıp gitmesi, yeni bir hayata başlaması bugün bile beni şaşırtıyor.

İtiraf edebilirim artık. Belki de babam olmasa, başka biri olsa bu hikaye bana ilginç gelirdi.

Ama sanırım o zaman gelmedi.

Çünkü birkaç ay sonra görünürde herhangi bir belirti yokken birdenbire yere düştüm ve mosmor kesildim. Konuşamadım, hareket edemedim. Beni hastaneye götürdüler ve birkaç saat sonra kendime geldim.

Belki de hastalığımın babamın gidişiyle ilgisi yoktu ama ben öyle inandım.

Ve birşeye inandığım zaman dünyanın en büyük saçmalığı da olsa ne yazık ki ne derseniz deyin benim için farketmez.

Ve elbette ne olursa olsun bir çocuk hastalandığında, korktuğunda, kendisini yalnız hissettiğinde babasının yanına geleceğine inanır ve bekler.

Yalnızlık dedim.

Artık bunca yıl sonra bunu söyleyebilirim, yalnızlığın ne olduğunu, gerçekte ne anlama geldiğini bilen pek az kişiden biriyim.

O zamanlar bütün bunların tam anlamıyla farkında değildim tabii... Hayat yine de devam ediyordu. Ama annesinin masal kahramanı, okulun en sevilen, kıskanılan başarılı kızı, gözlerine, saçlarına herkesin sokakta yürürken bile methiyeler düzdüğü Ebru'ya tıpkı o gereksiz yere hüzünlü masallardaki gibi birşey olmuştu, nazar değdi, büyü yapıldı dedikleri gibi birşey...

İyi ama o büyüyü bozacak, belki bir öpücükle herşeyi eski haline getirecek biri var mıydı?

Yoksa o, yalnızca biz küçük kızların, hayatı ne olursa olsun bir gün daha sürdürebilmesi için uydurulmuş bir masal mıydı?

Bence çok da önemli değil. Önemli olan böyle bir masala inanmak isteyip istemediğiniz çünkü.
Ben böyle bir masala inanmak istiyordum.

Ama daha önce anlatmam gerekenler var.

Birdenbire bütün hayatımız değişti.
Bizde masalın tersi oldu.
Herkesin gıpta ettiği prenses bir anda Külkedisi'ne dönüşüverdi.

Anneannem (ki ona herkes gibi benim de Sare Hanım dememi ister, anneanne, nene, abla gibi laflardan hoşlanmazdı) Emirgan'da tepeden denize bakan, ağaçların içinde, oldukça eski, iki katlı bir evde oturuyordu.

Bizim evle karşılaştırınca onun zengin mi yoksul mu olduğunu pek anlayamazdım. Çünkü evin kendisi gibi eşyalar da oldukça eskiydi. Hatta o zamanlar artık her eve giren televizyon bile yoktu.

Ama buna karşılık belki de gördüğüm en güzel tablolar, heykeller, porselenler, kristal avizeler, mobilyalar da oradaydı. Evet gardırop, komodinler kurt yenikleriyle doluydu, bazen oradan buradan sular damlardı ama evin tavanları bile inanılmaz güzellikte ahşap işlemelerle bezeliydi.

Sonradan o evin aslında çok ünlü bir mimarın evi olduğunu, öldüğü zaman dedemin satın aldığını öğrenmiştim.

Bazı haftasonları orada kalırdım. Bazen de yaz aylarında daha uzun süreliğine... O bakımsız bahçe benim için masal ülkesine açılan kapı gibiydi. Orada kendi kendime oyunlar oynar, kendime dair hikayeler uydurmaya bayılırdım.

Sürekli bahçede kaybolup bulunmak bu oyunların en hoşuma gideniydi. Ve ancak yıllar sonra evdeki telaşın aslında tümüyle beni kandırmak için kurgulandığını, kimsenin benim kaybolmamdan korkmadığını öğrenecektim.

Ama aslında bu evin özelliği kapının neredeyse sürekli açık olmasıydı. Gelen giden eksik olmazdı. Salondaki büyük masa hemen her akşam dolar, dönemin ünlü yazarları, sanatçıları gelir, yenilir içilir, sabahlara kadar sohbet edilirdi.

Ben onu anneannem olduğu için sevmezdim. Ona herkes gibi ben de hayran olduğum için severdim. O zaten tanıdığım kimseye benzemezdi. Bana da torunu ya da küçük bir kız gibi davranmazdı.

Annemden o kadar farklıydı ki nasıl olup da annemin onun kızı olduğunu bugün bile anlayamam.

Hani şu eski filmlerdeki gibi annemin başkasının kızı olup da evlatlık verildiğini duysam hiç şaşırmam.

Yan evdeki Yıldız Teyze anneannemden hiç çıkmazdı. Evin hizmetine bakan Saniye gelen gidenden bunalıp arada bir gitmeye kalkışır ama sonra yine kendiliğinden çıkıp gelirdi. Onun bu gidip gelmeleri eğlence gibiydi.

Sare Hanım arada mutfağa girip özel bir yemek yapmak istemezse elini birşeye sürmezdi. Evin içinde sürekli "Saniye, Saniye" diye seslenişi duyulurdu.

Artık kendisini bir anlamda evin sahibi gibi gören Saniye de bu duruma çok alıştığından, önce ortada görünmeyip onu bağırtır, anneannem ne istediğini unutursa ne ala, unutmaz da sesini yükseltirse, dalga geçerek, "Tamam tamam bir saniye," diye çıkagelirdi.

Gelip giden insanların hepsinin ayrı özellikleri, tuhaflıkları, hem de bana göre çok acayip huyları olmakla birlikte Saniye belki de bu evdeki en komik tiplerden biriydi.

Gelenlerin çoğunu sanki o da sanat ortamında yetişmiş gibi tanır, kim ne yer ne içer, kim hangi meyveyi sevmez, kim hangi gün gelir, kim kiminle karşılaşmak istemez, kimler biraraya gelirse kavga çıkar hepsini bilirdi.

Konuklar hakkında da kendi fikirleri vardı. Kimini hiç sevmez, kimine hayran, kimiyle uzun uzun sohbetler eder, kiminin dedikodularını anlatmaya bayılırdı. Hangisi sinsi, hangisi çıkarcı, hangisi iyi insan bunları kendince garip işaretlerden çıkartıp edebiyat eleştirmenlerinin karakter analizi yapması gibi ortaya atıverir, anneannemi çok güldürürdü.

Sare Hanım, babamla annemin evlenmesini istememiş, evlendikten sonra da pek görüşmemiş, ben doğduktan sonra araları biraz düzelmişti.

Babamın da ondan hoşlandığını sanmam. Çünkü ne zaman beni çağırtsa sinirlenir, göndermek istemez, "Kaç yaşında kadın, her akşam ayyaşları, komünistleri masaya topluyor, yakışıyor mu, küçücük çocuğun bunların arasında ne işi var," diye söylenir ama sonunda mecbur kalıp yollardı.

Kırk yılın başı karşılaştıklarında bu arkasından atıp tuttuklarını yüzüne söyleyemez, çıtı çıkmadan oturup onu dinlerdi.

Zaten Sare Hanım'ın böyle bir özelliği vardı. O açık yeşil, parlak gözleriyle baktı mı yerinize çakılıverirdiniz. Gözlerimi ondan aldığımı söylerdi hep.

Ayrıca onun kimseden çekinmesi yoktu, tepesi attı mı aklına geleni pat diye söyleyiverir ama sonra biraz zaman geçince bu sefer "Tüh ben ne yaptım, durup dururken ne diye kalbini kırdım, böyle de söylenmez ki," diye üzülür, hediyeler hazırlar, gönül almaya çalışırdı.

Belki de annemle aralarındaki en önemli farklardan biri de buydu.

Annem adeta tüm dünyayı bir düzene uydurmaya çalışır, daha doğrusu düzen bozulmasın diye uğraşır, herşey yolundaymış, iyiymiş gibi yapardı.

Özellikle haftasonları oraya gittiğimde akşamüzeri büyük kristal avizeler yanar, sofra yavaştan kurulmaya başlanır, Sare Hanım da içeri gidip giyinirdi.

Bu tören hiç değişmezdi.

Bazen yanına gidip onun giyinip makyaj yapmasını izlerdim. O zamanlar benimle sohbet etmeyi sever, bana kumaşların özelliklerini, hangi rengin hangi renkle uyacağını anlatırdı. Arada bir terzi Perihan Teyze gelir, elbiseler dolaptan çıkar, tadilat yapılır, yeniden özenle yerlerine yerleştirilir, birtakım dergilerden patronlar çıkartılıp senenin modasından kumaşlar sipariş edilirdi.

Bir keresinde bir kumaşı yüzüme sürerken yanıma gelip ne yaptığımı sordu. "Dokunuyorum," dedim. O zamanlar farkında değildim ama sonradan anladım ki garip bir biçimde dokunma ve koku alma duyum çok gelişmiş. Bunu ilk anneannem farketmişti. Kumaşları bugün bile bir uzman gibi ayırdetmemin, çoğu insanın duyamadığı kokuları duymamın ve herşeyi hatta insanları bile dokunuşla, kokularıyla tanımamın nedeni herhalde bu olsa gerek.

Anneannemin çoğu oldukça eski ama belli ki döneminin oldukça pahalı, gösterişli giysilerinin doldurduğu büyük gardırobu benim en büyük zevklerimden birini oluşturdu.

Onları giymesem de çıkartıp dokunmaya, sonra onlara bakarak biraz değiştirdiğim modellerini çizmeye başladığımda herhalde ortaokul sıralarındaydım.

Annem, küçük bir bebekken bile kumaşları ayrıdedebildiğimi, biraz sert ya da kaba giysiler giydirmeye çalıştıklarında ittiğimi, ağladığımı, yumuşak özel giysiler gördüğümde gülümseyip elimi yüzümü sürdüğümü söylemişti. Tabii eve gelip giden teyzeleri kokularına göre ayırdığımı da...

Sare Hanım gezmeyi pek sevmezdi. Genellikle herkesin ona gelmesini isterdi. Bu nedenle de en üzüldüğü şeylerden biri çok sevdiği şapkalarını kullanamamasıydı.

Ayda yılda bir, kıramayacağı birinin sergisine ya da oyununa gitmek için çıkar, ondan da pek memnun kalmazdı.

Bir keresinde ünlü bir şair öldüğünde cenazeye gitmesi gerekmiş, "Aman neyse fırsat çıktı, şu şapkamı takabilirim artık," diye sevinmişti.

Zaten onun yaşamla ve ölümle ilişkisi çok garipti. Biri öldüğünde onu sevse bile çok fazla üzülmez, "Eh zaten bin yaşına gelmişti, bu kadar içmeseydi, kazık kakacak değil ya," diyebilirdi. Bana öyle gelir ki hayatın içinde ne varsa onu öylece kabullenmiş ve hiç şaşırmazmış gibi bir hali vardı.

Kimbilir belki de bu onun hayata katlanma biçimiydi.

Çoktan ölmüş olanlar ve yabancılar da dahil ünlü sanatçıların, yazarların hayatı hakkındaki konuşmalar sanıyorum onu en çok heyecanlandıran konulardı.

Örneğin bir yönetmen geldiğinde eski, sevdiği bir filmini nasıl çektiğini anlattırır, en küçük ayrıntılara kadar sorar ve sanki o filmin içine girmiş, hatta orada oynarmış gibi herkesi unutur giderdi.

Kimi zaman hararetli tartışmalar olur, siyasi kavgalar çıkar, kimi zaman şarkılar söylenir ve gece geç saatlere kadar uzardı.

Bu gecelerde bana hiçbir zaman, "Hadi bakalım artık yatağa" ya da "Bunlar çocuklara göre şeyler değil kızım," filan demezdi. Ben canım ne zaman sıkılırsa o zaman gider yatardım. Annemin bütün tembihlerine rağmen...

İçkiyi ve sarhoşluğu sevmem. Sare Hanım küçük, renkli kristal kadehlerde şarap ve bazen de büyükçe bir kadehte konyak içerdi ama çok fazla değil. Bir anlamda içermiş gibi yapardı. Kadehi ağzına götürür ama sanki değdirip tadına bakıp geri koyar böylece bütün gece içermiş gibi görünürdü.

Galiba içmekten çok uzun zayıf parmaklarıyla o zarif kadehleri tutmak hoşuna giderdi.

Bazıları gecenin sonunda merdivenleri zor inerken o gayet sakin saat kaç olursa olsun Saniye'den kahvesini ister, Yıldız Hanım'la sohbet edip biraz dedikodu yaptıktan sonra yatardı.

Ne de olsa her akşam gelen gidenle ilgili konular olur ve bunlar sanki önemli bir toplantıdan sonra değerlendirilmesi gereken şeylermiş gibi tek tek ele alınırdı. Ayrıca gelenler bir anlamda sınavdan geçer, kimilerinin, Yıldız Teyze'nin deyimiyle, "ayağı kesilir"ken, bazıları yeniden davet edilir, bir süre uzak kalan biri varsa acaba kırıldı mı diye meraklanılırdı.

Haddini aşan, sesi biraz fazla çıkan, değer verilen bir konuk hakkında ileri geri konuşanlar da Sare Hanım'ın "biraz soğutalım arayı" sözüyle ortadan kayboluverirlerdi.

Çok kızdığı biri için, "münasebetsiz", "sersem" belki en fazla "hödük" sözcüklerini kullanırdı.

Şiirlerini okumaya uğraşan şairlerden ve kendini övüp duranlardan pek hoşlanmazdı.

"Kendini ne anlatıp duruyorsun yahu, yaşadığın tuhaf olayları anlat da eğlenelim münasebetsiz adam," diye kızardı sonradan.

Tabii güne başlama saati de bizim evdekinden çok farklıydı. Ancak öğle saatlerinde uyanır, kahvesini ister, Saniye önceden sarılmış sigaralarından birini uzun ağızlığa yerleştirip getirir ve ne yemek yapacağını sorardı ki işte her seferinde onu çileden çıkartan da bu soru olurdu.

"Görüyorsun bu kadın beni delirtmek için mahsus yapıyor, sabahın köründe akşama ne yeneceğini mi düşüneceğim, akılları fikirleri yemekte," diye söylenir ama kahvesi bittikten sonra neşesi yerine gelip akşama neler yapılacağına dair emirlere başlardı.

Zaten geçe kalmaz Yıldız Teyze de gelirdi. Akşama özellikle çağırılmış biri varsa ya da ilk kez gelen bir misafir, onun için mutlaka farklı yemekler düşünülürdü.

Bu arada anneannem genellikle ya yarım kalmış romanını okumaya devam eder ya da yeni gelen imzalı kitaplara ve sanat dergilerine göz gezdirirdi.

Dedem çok erken ölmüş ve ona fena sayılmayacak bir miras kalmıştı. Zaten okul yıllarından beri sanata, edebiyata çok meraklıymış. Annemi büyütüp evlendirdikten sonra evini yazarlara, sanatçılara açmış.

Hatta pek fazla dile getirilmese de şu garip şiirleri yazan ve sonra biraz komik bir biçimde ölen ünlü şairle de büyük bir aşk yaşamış.

Eğer doğruysa adamcağız bir gece sarhoşken kendi kendine aklına gelen bir şiiri mırıldanırken karanlıkta belediyenin açtığı çukura düşmüş ve kimse bulamadığı için de orada ölüp kalmıştı.

Aslında şimdi uzaktan bakınca daha iyi anlıyorum ki Sare Hanım bütün o ağırlığına, herkesin hem dostu hem hamisi gibi davranmasına karşın sık sık aşık olurdu.

Çünkü onun için aşk, hayatın bir gün daha sürmesi için gereken tek duyguydu.

Önemli olan o aşkı yaşaması değil, yalnızca hissetmesiydi.

Bunu, gelen kimi insanlara daha farklı bir ilgi göstermesinden, ertesi gün Yıldız Teyze'yle fısır fısır onun hakkında konuşmasından, o geleceğinde giyinirken biraz daha fazla özenmesinden ve tabii ki gözlerinden anlardım. Daha doğrusu o zaman bunu anlamazdım ama bir farklılık olduğunu bilirdim.

Çünkü o yemyeşil gözleri, bilmem makyajın da etkisiyle mi sanki birden başka biçimde parlardı.

Gece sona erdiğinde renkli giysilerini çıkartıp makyajını silerken onu görmemi pek istemezdi.

Uyandığı zaman bile hep bakımlıydı ve sanıyorum onu dedem bile gerçek haliyle tam olarak görmemiştir.

Ben görmüştüm ve bana aynadaki o birbirinden çok farklı iki yüz büyük bir hüzün vermişti.

Rimeller, pudralar, ruj silindikçe sanki hayatın güzel yüzü çekilip gidiyor ve geriye soluk, yorgun, bitmiş bir hayat kalıyor gibi gelmişti.

Gerçek hayatımız gibi...

Şimdi hala gecenin bitmesini sevmem.

Acaba neden?

Acaba neden kaybolmak isterdim? Neden hep gizli geçitlerin peşindeydim? Öğledensonra uykusundan uyandıklarında evin içinde bile neden bir yerlere saklanıp herkesin beni aramasını, meraklanmasını isterdim?

Anneannemin eviyle annemin evi benim için iki ayrı dünyaydı.

Ama asıl neden şu ki, burası benim gizli hayatım gibiydi. Burada başka bir Ebru'ydum. Evdekinden, okuldakinden farklı...

Ve ne garip, çok küçükken bile bunun farkındaydım.

Sare Hanım benim bu küçük oyunlarımdan hiç sıkılmaz, her seferinde "Ay şimdi düşüp bayılacağım, yine nereye gitti, kayboldu, Saniye bahçeye baktınız mı, bana biraz kolonya verin yine tansiyonum çıktı," diye numaralar yapar, ben artık bir süre sonra korkup ortaya çıkınca ya da bulununca da, "Ah yaramaz çocuk çok korkuttun beni, ya seni bulamasaydık, hiç mi acımıyorsun bu yaşlı kadına," diye beni kucaklardı.

Tabii ben de inanır, yaptığımdan utanıp onu öperdim. Kucağında yatarken yumuşacık giysilerine başımı koyar, o güzel kokuyu duyardım ve kendimi hiç hissetmediğim kadar iyi hissederdim.

Ben en çok akşamüstüleri severdim.

Çünkü o saatlerde ev canlanır, ışıklar yakılır, akşam için hazırlıklar başlardı. Kendisi gibi beni de mutlaka giydirir, saçımı örer, kurdela takar, annemi delirten ne kadar renkli, parlak kıyafet varsa giymeme izin verirdi.

Derdi ki, "Gündüzleri bizim beynimizde bir bekçi vardır, akşam olunca onun mesaisi biter, bizi de rahat bırakır, bu yüzden akşamlar güzeldir..."

Terzi geldiği zaman sevdiğim renklerden bana da etekler, bluzlar, elbiseler dikilirdi.

Ben de sanki gelen konuklardan biriymişim gibi havaya girerdim.

Zaten evin maskotu gibi her gelen de benimle ilgilenir, sohbet eder, hediyeler getirirdi.

Babamın gidişinin üstünden birkaç ay geçip ben bir gün ansızın düşüp bayılınca birşeyler değişti. Sanki birdenbire büyüdüm. Sare Hanım en unlu doktorları buldu, ama onlar bende birşey bulamadılar.

Bir sürü tetkikler yapıldı. Onlar pek bir sonuç vermeyince benimle uzun uzun konuşup babamı, annemi, nelerden korktuğumu, duygularımı sorup duran, bana garip garip şekiller, resimler gösteren doktorlarla buluştum.

Bazen dalıp gidiyordum ve başım çok ağrıyordu, bazen uyurken vücuduma dikenler batıyormuş gibi uyanıyordum, bazen sanki yere düşecekmişim gibi başım dönüyor ve oturduğum yerde kalakalıyordum. Bazen konuşmalar, çevredeki sesler inanılmaz derecede yükseliyor, kulaklarımı kapamak istiyordum.

Ve o zaman konuşamıyor, adeta kilitleniyor, olduğum yerde mümkünse karanlıkta öylece kalmak istiyordum.

Bazen uyandıktan sonra neler olduğunu hatırlamıyordum.

Aslına bakarsanız gördüğüm rüyalarla gerçekleri birbirine karıştırdığım oluyordu.

O sıralar tam olarak hissettiğim şey korkuydu.

Çok korkuyordum.

Bütün o doktorlar, psikologlar bana iyi gelmiyordu. Aksine onları görünce daha kötü hissediyordum. Annem sürekli ya ağlıyor ya "Mutlaka nazar var, kurşun mu döktürsek," gibi anneannemi delirtecek sözler söylüyordu.

Bir tek onu isterdim yanımda o anlarda. Çünkü anneannem elimi tutar, konuşmazsam konuşmaz, bazen bana ilgisiz hikayeler anlatır, saçlarımı okşar ve kötü birşey yokmuş, ben hasta değilmişim gibi davranır, ben sorunca da "Herkesin birtakım hastalıkları vardır, kimisi doğuştan, kimisi sonradan olur, bunlarla başa çıkacaksın, bunların seni yenmesine izin vermeyeceksin," derdi.

Ne garip belki de benim halime en çok üzülen oydu ama ben onun bunu hiç umursamadığını sanırdım. Sonra birden kalkar, "Hadi bakalım toparlan, bu akşam sana bir sürprizim var," derdi.

Genç bir oyuncu çağırır, sevdiği bir piyes alır, benimle karşılıklı oynamasını isterdi örneğin. Ve sanki bir yönetmen edasıyla, "Hayır hayır, onu öyle tonlamayacaksın şekerim, sözleri öyle üstüste sıralama, hisset, sessizlikler çok değerlidir, bir an bekle sonra söyle o cümleyi," gibi uyarılarda bulunurdu.

Sanırsınız ki birkaç gün sonra perde açılacak ve biz sahneye çıkacağız.

Sonra o an geçer, ben de hastalığı mastalığı unuturdum. Yeni atak gelene kadar...

Sanırım onun üzüntüye, acıya tahammülü yoktu. Bunları sıradanmış gibi konuşsa da görmek istemezdi. Sanki elinde sihirli değnek varmış ve herşeyi halledebilecekmiş gibiydi. Belki de bu yüzden anlı şanlı koca yazarlar, sanatçılar özel hayatlarındaki sorunları bile gelip ona anlatırlardı.

Pek anlatmazdı ama öğrenebildiğim kadarıyla bu tutumunun nedeni dedemdi. Dedem zamanında çapkınlıklarıyla ünlüymüş. Sare Hanım'ı çok üzmüş. Ve çok genç yaşta geçirdiği bir felç yüzünden yatağa bağlanmış. Anneannem yıllar boyunca ona bakmak zorunda kalmış. Tabii dedem bu durumu kaldıramadığı için de gün günden huysuzlaşmış. Ölümü de oldukça acılı ve üzücüymüş.

Biz annemle üst kata yerleştikten sonra da Sare Hanım alışkanlıklarını değiştirmedi.

Tabii ki annem bu evdeki yeni durumdan hoşnut değildi. Hem gelen gidenlerden hoşlanmaz, hem anneannemin otoritesine karşı gelemez hem de benim onların yanında oturmamı istemezdi.

Ama anneannem bir bahaneyle beni çağırır, ben de annemin "yine mi?" suratına ve "hayır bu kılıkta inemezsin aşağıya," laflarına aldırmadan aşağı koştururdum.

Galiba hem anneannemin bu kez feci şekilde haklı çıkmasından, hem elimizde kalan parayla artık geçinemeyeceğimizden, hem de bana olan düşkünlüğü nedeniyle aslında bütün bunlara katlanmak zorunda kaldı ve iyice kendi içine döndü.

Bir süre sonra da bu hayata alıştı.

Böylece bu evde iki ayrı hayat başladı.

Üst katta annemin yine eskisi gibi kurduğu özenilmiş, bezenilmiş, dış dünyanın kötülüklerinden uzak, temiz, sessiz dünyasıyla, alt katta daha aldırışsız, çok daha rahat, kalabalık, gürültülü ve renkli bir hayat...

Kimbilir belki zaten insanın hayatı da böyle olmalı...

İstediğinizde üst kata, istediğinizde alt kata gidebileceğiniz bir hayat.

O yılların içinden gelen iki kişi daha var.
Seda ve Tolga.

Babamın gidişinden sonra kendimi iyice derslere vermiştim. Hatta annem bile bu duruma şaşırıyor, eskiden her dakika ödevleri sorarken şimdi "Kızım yeter artık gözlerin kanlandı, biraz dinlen, yarın çalışırsın," gibi ona pek uymayacak sözler söylüyordu.

Her nedense o sıralarda okul birincisi olmak ve bursla yurtdışına gitmek gibi bir düşünce oluşmuştu bende.

Galiba anneanneme gelen bir yabancı dil profesörüyle konuşmalarımızın da etkisi vardı bunda. Vahit Hoca kendi alanında dünya çapında çalışmalar yapan birisiydi ve benim mutlaka çok iyi bir okula kabul edileceğimi, bu imkanı kullanmam gerektiğini söyleyip duruyordu.

Ama ne gariptir ki dil okumayı düşünürken beklenmedik bir rastlantıyla o sıralar kimsenin aklına gelmeyen bambaşka bir okula gidecektim.

O yıllardaki tek yakın erkek arkadaşım Tolga da benim gibi edebiyata, sanata meraklıydı. Şiirler, kısa öyküler yazıyor, günlük tutuyordu. Lisenin ikinci yılında onunla birlikte okul dergisi çıkartmaya başladık. Dergi dediysem tabii fotokopiyle çoğaltılan on, oniki sayfalık birşey.

İçinde kendi yazılarımız, başka yazarlardan alıntılar, resimler, desenler vardı. Birkaç kişi de yazılarını, kitap tanıtımlarını verirdi.

Hatta son sınıfta dergi epeyce havalı olmuş, dergiyi okuyanlar adeta bir tür klan gibi ayrıcalıklı bir havaya bürünmüştü. Öyle ki yazı ya da desen vermek isteyenleri ince bir elemeden geçiriyor, sıraya koyuyorduk. Dergi fazla sayıda basılmadığı için de en başta bizi izleyenler ötekilere binbir nazla okutuyordu. Hatta komik ama derginin korsanı bile çıkmış, bir arkadaşımız edindiği kopyayı çoğaltmıştı.

Tolga'yla bizi herkes sevgili sanıyordu. Ama değildik. Doğrusu o kadar yakın arkadaş olmuştuk ki artık birbirimize karşı ne hissettiğimizi tam anlayamıyorduk belki de.

Seda'ya kalsa Tolga bana kesin aşıktı ama bunu söylemeye çekiniyordu. Aramızda bir tür aşk vardı belki de çünkü her sabah onu görmek beni mutlu eder, geleceğini söyleyip gelmediği zamanlarda (ki bunu sık sık yapardı) içim sıkılır, evin içinde dolaşıp beklerdim.

Arada böyle sudan nedenlerle bozuşur, birkaç gün surat asardık. Sonra mutlaka bana bir mektup yazardı. Ben mektubun geleceğinden emin bir şekilde durumu uzatırdım. Ama neden böyle yaptığımı şimdi pek bilmiyorum, galiba bunu oyun gibi görüyordum çünkü aslında ona karşı o anlamda bir çekim hissetmiyordum ve bunu gayet iyi biliyordum.

Zaten nasıl hissedecektim ki. Tolga eşcinseldi.

Ve bunu hiçbir zaman açıkça söylemese de bana anlattığı kimi şeylerden hatta yazdıklarından gayet iyi biliyordum. Belki annesi ya da başkaları da hissediyordu ama onlara durumu hiç açık etmezdi.

Bir biçimde anladığımı biliyordu ve bu ikimiz arasında kabullenilmiş bir sırdı.

Yine de bu aşk oyunu beni mutlu ederdi, sanırım onu da...

Hatta kıskançlıkları vardı. Beni beğenen ya da görüşmek isteyen biri çıktığında mutlaka ona çeşitli kulplar bulur, çaktırmadan iğneler, oğlanın öyle açıklarını bulup çıkartırdı ki çocuk daha benimle ikinci buluşmasına kadar gözümden düşmüş olurdu.

Açıkçası kendimi onun yanında o kadar rahat ve iyi hissederdim ki başkalarıyla konuşurken zaten sıkılır ve bir an önce onun yanına gidip anlatmak isterdim. Hatta bir keresinde bizden büyük ve okulda pek beğenilen o çocukla birkaç hafta flört etmemin en önemli nedeni belki de buydu. Yani buluştuktan sonra gidip Tolga'yla onun dedikodusunu yapmak...

Üstelik çocuk hakkında sanki gerçek aşığımmış da beni delice kıskanıyormuş gibi öyle şeyler söylerdi ki gülmekten gözlerimden yaş gelirdi.

Gariptir, Seda en yakın arkadaşımdı ama onunla bu kadar rahat değildim.. Örneğin Tolga'yla aklımıza ne gelirse en açık şekilde konuşurduk ama Seda'yla bazı konular hep tabuydu.

Benzetmek gerekirse Seda biraz anneme, Tolga'ysa anneanneme benzerdi.

Zaten anneannem Tolga'ya bayılırdı. Tolga ona gelirken çiçekler alır, nereden buluyorsa antika kalemler, defterler, kitaplar getirirdi.

Tabii Sare Hanım'ın gözdesi olup ara sıra akşam yemeğine çağırılmak ve adeta taptığı yazarlarla, şairlerle tanışmak onun için çok büyük olaydı. Yani anneanneme olan düşkünlüğünün belki de asıl nedeni buydu.

"Ne ince ruhlu çocuk bu Tolga," derdi anneannem.

Sanırım o durumu çoktan anlamıştı. O yüzden de bir tek o hiçbir zaman bana aramızda aşk olup olmadığını sormadı.

Ne yapayım ki huyum böyle, birşeyi anlatırken birden aklıma başka konular geliyor ve böyle daldan dala atlayarak zamanı, mekanı, insanları birbirine karıştırarak, aslında çok iyi bildiğim ama karşımdakinin bir türlü anlayamadığı bir kurgu oluşturuyorum.

Daha doğrusu bir kurgu bile oluşturamıyorum.

Neyse ki yazar olmaya kalkışmadım. Herhalde kimse yazdıklarımdan anlam çıkartamazdı.

Gerçi şu da var ki ben hayata benzemeyen romanları sevmem. Çünkü hayatın o romanlardaki gibi düzenli, bizim istediğimiz gibi bir kurgusu yok.

Var mı?

Tolga yıllar sonra yazdığı romanında belki de benim dediğimi yapmaya çalıştı. Çocukluğumuzu, gizli oyunlarımızı, büyüyünce yüzümüzü kızartacak ayrıntıları, kendi ikili hayatını, belli belirsiz bir biçimde anlattı. Ama öylesine karmakarışıktı ya da öylesine gizlenmeye çalışmıştı ki okuyanlar anlamadı.

Galiba hayat romanlara benzemiyor.

Sokağa çıkıyorsunuz ve aniden hiç beklenmedik birşey oluveriyor.

Birine deli gibi aşık oluyorsunuz ve o birdenbire ortadan kayboluyor.

Birinin hep yanınızda kalacağını sanıyorsunuz ama işte akşamüstü bavulunu toplayıp yolculuğa çıkıyor.

Hayatınızın yolunda olduğunu, çok mutlu olduğunuzu, hep böyle devam edeceğini sanıyorsunuz ama bir gün düşüp bayılıyorsunuz ve hayatınız tümüyle değişiyor.

Yoksa bu herkes için böyle değil mi?

Belki değil.

Annemin söylediği gibi hep garip olaylar benim başıma mı geliyor?

Böyle sanki hayatının romanını yazar gibi kendi özel dürbünüyle zamanın ötesinden geçmişe bakınca insan tüm ayrıntıları anlatmak zorunda hissediyor...

Çünkü aslında bizi yakından tanıyanlar bile gerçek hayatımızı, sayısız ayrıntıyı, gizlenmiş duyguları, unutulmuş anları, kırıklıkları, gizli mutlulukları, kaçamak bir bakışı, bir yerde rastlayıp sonra hiç görmediğiniz ama her nedense yıllar içinde ara sıra hatırladığınız o gülümsemeyi bilmiyor...

Yavaşlıyor tren, görevli gelip biletlerimizi soruyor. Karşımdaki yolcu uykusundan uyanıyor. Ben dalgınlığımdan sıyrılıyorum. Ağaçların içinde sevimli bir köy mü, kasaba mı? Biraz duruyoruz.

Ferhat'ı ilk gördüğümde lisenin son sınıfındaydım. Bahar gelmişti ve artık dersler bitmek üzereydi. Bahçedeki büyük manolya öyle güzel kokuyordu ki... Karşı tepedeki korunun içinde mor salkımlar, erguvanlar yeşillerin arasında eşsiz bir manzara resmi gibiydi.

Korunun içinde yüksek kuleleriyle benim perili köşk dediğim eski evin camları açılmıştı. Temizlik başladığına göre yaz geliyordu.

Bir cuma akşamüstüydü.

Tolga'yla okuldan çıkınca eskicilerin olduğu sokağa gitmiştik. O yine hediyeler almış ben de anneanneme güzel bir sigara tabakası bulmuştum.

Geldiğimde Sare Hanım'ın bahçedeki hasır koltuklarda uzun saçlı biriyle oturduğunu gördüm. Adamın arkası bana dönüktü.

"İşte benim neşem de geldi," diye el salladı anneannem beni görünce. Yanlarına doğru yürürken bana döndü ve o zaman onu gördüm.

Eve gelip gidenlerden değildi. Onu ilk kez görüyordum. Beni görünce ayağa kalktı, elini uzattı, anneannem bizi tanıştırdı.

"Bu benim torunum Ebru, bu yakışıklı beyefendi de yakında resim tarihini değiştirmeye hazırlanıyor," dedi.

"Belki de resmi tarihi..." diye güldü o...

Garip ama nedense elimi sıkarken yüzüne bakamadım. Tuhaf, bugün bile anlatamayacağım bir bakışı vardı, derin, sert hatta vahşi denilebilecek bir bakış. Uzun boyluydu. Geniş omuzlu, elmacık kemikleri çıkık, geniş alınlı, uzun saçlı, büyük burunlu, avurtlar hafif çökük ve belki biraz yorgun...

Yaşı belli olmayan insanlardandı.

Geri dönüp eve çıkmak istedim ama anneannem durdurdu,

"Gel gel otur nereye gidiyorsun, bizimle çay iç, sonra çıkarsın."

Ne yapacağımı bilemedim ama üstümdeki formayla burada oturmak istemediğim kesindi.

"Ben çıkıp anneme haber vereyim bir de üstümü değişip geliyorum, hem sana sürprizim var," deyip fırladım.

Gerçekte insan birinden ilk görüşte neden etkilendiğini tam olarak bilir mi? Ben bilemem. Üzerindeki ceketin kumaşından, o bakıştan, durgun ve sakin bir halde, yumuşak ama güçlü sesiyle "Memnun oldum," deyişinden mi? Kimbilir.

Yukarı çıktım, anneme aşağı ineceğimi söyledim ve odama gidip üstümdekileri herhalde birkaç saniyede çıkartıp fırlattım. O yine sorular soruyordu, hepsine yine klasik cevapları yetiştirdim ki konuşma uzamasın.

Terlemiş miydim biraz? Ama vakit yoktu. Pamuğa parfüm sıkıp koltukaltımı sildim, rengarenk desenli uzun gömleğimle bol bir pantolon geçirdim üstüme. Bu pantolonu alırken altına giyecek ayakkabı bulamadığım için kendime kızdım. Sonra mantar topuklardan birini ayağıma geçirdim, saçlarımı biraz dağıttım, aynaya baktım, eh işte idare ederdi, zaten yapacak fazla birşeyim de yoktu.

Tabakayı aldım, annemin "Misafir kimmiş, fazla kalma, yemek yiyeceğiz," laflarını geçiştirip doğruca aşağı indim.

Anneannem tabakayı pek beğendi, beni öven sözler söyledi. Ferhat, gelen çoğu misafir gibi bana okulla ilgili, derslerle ilgili, nelerle uğraştığımla ilgili sıradan soruları sormadı. Ben geldiğimde aslında bir filmle ilgili konuşuyorlardı. Filmin sonundaki sahnede iki kişi tenis oynuyordu ama ortada tenis topu yoktu, filmi bilmediğim için ne anlattıklarını tam olarak anlamıyordum, anneannem "Evet bazen ben de bunları beğeniyorum ama doğrusunu söylemek gerekirse Alain Delon'un filmlerini izlemeyi tercih ederim, belki de ben sinemayı hayatın yansıması değil de daha güzel kurgulanmış hali olarak görmek istiyorum," dedi.

O zaman Ferhat güldü, "Haklısınız, aslında sanat için de aynısı söylenebilir, belki roman da doğada gezdirilen bir ayna değildir," deyip birden bana döndü, "Siz, nasıl filmleri seviyorsunuz?" diye sordu.

Onları dinlerken aslında dalmış onu izliyordum. Yakalanmış gibi kızardım.

Gözlerimi kaçırdım, fincanı masaya bıraktım, "Galiba rüya gibi olanları," dedim.

"Rüya gibi mi?"

"Evet, aslında olmayacak şeyleri biraraya getiren filmleri, beni başka bir yere götüren filmleri severim..."

"Ne güzel bir tanımlama değil mi Sare Hanım," diye anneanneme döndü. Döndü ama aslında bir yandan bana baktığını hissediyordum.

Şu salak gözlükleri gözümden çıkarmak istiyordum ama bu sefer de onu göremeyecektim.

"Yaa işte bizim Ebru böyledir, hem biliyor musun okulda çok güzel bir dergi çıkartıyor, sanat dergisi…"

"Yok yok bizimki fotokopi, zavallı birşey," dedim..

"Niye öyle söylüyorsun gayet de güzel, kendi arkadaşları da yazıyor, aa bak Ferhat'la bir röportaj yapsanıza dergiye, güzel olmaz mı?"

Bir an sustum.

"Kimler kimlerle yaptılar, pek havalı dergi canım,"

"Anneannemin sayesinde," dedim,

Bardağını yerine bırakıp arkasına yaslanırken döndü ve uzun parmaklarını içinden geçirdiği saçını arkaya attı. Sanki müziğin durduğu bir anda obuacının nefes alması gibiydi.

"Tabii memnun olurum, ne zaman isterseniz," dedi, gülümsedi.

Kısık bir sesle ciddi ciddi cevap verdim:

"Zaten son sayımız olacak, ben de sevinirim…"

İşte aynen böyle oldu. Onlar yeniden kendi konularına döndüklerinde acaba kaç yaşında, acaba evli mi, acaba sevgilisi var mı, bunları düşünüyordum. Belli etmediğimi sanarak gozucuyla ona bakıyordum ve bunları neden düşündüğüme kesinlikle anlam veremiyordum.

Çocukluğumdan beri bir köşede durup insanlara bakarım. Yüzlerini, konuşmalarını, bakışlarını incelerim. Kendimce onlarla ilgili hikayeler uydururum.

Onun yüzünde birşey vardı, bakışlarında mı, gülüşünde mi, konuşmasında mı bilmiyorum.

Bazı şeyleri hissederiz, düşünürüz, biliriz ama kimseye söylemeyiz.

Bunu ona asla söylemedim, başkasına da, hatta belki kendime bile ama o akşamüstü orada otururken sanki elimde olmayan bir güç beni ona çekiyordu ve bu duyguyu daha önce bilmiyordum.

Aklımda ne vardı, bir an önce onu Tolga'ya anlatmak ve en kısa zamanda onunla röportaja gitmek.

Anneannem birlikte gittiğimiz sergiyi anlatıyordu. Makara bantların sarıldığı kundura boyama sandıkları, bir araya getirilip altına şiirler yazılmış objeler, ahşap levhalara nakşedilmiş büyük harfler...

"İyi ama bunun neresi resim, insan en azından desen çizebilmeli şekerim, herhalde ben artık iyice yaşlandım, bunlardan anlamıyorum," diye söyleniyordu.

Ferhat, her zamanki yumuşak konuşma tarzıyla, "Böyle söyleseniz de aslında hep farklı şeyler yapan insanları destekliyorsunuz, ben de bunu merak ediyorum, neden?" diye sordu.

Biz çay içiyorduk, o kristal bardakta içki içiyordu. Konuşurken bardağın içindeki buzu yuvarlıyordu.

"Evet bakma sen benim böyle söylendiğime," dedi anneannem, "herkes deli deli şeyler yapmazsa hayat boyu aynı filmi izleriz değil mi? Bak benim evimde hep natürmortlar var ama meyve sebze de bir yere kadar..." Ve o ünlü kahkahalarından birini atıp ağızlığına yeni bir sigara taktı.

İçkisi bitmişti, anneannemin Saniye diye bağırmasına az kalmıştı, kalktım, bardağını aldım, "Yenisini getireyim ben size," dedim.

"Aslında kalksam iyi olur," dedi, "akşam oluyor, daha fazla rahatsız etmeyeyim."

"Aa, ne güzel sohbet ediyoruz, getir sen getir kimse gitmiyor," dedi anneannem.

Güldüm. Yakında öğrenirdi o da...

Sare Hanım istemezse kimse bir yere gitmiyor.

Gidip mutfaktan içkisini doldurdum, buzlarını koydum, geldim, ama verirken elim titredi, birden alttan elimi tuttu, gözgöze geldik, karnımdan başıma kadar içimden ateş geçti sanki, kısacık bir an, hayatın içinde anlamı olmayan bir an, ama anlamı vardı, o elimden bardağı alıp teşekkür ederken...

Evet o anda birşey oldu ama ne olduğunu ben anlamadım.

Onsekiz yaşımın yazı…

Belki de hayatımın en mutlu zamanı…

Artık kocaman bir kızdım ve üniversiteye gidecektim.. Hem de nereye…

Bir gün anneannemin bir arkadaşı gelmiş ve çizimlerimi görmüştü, sonra kumaşlara olan ilgimi dinleyince Londra'da moda okulunda ders veren ünlü bir modacıyı tanıdığını ve bazılarını ona yollamak istediğini söylemişti.

Seniha Teyze ülkenin en ünlü markalarından birinin sahibinin eşiydi ve aslında o markayı birlikte kurmuşlardı.

Anneannem buna pek sevindi. "Seniha öyle kolayına beğenmez, mutlaka bunun arkasından birşey çıkacak, bak görürsün ben sana hep söylemez miydim," dediyse de fazla üstünde durmadım. Hatta ertesi gün unuttum gitti. Zaten biraz aklım havalardaydı o sıralarda. Ne de olsa okul bitiyordu, o sıkıcı kış sabahları erkenden kalkıp eski, soğuk, karanlık okula gitmeyecektim artık.

Tolga'nın dediği gibi, "o pasaklı tuvaletlerde ellerimi yıkarken titremekten kurtuluyorum ya başka ne isterim…"

Annem benim yurtdışına gitmemi istemiyordu. Madem dil okuyacaktım burada da güzel okullar vardı. Aslında orada yalnız kalacağım düşüncesi onu huzursuz ediyordu.

Ama son zamanlarda kendimi daha iyi hissediyordum ve bayılmalar, kasılmalar, kendinden geçip sonra unutmalar azalmıştı.

Taner Amca'nın verdiği ilaçlardan mı, birden büyüdüğüm için mi, artık eskisi kadar karanlıkta babamla karşılaştığım anı kurup, ona neler söyleyeceğimi düşünüp ağladığım geceler azaldığı için mi bilmiyorum ama Tolga da bir yıl içinde çok değiştiğimi söyleyip duruyordu.

Tolga'nın annesi eğer yurtdışına gideceksek ikimizin aynı yere gitmesinin iyi olacağını söylüyor, buna göre tercih yapmamızı istiyordu. Orada ikimizin oturacağı küçük bir ev tutabileceklerini söylüyordu ki bu düşünce annemin aksine bizi sevinçten deliye çevirmişti.

Hatta oturup sanki yeni evlenecek çiftler gibi neler yaparız, evi nasıl döşeriz, onlara kadar düşünmeye başlamıştık.

Tolga'nın babası çok zengindi. Ben hiç yurtdışına gitmemiştim. O çocukluğundan beri kışları kayağa, yazları birtakım ünlü tatil kasabalarına giderdi. Ama aklındaki şehir Londra'ydı.

Zaten bana, "Sen ne okuyacağına karar ver okulu bul gerisi kolay," diyordu. Çünkü onun umurunda bile değildi üniversite okumak. Yalnız başına kalabilmek, kendi hayatını kurmak, yazar olmak istiyordu. Sırf babası istiyor diye okula yazılacaktı işte.

Ben de anneannemi işliyordum ki annemi ikna edebileyim.

Ama Sare Hanım'ın bazı konularda kimselere belli etmeden alttan alta bir plan yaptığını, kafasına koyduğunu ne olursa olsun gerçekleştirdiğini unutmuştum.

Bu konudaki tek hüsranı annemdi ve sanırım bu nedenle de ona hep kızgın kaldı.

"Annen de senin yaşındayken sözümü dinleyip dışarda okusaydı böyle manasız bir ev kadını olmayacak kadar akıllıydı, üstelik başına bütün bunlar gelmeyecekti..." diye bazen söylenmeye başlar, sonra birden, "Aman neyse bunlar geçmişte kaldı, ben geleceğe bakarım, geçmişle uğraşa uğraşa hayat geçiren budalalardan değilim..." diye kestirip atardı.

Sonra bir gün beni karşısına alıp, "Sana bugün büyük bir sürprizim var," dedi.

Ben meraklandım. Ama o kahvesini, sigarasını içmeye devam etti ve biraz sonra kapı çaldı.

Meğer o günden sonra Seniha Teyze'yle sürekli konuşmuşlar ve sözünü ettiği Londra'daki ünlü modacıyla bağlantıya geçmişler. O çizimlerimi gördükten sonra ve tabii şimdi anlıyorum ki Seniha Teyze'nin torpiliyle beni okula almayı kabul etmiş.

İçeri elinde koca bir dosyayla Seniha Teyze girdi. Her zamanki gibi enerjik, bakımlı, (bayılırdım onun saçlarını yapışına, sanki hiç yokmuş gibi duran makyajına, giysilerine...) yüksek perdeden sesiyle bizi selamladı.

Anneannem gerçekten heyecanlandı.

"Eee, herşey tamam mı Seniha?" dedi.

"Tamam tamam Sare Hanım, hepsi tamam, yalnız şu belgeler doldurulacak ve bir de özel mektup yazılacak, sonra kısa bir hazırlık dönemi o kadar..."

"Peki konuştuğumuz gibi de oldu mu?"

"Aynen öyle oldu benden kurtulur mu, tam burslu gidecek..."

Ben şaşkın şaşkın onlara bakıyordum.

Evet benden sözediyorlardı ama öyle kaptırmışlardı ki sanki orada olmayan biriyle ilgili konuşur gibiydiler.

Sonra Seniha Teyze bana döndü:

"Evet Sare Hanım işte geleceğin ünlü modacısı karşımızda oturuyor şu an..."

Anneannem bana sarıldı ama ben hala şoktaydım.

İşte böyle öğrendim hangi okula gideceğimi...

Şimdi o akşamüstünü, her zamanki gibi birilerinin gelmesinin beklendiği aslında sıradan bir akşamüstünü, tabii ki o an farkına varmadıysam da hayatımı tümüyle değiştiren bu iki olağanüstü kadının karşısında oturduğum o günü bütün ayrıntılarıyla hatırlıyorum.

"Saniye Saniye, gel gel, bize zarif bir alkol getir bakalım da kutlayalım yahu sabahtan beri fenalık geçirdim burada zaten beklemekten, bak yine tansiyonum fırlayacak..." diye içeri seslendi anneannem...

Ben tabii annemden bahisle, bu işin o kadar kolay olmayacağını söyledim ve Sare Hanım'ı iyice kızdırdım.

"İşte şekerim bu bizim milletçe huyumuzdur, güzel bir hadise olduğunda hemen arkasından ne fenalık çıkar diye düşünürüz, kızım bu huyu hemen bırak, önce güzel haberin tadını çıkart gerisini sonra düşünürüz..."

Annem aşağı gelip haberi aldığında yüzü asıldı, hem sevindi hem üzüldü, Seniha Teyze'nin heyecanla okulu anlatması karşısında pek itiraz da edemedi. Tabii benim de onlarla birlikte kadeh kaldırmama şöyle bir ters baktı ama ses etmedi.

Belki de aklından, kızının gerçekten ne kadar büyüdüğü, yaşadıklarımızdan sonra bunun aslında önemli bir başarı olduğu geçiyordu ama kaygıları her zamanki gibi ağır basacaktı.

Bana mı öyle geldi bilmiyorum ama kadeh tokuştururken gözleri dolmuş gibiydi.

Tolga haberi aldığında Ajda'nın son çıkan şarkısını dinliyordu.

Onun küçükken başlayan 45'lik merakı o haldeydi ki sanırım en büyük koleksiyonlardan birine sahiptir. O plakların başında ne çok zaman geçirirdi. Bir şarkı başladığı an hemen devamını söylerdi.

O sıralar okuldakilerin çoğu yabancı şarkılar dinlerken o daha çok Türkçelere meraklıydı. Ve tabii ki en sevdiği de Ajda'yla Sezen'di.

Yeni bir plak aldığında onu defalarca dinlemekten bıkmazdı.

Onun için ağırdan aldım, bir haberim olduğu belliydi ama ne?

En sonunda dayanamayıp söyledim. Neredeyse, kalkıp hani filmlerde piyango çıkınca göbek atarlar ya sevinçten öyle oynayacak sandım.

Sanki okulu tam burslu kazanan ben değildim de oydu.

Hemen koşup annesine haber verdi ve annemi ikna etme işi onun üstüne kaldı.

Okuldaki notlarım çok iyiydi ama yine de okul daha bitmemişti, Tolga da bana kızdı, niye sürekli kaygılanıyorum diye…

Ayaklarım yerden kesilmişti ama yine de inanamıyordum bütün bunlara.

Bizimki o andan sonra Londra'yla ilgili ne bulduysa getirip neredeyse gitmeden kentin her yerini bana öğretmeye başladı.

Komikti halimiz. Bir yandan sürekli aynı Ajda şarkısını dinliyor bir yandan kitaplara bakıp nerelere gideriz, hangi müzikali izleriz, hangi müzede ne var onları konuşuyorduk.

Ama işte diyorum ya hiçbir şeye tam sevinemem ben. Çünkü mutlaka çok mutlu olduğumda bir terslik olur. Hem de hiç beklenmedik bir terslik... Anneannem bu huyuma ne kadar kızsa da bu böyle...

Biz annemin çıkaracağı arızalarla uğraşırken asıl darbe Tolga'nın babasından geldi. Bu yaşta bir kızla erkeğin aynı evde kalmasının doğru olmadığı şeklinde bir ifadeyle...

Öyle ya biz bunu hiç düşünmemiştik. Çünkü tabii ki annesi de dahil hepimiz (söylemesek de) onun durumunu biliyorduk. Ama babası bilmiyor ya da kabul etmiyordu.

Zaten ölene kadar da etmeyecekti.

Ev tutmak yerine pansiyonda kalmamız düşünüldü önce.

Sonra şeytan Tolga'nın aklına daha parlak bir fikir geldi. Ev ona tutulacaktı. Ben de pansiyonda kalıyor olacaktım. Ama aslında birlikte oturacaktık. Babası gelirse de o zaman düşünürdü bir çare...

Hatta bir keresinde, "Canım en kötüsü, yakalanırsak, evleneceğiz deriz, buna da laf edecek hali yok, hatta hoşuna gider," demişti de şaşkın şaşkın yüzüne bakakalmıştım.

"Aman korkma uyduruktan..." diye güldü sonra...

O hayatı boyunca bir başkası gibi yaşadığı için sır saklamayı, yalan söylemeyi neredeyse oyuna dönüştürmüştü. "Yalan da sanattır, herkes söyleyemez, çünkü bir yalan mutlaka başka yalanları getirir ve birini unutursan domino taşları gibi bütün hepsi üstüste yıkılır," der hatta bununla övünürdü.

Ben yalan söylemeyi pek bilmem. Utanırım söylemek zorunda kalınca. Gözlerimi kaçırırım, kızarırım, anlaşılır yani ne çevirdiğim. Aslında sonradan çok düşündüm bunu. Korktuğumdan değil, neden yalan söylemem gereksin diye düşünürdüm. Karşımdaki kim oluyor da ona yalan söylemek zorunda kalıyorum diye kızardım kendime.

Yalan söylemem ama çok şeyi gizlediğim doğrudur. Hayatımı da doğru söyleyeceğim diye herkese açıklamak zorunda değilim. Belki anneme duyduğum tepkidendi bu. Çünkü annem sürekli yalan söylerdi ama anlamsız yalanlar. Biri geleceğinde istemiyorsa, istemem demez, "Akşam bir akrabamız geliyor," gibi mazeretler uydururdu. İnsanları kırmamak için böyle davranmak gerektiğini söyler, bunu bir nezaket kuralı gibi görürdü.

Anneannemse tam tersi… "Kimseyi memnun edecek halim yok, isteyen gelir benimle oturur, istemeyen oturmaz, kocama yalan söylememişim, elin adamına ne diye söyleyeyim?" derdi.

Tolga eğer günün birinde babasına gerçeği söyleseydi belki de hayatı bambaşka olabilirdi. Ama söyleyemedi.

İşte biz o günlerde böyle bir ruh hali içindeydik. Gelecek planları yapıyor, yakın gelecekteki gizli saklı hayatımızı nasıl kuracağımızı düşünüyor, geceyarılarına kadar kendi kendimize kurduğumuz bu oyunla belki de gerçekte olacağımızdan daha mutlu oluyorduk.

İşte Ferhat'ın bizim eve geldiği akşamüstünün hemen ertesinde oldu bütün bunlar.

Belki komik ama ben onun bana uğur getirdiğine inanıverdim.

Birkaç gün sonra Tolga'yla birlikte onun evine gittik. Tolga beni almaya geldiğinde şöyle baştan aşağı süzdü. Kızardım. Aslında epey denemeden sonra kendimce son derece sıradan giyinmiştim. Bir iki yerinden yırtık son moda bol paça pantolon, üstüne bol ipek gömlek ve püsküllü güderi ceket, ayağımda da salaş, bağlanmamış botlar vardı. Ve gömleğin açık düğmelerinden görünen büyük, renkli taşlardan kolye...

"Pek havalıyız bugün," dedi sadece ama şeytanın kuşkulandığına emindim.

Bahçedeki konuşmayı anlatırken o kadar da dikkatli davranmıştım oysa ki...

Büyük taş merdivenlerden çıkıp daracık çıkmaz sokağa girdik. Birkaç küçük kız lastik oynuyordu. Sessiz, eski, yoksul bir mahalleydi. Yalnızca kızların oynarken bağırışları duyuluyordu.

"Evet işte burası," dedi Tolga, demir bahçe kapısının önünde durup.

Kapıyı itti, içeri girdik. Bakımsız bahçede heykeller, garip ahşap parçaları, eski ve herhalde kullanılmayan bisiklet, hafifçe esen rüzgârın getirdiği çiçek kokuları, büyükçe bir malta eriği...

Bahçenin içinde tek katlı, gecekondu gibi bir evdi.

Kapıyı çaldık.

Ses çıkmadı.

"Burası olduğuna emin misin?" dedim.

"Evet, tam da uçuk ressama göre değil mi, 8 numara yazıyordu adreste..."

Yeniden çaldık.

Üzerinde uzun beyaz gömlek ve ıslak saçlarla açtı kapıyı... Boynunda bir havlu vardı.

"Gelin gelin, hoşgeldiniz, kusuruma bakmayın..."

Girdik ve bizden izin isteyip saçlarını kurulamaya gitti.

Şöyle bir etrafa baktım. Hayatımda bu kadar çok eşyanın olduğu bir yer sanırım hiç görmemiştim.

Ama ne gariptir ki bütün bu kalabalık insanın gözünü rahatsız etmiyordu. Özellikle uğraşılmamış olsa da belki seçilmiş eşyanın niteliğinden ötürü bütün bu birbirine benzemez parçalar yerli yerinde gibi görünüyordu.

Benim doğup büyüdüğüm ev, annemin mükemmellikle donattığı, herşeyin birbiriyle uyumlu olduğu klasik senfoni gibiydi.

Anneannemin evi, biraz daha karmaşık ve eski de olsa yine de kulağınızı rahatsız etmeyen modern bir eser gibiydi.

Ama burası hayatımda hiç görmediğim, birbirine hiç uymayan parçaların biraraya getirildiği, ahşapla camın, mermerle kağıdın, dev insan figürleriyle ne olduğu anlaşılmaz küçük bibloların, eski bir film afişiyle astronot giysilerinin, kırık bir bisikletle teneke bir arabanın, bilinmeyen yerlerin eski haritalarının, hani o şairin "Kardeşim su versin ona, susamış," dediği tahta atın, korkunç yüzlü kuklalarla canlı gibi duran bebeklerin, azraille meleğin, kavanozların içindeki ceninlerle kadim uygarlıkların ölüm törenlerinin, rönesans duvar resimleriyle çizgi filmlerin içiçe geçtiği dünyadışı bir yer gibiydi.

Asıl olanla taklidin, yaşamla ölümün, iyilikle kötülüğün, masumiyetle sapkınlığın, gerçekle rüyanın içiçe geçtiği, ancak sizin bakışınızla, o anki algınızla anlam kazanan bir sanat eseri gibiydi.

Adeta bir rüya gibi...

Çünkü rüyaları biz biçimlendiremeyiz. Birbiriyle ilgisiz, zamandan, mekandan kopuk, görülmüş ya da hiç bilinmeyen şeyler biraraya gelir ve kendimizi çekilmesi imkansız bir filmin içinde buluruz.

Sarhoşluk gibi...

Sınırların kalktığı, bilinen bütün biçimlerin bozulduğu, sözcüklerin artık ne anlama geldiğinin bile anlaşılamadığı, başka dünyaya geçmiş gibi hissettiğiniz başka bir ruh hali...

Tam da benim gibi...

Rüyadan uyanırken hep huzursuz olurum. Çocukluğumdan beri... Sanki bir yere gitmişim ve yeniden bu dünyaya geri geliyormuşum gibi... Çoğu zaman çarpıntıyla uyanırım ve orada bıraktığım puslu görüntüleri, insanları unutup yeniden uyandığım, tanıdığım, bildiğim gerçeğe dönmek için biraz zaman geçirmem gerekir.

Ben aşık olmak nasıl birşey bilmiyordum.
Üstelik bunu bilmediğimi de bilmiyordum.

O uçuşan kelebekleri, birini görünce heyecanlanmayı, kalp çarpıntısını, yüz kızarmasını filan aşk sanıyordum ben.

Bir de tabii elele tutuşup gezmeleri, akşam olup gitmesin diye ikide bir saate bakmaları, olur olmaz konuşmalarla hiç sıkılmadan oturmaları...

Birine yalnızca bakmanın, onun kokusunu hatırlamanın, gün içinde yanımdayken birşeyi söyleyiş biçiminin, elinin basit hareketinin, gömleğinin kırışıklığının, saçlarını karıştırmasının, olur olmaz anlarda yeniden aklına geleceğini bilmiyordum mesela.

Ya dünyanın öteki ucundan hatta yılların içinden bile onun kokusunu duymayı?

Ve bütün bunların beni garip bir biçimde heyecanlandırmış olmasını, sabahları sanki birşey olacakmış gibi uyanmamı, yüzümde durduk yerde beliren saçma gülümseyişi, birileriyle konuşurken dalıp gitmelerimi ve söylenenlerin umurumda bile olmayışını anlayamıyordum.

Sonra o geri geldi...

Saçları hala biraz ıslaktı. Yine uzun beyaz bir gömlek giymişti. Ayakları çıplaktı. Bize kahve yaptı. Oturup sigara yaktı.

"Evet," dedi, "şimdi, soru mu sormak istersiniz, sohbet etmek mi?"

Ne diyeceğimizi bilemeden birbirimize baktık Tolga'yla...

Sanki bana fazla sormayın, ben soruları sevmem, der gibiydi.

Tabii yine de bir sürü soru sorduk. Çünkü gelmeden önce onun hakkında birbirinden çok farklı hikayeler anlatıldığını duymuştum. Daha ilk resimleriyle birdenbire büyük olay yaratan, bir anda ünlü ressamların önüne geçen ama kendi sergisinin açılışına bile gelmeyen, ortada görünmeyen bu adam hakkında herkes konuşuyordu.

Kimine göre bütün bunlar planlanmıştı. Böyle gizemli bir hava yaratarak resimlerine çok daha yüksek fiyatlar koyacaktı. Kimi onun çılgınca resimler çizen ve ne çizdiğinin farkında bile olmayan delinin biri olduğuna inanıyor, kimi, düzene karşı bir anarşist olduğunda ısrar ediyordu.

Annesi çok küçükken ölmüş ve ona teyzesi bakmıştı. Babasının tek başına hem ona hem hasta kardeşine bakacak durumu yoktu.

Erkek kardeşi zihinsel engelliydi. Babası Erzurum'a tayin olunca o Van'da teyzesinin yanında ilkokulu okumuş ve onca yıl babasını ve kardeşini belki bir ya da iki kez görebilmişti.

Annesini çok hatırlamıyordu. Ama teyzesini annesi kadar çok sevmişti.

Yoksullardı.

"Aslına bakarsanız uzun zaman bunun farkında değildim," dedi. "Herkes yoksuldu çünkü, sonuçta yemeğimiz vardı, okula gidiyorduk, sokakta oynuyorduk, yazın nehirde yüzüyorduk, kırlarda dolaşıyorduk, bir eski radyo vardı, oradan dinlediklerimiz de bize masallar dünyasından öyküler gibi gelirdi... O kadar uzaktı bizim gerçeğimizden..."

Durup bir an sanki o günler gelmiş, şu an yanıbaşımızdaymış gibi baktı ve gülümsedi, "Ne zaman ki insan başka şeyler görüyor o zaman çaresizliğin, yoksulluğun ne demek olduğunu anlayabiliyor, ne zaman ki başkalarının evlerini görüyor, kendi eşyalarının ne kadar zavallı olduğunu farkediyor."

Tolga'yla birbirimize baktık. İki şımarık çocuk. Hep bir eli yağda bir eli balda büyümüş. Şimdi böyle bir adamın karşısında oturmuş ona sorular mı soruyorduk?

"Ben ortaokulu bitirdiğimde babam yeniden evlendi. Ölen eşinden yüklüce mirasa konmuş bir kadınla. Beni de yeniden yanına almaya karar verdi tabii. Bu kez teyzem deliye döndü, aslına bakarsanız biraz deliydi de gerçekte ama pek belli olmazdı, sakin, içine dönük, durduk yerde ağlayan kadınlar vardır ya öyle bir kadındı zaten. Benden ayrılacağını duyunca artık ağlaması hiç kesilmedi. Sonunda ben de bir karar verdim ve onun yanında kalacağımı, yazları ya da tatillerde de babamın yanına gideceğimi söyledim. Sanırım yeni anne de buna pek üzülmedi."

Bir an aklıma babam geldi.

"Babanızın evlenmesini nasıl karşıladınız?" diye sordum.

Kahvesinden bir yudum aldı. Kafasını kaşıdı. Bana değil uzak bir noktaya bakarak cevap verdi:

"Bilmem, galiba o zaman bunu çok önemsemedim, sanki içimden ben ona zaten küsmüştüm ve duygusal anlamda o konu benim için kapanmıştı, daha doğrusu ben öyle sanıyordum. Bir oğlanın babasıyla böyle bir konusu tabii asla kapanmıyor yalnızca saklıyorsun ve orada seni bekliyor, yıllar sonra yeniden beklenmedik biçimde karşına çıkmak üzere..."

Belki bir kızın da babasıyla... diye geçirdim içimden... Devam etti, "Onlar İstanbul'daydı ben Van'da. Ama artık parası vardı babamın yani daha doğrusu karısının... Onun için de ilk tatilde onların yanına gitmem için otobüs bileti geldi. İlk kez bu kadar uzun bir yolculuğa çıkmıştım ve tek başıma pencereden yollara, sanki bırakılmış, terkedilmiş gibi görünen uçsuz bucaksız topraklara, ekili tarlalara, telefon direklerine, yoksul evlere, güzel evlere, kimi zaman insanın içini burkan bozkıra, kimi zaman yemyeşil küçük köylere bakarak ve elimdeki deftere gördüklerimi çizerek geldim.

O yolculuğu hiç unutmam. Belki ilk uzun yolculuğum olduğu için, belki kısa da olsa tüm hayatımı ilk kez kendi başıma yeniden gözümde canlandırdığım için, belki birçok hayatın içinden geçerken aslında kendi yaşadıklarımın öyle çok da acıklı, çok da bana özgü olmadığını ilk kez anladığım için, bilmem..."

Sanki sesi titredi gibi geldi bana... Tolga hayranlıkla ona bakıyordu.

Birden kalktı, "Burası fazla sessiz," dedi, gözlerini mi sildi acaba, eski bir pikaba bir plak koydu, sert, sigaradan kalınlaşmış sesli adam Fransızca şarkı söylemeye başladı. Sürgün edilmekten, bir bavulla yaşamaktan ya da ülkesinin artık o bavul olduğu gibi şeylerden sözeden bir şarkıydı.

Sanki tüm bunları anlatmak için yıllardır bizi beklermiş gibi, sanki az önce soruları sevmem diyen o değilmiş gibi, sanki biz yokmuşuz ve kendi kendine konuşuyormuş gibi kaldığı yerden anlatmaya başladı.

Öylesine canlı anlatıyordu ki sanki o ana, o zamana birlikte gitmişiz, biz de onunla oradaymışız gibi hissediyorduk.

Çok sonra bana o gün bütün bunları gerçekten de yıllar sonra ilk kez bize anlattığını söyleyecekti.

"İstanbul'da beni otogardan babam aldı. Henüz benim için yeni olan, farklı olan tek şey inanılmaz kalabalıktı. Sanki herkes üstüme geliyormuş gibi korkmuştum. Bu kadar çok insanın aynı anda yollarda yürümesi, bu kadar çok arabanın dolaşması hiç filmlerdeki gibi değildi...

Hem ürkütücü hem de heyecan vericiydi.

Aslına bakarsanız çok fazla film de izlemiş değildim. Kasabadaki sinemaya bir ya da iki kez gitmiştik. İstanbul'u da ilk izlediğim o siyah beyaz filmde görmüş ve aşık olmuştum. Sanki benim için dünyadaki en eşsiz yer gibiydi."

Kahve getirdi. Müziğin sesini biraz kıstı.

Sonra devam etti.

"Babamın yeni evi bizimkine benzemiyordu. Bilmemne palas diye havalı, yeni bir apartmanın bahçe katındaydı. Oldukça büyüktü ve benim için de ayrı oda hazırlanmıştı. Kardeşim beni yadırgadı, huysuzlandı, belki gerçekten hatırlamadı belki de içinden bana küsüp unutmuştu... Köşede oturup bu yabancıya yadırgayan gözlerle bakıp elindeki ipliklerle oynamaya devam etti.

Cici annemiz babamın yaşlarında, giyimine meraklı, süslü, püslü bir kadındı. Gür bir sesi vardı. Kendinden emin, kesin cümlelerle konuşuyordu.

Babamın onunla sırf parası için evlendiğini herkes gibi herhalde o da biliyordu. Ama ben bugün bile onun niye babamla evlendiğini anlayabilmiş değilim."

Ne garip diye düşündüm, bambaşka insanlar benzer şeyler düşünüp, beklenmedik biçimde benzer şeyler yaşayabiliyor, hissedebiliyor demek ki...

"Çünkü babam neredeyse hiç konuşmayan, saatlerce gazetenin verdiği bulmacaları çözüp sıkılmayan, sonra uyuyakalan biriydi. Evlendiği için ona kızmadım, en azından kardeşimle ilgilenen biri var diye düşündüm..."

O insana huzur veren, yumuşak ama etkileyici sesiyle bunları anlatırken ben sanki radyo tiyatrosu dinler gibi garip bir ruh haline girmiştim.

Bir an, hiç beklenmedik biçimde, normalde herkes sorularıma son derece basit, sıradan cevaplar verirken onun yıllardır beni tanırmış gibi böyle hayatını anlatması beni irkiltti. Sanki gizlice onun çekmecelerini karıştırmış, günlüğünü okumuş gibi suçluluk duydum.

"İşte orada ilk akşam yemeğimizi yerken galiba ilk kez yoksulluğun farkına vardım. Masanın üstünde sallanan kristal avize bile gözümü alıyordu. Elimi, ayağımı nereye koyacağımı şaşırdım. Bir sürü çatal bıçak, bardak, üstüste konmuş tabaklar, porselen takımlar, sanki kadıncağız eski bir ihtişamı sürdürmeye çalışır gibiydi."

Aklıma annem geldi tabii...

"Aslında o gece hemen oradan çıkmak ve geri dönmek istiyordum. Kendimi hiç bir zaman bu kadar rahatsız, bu kadar yabancı, bu kadar ait olmadığım bir yerde bulmamıştım. Karşımda oturan bu adam benim babamdı ama aslında onu hiç tanımıyordum, bu benim kardeşimdi ama o da beni tanımıyordu, bu kadınsa tümüyle yabancıydı. Bana sorulan sorulara (ki babamdan çok kadın soruyordu) kısa kısa cevaplar veriyordum. Şimdi size verdiğim cevapların tam aksine..."

Gülmesiyle birden sanki bir rüyadan uyandım.

"Siz tabii benim doğup büyüdüğüm yerleri bilmezsiniz," dedi.
"Hayır," dedi Tolga benim yerime, "gitmedik hiç..."
"Bir yere gitmekle, orada yaşamak, bazı şeyleri görmekle onu anlamak çok farklı, her gün sokaklarda dilenen çocukları görürsünüz ve belki üzülürsünüz ama onların aslında ne yaşadığını asla bilemezsiniz, tıpkı benim de bunca zenginliğin içindeki insanların bir resme dünyanın parasını verip, yanlarında çalışan bir işçinin zar zor geçindiği maaşını düşürmek için uğraşmasını anlayamamam gibi..."

Çocukken bir odun parçasını yontarak heykeller yaptığını anlattı. Bazen bir koyun, bazen ağaç, bazen neye benzediğini kimsenin anlamadığı figürler yontuyordu.

Okuldaki öğretmenlerden biri yaptıklarıyla ilgilenmiş, onu resim çizmesi için yüreklendirmişti.

"İyi bir öğrenciydim, çünkü yapacak pek işim yoktu, yılbaşında okul kitapları alındığı zaman hepsini okurdum, anlamasam da okurdum, ilgimi çeken cümlelerin altını çizerdim, şiirleri, hikaye parçalarını ezberlerdim, anlamadığım bir formül olduğunda sayısız kez yeniden çözmeye çalışır ve sonunda kendime göre çözerdim. Sonra karpuzlardan, kabaklardan bile heykeller yapmaya başladım. Öğretmenim onları alıp okulda sergiliyordu. Bir gün bana büyükçe bir defterle siyah, kalın kalemler getirdi. Ben de çizdim. Öyle çok çiziyordum ki defter hemen bitti. O zaman gidip okuldaki teksir kağıtlarını alıp onların arkasına çizerdim.

Benden manzarayı, keçileri, çobanları, uçsuz bucaksız otlakları çizmemi isterlerdi. Onları da yapardım ama neye benzediği bilinmez garip şeyler çizmek daha çok hoşuma giderdi ya da ne bileyim içimden öyle gelirdi."

"Neye benzediği bilinmez mi?" diye sordu Tolga...

"Evet, onlar benim rüyalarımdı..."

Sonra büyük masaların üzerinde üstüste yığılmış bir sürü çizim gösterdi bize. İnsanı öyle hemen içine alan, renklerini beğendiğiniz ya da size alıp evinize asma isteği veren resimlerden değildi bunlar... Şaşırtıcı, karışık, içiçe geçmiş figürlerle, renklerle, yazılarla dolu, o güne kadar pek de görmediğim türden şeylerdi. İlk bakışta tam olarak ne olduğunu anlamıyordu insan. Hani bir buluta bakıp ondan biçimler oluşturmaya çalışmak gibiydi.

Bir köşede tahtadan yontulmuş bir araba üzerine paslı bir tel takılmış. Yanında, çiviler çakılmış, üzerine futbol sahası çizilmiş bir tahta parçası...

"Bunlar sizin gerçek oyuncaklarınız mı?" diye sordu Tolga.

Güldü.

"Evet," dedi, "top alamadığımız için bozuk parayla bu tahta sahada maç yapardık. Bu arabayı da ben yaptım. Kılıçlar, tüfekler daha bir sürü oyuncak yaptım ama birçok şey gibi onları da bir yerlerde bıraktım ya da belki birilerine verdim... Bende kalan bunlar..."

Anneannem Ferhat'ı ilk gördüğüm akşam sonradan bana onun tutuklandığını, kısa bir süre önce hapisten çıktığını söylemişti.

Sormak istedim.

"Önemli değil," dedi, "bizim gibi ülkelerde farklı görüşleri savunan herkes neci olursa olsun bir gün devlet zulmüne uğrar, hatta devleti yönetenler bile..."

Ve daha fazlasını soramadan sözü değiştirdi, o bize sorular sormaya başladı.

Tolga'nın makinasıyla birlikte ilk fotoğrafımız çekildi. Hala duruyor o fotoğraf. Ben yanında biraz küçük kalmışım, o da elini omuzuma koymuş ve biraz eğilmiş, o gülüyor bense şaşkın şaşkın bakıyorum.

Çıktık. Akşam biraz serinlemişti. Yürürken Tolga bana döndü, "Nasıl adam bu, resmen çarpıldım," dedi.

"Bilmem," dedim, "resimleri gibi galiba..."

Yoksa... Rüyaları gibi mi?

Ama o gün kısa kısa resim parçaları gibi anlattığı çocukluğunda çok daha fazlasının olduğunu ancak uzun zaman sonra öğrenebilecektim.

Evet bir anda hayatım değişmişti. Büyümüş müydüm? Bence öyleydi. Bu, sabah akşam, uyandığımda, yattığımda içimde hiç kesilmeyen çarpıntı büyümenin heyecanı mıydı?

Annem her ne kadar anneannemin bu yaptığından hiç memnun olmasa da yavaş yavaş ikna olmuştu. Belki de ona böylece yeni bir uğraş doğmuştu.

Tabii ki onun da Londra'ya gelip en azından bir süre bizimle kalacağından hiç kuşkum yoktu. Ama buna da razıydık.

Çünkü bu sayede Tolga'nın babası da itirazlarından vazgeçmiş, ona yalanlar uydurmamıza gerek kalmamıştı.

Zaten evde Meral Teyze'nin sözü geçerdi.

Ev nerede tutulacak, nasıl olacak, nasıl döşenecek bunları ikisi uzun uzun konuşuyor hatta bazen iki kaynana gibi bozuşuyorlardı.

Meral Teyze, o eski püskü Londra evleri olmaz, mutlaka yeni ev olmalı, ısınmalı, her tür konforu olmalı diyordu.

Annem üç oda olmasında ısrarcıydı. Tabii ki bir odaya onlar geldiklerinde yerleşeceklerdi.

Ayrıca okula yürüyüş mesafesinde olmalıydı. Öyle geceleri filan güvenilir bir semt olması şarttı.

Sare Hanım bu işlere hiç karışmadı. "Meral bilir ne yapacağını, uzatmaya gerek yok, bulur o, becerir," diye kestirip attı. Onun için hedefe ulaşılmış, mesele kapanmıştı.

Onun asıl ilgilendiği başkaydı. Eski dergiler çıkartıyor, bana modeller gösteriyor, kumaşlar hakkında bilgi veriyor ve daha çok çizmemi istiyordu.

Hatta ona kalsa terzi Perihan Hanım geldiğinde biraz dikiş öğrensem iyi olacaktı.

Bense dediğim gibi bütün bunlar sanki benim hayatımın dönüm noktası değilmiş gibi aldırışsız bir havadaydım.

Zaten Tolga söylemişti, biz kendi isteklerimizde ısrar etsek de işe yaramayacaktı.

"Bırak annem istediğini yapsın sonra biz yerleşince kafamıza göre değiştiririz," diyordu.

Benim aklımsa o resimlerin içindeki adamdaydı.

Bunu kimseye söylemeye cesaretim yoktu hatta belki kendime bile ama böyleydi.

Şimdi artık bunca yıl sonra rahatlıkla söyleyebilirim.

İlk gördüğümden beri onu düşünmeden geçen tek günüm bile olmadı.

Aslında bu eve gelip giden yazarların, sanatçıların hepsi değişik, çekici, ilginç insanlardı. İçlerinde çok etkileyici olanlar hatta hayran olduğum insanlar da vardı. Ama o güne kadar ara sıra öylesine aklıma gelse de hiç birine karşı böyle hissetmemiştim.

Örneğin çok hayran olduğum bir oyuncu vardı. Oyunlarına da gitmiştim, yemeğe geldiğinde o davudi sesiyle konuşurken hayran hayran ona bakarken yakalardım kendimi.

Anneannem de benimle eğlenir, bazen öylesine sorar gibi, "Akşama kimler geliyor?" dediğimde, "Ayol sen asıl soracağını sorsana hadi iyisin seninki geliyor akşam," diye gülerdi.

Ben de utanır kızarıp bozarırdım ve "Canım ne var bunda pek hoş adam doğrusu ben de olsam beğenirim ama daha senin sıran değil bu işlere..." diye cümleyi bağlardı.

Sonunda o da bir gün yanında pek havalı oyuncu bir kızla gelmiş ve ben de kendimce ona küsüp bu hayale bir son vermiştim.

Sonra o kadınla evlendi. Kadın çok ünlü bir oyuncu ve şarkıcı oldu. O yakışıklı adamsa oldukça genç yaşta kansere yakalandı ve kısa sürede öldü.

Ne garip, o akşamı, ona kendince aşık olmuş ve sonra da kendince küsmüş küçük kızı belki de hiç hatırlamadan...

Böyle ne çok hayat var aklımda.

Eve gelenlerin çoğu tanınan insanlar olduğu ve gelecekte daha da ünlü olduklarından onların hayatını, neler yaptıklarını sonraki yıllarda izleme şansım oldu.

Bazılarının bir köşede ezik büzük oturup söze bile giremezken yıllar sonra üst perdeden atıp tutan, kimseleri beğenmeyen insanlar olduğunu, bazılarının hararetle savunduğu tüm düşüncelerin tam tersi bir yere savrulduğunu, bazılarının geçmişlerini anlatırken aslında bambaşka yalanlar uydurduğunu, kendilerinden çok şey beklenen bazılarının da yokolup gittiğini gördüm.

Şimdi düşünüyorum da bir çocuk, bir genç kız için çok farklı bir ortamdı bu. Hepsi, yaratan, çılgınca düşünceleri olan, çoğu zaaflarına kapılmış ve sanki bununla mutluymuş gibi davranan, dünyanın her yerinden, tarihin her döneminden bilgiler getiren ulaklar gibi insanlarla oturmak, onların kendi aralarındaki tar tışmaları, konuşmaları, dedikoduları dinlemek gerçekten de çok garipti. Ama o sıralar bu benim sıradan hayatımdı, bütün bunların farkında bile değildim.

Bir yılbaşı akşamı annemle yemek yedikten sonra aşağı indim. Tabii ki annem gelmeyecekti ama anneannem için yılbaşı önemli bir gündü.

Bu kez oldukça kalabalıktı. Hatta kapı açıktı ve birileri geliyor, birileri gidiyor, sürekli içkiler yemekler geliyor, herkes birileriyle sohbet ediyordu.

Daha onyedi yaşındaydım ama üzerimdeki gece elbisesiyle, topuz yapılmış saçlarımla pek havalı hissediyordum kendimi. Hatta oldukça parlak, kırmızı ruj da sürmüştüm.

O gece genç bir şairle ve arkadaşlarıyla uzun uzun sohbet ettim. Hatta biraz da sarhoş oldum. Benim çok sevdiğim yazarlardan, şiirlerden sözediyordu.

Kimi çok ünlü yazarların hayatlarına nasıl son verdiğinden açıldı sonra konu. Birinin damarlarını keserken son şiirini yazdığından, birinin tüm istediklerine sahipken artık bu dünyaya bunca acıya daha fazla dayanamıyorum diyerek suyun içinde yürüyüp gittiğinden, bir başkasının günlüklerinin sonunda intihar ettiği için kitabın yarım bir cümleyle bittiğinden sözediliyordu.

Hatta bir ara anneannem yanımıza gelip biraz dinledikten sonra, "Ah tabii gençler toplanmış ölümden sözediyorlar, yaşlılar ölümden hiç sözetmez, hatta duymak dahi istemez, içim sıkıldı," diyerek gitti.

Ben o akşam o şaire de aşık olmuştum.

Ama iki gün sonra ondan bir haber geldi.

Akşamüstü evinde arkadaşlarıyla otururken kalkıp içeri gitmiş ve pencereyi açıp aşağı atlayarak intihar etmişti.

Bu beni beklenmeyecek biçimde etkiledi. Nasıl olur da böyle hoş, bilgili, yetenekli, herkesin çevresinde pervane olduğu genç adam böyle bir delilik yapardı?
Yoksa o gece bunu yapacağını bilerek mi bu konuları açmıştı?
Acaba o gece cesaretimi toplayıp onunla görüşmek istediğimi söylesem intihar etmekten vazgeçer miydi?

Şöyle yazmıştı öldükten sonra masasının üstünde bulunan son şiirlerinden birinde:

Zamandan bir parça daha koptu
Akşam bana, yarın da böyle olacağını söylüyor
Nedensiz bir hüzün
Belki de bu yüzden
Nedensiz bir ben
Belki de bu yüzden

İnsan arkadaşlarıyla oturup sohbet ederken, gülüp eğlenirken birdenbire içeriye gidip pencereden atlar mı?
Bunu düşünmek bana derin bir hüzün vermişti. Hala da veriyor.
Üstelik acıklı olan, uzun süre içeride kahkahalar atıp eğlenen arkadaşları ne olduğunu farketmemiş ve ancak kapıya polis gelince anlamışlardı.

Hayat bütün bu sorulara cevap vermeyi zorlaştırıyor. Ama ben o zaman ona kızdım. Ne olursa olsun bir daha istediklerimi ertelememeye de belki o an karar verdim.

Belki de Ferhat'ın atölyesine yeniden gidecek cesareti toplamamın aslında bununla ilgisi vardı.

Söyleşinin çıktığı dergiyi alıp Ferhat'a gidecektim ama Tolga da gelmek istiyordu tabii. Hatta olur olmaz zamanlarda ondan sözedip canımı sıkıyordu. "Acaba gerçekte nasıl biri, sevgilisi var mı, çok mu çapkın, gerçi evde bir kadın yaşıyormuş gibi gelmedi bana ne dersin, bence çok sevgilisi vardır, kesin birşey," diye iyice sinirlerimi oynatıyordu.

Sare Hanım da birkaç kez, "Ferhat nerelerde acaba epeydir görünmedi, arayıp çağırmak lazım," demişti ama ben onun adı geçince hemen lafı değiştiriyordum. Kızardığım anlaşılacak diye ödüm kopuyordu.

Tolga'yla annesinin eve bakmak için Londra'ya gittikleri zamana kadar oyalandım.

Niye beni beklemedin derse, aman ne bileyim aklıma esti gittim işte, diyecektim.

O cuma gecesi neredeyse hiç uyumadım. Hatta gitmekten vazgeçecektim. Kalbim şimdiden böyle atıyorsa onu görünce ellerimin titreyeceğinden emindim.

Saçlarımı nasıl yapsaydım, toplasam mı açsam mı, yeni aldığım yazlık elbisemi mi giysem yoksa daha derli toplu pantolon gömlek gibi mi? Makyaj yapmasam daha iyiydi bence, böyle şeylerden pek hoşlanacak birine benzemiyordu.

Aman belki de dergiyi elimden alıp bana güle güle diyecekti. Belki de evde birileri olacaktı.

O zamandan beri kalkıp Sare Hanım'ı ziyarete gelmediğine göre tabii ki benim düşündüklerimden habersizdi.

Ama ne komik, kendi kendime film kişisi gibi rol yazıyordum, belki de onu şaşırtacak şeyler yapmalıydım, insanlar önce beğenmese de şaşırdıkları şeylerle daha çok ilgilenir. Biraz serseri, biraz umursamaz, rahat bir kız gibi mi olmalıydım acaba? Yoksa aksine daha ağır, hanım hanımcık mı?

Eh aslında ikisi de bendim. O yüzden fazla rol yapmaya gerek kalmayacaktı. En önemlisi açık mı olmalıydım –ki buna çok şaşıracağı kesindi– yoksa gizemli biçimde onun beni merak etmesini mi sağlamalıydım?

Evet bu ikincisi daha iyiydi.

Bir yandan bunları kuruyor bir yandan da "Ne aptalsın adam kimbilir kaç kadın tanımıştır, senden kaç yaş büyük, anında anlayacak niyetini ve gülüp geçecek," diyordum.

Sonra bu düşünceyi hemen kovalıyordum çünkü kendi kendime yazdığım romanı bozuyordu.

Hem aşk zaten hayallerden oluşmaz mı?

Aşk ne zaman biter diye kitaplar yazıyorlar bir de... Ne zaman bitecek, hayal kurmayı bıraktığınız zaman... Hayal gerçeğe döndüğü zaman...Kırıldığı zaman...

Aman çok biliyorum sanki...

Kendi kendime dedim ki (galiba artık sabah oluyordu ve bayılmak üzereydim) madem ki sen günlerdir anlamsız biçimde mutlu sun, onu düşünmek sana iyi geliyor, kendini böyle rollere sokup ilk kez nasıl bir kadın olduğunu düşünüyorsun ve bu seni bugüne dek olmadığı kadar heyecanlandırıyor, bunu yaşayacaksın.

Hem en kötü ne olabilir ki? Bana kötü kız gözüyle mi bakar? Utanmaz küçük liseli mi der? Hiç sanmam. Yalnızca korkabilir.

En önemlisi korkmamasını sağlamak...

Hem ne yapıyordum ki, dergiyi götüreceğimize ona söz vermemiş miydim o gün?

Kapıdan bırakacaktım işte... Davet etmezse zaten biriyle buluşmaya giderken uğradığımı söyleyecektim.

İşte sabaha kadar böyle gelgitlerle uğraşırken yine gerçekle düş birbirine karıştı.

Ne güzel bir cumartesi günüydü.

Denizin kokusu, martıların neşesi, ışığın dünyaya sanki yeni bir ruh veren canlılığı, çiçek kokuları...

Tabii yola çıkmam epey zamanımı aldı. Öğlene doğru uyanabildim ve gözlerimin şişi gitsin diye Sare Hanım usulü çay banyosu yaptım.

Sonra aşağı indim. Sare Hanım her zamanki gibi uzun, renkli çiçekli sabahlığıyla oturmuş kahvesini içiyor.

"Gel bakalım gel, bu ne güzellik böyle hayrola nereye?" diye sordu.

"Arkadaşlarla buluşacağız," diye belki de ilk kez yalan söyledim ona.

Şöyle bir süzdü beni sonra "Git içerden benim ilk çekmecemden kırmızı küçük kutulardan birinde yeşil küpeler var biliyorsun, onları getir," dedi.

Getirdim. Kulağıma taktı.

"Hah şimdi oldu," dedi, "çok yakıştı..."

Kızardım.

İncecik ipekliden kısa bir elbise vardı üstümde, renkli geometrik desenler, yeşiller, maviler, bejler, çok severek almıştım.

"Aaa ama bu ayakkabılar olmamış ki bunun altına," dedi.

"Uff biliyorum ama bulamadım başka birşey," dedim.

"E, hani sana lacivert beyazlı üstünde kurdela olan ayakkabılar almıştık onları giysene..."

"Gündüz gündüz mü?" dedim. Hem çok özenmiştim hem de özenmiş görünmek istemiyordum çünkü. Düz basit bir ayakkabı giymiştim.

"Canım ne gündüzü akşamüstü artık giyebilirsin, yalnız çantasını da al, geç kalmazsın değil mi akşam misafir var."

Onu yanağından öptüm. "Kalmam kalmam," dedim.

Arkadaşlarımla sinemaya bu kılıkta gitmeyeceğimi biliyordu bence. Belki de okuldaki çocuklardan biriyle buluşacağımı düşünmüştü.

Mor salkımlı eski duvarların önünden geçip evine geldim.

Elimde dergi ve çantamda da küçük bir hediye vardı.

Nedense ona yakışacağını düşünmüştüm. Çok sevdiğim rengarenk ipek fular. Beyaz gömleğinin üstüne takar mıydı?

Sonradan öğrenecektim ki yaşlı mahalle terzisi dikiyordu gömleklerini. Ve hepsi beyaz, uzun, çok güzel ince pamukludan.

Evin önünden geçtim, biraz yürüdüm tekrar geri döndüm.

Sokak duvarlarından birine o sakallı, kızıl yıldızlı beresiyle Che Guevara'yı çizmişlerdi. Kocaman bir duvar resmi… Altında sloganlar… Kahrolsun…

Kapıyı çaldım. İçerden yüksek sesle klasik müzik geliyordu. Kapıyı açtı, pek de şaşırmış gibi değildi.

"Ben," dedim, "dergiyi getirecektim ya…"

"Hoşgeldin," dedi ve girmem için yana çekildi.

"Arkadaşın yok mu?"

"Tolga mı? A, hayır o Londra'ya gitti..."

Gelince bakalım bu yaptığımı ona nasıl anlatacağım…

Yine kahve kokusu...

İlk oturduğum eski koltuğa oturdum.

Birşey yapmam gerektiğini düşünerek hemen dergiyi uzattım.

"Güzel kahvem var, ister misin?" diye sordu.

İsterim.

"Sade?"

Sade.

Saçımla oynuyordum yine. Saçınla oynama Ebru diyordum ama oynuyordum.

Kahveleri getirdi, beyaz düz porselen fincanlar...

"Ne güzel kokuyor," dedim.

"Ben de seviyorum, belki tadından çok kokusunu..."

Dergiyi karıştırdı.

Fincanı alırken elim titredi, yerine bıraktım.

Gördü.

"Sıcakmış biraz," dedim.

Bir an hemen çıkıp gitmek istedim.

Sessizlik olmasın diye, "Sokakta, duvardaki resmi siz mi çizdiniz?" dedim.

Kalkıp müziğin sesini kıstı.

"Guevara'yı mı? Hayır, ben kahramanlarla pek ilgilenmem... Ve zaten sonunda kahrolan sistemler olmaz. Hep insanlar kahrolur..."

Koltuğun ucuna doğru oturdu. Yakın.

"Sare Hanım nasıl, uzundur göremedim onu," dedi.

"İyi, o da sizi soruyordu..."

Bakalım buraya geldiğimi duyunca ne olacak? Umarım görüşmezler...

"Çok şanslısın biliyorsun değil mi," dedi, anlamadım, "böyle bir anneannen olduğu için..."

"Ah evet, biliyorum," dedim, "belki de tek şansım..."

"Onunla oturup konuşmak bile insanı rahatlatıyor," dedi sonra durdu, "tek şansım mı dedin?"

"Evet..."

"Belki başka şansların da vardır da henüz farkında değilsindir," dedi.

Utandım. Ne demek isteğini anladım.

Ne garip, böyle karşılaşmalarda, "Ee nasıl gidiyor," filan gibi sorular sorulur. O sormuyordu.

Ne diyeceğimi bilemedim. Çantamdan fuları çıkarttım.

"Size bunu getirdim ama bilmem takar mısınız?"

"Bana mı?" Aldı, okşadı, sonra hemen boynuna taktı...

"Takarım tabii çok güzelmiş, teşekkür ederim, galiba beni fazla renksiz buldun..?"

Güldük.

"Sadece beyaz gömleğin üstünde güzel durur diye düşündüm..."

"Durdu mu?" diye sordu...

"Evet, çok güzel, nedense size vermek istedim," dedim.

"Bir ressama verilecek en güzel hediye... Renkler ve desenler..."

"Her gün çiziyor musunuz yoksa aklınıza esince mi?"

Soruya bak! Neden resim diye sorsan daha iyiydi... Oynama su saçınla...

"Her gün çizerim bazen deftere bazen tuvale gençlikle karalamalar yaparım..."

"Yolda gelirken aklıma bir soru geldi?" dedim.

"Öyle mi?"

"Sen neşeli bir ilkyaz cumartesisinin resmini yapabilir misin Ferhat?"

İlk kez kahkaha attı.

Ve ben de ona ilk kez "sen" demiş oldum.

"Bak bu resmin adı bile yeter, hemen yapmalıyım..."

Kahveden bir yudum aldım, elim titremedi. Biraz rahatladım.

En sevdiğim fularım boynunda, karşımda oturmuş gülüyordu.

Sonra nasıl oldu bilmiyorum ama kendimi ona Londra planlarını, yeni okulu, tasarım merakımı, kokuya ve dokunmaya olan zaafımı anlatırken buldum.

İkinci kahvenin yanında birer küçük kadeh konyak geldi.

Çok mu konuşuyordum?

"Galiba şöyle bir resim geldi aklıma, erguvanlar, mor salkımlar, ayva ağaçları, çocuklar, yerde yuvarlanan bir kedi, ona ağacın üstünden bakan bir karga, denizle içiçe girmiş bahçeler ve bu fuların renklerinde boyanmış bir bisiklete binen sen... Ne dersin?"

Ne mi derim? Bu adam benim aklımı mı okuyor?

"Belki de resmin içinde resmi çizen ve çizerken gülen ressam..."

Neydi bu?

"Madem ki resmi sen ısmarladın istediğini söyleyebilirsin," güldü, "Da Vinci de siparişle resim çiziyordu.."

Neydi?

Herhangi bir cumartesi günü, koskoca bir adamla sıradan bir konuşma mı?

Hiç tanımadığım biriyle ilk kez yalnız konuşurken aniden hayallerin içine girmek mi?

Sanki o kapı kendiliğinden açılmıştı. Düşünmeden, dün geceki gibi planlar yapmadan, öylesine, kendiliğinden... O kadar kendiliğinden ki, düşünsem aklıma gelmeyecek şeyler söylüyordum ve o da sanki beni yıllardır tanırmış gibi onlara benim beklediğim cevapları veriyordu.

Ya da hiç beklemediğim...

Evet orada onun yanında otururken, hatta daha gelmeden önce bile sanki bütün bunların böylece, kendiliğinden olacağını hissetmiştim.

Ben buraya gelirken ne istediğimi biliyordum.

O bilmiyordu.

Konuşurken, geçmişten, birbirinden çok farklı hayatlarımızdan, komik anılardan sözederken, o gözlerime bakarken, ben onun gülüşüne, eski şarkılar çalarken, yavaş yavaş akşam olurken tek bildiğim zamanı durdurabilmeyi, burada bu anın hiç geçmemesini istediğimdi.

Ve ne gariptir ki bundan böyle de hep bunu isteyecektim.

Sanki yıllardır böyle oturup konuşuyormuş gibi…

Bütün bu karmaşanın içindeki huzuru sanki önceden bilirmişim gibi…

Öyle bir an geldi ki kucağına uzanmak ve hiç konuşmadan öylece kalmak istedim.

Beni öpmesini istedim.

Bunları ve itiraf etmeliyim, daha fazlasını da…

Akşam oluyor, gitmem gerekiyor.

Bir an önce buradan kalksam iyi olacak diyordum kendi kendime.

O güne kadar böyle şeyler hissetmemiştim.

Hem şaşkındım hem de bu duygunun kaybolmasını istemiyordum.

Tıpkı bahçedeki gizli dehlizde ilk kaybolduğum günkü gibi... Hem korkuyordum hem de devam etmek, başka neler olduğunu görmek istiyordum.

Oraya ne zaman girsem gizemli, bana ait, kimsenin bilmediği bir dünyaya girmiş olurdum. Sonra oradan gerçek dünyaya dönerdim.

Belki de bu iki dünya arasındaki gidiş gelişler benim sonraki hayatımı belirledi.

Nasıl bir duyguysa, bütün düşünceler, kaygılar, korkular silinip gitmişti aklımdan, buradaydım, sanki her zaman olduğu gibi birlikteydik, bir an onun da benimle aynı şeyleri düşündüğünü, istediğini sanıyor sonra kendimi toparlayıp konuşmaya devam ediyordum.

Hiç tanımadığı biri insanda nasıl böyle bir etki yaratabilir ki?

Ama durumu idare ettiğimden, içimden geçenleri ona belli etmediğimden emindim.

İşte karşısında oturmuş kendinden emin genç bır kadın olarak onunla her konuda konuşuyor, sohbet ediyordum.

Söz bir türlü dönüp dolaşıp ikimize gelmese de...

Önce gözleri gülen insanlar vardır. O da onlardandı. Bazen çok ciddi birşey söylüyor, zaten konuşurken doğruca gözlerime bakıyor ve ben o gözlerin içinde kaybolup gidiyordum, susuyor ve gözlerinden aslında şaka yaptığını anlıyordum. Arkasından gülmeye başlıyor, kendi söyledikleriyle alay ediyordu.

Kendi kendime bir yandan konuşmayı sürdürürken bir yandan hayaller kuruyordum. Onunla uzakta, bizi kimsenin tanımadığı yerlerde olduğumu düşünüyordum. İçimden de gülüyordum tabii... Hem kendi halime hem onun bütün bunlardan haberi olmayışına...

Aslında birdenbire aklımdan geçenleri olduğu gibi söylesem bence çok gülerdi.

"Ben çok şey anlattım ama sen bana anlatmadın," dedim birden. Aslında anlattıklarının çok daha derininde olanları duymak istiyordum.

"Benim hayatım pek de neşeli değil," dedi, "anlatırsam sıkılırsın..."

"Hayır, sıkılmam, benimki de öyle sayılmaz aslında..."

Sonra anlatmaya başladı.

Aslında beş kardeşlerdi ama üç kardeşi ondan önce ölmüştü.. Onun hatırladığı ağabeyi de altı yaşındayken hayatını kaybetmişti. Anne babası akraba evlliği yaptığı için...

"Bir tek ben ve kardeşim hayatta kaldık. Ama kardeşim de zeka özürlüydü. Bizim oralarda dedikleri gibi moron..."

Birdenbire aklındaki herşey uçup gitti. Bütün o konuşmalar, sanatla, ünlü isimlerle ilgili söylediklerimiz bitti. Dalgın dalgın anlatmaya devam etti...

"Evet insanlar acımasızdır. Ne tuhaf, çocuklar da öyle.

Bazen insan kendisine bile doğruları itiraf edemez. Tek başına kaldığı anlarda bile bazı şeyleri başka türlü görmeye ya da gördüğünü düşünmeye çalışır.

Ama aslında yıllar boyu Mehmet'ten utandım. Yanımda bir yere gönderdikleri zaman ondan nefret ettim. Yürürken önde giderdim ki kalabalıkta birlikte olduğumuzu anlamasınlar. Ama o tek başına kalakalırdı ve dönüp onu almak ve elini tutmak zorunda kalırdım.

İnsan kardeşinden utanır mı? Utanılacak birşey yaparsa utanır değil mi?

O ne yapmıştı ki?

Yalnızca anlatmaya çalışırken, sevinince, üzülünce, başka çocuklar gibi heyecanlanınca, onlar gibi sözcükleri kullanamadığı için garip sesler çıkartır, elleriyle garip hareketler yapar, bazen kendine zarar verir, bazen bir yerlere saldırırdı ve insanlar ondan korkardı.

Çocuklardan birinin yanına giderdi örneğin, bir kızın, bir bebeğin ve aslında istediği onu sevmek ya da onunla ilişki kurmaktı ama korkuturdu onları.

Kim korkmazdı ondan biliyor musun?

Hayvanlar."

Ansızın buradan bambaşka bir yere, onun hayatına, onun gizli tüneline girmiştik sanki ve ben yalnızca dinliyordum.

"Hayvanlar mı?" dedim.

"Evet," dedi, "çünkü hayvanlar bizim gibi acımasız sözdizimini bilmez. Birinin renkli, birinin çirkin, birinin şişman olduğunu bilmez. Belki zayıf olan orada zaten yaşayamadığı için..."

Gözlerinin dolduğunu hissettim. Elini yüzünde gezdirdi, bana bakmadan anlatmaya devam etti:

"Köpeğimiz vardı küçükken. Mehmet en çok onunla anlaşırdı. Sanki o köpek, Panço, onun her halini bizden iyi anlardı. Üzgünse yanına gider, kucağına kafasını koyar, kendisini sevdirir, neşeliyse onunla koşar zıplar, gülüyor ve deli deli hareketler yapıyorsa o da havlayıp bağırarak ona eşlik ederdi.

Çok küçüktü daha. Belki beş yaşında ya var ya yoktu. Bir gün okuldan dönüyorduk. Her yer kar içindeydi. Öyle çok kar yağmıştı ki ertesi gün, sonraki gün hep okullar tatil edilmişti. Yolda yürürken biz kartopuna daldık ve ben Mehmet'i unuttum. Neden sonra baktım ki ortada yok. Deliye döndüm. Her yere baktık bulamadık. Mehmet yok. O an bunun ne olduğunu anlamamıştım. Sorumluluk muydu? Babama ne söyleyeceğim miydi? Hayır. Kalbim deli gibi atıyordu ve hayatımda belki de hiç böyle korkmamıştım. Ölecek olduğum zaman bile böyle korkmadım hayatımda. O zaman tabii bilmiyordum ama onu gerçekten sevdiğimi anladığım an, o andı bence.

Sonra onu bir ağacın altında bulduk. Neredeyse donmuş halde oturmuş elindeki karı yemeye çalışıyordu hala."

Onu dinlerken düşünüyordum. Nasıl olmuştu ya da ne zaman, birilerini güzel, birilerini çirkin, birilerini bize uygun, başkalarını farklı görmeye başlamıştık? Nasıl olmuştu da onları hep yoksaymaya hatta yoketmeye çalışmıştık? Bu hep böyle miydi?

"Nerede şimdi, ne yapıyor?" diye sordum.

"Babamın yanında, zaman zaman gidip görürüm onu... Ne yazık ki onu görmek hala beni üzüyor... Ve o da benden uzak duruyor."

Sonra yine zamanın içinden geçti, buraya geldi. Bana baktı, gülümseyerek, "Ne yaptın sen bana böyle, çenem düştü, seni evden merak ederler..." dedi...

Evet ederler... Kalktım.

Kapıdan çıkmadan önce karşılıklı durduk. Birden sarılıp onu dudaklarından öptüm. Şaşkın kalakaldı sonra beni kucakladı ve öpmeye devam etti. Ve ben merak edenleri, nereye gideceğimi, nereden geldiğimi, bundan sonra olacakları hepsini unuttum…

Hayır, tabii ki böyle olmadı. Bu sadece aklımdan geçti.

Karşılıklı durduk, elimi sıkıp beni yanaklarımdan öptü, kokusunu duydum ve bir daha hiç unutmadım, gülümsedi, birşey söylemeyecek miydi, ben söylese miydim, söylemedi, ben de söyleyemedim.

Öylece arkamı dönüp yürüdüm.

Tren sallanarak ilerliyor, karşımdaki adam uyukluyor, hatta ara sıra derin bir iç geçiriyor rüyasında, ben yine pencerelerden dışarı bakıyorum ama dışarıdakileri görmüyorum da sanki trenin camlarında kendi kısa hayatımın filmini izliyorum.

Kısa dedim evet ama bu kadar kısa zamanda neler olmuş.

Üstüste yaşananlara böyle uzaktan bakıp düşünmeye sanki fırsat olmamış…

Bu anlattıklarımın üzerinden yıllar yıllar geçmiş…

Buraya gelirken kararlıydım.

Bütün bunlar olmasa kimseyi dinlemeyip bu ameliyata girmeye kesin karar vermiştim.

Ama şimdi içimde başka bir duygu var. İlk istasyonda inmek, geri dönmek, onun yanına gitmek istiyorum. Belki de bu garip rastlantıların bana söylemek istediği birşey var.

Yazık ki onun ne olduğunu hala anlamıyorum.

Doktor bana bir keresinde, "Tam olarak ne hissettiğini anlatabilir misin?" demişti.

"Yorgunum," demiştim, "sanki çok yaşlıyım ama genç bir kadının bedenindeyim."

Ve böyle daha fazla sürdüremeyeceğimi biliyorum. Bunu biliyorum.

Onun için buraya geldim. Onun için bunu yapmalıyım.

Kucağımda çocukluk arkadaşım Puska var. Adının neden Puska olduğunu benim bile hatırlamadığım, küçük tüylü oyuncağım...

Bazıları geçmişini unutmak ister, anıları siler, onların yerine başka anıları, belki başkalarının anılarını koyar, kendisine tıpkı bir roman kahramanı gibi farklı, yeni bir geçmiş yaratır.

Bazılarıysa benim gibi çocukluğuyla yaşar.

Gülüyorum bazen kendi halime.

Tıpkı küçük bir kızken Puska'yı nasıl her yere götürdüysem, nasıl onu unuttuğum anda geri dönüp almak için kıyametleri kopardıysam, şimdi de çocukluğum sanki onun gibi yanımda her yere benimle geliyor, benimle oturup kalkıyor, benimle uyuyor, uyanıyor.

Kızardı babam, Puska'yı sanki aileden biriymiş gibi yemeğe otururken bile baş köşeye yerleştirmeme, onu her yere götürmeme...

"Koca kız oldu hala elinde bu ne idüğü belirsiz oyuncakla dolaşıyor..." derdi.

Ne idüğü belirsiz mi? Puska'ya bakardım ama biz onunla anlaşmıştık, büyüklerin söylediklerine aldırmayacaktık, onun için üzülmediğini bilirdim.

İşin tuhaf yanı, onu bana kimin aldığını, onu nereden bulduğumu kimse hatırlamıyor...

O kadar oyuncağım varken bu boz renkli, fil mi köpek mi, kedi mi tavşan mı olduğu belli olmayan tüyleri tiftik tiftik olmuş hayvana neden böyle düşkün olduğumu da kimse bilemiyordu zaten.

Çok da derdim değil. Kaç yaşına gelmiş kadının hala yanında oyuncakla yatmasını garip bulan varsa da bulsun. Yaptığım pek çok şeyi de garip buldular, onlara da aldırmamayı çoktan öğrendim.

Ben kimseyi yargılamam, kimseye neden böyle yaptın, neden öyle yaptın diye sormam, birilerine zarar vermiyorsa, kötülük etmiyorsa kimsenin saçmalıklarını çekiştirmekle zaman geçirmem. Baktım ki çok sıkıldım, ondan uzaklaşırım olur biter.

Bunları kimden öğrendim? Tabii ki anneannemden.

Belki biraz da tam ne olduğunu anlamadığımız ama hepsini izlediğimiz ilk gençlik yıllarımın Fransız filmlerinden…

Yaşlılık nasıl birşey diye sormuştum Sare Hanım'a bir keresinde…

"Ben nereden bileyim, yaşlı değilim ki," diyecek sandım her zamanki gibi şakaya vurup ama öyle yapmadı. Bir an durdu, yüzü asıldı,

"Şöyle birşey, önce etrafındaki konuşmalardan sıkılıyorsun, sonra eşyalar, eskiden çok değer verilen ıvır zıvır saçma gelmeye başlıyor, sonra ertelenmemesi gerekenler, yapılması gerekenler, uyulması gerekenler saçma geliyor, sonra giyinip kuşanıp bir yerlere gitmek saçma geliyor, sonra bu aşk meşk meseleleri saçma geliyor ve sonra hepsi saçma gelmeye başlıyor. Hiç birşey yapacak takatin kalmıyor."

Ona baktım. Birden canlandı, eski haline döndü,

"O yüzden ben her gün böyle giyinirim, her akşam insanları çağırırım, bütün ışıkları yakarım, başka şeyler düşünmeye zamanım kalmayacak kadar meşgulüm… Ha bir de yavaş yavaş unutursun ama ben bundan şikayetçi değilim, unutmak hiç de fena sayılmaz…"

Zaten bana her zaman derdi ki, "Sakın oturup da kafana takılanları fazla düşünme, hep uğraşacak birşeylerin olsun, insanlar bazen seni yalnız bırakır, o zaman kendi kendine oyalanmayı bilmelisin, böylece hiç sıkılmazsın…"

Ben de öyle yaptım. Düştüğüm zaman, sabah kalkıp yürüyemediğim zaman, olup bitenleri hatırlayamadığım zaman, ışığa bakamayıp günlerce karanlıkta oturmak zorunda kaldığım zaman, çok canım yanıp ağlasam da güçlü olmaya çalışarak geçen zamanlarda hep bunlar geçecek, bir kere daha olmuştu, yine oluyor, korkmayacaksın, dedim…

Aslında hayatı fazla ciddiye almadığımı, aldığım zamanları gençlik döneminde geride bıraktığımı, sonra da her zaman herşeyin üstesinden gelebilecek bir gücüm olduğunu düşündüm.

Çünkü eğer içinde o güç varsa, olup bitenlere ne olursa olsun direnerek çıkıp gidebiliyorsan, vazgeçmeyi öğrenmişsen sonunda istediğin gibi yaşamayı başarıyorsun ve artık seni kimse çok fazla değiştiremiyor.

Sonra doktor bana, "Bazen hepimiz böyle hissederiz aslında," dedi, "derken birşey olur ve yeniden gençleşiriz, bu kararı verdikten sonra çok güçlü olmalısın, sen inanmazsan bizden fazlasını bekleme…"

Evet güçlü olmalıyım. Buraya kadar gelirken nasıl olduysam öyle… Ve üstelik oldu, beklenmedik birşey oldu ve gidip o çiçeği, yılanbalığına kaptırmadan almam gerekiyor, ölümsüzlüğün o gizli çiçeğini… Kimseye söylemek yok.

Hadi gel Puska, yine hatırlamaya çalışalım unuttuklarımızı, kimbilir belki görmediğimiz daha çok işaretler vardır orada…

Tolga Londra'dan heyecanla döndü. Yeni evi, oturacağımız semti, hemen yakında her sabah kahvaltı edeceğimiz küçük kafeyi, hatta oradaki sempatik garsonu anlatıp duruyordu. Epeyce alışveriş yapmıştı, odanın her tarafına aldıklarını yaymış bana gösteri yapıyordu. Tabii bana da yeni moda rengarenk gömlekler, pantolonlar, kocaman taşlı kolyeler, kitaplar almıştı.

Çok komikti gerçekten de... "Okuldakilere söylemeyelim gözleri kalır," diye beni ciddi ciddi tembihliyor, tahtalara vuruyordu.

Üşenmedi bana aldıklarını tek tek denetti. Bazılarını çok beğendi bazılarına burun büktü. "Senin de biraz göğüslerin mi büyüdü ne, bunu kaldır, değiştiririz gidince," diyordu.

"Keşke benim kardeşim olsaydın," dedim.

"E zaten öyle sayılırım," diye bana sarıldı.

Ev aslında eşyalıydı ama yine de annesine bir sürü şey aldırmıştı tabii.

"Biraz eski püskü ev ama yeri şahane," diyordu, "yürüyerek her yere gidebiliriz, bisiklet alsam mı dedim ama o da havamı bozar, ne diyorsun?"

Gülüyordum, ne diyeceğim...

"Evet bence de bu kıyafetlerinle bisiklete binip paçana halka takman hoş olmaz..." dedim...

"Eee sen neler yaptın?" dedi sonunda o uzay stili yuvarlak koltuğuna gömülüp.

"Hiiç," dedim, "aynı şeyler işte, ha Ferhat'a dergiyi götürdüm bu arada..."

Gözleri açıldı birden...

Gömüldüğü koltuktan zor fırladı.

"Ferhat'a? Dergiyi mi götürdün? Şimdi hemen hemen anlatıyorsun herşeyi..."

"Ne var canım, dergiyi götürdüm işte... İstemişti ya..."

"İstemişti ya... Tabii tabii... Seni şimdi parçalarım. Hemen anlat diyorum!"

Kızacağını düşünmüştüm ama gülmeye başladı.

"Çabuk diyorum..."

Resimleri, anlattıklarından bazılarını... Tam anlatıyordum ki, eliyle ağzımı kapadı...

"Sen benim gözlerime bir baksana," dedi, "başlatma şimdi resimlerden mesimlerden..."

"E ama bunları konuştuk..."

"Koca adam oturup sana saatlerce bunları niye anlatsın, zaten ben ilk gün anlamıştım,"

"Neyi anladın canım, oturduk sohbet ettik işte ne olacak..."

"Oturduk sohbet ettik, ne olacak," diye taklidimi yaptı.

"Off çok heyecanlı... Biraz ayrıntı rica etsem..."

"Tolga" dedim, "bırak ayrıntıyı filan, beni dinle, kimseye söylemek yok, gülüp dalga geçmek de yok... Birşey oldu..."

Birden o da ciddileşti.

"Ne oldu? Çabuk söyle?" dedi.

"Galiba, ben aşık oldum.."

"Sen insanı delirtirsin sahiden, onu anladık, bilmediğimi söyle, adamdan haber ver..?"

"Ne haberi vereyim bir şey bilmiyor ki…"

"Aman ne komik! Küçük hanım giyinip süslenmiş çok lazımmış gibi koştura koştura dergiyi götürmüş, beş saat oturup sohbet etmiş adam da anlamamış… Delirdin herhalde!"

"Ya sahiden de böyle oldu, çıkarken yeniden görüşür müyüz diye bile sormadı..."

"E sormamıştır tabii, ortada Sare Hanım var, çekinmiştir…"

"Öyle midir?"

"Yok değildir, senin vazgeçilmez sohbetinle çok eğlendiği için oturmuştur o kadar saat…"

"Dalga geçmek yok dedim, ne bileyim belki de ayıp olmasın diye öyle yaptı… Zaten sonunda seni evden merak ederler deyip sepetledi…"

"Korkmuştur," dedi.

"Benden mi?"

Onun kaş kaldırma hareketi vardır… Aslında komik olur ama o ciddi konuşurken yapar. Bir kaşını kaldırdı:

"Bilmem," dedi, "belki de kendisinden…"

Neden bütün bunları hemen Tolga'ya anlatırdım da Seda'nın haberi olmazdı?

Çünkü o herşeyi yargılardı.

Küçük, düzenli bir dünyanın içinde kalmak isterdi, belki de kendisini orada güvende hissettiği için...

O kadar çok konuşurdu ki sonunda herkesi yanından kaçırmayı başarırdı.

Küçükken bile çok bilirmiş gibi ahkam keserdi. Üstelik bunları öyle keskin söylerdi ki cevap da veremezdiniz.

Herkes hakkında kesin yargıları vardı. O kız içten pazarlıklı, o oğlan sinsi, öteki kompleksli, bu ruh hastası...

İnsanların kağıttan kesilmiş formlar olmadığını, herkesin içinde, kendisi de dahil, çok farklı insanlar olduğunu, kimsenin aslında ne kötü ne de iyi olduğunu anlamak istemezdi.

Böyle davrandığı için kimse de onu sevmezdi. Neredeyse tek arkadaşı bendim. Ben onu olduğu gibi kabul etmiştim. O benim tuhaf kızkardeşimdi. Ne yapalım ki böyleydi. Dediklerini pek umursamaz ama değiştirmek için de çabalamazdım. Garip bir biçimde beni sahiplenmişti. Herkesin bana zarar vereceğinden, beni inciteceğinden korkardı.

Anne babasını bir kazada kaybetmiş, o arabadan bir tek o sağ çıkmış, sonra da bütün hayatını dul teyzesiyle geçirmişti.

Neyse ki o kazayı hatırlamayacak kadar küçüktü.

Daha ilkokulda bile tombuldu. Sonraki yıllarda iyice şişmanladı ve neredeyse bütün hayatını o kilolarla uğraşarak geçirdi.

Belki kimse bilmezdi ama hayatı çok zordu. Aksi, huysuz, otoriter bir teyzeyle, kıt imkanlarla tek başına ayakta durmaya çalıştı her zaman. Kendisini orada sığıntı gibi gördü. Belki gerçek bu değildi ama önemli olan onun öyle hissetmesiydi.

Ve üstelik ne olursa olsun güçlü görünmeye, erkek gibi davranmaya çalışırdı. Kıvırcık kısa saçları ve iri yapısıyla zaten hep erkek fatma'ydı o.

Bir keresinde ona çok kızıp, "Yeter artık, herkes kötü değil, sen de mükemmel değilsin, kimse mükemmel değil, başkalarını değil, kendini değiştir yapabiliyorsan," diye bağırmıştım.

Birkaç hafta benimle konuşmadı. Sonra bu söylediklerimin bir anlamı olmadığını düşünüp ona küçük porselen bir biblo aldım. Çünkü kendisiyle başbaşa kalıp mutlu olduğu anlar porselen koleksiyonuyla geçirdiği zamanlardı. Bir *tinker bell* biblosuydu ve kurduğunuz zaman müzikle birlikte dansediyordu.

Onu koleksiyonunda özel bir yere koydu ve çalan müziği de hiç unutmadı.

Bazen insanlara dışardan bakıp onlarla ilgili yargılara varırız. Ben Seda sayesinde kimseyi böyle yargılamamayı, o görüntünün altında hiç bilmediğimiz bir hikaye olabileceğini öğrendim.

Onun altın gibi bir kalbi vardı aslında. Yalnızca kendini korumak için onu ortaya çıkartamıyordu. İncinmekten korkuyordu. O yüzden ne lastik ya da ip oyunlarına ne yakartopa katıldı. Bence çok istese bile köşeye oturup kitabını okumayı tercih etti.

Niye ona anlatmadım yaşadıklarımı? Çünkü hemen neyin yanlış neyin doğru olduğunu söylemeye başlayacak, kaygılanacak, başımın etini yiyecekti.

Ne işim vardı koca adamla… Üstelik sanatçı... Mutlaka beni "kötü niyetlerine" alet edecekti. Başka ne olabilirdi ki? Beni kullanıp, hahaaha, buruşturulmuş mendil gibi kenara atacaktı…

Onu asla görmemeliydim, arasa bile telefonuna çıkmamalıydım.

Elbette bunları söyleyecekti. Tıpkı annem gibi. Sanki ben bilmiyorum da…

Onun için ona söylemedim.

Bu Tolga'yla aramızda sır olarak kalacaktı.

Biz onunla çocukluğumuzdan beri en gizli şeyleri bile paylaşmıştık ve kimseye söylememiştik. Ben bir erkeği o da bir kızı ilk kez çıplak görmüştük. Birbirimize dokunmuştuk. Hatta öpüşmüş ve bunun çok anlamsız olduğunu düşünüp çok gülmüştük.

Sahiden de kötüydü.

O benim doktorculuk arkadaşımdı.

Bir keresinde poposuna sahiden de iğne batırmıştım.

İlk sigarayı da ilk içkiyi de onunla içmiştik.

İlk çıplak fotoğraflara onunla bakmıştık.

Okulda otururken birden içimden birşeyler aktığını hissedince öğretmenin kulağına söyleyip tuvalete gittiğim gün de önce onun haberi olmuştu.

Artık büyümüştük ve bunları hiç konuşmasak da birbirimizi çok iyi tanıyorduk. Ve artık o da bana sempatik garsonu rahatlıkla anlatıyordu.

Evet sahiden de büyümüştük…

Şimdi mezuniyet zamanıydı, sonra…
Sonra hayat yeni başlıyordu…
Yeni bir hayat…

Şimdi dönüp bakınca diyorum ki bütün bunlar yalnızca basit rastlantılar olabilir mi?

Herhalde bir hafta sonraydı. Tünel'e çizim için kağıt, kalem almaya gitmiştim.

O eski otelin önünden geçiyordum ve birden pencereden onu gördüm.

Otelin lobisinde, pencerenin önünde bir masada oturmuş birşeyler çiziktiriyor ya da yazıyor ve kahve içiyordu.

Yok bu herhalde bir yanılsamaydı.

Geçtim biraz yürüdüm. Geri döndüm.

Gerçekten o muydu? Öyleyse o da beni görmüş müydü? Gördüyse şimdi yeniden oradan geçmem doğru olmayacaktı...

Elimde kocaman resim defterleri, boyalar, otele döndüm.

Kapıdaki adam bana gülümsedi, ben de gayet rahat içeri girdim. Sola döndüm ve onun oturduğu yere geçtim. Evet oydu.

En köşede, pencerenin önünde tek başına oturuyordu. Zaten içeride bir başka masada üç kişi oturuyordu. Başka kimse yoktu.

Sanki çok gizli birşey yapıyormuşum ve o da bunu biliyormuş gibi titriyordum ama onu görmemiş gibi başka bir masaya yöneldim, elimdekileri masaya koyup oturdum.

Dalmıştı. Her ne çiziyorsa onunla meşguldü.

Gizlice onu izliyordum. Sonra bir an önündeki kadehten bir yudum aldı ve alırken beni gördü.

Gözgöze geldik.

Ne yapmalıydım?

Evet biliyorum aşk, insanların kalbine ok atan tombul, küçük melekle tasvir edilir.

Bebek aşk tanrısının haşarı bir biçimde gülümseyerek attığı ok günün birinde kalbinize saplanır.

Ama kimse kalbine saplanmış görünmez ok yüzünden çektiği acıyı anlatmak için doktora gitmez. Sanki tıpkı o simgedeki gibi acının da mutlulukla birlikte geldiğini herkes bilir.

Ani bir kalp çarpıntısı, yürek sancısı, göğüs sıkışması... Sıradan bir günde paniğe kapılmanız gerekir değil mi? Ama şimdi hiç de öyle gelmiyordu.

Aksine ben şimdi kendimi başkalarından çok farklı, özel bir duyguyla ödüllendirilmiş gibi hissediyordum.

Yoksa kalkıp bana doğru yürüyor mu?

Başım dönüyor. Bulutların üstündeyim ama kalbim sıkışıyor, ayağa kalkıyorum ve "Hemen kendine gel Ebru," diyorum, ne güzel rastlantı, ne rastlantısı, bu saatte kimselerin gelmediği otelin lobisinde, artık işarete gerek var mı, bir kanıta? Kendimi yokuştan aşağı son hızla gider gibi hissediyorum işte. Başka kanıt gerekir mi?

Ve bunun adı yok. Korku mu? Mutluluk mu? Yalnızca heyecan mı?

Gülümseyerek karşımda duruyor. Ayağa mı kalksam, ne yapsam diye düşünüyorum ama kıpırdayamıyorum.

Önümdeki boyalara, kağıtlara baktı ve "Ne o sen de mi resim çiziyorsun yoksa?" diye sordu.

Merhaba, nasılsın, burada ne arıyorsun filan yok.

Biraz sonra kendimi orada küçük bir masada bu hiç beklenmedik anda onunla yine sanki yıllardır tanışıyormuşuz hatta sözleşip buluşmuşuz gibi konuşurken buldum.

Onu tanıyorlardı çünkü pek kimselerin olmadığı saatlerde buraya gelip oturuyor, birşeyler karalıyordu.

Birden dedi ki, "gel yukarı çıkalım, otelin terasında inanılmaz bir manzara vardır bu saatte..."

Yukarı çıktık.

Gün batıyordu.

Eski İstanbul'un üzerinde.

Karşı kıyıdaki camlara güneş vuruyordu.

Anneannemin en sevdiği şiiri hatırladım.

"Başkadır bu akşam bütün akşamlardan / güneşin vehmi saraylar yaratır camlardan".

"Bütün bunlar bir ressam için bulunmaz şeyler değil mi," dedim.

"Bilmem," dedi, "akıl hastanesinin küçük penceresinden inanılmaz bir gökyüzü çizen ressamlar da vardır. Galiba önemli olan ne gördüğün değil, ona nasıl baktığın..."

Söylediği resmi hatırladım. Ama söylemedim. Dünyanın en ünlü ressamlarından birinin benim çocukluğumda çizdiğim resimlere benzer bir resmiydi. Lacivert gökyüzü, sarı ay, hepsi yerli yerinde ama ressamın gördüğü gibi...

"Acaba bende ne görüyorsun?" diye sordum.

Kızardım.

O manzaraya baktı. Sonra bana döndü, elini uzattı, gözlüğümü çıkardı.

Şaşırdım.

Gözlerime baktı.

"Bazen birine bakarsın ve yalnızca onu görürsün, güzeldir, çirkindir, şişmandır, zayıftır... Bazen gözlerine bakarsın ve onu değil kendini görürsün... Aslında insan neye bakarsa baksın kendini görür. Onun için aynı yerle ilgili herkesin farklı izlenimi vardır."

"Ama," dedim, "soruma cevap vermedin..."

"Belki de vermesem daha iyi," dedi.

Sessizlik oldu. Garson gelip birer kahve daha getirdi.

Niye, diye sormalıydım, sormadım.

Saçlarımı yüzümden çekti, yüzümü okşadı, ben de onu öptüm.

Evet bu kez gerçekti.

İnsanın kalbine bir ok saplanması ve aynı anda acıyla mutluluğu birlikte hissetmesi...

Hayır, bu kez doktora gitmeme gerek yoktu.

Bir sabah... Bütün pencereler açık... Tüller uçuşuyor... Serin, güzel bir ilkbahar günü. Bahçede kuşların neşesi... Uzaktan bir gemi gür sesiyle selam vererek geçiyor.

Sare Hanım üstünde ipekli, çiçek desenli sabahlığıyla koltuğunda oturuyor.

Annemle mezuniyet için ne yapılacağını, bana nasıl bir elbise dikileceğini konuşuyorlar.

Galiba konuyla en az ilgilenen benim.

Zaten bana soran da yok.

"Bütün kızlar pembe giyecekmiş, çok güzel kumaşlar getirdi Perihan, muhakkak ince olmalı şöyle dökümlü yerlere kadar..." dıyor anneannem.

Kahvesini içiyor annem, "Bilmem ki acaba kabarık mı olsa etekleri pek severim ben..."

"O ne öyle gelinlik gibi, evlenmiyor ya kız, mezun oluyor, kabarık etek olmaz..."

Annem susuyor.

Yıldız Teyze, "Kapatsana sen de fincanını, senin de falına bakayım..." diyor.

Kapatıyorum.

"Yarın sen ortadan fazla kaybolma," diyor anneannem, "Perihan gelecek, hem kumaşlara bakalım hem de ölçünü alsın hemen başlasın.."

"Zaten ne kaldı şunun şurasında..." diyor annem, "acaba hazır mı alsak, çok güzel elbiseler var Nişantaşı'nda... Artık kimse elbise diktirmiyor..."

"Ben diktiriyorum efendim," dedi anneannem, "herkese göre yapılmış elbiseden ne hayır gelecek, olmaz öyle, tam üstüne göre ölçülüp biçilir dikilir, modeline de insan kendi karar verir.."

Sare Hanım varken tabii annemin sözü geçmeyecek, Perihan Teyze gelecek, yine her zamanki gibi annem söylenecek ama boşuna...

O çoktan elbisenin modelini bile kafasında seçmiştir.

"Ama siz gidin bir ara da ayakkabı bakın, en mühimi o... Vakıa önce renge karar verelim..."

"Var ayakkabım anneanne," diyorum, "yeni aldık daha..."

"Kadında ayakkabı en mühim şeydir. Bir ayakkabı bir kadını alır başka bir kadına çeviriverir. O topuğun iki santimi insanı değiştirir. Ayakkabı seçemeyen kadından hayır gelmez, ben bunu bilir bunu söylerim, değil mi Yıldız?"

"Evet evet hep söylersiniz Sare Hanım," diye onayladı Yıldız Teyze.

Ben güldüm.

Annem bozuldu çünkü çoğu zaman düz ayakkabılar giyer ve anneannem ona "Sanki selvi boylusun bir de bunları giyiyorsun, cüce gibi geziyorsun ortalıkta, bilmem kime çektin..." diye söylenirdi.

Birden dedim ki, "Ben mezuniyet elbisemi kendim çizmek istiyorum..."

Sare Hanım öksürdü, suyundan bir yudum aldı, elindeki sigarayı söndürürken şöyle bir bana baktı.

"Aman kızım olur mu öyle, Perihan getirince modellerin içinden sen seçersin..." dedi annem.

"Dur dur bakayım," dedi Sare Hanım, "nasıl gelmedi bu benim aklıma, çok iyi fikir, tabii ya, kızı moda mektebine yolluyoruz, sonra burada terzilere elbise çizdiriyoruz..."

"Zaten çizdiğim bazı modeller var onların üstünde biraz daha çalışırım tabii Perihan Teyze bana yardım ederse..."

"Aman bayıldım bu fikre, hem de ilk modelini kendin giymiş olacaksın..."

Sonra bana baktı, ne düşündüyse, "Gelsene bakayım sen benim yanıma," dedi, gittim, eliyle uzandı gözlüğümü çıkarttı.

Bir an şaşaladım. Sanki daha dün yaşadığım an gibi... Sanki o anı o da görmüş gibi kızardım...

"Artık bu gözlükleri de atalım gitsin, kızın dünya güzeli gözleri görünmüyor, lens diye birşey çıktı biz hala gözlükle dolaştırıyoruz, bir ara Metin Bey'e gidin de halledin şu işi..."

"Gözlük yakışıyor ona, değil mi Ebru?" dedi annem.

"Bilmem ki..."

"Sen benim dediğimi yap canım, gözlük kimseye yakışmaz, yaşlanınca takılır o kadar, artık o genç kız oldu dörtgöz diye dalga geçilecek zamanı geçti, hatta yarından tezi yok ben de geleyim beraber gidelim benim de yakına baktırmam lazım, bahane olsun..."

Güldüm. Sahiden de ilkokulda ne çok dalga geçerlerdi benimle dörtgöz diye...

Ama asıl garip olan bir gün önce Ferhat'ın da aynı şekilde gözlüğümü çıkartıp gözlerime bakmasıydı.

"Gel bakalım falın neler söylüyor," diye fincanı eline alıp bakmaya başladı Yıldız Teyze.

"Saniye, bana biraz daha su getir kızım, ilacımı da ver," diye içeri seslendi anneannem. Kesik kesik öksürüyordu.

"Burada sanki kış geçmiş gibi bulutlar dağılmış, bak nasıl güzel bir parlaklık doğmuş... Aaa maaşallah pırıl pırıl olmuş her yer..."

"Sen manzarayı geç de başka ne var ondan haber ver," dedi anneannem bana göz kırpıp. İçimden, ne biliyor, yoksa Ferhat ona söyledi mi diye bir ürperti geçti. Ama ne zaman söyleyecekti ki? Telefon etmişse? Yok yok söylemez.

"Bak şurada, görüyor musun?"

Eğilip baktım fincana birşey göremedim, "Şurada hemen uzun boylu zayıf biri var..."

Sare Hanım'a baktım. Annem pek ilgilenmemiş, elindeki gazeteyi okuyordu, "Havalar daha da ısınacakmış, bahar günü çöl sıcakları geliyor yazmışlar..."

Anneannem ona şöyle bir baktı, "sen de gazeteye mi inanıyorsun, Noel Baba'ya inanmak gibi yahu gazeteye inanmak... Gelmez, birşey olmaz, sen devam et Yıldız..."

"Biraz uzaktan gelmiş ya da uzağa gidecekmiş gibi... Ama elini de sana uzatmış. Bak sen de buradasın işte gördün mü?"

Baktım sahiden de bu sefer gördüm. Buyurun bakalım. Her gün bakılan falla dalga geçer misin?

"Ee nasıl uzaktaymış peki anlamadım..."

"Orasını bilemem, uzakta işte, hem uzak hem yakın, geliyor mu, gidiyor mu anlayamadım..."

"Tolga'dır o canım," dedi annem lafa karışmış olmak için...

"Tolga mı? Ayol ne Tolga'sı, duymuyor musun uzun ince adam diyor..." dedi anneannem...

Saniye ilaçla suyu getirdi. O da meraklandı, "Kısmettir kısmeti çıkmış besbelli..." dedi.

"Ne kısmeti canım, nereden çıkartıyorsun," diye sinirlendi annem, zaten onun söze girmesinden hiç hoşlanmaz, anneannemin onu çok şımarttığını söyler dururdu.

"Başka ne olacak?" dedi Saniye ona hiç aldırmadan giderken, "Koca kız oldu kısmettir o kısmet..."

İşi dalgaya vurdum, "Kısmetse de var mı yok mu belli değil anlaşılan daha karar verememiş..."

Gülüştük.

Fal faslı da böylece kapanmış oldu.

Kapanmış oldu ama ben şaşırmıştım. Hala anneannemin birşeyler öğrendiğinden kuşkulanıyordum.

Önce gözlük sonra uzun, ince adam...

Tam da ona rastladığımın ertesi günü...

Belki de insanın aklı neye takılıysa birileri onu anlayabiliyordur.

Kalkarken fincanları alıp içeri götürdüm. Saniye küçük masaya oturmuş yaprak sarıyordu.

"Ooo akşama yaşadık desene," dedim, bayılırdım sarmaya...

"Güzel kızım sana yapıyorum zaten şimdi anneannene sorsam yine kızacak bu saatte bana akşamı soruyorsunuz diye, en iyisi dedim ben bildiğimi okuyayım, beğenmezse de artık köfte patates ne varsa yersiniz..."

İçerden Sare Hanım'ın sesi geldi, "Bak duyuyorum buradan seni Saniye, daha sağır olmadım şukur..."

Saniye fısıltıyla, "Maşaallah bilmez miyim ondaki kulak filde yoktur..." diye beni güldürdü.

Tam fincanları musluğun yanına koyuyordum ki yeniden bakmak geldi içimden.

Fincanı aldım baktım. Sonra bir daha baktım. Bu nasıl şey?

Ben duruyordum ama o yoktu.

Faldaki adam bir anda silinip gitmişti.

O akşam ünlü bir şairle eşi de geldi yemeğe. Fransa'da uzun yıllar yaşamış olan bu adam ilgimi çekmişti çünkü alışılmadık şeyleri son derece normalmiş gibi söyleyiveriyordu.

Konu elbette onun unutulmaz aşk şiirlerine ve aşka geldi sonunda...

Saçlarını hep kocaman topuz yapıp, kalın dudaklarını da koyu kırmızı boyayan romancı Nazlı Hanım,

"Şiirlerinizde hep aşk var ama sanki daha çok aldatma var, ikisi hep birlikte midir?" diye sordu.

"Öyle değil midir?" dedi Cemal Bey, "Daha en baştan bile birbirini aldatmaz mı aşıklar? Hatta kendilerini de... Aşk birini olmadığı gibi görmektir..."

"Ama ben daha çok ihanetten sözediyorum," dedi Nazlı Hanım.

"Kadınlarla erkeklerin aldatması farklıdır," dedi Cemal Bey, "erkekler için aldatmak yoktur aslında, onlar oyun peşindedir, öyle ki bunun sonuçlarının ne olacağını bile fazla düşünmezler..."

"Ama aldatılmak vardır değil mi?" dedi bir başkası...

"Erkekler için mi? Evet, boynuzlanmak dediğiniz şey... Orada anlarlar ne olduğunu ancak..."

"Peki, kadınlar için nedir?" dedi şairin eşi…

Sessizlik oldu, herkes cevabı bekledi. Şair sakin sakin suyunu içti, sigara yaktı…

"Kadınlar için sevgi isteğidir, kaçıştır, yeni bir başlangıçtır, aşktır… Bir kadın asla yatağa girerken kaçamak yapmak, çapkınlık yapmak için girmez…."

"Yok ben buna inanmıyorum, pek çok kadın var yalnızca seks için yatağa giren ve ertesi gün ortadan kaybolan…" dedi Nazlı Hanım.

"Çok sarhoştur hatırlamıyordur," dedi biri, gülüştüler.

"Belki başka ülkelerde örneği çoktur. Ben daha çok bizdeki durumu söylüyorum," dedi şair, "bizim kadın erkek rollerimiz farklı… Misal, ben küçükken asla bir kızla yatabileceğime inanmıyordum. Anahtar hep kadınların elinde çünkü. Onlar da biz de bunu biliyoruz. Onun için de erkek fırsatını bulduğu an, en istenen, beğenilen erkek bile olsa o geçmişteki eksiği kapatmaya çalışıyor…"

Şairin eşi biraz bozuldu galiba… "Sen de öyle mi yapıyorsun Cemal Bey," dedi.

"Fırsatını bulsam ben de yaparım emin ol," dedi adam gayet rahat.

"Hem herkes bilmez mi bunu," dedi, "ilk kez bir kadınla yattığınızda eğer herşey iyi gitmiş bile olsa, ertesi sabah erkek oradan kaçmaya çalışırken kadın şimdi ne olacak diye düşünmeye başlar…"

Bunu masadakilerin bazıları doğruladı, bazıları karşı çıktı.

Nazlı Hanım, "Peki ya aşk Cemal Bey, siz ki en güzel aşk şiirlerinin şairisiniz…"

"Evet ama aynı zamanda, çok aşık bir kadın, erkeğin felaketidir, diye yazan da benim.."

"Yani aşk kadınlara ait birşey mi?"

"Böyle de denebilir, çünkü bir içgüdüyü, yalnızca doğanın bizden beklediği bu eylemi ancak kadınsı bir incelik böylesine özel, böylesine eşsiz hale getirebilir. Ancak bir kadın yanındaki çirkin, sevimsiz, huysuz adamı böylesine yüceltebilir…"

Karısı içkisinden bir yudum aldı… Yüzü asıldı. "İşte Cemal Bey'in dahiyane fikirleri böyle…"

Bozulmuştu belli ki.

"Niye hayatım, sana iltifat ediyorum, benim gibi çirkin, sevimsiz, huysuz bir adama bile aşık olabildin diyorum…"

Siyah kalın çerçeveli gözlükleri ve hep siyah takım elbisesiyle gezen genç yönetmen,

"Aman üstad," dedi, "şaşırtıyorsunuz bizi, siz hiç aşık olmadınız mı, erkekler aşık olmaz nasıl denebilir, ya Romeo ne olacak, ya Abelard?"

Şair gülümsedi, "Aşkı için dağları delen Ferhat'ı da örnek verebilirdiniz genç dostum," dedi, "elbette ben de aşık oldum ve diyorum ki erkekler aşık olduklarında kadınsı yanları öne çıkar, onları o hale getiren içlerindeki kadındır…"

Büyük bir ilgiyle dinliyordum.

Ferhat deyince ürperdim.

Sare Hanım, "Bakın bu hoşuma gitti," dedi, "bence haklısınız, bu erkek milleti ancak aşık olduğu kısa zaman içinde adama benzer…"

Kahkahalar patladı.

Cemal Bey, "Biliyor musunuz dünyada en çok kullanılan simge nedir?"

Markalar söylendi, tarihten örnek verenler oldu…

O ana kadar hiç konuşmamıştım. Kendimi tutamadım.

"Kalp mi?" dedim…

Bana döndü, "Bravo," dedi, "genç hanım doğru söylüyor, evet tabii ki kalp... Okul sıralarının üzerinde, ağaçlarda, parklardaki banklarda, duraklarda, duvarlarda, kartlarda, aklınıza gelecek her yerde ona rastlarız. Kimi bir okla yaralıdır ve üzerinde iki ismin baş harfleri yer alır. Kimi ne yazık tam ortadan kırılmıştır. İnsanlar birbirlerine seni seviyorum yazmak yerine kalp işareti yapılmış kartlar atarlar."

Birden aklım başka yere gitti.

Küçük bir kız çocuğuyken kalbim babama aitti. Çok sürmedi. Ortaokula gittiğim ilk yıl birkaç sıra uzağımda oturup kağıtlara kalpler çizen ve üzerine ismimi yazan, şimdi yüzünü bile hatırlamadığım o çocuk sayesinde kalbimin yerini tam olarak belirleyebildim. Göğsümün solundaydı ve anlaşılmaz biçimde bu çocuğun dönüp bana baktığı her an deli gibi atmaya başlıyordu.

Bu duygu yıllar içinde gelip gidecekti. Her keresinde onun gerçek olup olmadığını, birini gerçekten sevip sevmediğimi kanıtlayan bir işaret gibi kalbim sıkışacak, nefesim hızlanacaktı.

İnsanlar bazen birbirine "Acaba ona aşık mıyım?" diye sorar. Oysa aşkın kanıta ihtiyacı yok. Birini gördüğünde yokuştan aşağı çılgınca koşar gibi bir duygu hissediyorsan, kalbin yerinden fırlıyorsa aşıksın...

Hatta kimi zaman onu görmeye bile gerek kalmaz. Yalnızca telefonun başında ondan haber beklerken de aynı duyguyu yaşayabilir insan...

Bu duygu mutluluk, heyecan, coşku gibi özlediğimiz isimlerle ifade edilebildiği gibi beklenmedik bir anda birdenbire hüzün, keder, acı gibi sözcüklere de dönüşebilir.

Hepimiz şaşmadık mı? Kısa süre önce kalbimizin çılgınca çarpmasını sağlayan şu adam, şu kadın nasıl olup da şimdi yalnızca kalp ağrısına dönüşüverdi?..

Nazlı Hanım onun sözlerine ekleme yaptı.

"Hatırlar mısınız, okul yıllarında sevgililer birbirine kalple birlikte aynı zincire takılmış küçük bir anahtar verirlerdi. Bilmem hala veriyorlar mı? Kalbimin anahtarı sende demekti bu."

"Ah," dedi şairin eşi, "ne yazık pek az erkek o anahtarı doğru kullanma yeteneğine sahip..."

"Aksine çoğu kalbinizi açacak yerde öylesine kilitler ki artık açmak için çilingir gerekir..." diye güldü Nazlı Hanım.

"Kalbimin anahtarı sende" kolyesi mi.. Ne şeker... Hiç görmemiştim...

Sare Hanım, birden uzun süredir herkesi dinleyip konuşmayan, sürekli masadaki mezelerden tırtıklayan kel, şişman adama döndü, "Ama Fazıl Bey siz hiç konuşmuyorsunuz halbuki bu sizin alanınız..."

Fazıl Bey kalp doktoruydu.

"Aman efendim," dedi, "bizim için kalp beyefendinin şiirlerindeki gibi değil, emme basma tulumba... Bizim için önemli olan çarpması, artık çarpsın da ne sebeple çarparsa çarpsın..."

Herkes güldü.

Genç yönetmen, "Aztekler kurbanların kalplerini canlı canlı söküp çıkartıyorlardı. Bugün onlara acımasız katiller gözüyle bakabiliriz ama kalbin önemini anladıklarına şüphe yok..." dedi...

"Bugün de yüz yıllar sonra kalpleri söküyoruz," dedi Fazıl Bey, "ama bir başkasına takmak ve onu yeniden hayata döndürmek için...Yine de bazı hastalar kimin kalbini taktığını merak ediyor ve onun huylarını edindiğine inanıyor..."

"O zaman söyleyin bakalım sevgili doktor, madem kalbin bu duygularla ilgisi yok, neden sevgiliyi görünce kalbimiz yerinden fırlayacak gibi çarpıyor...?" dedi anneannem.

"Kalpten değil de beyinden gelen emir nedeniyle... Heyecan, korku, öfke gibi duygularda da olduğu gibi... Gelip de sigara içmiyorum, her gün spor yaparım, sapasağlamım ama bakın kalbimde görünmez bir ok var ve canım yanıyor diyen hasta görmedim. Ama geçmiş zamanda bu yüzden doktora giden çok kadınlar varmış.?"

"Peki gelse ne ilaç verirdiniz?" diye sordu Nazlı Hanım.

"Aşkın ilacı mı? Hanımefendi siz söyleyin, böyle bir ilaç olsa da onu içmek isteyen hasta çıkar mı? Dünyada o kalp çarpıntısından daha güzel ne vardır?"

Doktorun bu sözleri beğeni topladı.

"Ancak kadınlarla erkeklerin çarpıntısı biraz değişiktir," dedi Cemal Bey, gülerek, "alın size örnek, bir kadının kalbi bir kağıda bakarken çarpar mı?"

"Kağıt mı?"

"Evet, belki bir aşk mektubuysa, ya da ayrılık..."

"Peki ya erkeklerin?" diye sordu yönetmen...

"Erkeklerin kalbi kağıda basılmış çıplak kadın resmine bile deli gibi çarpmaya başlar, işte aradaki fark bu kadar açık..."

Herkes gülüşmeye başladı, konu dağıldı...

Ben dalmıştım. Hepimize okullarda gösterdikleri gibi, damarların içine girip çıktığı, kanla beslediği, kanı pompalayarak hayatı devam ettiren bir kas yumağı..

Hepsi bu mu gerçekten?

Peki bunca makina, içimizi gösteren filmler, herşeyi ölçen aletler bizim için özel olan birini gördüğümüzde saatlerce koşmuş gibi atmasının nedenini söyleyemiyor mu?

Ya da beklenen telefon gelmediğinde duyduğumuz o tanımsız yürek sıkışmasının nedenini?

Evet burada her akşamki gibi konuşmaları dinliyordum ama şimdi tıpkı benim gibi Ferhat'ın da içinde kendiliğinden bir çarpıntı duyduğunu ve hem huzursuz olup hem de gülümsediğini düşünüyordum.

Sonra anneannem kendisine imzalı gelen şiir kitabını açtı ve okudu: "Bakın ne güzel yazmış şair, bence aşk mevzuunu bununla kapatalım: *"Ah aşkların çocuk bahçesi neden ömrün çok kısa?"*"

Gerçekten öyle mi?

Çok mu kısa?

O gece sabaha kadar oturup birşeyler çizdim. Az çok herkesin ne giyeceğini biliyordum. Birbirine benzer uzun elbiseler... Etekleri yerlerde sürünecek.

Bütün kızlar kalın tafta etekleri elleriyle tutarak masal prensesi havalarında gezinecek...

Birkaç oğlan baloya benimle gitmek istemişti ama ben Tolga'yla gidecektim. Tolga kendisine Londra'dan yakaları kırmızı, siyah bir smokin almıştı. Üstünde aynı o renklerde kelebekler olan papyon. Çok şekerdi. Tam ona göre.

"Emin ol hepimizden çok sen ilgi çekeceksin," dedim.

"Babam ceketin yakasına ne der bilmiyorum ama papyonu görünce kesin delirecek... Artık bu yılın modası buymuş filan diyeceğim. Neyse ki annem bayıldı..."

Bir sürü şey çizdim, bir sürü modele baktım ama yine de asıl istediğimi bulamadım.

Sonunda tül etekleri yerlere kadar inen, üstü omuzları ve göğüsleri kapatan bir elbise çizdim.

Mezuniyetten çok sanki kendi çizdiğim elbiseyi giyecek olmak beni heyecanlandırmıştı.

Aslında bir dönem bitiyordu hayatımda.

Buna bu kadar sevinmeli miydim, bilmiyordum.

Her gün okula git, öğretmenlerle iyi geçin, derslerine çalış, böylece günler geçip gidiyordu.

Annem hele ki anneannem varken benden rahatı yoktu.

Artık büyümüş, akşam sofralarında ünlü yazarlarla, sanatçılarla birlikte oturuyor hatta söze bile karışıyordum.

Ben konuşmasam bile çoğu zaman onlar bana sorular soruyordu zaten.

Şimdi bir anda kendimi yalnız, güvensiz, boşlukta hissediyordum.

Hiç bilmediğim bir kentte, yabancıların içinde yeniden başlayacak olmak bir yandan heyecanlandırsa da aslında korkutuyordu beni. Neyse ki Tolga vardı.

Sanki son hazırlıklarını yapıp bilinmeyen yerleri keşfe çıkan kaşifler gibi hissediyordum kendimi.

Farkettim ki ben öyle maceraların, keşiflerin insanı değilim. Ben herşeyin istediğim gibi, alıştığım gibi olmasını seviyorum.

Dünyayı gezip her yeri görmek isteyen değil, olduğu yerde kendisine yeni dünyalar kuran biriyim ben.

Böyle masanın başında uyuyakalmışım, sabah bir ara gözümü açıp kendimi elbiselerle yatağa attım.

Ertesi gün Perihan Teyze geldi. Ona birkaç model gösterdim ama kendi istediğimi söyledim.

"Çok güzel olmuş, bayıldım ama bilmem annenler ne der, bunun göbeği açık," dedi.

"Aman sen annemi karıştırma Perihan Teyze," dedim, "anneanneme sorarız..."

"Çok müşterim oldu ama Sare Hanım gibisini hiç görmedim," dedi, "o kumaşı bilir, neyin neyle giyileceğini, hangi rengin neyle gideceğini, nereye ne seçileceğini hepsini bilir, sen de ona çekmişsin..."

"Kimmiş o çok bilmiş bakayım," diye Sare Hanım salona girdi.

Çizimler yerlere saçılmış, kumaş örnekleri...

Gözlüğünü taktı, önce çizimlere baktı. İki tanesini eline aldı, oturdu.

"Ne diyorsun Perihan," dedi, " bu daha okula gitmeden olmuş, bunların ikisi de birbirinden güzel..."

"Ben birini seçtim aslında ama.."

"Seçtiysen ne soruyorsun?"

Böyleydi işte o.

"Dur bakayım ben bileyim hangisini seçtiğini..."

Biraz daha baktı ve benim seçtiğimi ayırdı.

"Bunu mu?"

"Yaaaa," dedim, "evet, beğendin mi?"

"Bu omuzlardan arkaya dönerse böyle durur mu, hareket edince bozulur mu Perihan?" dedi.

"Yok bozulmaz da..."

"Eee..?"

"Bilmem ki mezuniyet gecesi ya, bunun göbeği açık..."

"Ne olmuş göbeği açıksa?"

"Yani bilmem ki pek böyle elbise dikmiyoruz mezuniyetlere..."

"İyi ya şimdi dikersin işte... Bayıldım ben buna... Benim göbeğim güzel olsa ben bile giyerim..."

Sonra çizimi ona uzatıp içeri seslendi, "Saniye Saniye kızım, her sabah kahveyi yeniden mi söyleyelim, bugün de kahve içiyorum, birdenbire bu sabah çay içmeye karar verecek değilim..."

Sonra gözlüklerini çıkartıp arkasına yaslandı, "Belki," dedi, biraz daha o bandı genişletirsin göbek kısmı daralır anladın mı?"

"Anladım," dedi Perihan Teyze…

"Bu omuzlardan gelişini ne güzel çizmişsin, Sophia Loren'in buna benzer elbisesi vardı bir filmde, sen ver bakalım şu kumaşları şimdi onu seçelim…"

Perihan Teyze pembenin neredeyse her tonundan kumaş parçalarını ona uzattı.

"Böyle uçuşan bahar gibi olmalı, giydirirler kızları şimdi ağır ağır kumaşlarla yürüyemezler, hışır hışır taftalarla, yok yok uçuşsun şöyle gençliği, ilkbaharı anlatsın, yürüdükçe uçar gibi görünsün… Meleklere benzesin benim kızım…"

Saniye kahveyi getirdi.

"Durun şunu içeyim de kendime geleyim, daha afyonum patlamadı, annen şimdi göbek diye konuşur durur, bana bak sakın gevşeme, bu elbise olacak o kadar… Bir de bunun altına ayakkabı seçelim gidip offf çok işimiz var daha göz doktoruna da gideceğiz, neyse aynı yerde ikisi de birarada çıkar, hemen sen ölçü al Perihan, başla… Saniye Saniye ilacım evladım, ilacımı da ver.."

"Getiriyorum büyük hanım.."

Saniye'nin böyle huyları vardı, anneannemi delirtmek için özellikle yapıyormuş gibi…

"Büyük hanım mı? O ne yahu, o nereden çıktı? Ne büyük hanımı… Nereden öğreniyorsun böyle acayip lafları, hanımın büyüğü küçüğü ne, saray mı burası? Haşmetmeap de bari… Hey Allahım sen bana sabır ver…"

Onların ikisinin bu hali beni öyle güldürürdü ki, yalnızca her sabah konuşmalarını dinlesem keyfim yerine gelirdi.

Ama yakında gidecektim ve artık bu sabah keyfi olmayacaktı. Bir an içim burkuldu. Ya gidersem ve anneannemi bir daha göremezsem…

Zaten aklıma iyi birşey gelmez ki…

Ne çok zaman geçti. Ne çok şey unuttum. Ne çok şeyi artık hatırlamadığım için üzüldüm.

Ama elbette o günü, o sabahı, o akşamı, o geceyi en küçük ayrıntılarına kadar hatırlıyorum.

Elbisem bir akşam önce geldiğinde Perihan Teyze hala üzerinde düzeltmeler yapıyor, anneannem fenalık geçiriyor, annem yine "hazır alsaydık keşke"lerine devam ediyordu.

O akşam evin içinde Yıldız Teyze ve Saniye'nin de katılmasıyla tam bir kadınlar partisi vardı. Sonra Tolga'yla Seda uğradılar. Seda'nın elbisesi daha düz, kapalı bir elbiseydi. Benimkine biraz şaşırdı. Tolga'nın övgüleri karşısında biraz da bozuldu gibime geldi. Ama o sırada bunun üzerinde pek fazla durmadım.

Neyse ki geceyarısını geçerken elbise hazırdı.

Annem bana çok güzel, üzeri minik taşlarla süslenmiş küçük bir saat hediye etti.

Sare Hanım da eski, küçük incilerden kolye ve küpelerini...

Sonra içeri gitti, o çok sevdiğim yakut yüzüğü alıp geldi. Parmağıma taktı.

Evet birşey eksikti.

Hiç düşünmediğimi sandığım halde aslında sürekli bir burukluk gibi içimde birşey eksik...

Ne olduğunu hepimiz biliyoruz ama söylemiyoruz.

Yarın herkesin babası orada olacak.

Benim babam tabii ki gelmeyecek.

Yoksa gelir mi?

O sıralar belki de gelir diye düşünmüş müydüm? Evet itiraf etmeliyim ki düşünmüştüm.

En azından kızının mezuniyetine gelir belki diye...

Bunca doğumgünümde, yılbaşında aramış mıydı ki?

Ama kimbilir belki haberi bile yoktu. Belki zamanlamayı bile hatırlamıyordu.

Yine de o gece orada hem söylenip duran, hem gülüp eğlenen, başta annem, o elbisenin içinde beni gördükçe ağlayan kadınların arasında kendimi mutlu hissettim.

Ertesi gün saçlarımın toplanması, o gergin topuzun yapılması ne kadar sürdü bilmiyorum ama bir ara neredeyse imdat diye bağıracaktım.

Sonunda hafif bir makyajla herşey tamamlandı ve hep birlikte deniz kenarındaki otele doğru yola çıktık.

Hem kendimi çok güzel hissediyordum hem de niye bu kadar heyecanlı olduğumu anlamayıp kendi kendime gülüyordum.

Sanki bir mucize olacakmış gibi...

Oldu da...

Denizden ılık rüzgar esiyor, gün henüz batmamış, güneş ilerde kızıla dönmüş bir top gibi boyuyor gökyüzünü... Otelin bahçesinde pembeler içinde genç kızlar, siyahlar içinde genç erkekler...

Daha bahçeye girer girmez, heyecan hissediliyor. Anne babalar, öğretmenler kendilerine ayrılan masalarda oturuyor, birtakım duygulandırıcı konuşmalar yapılıp derece alanlar açıklandıktan ve tabii bitmek bilmez fotoğraf çekimlerinden sonra onlar gidecek ve burası bize kalacak.

Tolga heyecandan yerinde duramıyor, oradan oraya koşturuyor, kim kiminle gelmiş, kim ne giymiş, kimin saçları çok komikmiş anlatıyor, "Bu gece sarhoş olacağız ona göre, tam dağıtmak niyetindeyim," diyordu.

Üstüne biraz dar gelen pırıltılı kırmızı yakalı smokini ve rugan ayakkabılarıyla hemen ilgi odağı olmuştu.

Yıllardır okuldaki tüm kızların korkulu rüyası Nedret Hanım bir ara yanıma gelip beni şöyle bir süzdü, "Son moda mı bu elbise?" diye sordu.

Ama artık tırnaklarıma bakacak, küpelerimi çıkartacak, saçlarıma karışacak zaman geçti Nedret Hanım...

"Hayır," dedim, "ben çizdim, yakında moda olacak daha olmadı..."

Suratını asıp gitti. Seda'yla Gülgün daha gitmesini beklemeden kahkahayı patlattı.

"Aman bundan kurtulduk, bak ben bunu unutmuştum," dedi Seda...

"Tabii unutursun," dedi Gülgün, "sana hiç karışmazdı da ondan, tam istediği öğrenciydin..."

Seda bozuldu. Şu anda da herhalde Nedret Hanımın en beğeneceği kılıkta gelmişti. Boğazına kadar kapalı uzun bir elbise, kısacık topuklar, kısa saçlar... Makyaj yok.

Gülgün durumu toparlamak için, "Aman hadi gel biraz dolaşalım, bizim gibi yalnız gezen yıldızlar var, herkes çift gelmedi..." diye elinden tutup onu sürükledi.

Sare Hanım ön masaların birinde kraliçe gibi oturmuş, etrafı inceliyordu. Annem elinde mendil sürekli ağlıyor, onu sinir ediyordu.

İşin kötüsü Saniye de anneme uymuş, beni gördükçe "Ah benim güzel kızım bugünleri de mi görecektik, daha dün erik isterim diye okuldan gelen bücürün haline bakın," diye o da ağlıyordu.

Söylemem gerekir ki evden çıkmadan aynada kendime bakmak hoşuma gitmişti. Artık gözlüklerim de yoktu. Tolga'nın demesine bakılırsa bütün oğlanlar benden sözediyordu.

"Ohooo, farkında değil misin kızım, herkesin radarındasın, yanına gelmeye çekiniyorlar ama merak etme şu tören bitsin burada kuyruk olacak bak iddiaya giriyorum... İstersen eski zamanlardaki gibi kendine dans defteri yap..."

"Aman eğlence çıktı sana, sen kendine bak, şu kılıkla bizi gölgede bıraktın, asıl herkes sana bakıyor..."

"Herkesi bilmem de sen babamın suratına bak, birşey de söyleyemedi, ala ala bunu mu aldınız Londra'dan demekle kaldı ama neyse ki notlarım iyi..."

"Bana bak sen keşfetmişsindir her yeri, gizlice birer sigara içelim mi, var mı öyle bir yer?"

"Olmaz olur mu, gel benimle, garsonların çaktırmadan sigara içtiği bir balkon buldum bile çoktan..."

Annemlere, ellerimi yıkamaya gidiyorum dedim, kalabalığın arasından kimileriyle selamlaşarak, kimileriyle biraz konuşarak, kimileriyle sadece gözgöze gelerek geçip arkadaki balkona gittik. Tam oraya giderken elinde tepsi dolusu şampanyayı taşıyan garsonla karşılaştık, "Hah işte biz de seni arıyorduk," dedi Tolga, hemen iki bardağı kapıverdi.

"Delisin sen," dedim.

"Biz kendi kutlamamızı yapalım da önden, gerisine bakarız," dedi.

Denizin kenarında, gün batarken, kırmızı renkler yavaş yavaş laciverde, mora dönüşürken, hafif bir esintiyle boğazdan geçen gemilere, teknelere bakarken, elimizde geniş şampanya kadehleri...

"İşte sonunda büyüdük..." dedim.

"Evet, sonunda..." dedi Tolga ve kadeh kaldırdık...

Konuşmalar yapılırken, müdür, okul aile birliği başkanı, vakıf başkanı, birincilikle mezun olan oğlan, ağlayanlar oldu. Doğrusu ben pek duygulanmadım bu konuşmalardan. Bir dönem kapanmıştı hayatımızda ama çok da umurumda değildi. Bir keresinde gelecekte okulun ortadan kalkacağını, insanların evlerinde istediklerini öğreneceğini anlatan bir ödev yazmıştım.

Her ne kadar babamın gitmesinden sonra kendimi derslere verdiysem de okulu hiçbir zaman sevmedim.

Uyulması gereken kurallar, hiç sevmesem de ezberlenmesi gereken şiirler, hiç anlamasam da öğrenmem gereken formüller, sabahın körü kalkıp yola düşmek, seni inciten, aslında hiç biraraya gelmek istemeyeceğin öğrencilerle birlikte yıllar geçirmek zorunda kalmak, bazı öğretmenlerin senin üzerinde otorite kurmaktan duyduğu zevki görmek ve ses çıkartamamak, sürekli sınava çekilmek, sürekli kendini kanıtlamak zorunda olmak, aklına gelen ama söylememen gereken sözleri yutmak, birilerinin senden şanslı olduğunu, birilerinin senden zengin olduğunu, birilerinin senden güzel ya da başarılı olduğunu öğrenmek…

Hayatın küçük modeli miydi bu?

Öyleydi.

Ama ben zaten hayatın bu halini de sevmiyordum ki...

"Buraya, bütün bu formülleri öğrenmeye gelmiyoruz aslında," demişti Tolga bir keresinde, "buraya gelecekte kimseyi rahatsız etmememiz için istenen kalıba girmeye geliyoruz..." Haklıydı belki de...

"Mezuniyet ödevinde, okulun artık anlamını yitirmiş bir yer olduğunu uzun uzun anlatmasaydın belki birincilik konuşmasını sen yapıyor olurdun," diye burnumu sıktı Tolga...

Güldüm.

"İyi ki olmamışım çünkü herkese teşekkürle dolu bu sıkıcı konuşmayı yapamayacaktım..."

"Aman iyi oldu, yoksa rezalet çıkabilirdi..."

Sonunda tören bitti, annem yine ağlayarak beni öptü, onları uğurladık. Tolga, Seda'yla ikimizi eve bırakacağını söyledi.

"Ama bu bizim gecemiz, biraz eğleneceğiz, geç kalırsak merak etmeyin," dedi..

Ama annem tabii ki uyumayacaktı. "Çok geç kalmayın," diye tembihlemeyi unutmadı.

Ara sıra başkalarıyla biraraya gelip sohbetler ettik, belki biraz geçmişten ama daha çok gelecekten...

Bazıları bizim gibi yurtdışına gidecek, bazıları üniversite sınavının sonuçlarını bekleyecekti.

Önce epeyce tepindik. Geç saatlerde orkestra biraz daha yumuşak, eski şarkılar çalmaya başladı.

Biraz sarhoş olmuştum galiba. Ama başım dönmüyordu. Bir iki çocukla dans etmiş, iltifatlar hatta buluşma teklifleri almıştım. Galiba herkese mavi boncuk dağıtıyordum. Seda arada yanıma gelip yine polislik yapıyor, fazla içme, bu çocuk sana fazla sarıldı, herkes sana bakıyor gibi klasik cümlelerini kuruyordu.

Tolga nasıl becerdiyse okulun en komik çocuklarından Fıy fıy Uğur'u alıp yanımıza getirdi ve Seda'yla dans etmesini sağladı.

"Başka türlü seni kurtaramayacaktım," dedi ve biz de dansa başladık.

Keyfim o kadar yerindeydi ki o an beni ancak gecenin bitmesi üzebilirdi. Hani çocukken arkadaşınız gelir, önce ne oynayacağınızı bilemezsiniz, o bir oyun ister, siz bir başkasını, sıkılırsınız, sonra gün biterken tam ne yapacağınızı bulmuşken ve mutluyken anneniz gelip onun gitmesi gerektiğini söyler, işte böyle bir ruh halindeydim.

Gerçi dans ettiğim Tolga'ydı ama bu gece hiç bitmesin istiyordum.

Evet babam tabii ki gelmemişti. Sırf bir kadehi bu yüzden kafaya dikmiştim. Bunu unutmak istiyordum artık.

Başımı Tolga'nın omuzuna koymuş onun ritmine uyuyordum. Yavaş yavaş dönüyorduk. Herkes etrafımızda dönüyordu. Işıklar dönüyordu.

Yine dalmış gitmiştim.

"Bir tek dönmeyen bana sensin..."

Şarkıyı dinliyordum, "Yok artık," dedi Tolga birdenbire...

Başımı kaldırdım. "Ne oldu?" diye sordum.

"Şuraya bakar mısın sen biraz," dedi ve beni çevirdi.

Dans ettiğimiz terasın arkasında düzenli kesilmiş çalılar ve sonra da çim bir alan vardı.

Çalıların arkasında öylece durmuş elleri ceplerinde bize bakıyordu.

Önce hayal görüyorum sandım.

Onu çevirdim.

"Gerçekten o mu?" dedim.

"Asıl ben sana sorayım, gerçekten o mu?"

"Yok olamaz," dedim.

"Sakın bana haberin olmadığını söyleme…"

"Yemin ederim yok."

Nasıl olabilirdi ki? Herhalde içimden geçen ama aklıma gelecek en son şeydi bu.

Yok canım benim için gelmiş olamazdı. Herhalde yine oteldeki başka bir davete gelmişti. Belki de benim burada olduğumu da bilmiyor, öylesine bu eğlenceyi izliyordu.

"Neler saçmalıyorsun," dedi Tolga, "gelmiş adam bildiğin, seni arıyor…"

"Beni oraya doğru götür ama belli etme," dedim.

"Aman yarabbim," dedi, "tarihe tanıklık ediyorum şu an…"

Sonra beni yavaş yavaş kenara doğru götürdü.

"Sakın beni çevirme," dedim, "sakın…"

"Gördü galiba," dedi, "bu kadar aynı renkte giyinmiş kızın içinde seni görmesi de ayrı mucize ya…"

"Sakın sakın, çevirme beni," dedim.

Birden beni bıraktı. Birkaç adım attı. Öylece kaldım, ne yapmam gerektiğini bilemedim, mecburen ona doğru döndüm.

Doğruca onun yanına gitti ve elini sıktı.

Ben de şaşırmış gibi arkasından yürüdüm.

"Ne güzel rastlantı," dedi Tolga, "siz misiniz, değil misiniz diye bakıyorum ben de…"

"Evet ne güzel rastlantı, otelde bir sergi vardı ona gelmiştim, biraz hava alıp sigara içmeye çıkınca bu eğlenceli topluluğu gördüm, hangi okul diye sordum, söylediler, o yüzden bakıyordum belki sizi de görürüm diye.."

Yanına gittim, elimi sıktı.

"Ne güzel elbise, çok hoş görünüyorsun…" dedi.

"Kendisi çizdi," dedi hemen Tolga…

"Gerçekten mi? Tebrikler... Bir periye benzemişsin.."

O an gerçekten peri gibi kanatlanmış mıydım, utancımdan kızarmış mıydım, evet tabii ki, ne yapacağımı şaşırmış halde elim ayağıma mı karışmıştı bilmiyorum. Hem onunla konuşmayı sürdürmek istiyordum hem de sanki herkes bizi görüyormuş gibi bir an önce geri dönmem gerektiğini düşünüyordum.

Ama zaten karanlıktı, kiminle konuştuğum şu an kimsenin umurunda bile değildi.

Bir an sessizlik oldu. O yalnızca bana bakıyordu.

"Ben Seda'ya bakıp geliyorum," dedi Tolga ve birden ortadan kayboldu.

Biz karşılıklı kalakaldık. Aramızda bodur bir çalılık vardı.

Neydi bu? Gerçekten bir sergiye mi gelmişti? Herhalde benim mezuniyetime gelmiş olamazdı. Bundan haberi bile olamazdı.

Belki de biraz sarhoş olmasam soramazdım ama sordum.

"Burada ne arıyorsun?" dedim.

Hiç duraklamadı.

"Seni arıyorum," dedi.

"Beni mi?"

Çalılıklar aramızda yasak gibi duruyordu. Ayışığında orkestra yavaş, eski aşk şarkıları çalıyordu, artık kimse hoplayıp zıplamak istemiyordu, yalnızca sarılmak istiyorlardı çünkü dans ederken...

"Bu bizim güzel sırrımız, hiçbir zaman unutulmayacak..."

Güzel sırrımız...

"Seni buradan kaçırmaya geldim," dedi sonra. Şarkı devam ediyordu yüksek sesle...

"Kimse bilemez kalbin içindekileri çünkü..."

"Kaçırmaya mı, nereye?"

"Bilmem, ister misin? Sen onu söyle..."

İstemek mi? O an aklımda ne varsa uçup gitti. İstemez miyim? Bu, herhalde bu gece isteyip de gerçekleşeceğini düşüneceğim son şeydi. Ama nasıl yapacaktım ki…

Tolga geldi. Birden kafamı topladım.

"Ben dedim, Ferhat'la sergiye bakmaya gideceğim, birazdan gelirim…"

Kulağıma eğildi, "İki saat sonra burada ol, seni bekleyeceğim, Seda'yı ben idare ederim," dedi.

"A tamam," dedi sonra yüksek sesle, "biz daha buradayız, görüşürüz…"

Çalıların bittiği yere kadar eteklerimi tutarak yürüdüm, dönüp onun yanına gittim, birlikte yürümeye devam ettik konuşmadan.

Nereye gidiyorduk? Ne yapmak istiyordu? Bunları soracak halde değildim.

Rıhtıma doğru yürüdük. İskelenin yanında küçük, külüstür bir balıkçı motoru çalışır halde bekliyordu. Şaşkın şaşkın bakıyordum. Kaptan bizi görünce halatı çekti, tekne iskeleye yanaştı, elini uzattı, Ferhat öteki elimi tuttu, kendimi teknede buldum.

Kimse bilemez kalbin içindekileri…

Ay, kenarından ısırılmış parlak bir elmaya benziyordu. Denizin üzerinde kıpırdayan ışıklar.

O şarkı hala çalıyordu biz uzaklaşırken…

Sonra yalnızca motorun gürültüsü kaldı.

Sallana sallana gidiyorduk.

Yine beyaz gömleği, üstünde eskimiş keten haki ceket. Rüzgarda saçları yüzüne düşüyor. Eliyle geriye atıyor sürekli.

"Nedenini bilmiyorum ama bu gece seni görmek istedim," dedi.

"Sen her istediğini istediğin zaman yapan biri misin?" dedim.

"Eğer elimden geliyorsa evet…"

Ben de bu gece seni görmek isterdim. Ama bunun olacağını hiç düşünmemiştim. İçimde bilmediğim bir duygu vardı. Birşey olacağını biliyordum sanki ama ne olacağını değil.

Beklediğim biri vardı ama o gelmedi.

Sen geldin.

Aklıma en son gelen şey geldi. Yoksa başıma mı demeliyim? Çünkü bu gece ayışığında, bu şarkı çalarken, ben artık dedikleri gibi "kocaman bir kız olmuşken" sanki masaldan çıkıp gelen prens elimden tutmuş gibi, beni bilmediğim yerlere götürecekmiş gibi…

Aslında bilmiyorsun ama çoktan beni bilmediğim yere götürdün bile diyorum içimden.

Ben şimdi oradaydım, bilmediğim o ülkede, belki de varolmayan, kimsenin bilmediği, gizlenmiş, dokunulmamış bir yerde...

Elimi tuttu. "Üşüyor musun?" dedi.

"Hayır," dedim, aslında üşüyordum hatta titriyordum ama aynı anda o kadar yanıyordum ki neden titrediğimi anlayamıyordum.

Ceketini çıkartıp omuzuma koydu.

Aslında söylemek istediğim ne çok şey vardı, bu gece ne çok konuşmuştum ama şimdi konuşamıyordum. Ne diyeceğimi, ne demem gerektiğini bilemiyordum.

Daha biraz önce dedikodu yapan, Tolga'yla dansederken yakışıklı oğlanları, havalı kızları çekiştirirken kahkahalar atan kıza ne olmuştu birdenbire?

"Demek nedenini bilmiyorsun?" dedim sonra.

Duymamış gibi, "Gözlüklerini çıkartmışsın," dedi.

Evet bu daha iyiydi. Başka şeylerden sözetmek.

"Evet anneannemin ısrarıyla..."

Aklıma onun da Sare Hanım'ın da gözlüklerimi çıkartması geldi. Bilemezdi tabii...

Işıklar içindeki yalıları, karanlıkta dev gölgeler gibi geçip giden gemileri, yaz gecesi eğlencelerinden gelen şarkıları arkamızda bırakıp sakin, sessiz bir koya geldik.

Kaptan motoru susturdu.

Sanki birden başka bir ülkeye gelmiş gibi olduk.

Arkaya gelip bize birer kadeh doldurdu. Benimle tanıştı. Sonra yerine geçerken radyoyu açtı.

Yalnızca ayışığının aydınlattığı sessiz koyda yalnız biz vardık şimdi.

Artık titremiyordum. Buradaydım. Onun yanında. Neresi olduğu umurumda bile değildi. Hatta şu an buradan daha uzaklara, bizi kimsenin bulamayacağı bir yere gidiyoruz dese gider miydim? Evet, bence giderdim.

Tekne durgun suda sallanıyordu. Yanımda oturmuş birlikte radyodan gelen müziği dinliyorduk.

Dün gece son anda elbisenin son düzeltmeleri yapılırken, bugün kuaförde, sonra Tolga'yla dans ederken aslında herşey olması gerektiği gibiydi. İşte biraz sonra Tolga, Seda ben eve dönecektik, belki Tolga biraz bizimle oturup gecenin dedikodularını anlatacaktı ve sabah hepsi bitmiş olacaktı.

Ama öyle olmadı.

Sonra birden o çıkıp geldi.

Demek sabahtan beri içimde hissettiğim adeta bana gizlice haber verilmiş olan buydu…

Artık ben o pembeli kızlardan biri değildim.

Yanımda öylece oturuyordu. Elimi tutuyordu hala. Elim ısındı elinde. Kulağına uzandım, "Beni yine öpsen ne olur?" diye sordum.

Bir rüya görmüştüm.

Dalgaların kıyıya çarptığı kıyıda hemen kumların üzerinde bir evde oturuyorum, Ferhat var yanımda, kalabalık, annem sürekli emirler yağdırıyor, yemekler geliyor, insanlar eğleniyor, sonra kıyıya eski büyük bir vapur geliyor ama iskele yok, yolcular doğruca suya iniyor, yürüyerek aramızdan geçip gidiyorlar, annem sinirleniyor, nasıl olur da tanımadığımız bunca insan evimizin içinden geçer diye, anneannem onu susturuyor, bak diyor ne güzel vapur, benim çocukluğumdaki vapurlardan, meraklanma kimse bize birşey yapmaz, bırak geçsinler, hatta isteyenler gelip bizimle otursun, birden deli gibi yağmur bastırıyor, herkes içeri kaçışıyor, ben diyorum ki, denize girelim, bizi yağmurdan da, fırtınadan da deniz korur, ikimiz suya giriyoruz ve suyun ne kadar sıcak olduğuna şaşırıyoruz, suyun altında çıplak olduğumu hissediyorum ve çok utanıyorum, neyse ki anlamadı diyorum, ama bir dalga geliyor, o beni tutuyor, çok su yutuyorum hep başıma gelir bu diyorum, gel diyor, şurası daha karanlık bizi kimse görmez, niye gizleniyoruz, gizlenmemiz gerekir evet hatırlıyorum, kucağındayım, çıplağım, beni bir mağaraya götürüyor, denizin içindeki mağarada, korkuyorum biraz, artık sesler yok, kimseyi duymuyoruz, karanlıkta, mağaranın içinde, dev bitkiler var, suyun içinde büyümüş, çizgi romanlardaki garip canavarlara benzetiyorum onları, suyun gelgitiyle canlı gibi hareket ediyorlar yavaşça, kaygan kayaya yaslanıyor, ben ona sarılıyorum, dudaklarından öpüyorum, büyük bir dalga geliyor ve birden kendimi başka kayalara çarparken buluyorum, suyun içine batıyorum ve korkuyla uyanıyorum.

Onun cevap vermesini beklemedim. Gözlerimi kapadım ve onu öptüm.

Bildiğim tek şey, hiç kimse için böyle hissetmediğimdi.

Herhalde dans devam ediyordu, önce Seda sonra Tolga paniklemiş olmalıydı, saatler geçmişti, artık saati bilmiyordum, sonra annem kaygılanmaya başlayacaktı, başım dönüyordu ve bütün bunları aynı anda düşünmek istemiyordum, bu o garip rüyalarımdan biriydi belki ama uyanmak istemiyordum.

Yüzümü tuttu iki eliyle, beni öptü. Saçlarımı okşadı.

Ne garip, benim gibi onun da tedirgin olduğunu anlıyordum artık.

Hatta benden daha çok.

En kötü ne olabilir ki diyordum. Kısa hayatım boyunca yaptığım en acayip şey bu muydu? Öyle olsun. Bir kez de ben böyle birşey yapsam ne olur?

Kötü kız mı olurum?

Birine aşık olmanın nesi kötü?

Hem üstelik kim beni suçlayabilirdi ki?

Aşk öyle sizin karar verdiğiniz birşey değildi.

İnsanın başına gelen birşeydi.

Kaza gibi birşey...

Belki şimdi birdenbire fırtına kopar ve bizi açık denize atabilir, geri dönemeyeceğimiz bir yerde denizle gökyüzünün birleştiği karanlık bir anda yokolup gidebilirdik.

Bunu belki kimseye anlatamazdım ama aslında anlatsam anlamazlar mıydı? Herkes bilmez miydi bunu?

Tam da buydu işte... Öpmek istemek ve öpünce neden istediğini anlamak. Çünkü onu öpseydim ve bu beni mutlu etmeseydi aşık olmadığımı anlayacaktım. Gerçek böyle birşeydi.

Ona sormak istediklerim var mıydı? Vardı. Ama şu an hepsi anlamsız geliyordu bana. Hem sözler neye yarar ki? Yanımdaydı işte. Üstelik de beklemediğim bir anda. Onunla konuşmak, merak ettiklerimi sormak, aklımdan geçenleri anlatmak... Hayır, ilgilendirmiyordu beni bunlar.

Onu gördüğüm ilk günden beri öpmek istiyordum ama bunu kendime bile itiraf edememiştim.

Sözler, gülüşler, anlatılanlar, anılar, yüz ifadeleri... Hayır, benim için gerçek olan yalnızca kokular ve dokunuşlardı.

Boynunu kokladım ve dudaklarını öptüm.

Başka hiç birşey...

Koku ve dokunuş... Beni hiç yanıltmadı...

İnsanı düşünceler yanıltır, duygular değil.

Karanlık denizde, sallanan küçük teknede, yalnızca ayışığının pırıltıları, eski şarkılar, yapılması gerekenler, uzak durulması gerekenler, bize öğretilmiş olanlar, üstümde pembe tüllerden bir elbise, bana şimdi buradan gidiyoruz ve geri gelmeyeceğiz dese hayır demeyeceğim bir adam, büyük bir hata mı, korkulması gereken birşey mi, bilmiyorum, bildiğim yalnızca kalbimin nasıl çarptığı, ona kimse kural koyabilir mi, kimse kalbimin yalan söylediğine beni ikna edebilir mi, ama asıl önemlisi onun beni öperken yalan söylemediğini anlamam...

Nasıl mı? Bunu o an benim yerimde olmayan kimse bilemez. Ben biliyorum artık.

Geri dönmeliyim. Niye? Dönmek istemiyorum. Ama dönmelisin. İçimdeki polis mi bu? Akıllı yanım mı? Yarın böyle düşünmeyecek miyim? Kendimi yarın kötü mü hissedeceğim? Ama o bana ne yapıyor ki... Yalnızca sarılmış öpüyor. Bunu ondan ben istedim.

Kendi kendime diyorum ki, bu nasıl bir öğreti? Gerçekte ilk günden beri istediğin adamla öpüşüyorsun ama kafanda hala bunlar var. Bunları silebilir miyim? Hepsinden kurtulabilir miyim?

Bir dalga geliyor ve tekne sallanıyor. Ayrılıyoruz. Ellerim hala ellerinde.

"Gemi geçti, aldırmayın," diyor kaptan.

Beni omuzlarımdan tutuyor. Yüzüme bakıyor. Sanki içimden geçenleri anlamış gibi...

"Tolga seni bekliyor," diyor, "dönsek iyi olur..."

Evet dönmemiz gerekiyor.

Rüyalar biter. En sevdiğimiz, uyanmak istemediğimiz rüyalar da korkunç kabuslar da..

Bu bir film değil. Buradan çıkıp denize açılıp, kimsenin bilmediği yerlere gidip bir hayat kurmak ancak filmlerde olur. Çocukken çok sevdiğim kitaplardaki gibi... Bilinmeyen uçsuz bucaksız buz kütlelerinin üzerinde ya da sıcacık gizli bir koyda, kendi halinde yaşayan ve dünya umurunda olmayan insanların unutulmuş kasabasında...

Eğilip yeniden öpüyor.

Olsun, belki de filmlerde olmadığı kadar uzağa gittim bu gece, belki masallarda olmadığı gibi garip şeylerle karşılaştım, belki rüyalarımda görmediğim kadar eşsiz bir duygu yaşadım.

Ne olmuş!

Kıyıya yanaştık. Gece bitmişti. Karanlıktı.

Biraz geç kalmıştık.

İyi ki de kalmıştık.

Ben, Ebru, pembe, biraz ıslanmış tüllerden elbisemle, aydedenin gülümsediği karanlık denizde, kimselerin olmadığı, kimselerin bizi görmediği bir yerde, hayatımın yeni bir dönemine girdiğim bu gecede, hayatımda ilk kez istediğimi yaptım. Kimseye sormadan, kimseyi umursamadan, ne istiyorsam onu yaptım.

Biraz üşümüş, biraz ıslanmış, elini tutarken, boynuna başımı koymuş, dalgalara karşı geri dönerken, biraz başım dönerken, kendi kendime dedim ki bunu yaptığın için pişmanlık duymayacaksın.

Duymayacağım.

Kim ne derse desin.

Söz mü?

Söz.

Nasıl becerdiyse Tolga, Seda'yı birileriyle yollamış, benimle sonra buluşacağını söylemiş ve herkes gittikten sonra tek başına otelin barında oturup beni beklemişti.

Ve tabii ki zil zurna sarhoş olmuştu.

Yine de geldiğimiz zaman bizi karşıladı.

Garip smokini, çözülüp sallanan komik papyonu ve jöleli saçlarıyla hem de sallanarak o kadar komik görünüyordu ki, gecenin bu saatinde gülmeye başladım.

Ferhat bizi eve bıraktı.

Tolga'ya, "Bana bak sen de geliyorsun, beraber oradan bir yere gittik, biraz fazla kaçırdık, tamam mı?" dedim.

Annem tabii ki uyumamıştı.

Ama her nasılsa söylenmedi.

Tolga dili dolaşarak, "biraz geciktik kusura bakmayın, ne de olsa mezuniyet," diye içeri girdi.

"Ben kahve yapayım," dedi annem.

"Sen yat anne," dedim, "ben yaparım."

Önemli olan "sağ salim" gelmemizdi. Annem gidip yattı.

Kahveleri getirdim.

Tolga ceketini, kelebekli papyonunu çıkartmış, salondaki koltukta yayılmıştı.

"Kahve filan istemiyorum," dedi, "iki saat tek başıma barda içki içtim, şimdi bana değişik bir hikaye anlatsan iyi olur..."

"Ne anlatayım," dedim, "beni balıkçı teknesiyle gezdirdi, çok güzeldi.."

"Gezdirdi mi? Sen bana baksana, sarhoşum diye benimle dalga geçme istersen, ne oldu diyorum..."

Gülüyordum.

"Ne olduğunu bilmek mi istiyorsun?"

Bir sigara çıkardı, yaktı, neredeyse yere düşecek gibiydi...

"Söyleyeceğim ama zaten yarın hatırlamayacaksın..."

"Bana bak, bütün gece seninle uğraştım, o şapşal Seda başımın etini yedi, ayrıca annemlere de hep beraber Ebru'ya gidiyoruz, orada kalacağım diye yalanlar uydurdum, bana güzel birşey söylemezsen rezalet çıkartırım, herkesi uyandırıp ne haltlar karıştırdığını söylerim anladın mı?"

Bunları ağzı dolaşarak söylüyordu, o kadar tatlıydı ki gülmemek için zor duruyordum.

Ama o anda birine bunu söylemek istediğimi farkettim.

"Ben," dedim, "onu öptüm..."

"Onu mu soruyorum," dedi, "çizgi filmlerde de herkes birbirini öpüyor."

"E, ne soruyorsun?"

Çok sarhoştu. Birden değişti yüzü, "O yaşlı çapkın seni kullanacak, keşke gitmene izin vermeseydim, keşke suratına yumruk atsaydım..."

"Aaa, ne o, kıskandın mı yoksa?"

Sigarasını söndürdü.

"Oraya gittiğimiz gün biliyordum. Anlamıştım ben bakışlarından. Şimdi söyle bana sahiden ne düşünüyorsun?"

"Ben ona aşık oldum," dedim, "hatta ben olmadım, ne olduysa kendiliğinden oldu, o beni öpmedi, ben onu öptüm, asıl sen şimdi söyle bana ne olacak?"

"Ne demek ne olacak? Adam kalkmış senin mezuniyetine gelmiş, tekne tutmuş, dünyanın en adi adamı değilse..."

Bir an durdu...

"Ki değil..."

"Eee...?"

"Sana bir tek şey söyleyeceğim... Keşke bu gece bütün bunlar benim de başıma gelseydi..."

Ben anlatmaya devam ediyordum ama baktım sızmış bile...

İçerden battaniye getirdim. Üstünü örttüm.

Gidip saçımı açtım. Takılarımı çıkardım. Makyajımı sildim. Soyundum. Aynada dantel çamaşırlarımla kendime baktım.

Gülümsedim.

Ben artık büyük bir kızım.

Şimdi ne yapıyor diye düşündüm. Acaba onun aklından neler geçiyor. Onun yanında olmak istedim.

Ve o an farkında değildim belki ama birinin hep yanında olmak istemek hiç de sandığımız kadar iyi değildi.

O gece uyuyamam sandım ama yorgunluktan mı, deniz havasından mı, biraz içkiden mi bilmem daha kafamı yastığa koyar koymaz uykuya dalmışım.

Hem ne uyku.

Rüyamda Seda beni arayıp televizyondaki filmi izlememi istiyordu ısrarla... Açıp filmi izliyorum. Filmin sonunda adımın geçtiğini duyuyorum. Yabancı bir filmin içinde benim adımın geçmesi çok garip. Sonra Seda gelip beni alıyor ve tanımadığım bir yere gidiyoruz. Beni neden oraya getirdiğini soruyorum ama cevap vermiyor.

Küçük bir eve giriyoruz. Hiç tanımadığım insanlar var salonda. Eski eşyaları olan, orta halli bir ev. Yerdeki halılar yer yer yolunmuş, yırtılmış. Yaşlıca bir adamla kadın oturuyor. Bunları tanıyor musun diye soruyor Seda. Tanımıyorum. Bak diyor, onlar senin gerçek annenle baban. Ürperiyorum rüyamın içinde. Şaşkın şaşkın bakıyorum. Kadın ağlıyor, adam hüzünlü. Nasıl olur diyorum? Bunca yıl benden gizlendi mi bütün bunlar? Arkada orta yaşlarda, toplucu, yeşil gözlü bir kadın oturuyor. "Peki beni tanıyor musun?" diye soruyor. Tanımıyorum. Hiç görmedim bu kadını. "Hayır," diyorum.

"Ben gerçek Ebru'yum," diyor.

Çarpıntıyla uyandım. Ne biçim rüya bu böyle dedim kendi kendime... Gerçek Ebru mu? Gerçek anne babam mı? Kadının yüzü uzun süre gözümün önünden gitmedi.

Saate baktım. Öğlen olmuş.

Uyandım ama hala sersem gibiydim. Sıcak suyun altına girdim ve yere taşın üstüne oturdum. Suyun altında durmaktan çok ne sakinleştirebilir beni? Kafamı toplamaya çalıştım. Rüyanın etkisinden çıkıp dün geceyi düşündüm. Tolga? Uyanmış mıydı? Ya uyku sersemi anneme ağzından birşey kaçırırsa? Yok yok yapmaz öyle şey...

Bütün bunlar nasıl olmuştu?

Sanki bir film sahnesi gibi...

Böyle şeyler gerçekte olur muydu?

Ama rastlantı değildi bu kez. Hepsini önceden ayarlamıştı.

Bunu yapmasını hiç beklemiyordum. Hem nasıl cesaret etmişti ki? Ya gitmeseydim? Anneanneme söyleseydim?

Üstelik ayrılırken bana kimse bilmesin, gizli kalsın filan bile dememişti. Belki de umursamıyordu.

Bir pantolon gömlek geçirdim üstüme...

Tolga çoktan gitmişti. Annemin pek kuşkulanmış bir hali yoktu. Benim gecenin en güzel, en zarif kızı olduğumdan sözediyordu. Belli ki babamın gelmeyişinin, hiç konuşmasak da beni üzdüğünü düşünüyordu. Bu halini bilirim. Eğer öyle olmasa mutlaka göbeğimin açıklığından topuklularla zar zor yürüyüşüme, yemeklerin kötülüğünden müziğin yanlış seçilmesine kadar laf ederdi şimdi.

Tam sorulara başlayacakken aşağı anneanneme kaçtım.

Kahvesini almış, gazetelere göz gezdiriyor. Beni görünce yakın gözlüklerini çıkardı.

Gittim onu öptüm.

"Aman aman prensesimiz nihayet uyanmış, sen de bana benzemeye başladın galiba artık, kahvaltı ettin mi, getirsin Saniye..."

"Ben alırım," dedim, mutfağa gidip kendime kahveyle çörek aldım.

"Olur mu bunla, ye biraz bak geç olmuş, güzel kahvaltı et..."

"Yok yok, yeter bu bana şimdilik," dedim.

Gazeteleri katlayıp kaldırdı. "Tek iç açıcı haber yok. Ne diye okuyorum hala bunları bilmem..."

Kahvemden bir yudum aldım. Galiba olup bitenler bizi ya da beni hiç ilgilendirmiyordu. Gazete de okumuyordum zaten.

"Eee, neler yaptınız bakalım bizden sonra, aldığım haberlere göre kafalar bulunmuş..."

"E işte dans filan derken... Hele Tolga düz yürüyemiyordu, görmeniz lazımdı, çok komikti hali..."

"Bakıyorum gözlerin parlıyor hala, dün akşam bütün iltifatları topladın değil mi?"

"Bilmem..." dedim.

Gözlerimin parladığı anlaşılıyor muydu sahiden?

"Yalnızca dans edip eğlendiniz mi, başka değişik hadise yok mu?" dedi birden, az daha kahveyi döküyordum.

"Yok, ne olsun ki başka?"

"Bilmem, sordum yani ne bileyim, mesela bugün buluşacağın biri var mı?"

Gözlerine baktım. Yoksa biliyor mu?

"Yoo, belki Tolga'yla Seda'yla buluşuruz..."

"Aman Seda dedin de, yazık aklımıza gelmedi, onun elbisesini de biz diktirseydik keşke neydi o acayip elbise Victoria döneminden gelmiş gibi..."

Rahatladım.

"Evet benim de aklıma geldi görünce ama ne bileyim kendisi bulmuş, hiç de sormadı..."

"Nasıl sorsun zavallı, imkanları da yoktur ki, sana daldık onu unuttuk..."

Bu yaşta bunları bile atlamıyordu. Gerçekten de onun için üzüldüğünü hissettim.

"Bazen yakın arkadaşlar arasında da kıskançlıklar olur, biliyorsun değil mi?"

"Seda mı? Yok canım o beni kıskanmaz. Hem bütün gece dans etti durdu. Keyfi yerindeydi yani... Siz eğlendiniz mi?"

"O manasız konuşmalarla mı eğleneceğiz. İçim kıyıldı. Bizim milletin mikrofon bulunca birden dünyayı kurtarma çabası nedir bilmem... Ama zaten sizin gecenizdi, ben senin yaşında olacaktım ki bak bakalım dans nasıl ediliyor..."

Aklım tabii ki başka yerdeydi ama her zamanki gibi onunla konuşmak beni rahatlattı. İçimdeki suçluluk duygusu uçup gitti. Benim yerimde olsa aynını yapacağından emindim. Hatta delirip olan biteni ona anlatmayı bile düşündüm.

Tabii yapmadım.

Ne olacaktı şimdi?

Beni evden arayamazdı. Ben de sersem gibi telefonunu almamıştım. Çat kapı evine gidecek halim de yok. Off ne salağım. O tüllerin içinde ayışığının altında Külkedisi gibi dolaşırken bütün bunları unutmuştum.

Al bakalım sana, atlı araba kabağa dönüşüverdi.

Ben dalmışım.

"Bu Yıldız da kayboldu ortalıktan, akşama misafir var, aa bil bakalım kim geliyor akşam?" dedi.

"Kim?" dedim.

"Hani Ferhat vardı ya sizin röportaja gittiğiniz ressam..."

Herhalde o an domates rengini almış olmalıyım. Kalbim çarpmaya başladı ve göğsümden başıma kadar bir sıcaklık yükseldi.

"Aa öyle mi?" diye kekeledim.

"Evet. Ne zamandır yoktu ortalarda. Senin pek sevdiğin şairimiz de geliyor... Akşam kaybolma yani...Sen de geliyorsun..."

Hayır bilmiyor. Off neyse...

Yüzüme şapşal bir gülümseme geldi oturdu. Bu adam hep böyle şaşırtacak mıydı beni? Deli. Tam da onu nasıl göreceğimi düşünürken...

Hiç gelmez olur muyum?

İşte bu yolculukta yanımdan geçip giden görüntüler gibi, o günleri hatırlarken de böyle hızla, üstüste nasıl geçtiğini düşünüyorum.

Öyle hızlı ki ayrıntıları tutamıyorum. Günler birbirine karışıyor. Küçük bir an bazen büyük resmin önüne geçiyor nedense...

Ne garip, güzel şeyler hep çabucak geçip gidiyor da acılar hayat boyu bizimle kalıyor.

Belki insan hayatın içindeki güzel anları toplayıp bir bavula koyabilseydi o zaman gittiği en kötü yerlerde bile mutlu olabilirdi.

Şimdi aradan geçen bunca zamandan sonra herşey çok farklı.

Şimdi artık bana ulaşabilir. Burada uzak bir ülkenin uzak kasabasına giderken herkesle konuşabilirim. Tabii ben istersem.

Cep telefonum yanımda ama kapalı.

Orada bu tuhaf yolculuğun sonunda yalnız olmalıyım.

Bu kararı kimseye sormadan verdim. Onun için kimseden yanımda olmasını isteyemem.

Herkese birkaç günlüğüne arınma merkezine gittiğimi, biraz yalnız kalmak istediğimi söyledim.

Şimdi biraz pişman mıyım? Evet. Ama hala zamanım var.

Galiba bu, trene ikinci binişim. Zar zor hatırladığım ilk keresinde İstanbul'dan Ankara'ya gitmiştik. Annem, babam, ben. Bir akrabanın düğününe mi? Cenazesine mi? Hatırlamıyorum.

Biri gelip yatakları açmıştı. O küçük kompartımanda sallanan vagonda dolap gibi yatağın içinde uyumak heyecan vericiydi.

Pencereden hiç bilmediğim, tanımadığım yerlere, evlere, gazete isteyen yoksul çocuklara, uçsuz bucaksız çayırlara, tarlalara, tek tük evlere, geçip giden telefon direklerine bakmıştım saatlerce büyülenmiş gibi...

Kucağımda yine Puska vardı.

Babam gazetelerini okuyordu. Annem kah uyukluyor kah bana birşeyler soruyordu. Bense hayatımın bu ilk garip macerasında bambaşka bir dünyadaydım.

Tren durduğunda gazete isteyen çocukların yoksulluğunun da, bu köylerin, kasabaların yalnızlığının da, hayatın aslında nasıl farklı, nasıl akıl almaz biçimlerde yaşandığının da farkında değildim...

Yalnızca toprağın (yağmur yağıyordu) kokusunu duyuyordum. Ve biz bütün bu hayatların, bütün bu unutulmuşluğun, bütün bu çilenin içinden öylesine geçip gidiyorduk.

Ben tüm bunları masal sanacak bir yaştaydım ama aslında hiç birşey masallardaki gibi değildi.

Ne olmuştu bana birdenbire böyle?

Daha akşam onun geleceğini duyduğum an ne giyeceğimi düşünmeye başlamıştım.

Sanki önemli olan buymuş gibi...

E hani ben böyle şeyleri umursamazdım. Umursuyordum işte ne yapalım...

Zaten kışlıklar yazlıklar, Londra'ya gidecekler, annem bütün dolaplarımı altüst etmişti.

Tolga'yı aradım, çarşıya çıktık. Seda'yı bir iki gün görmesem daha iyiydi çünkü soracağı sorulara ne cevap vereceğimi kestiremiyordum.

Nişantaşı, Şişli bütün gün dolaştık. Sonunda çizgili renkli incecik bluzla pilili kısa bir etek aldım. Aslında bol dökümlü bir pantolon beğenmiştim ama Tolga itiraz etti.

"Ne bu erkek çocuğu gibi pantolon giyip duruyorsun," dedi.

Ne bileyim oldum olası etekle kendimi çıplak hissederim.

"Bizde zaten mini etek yastıkla moda oldu," diye güldü.

"Ne demek o?"

"Mini etek giyen kızlar otururken bacaklarının üstüne yastık koyuyor ya..."

Öyle bir kahkaha attım ki herkes dönüp bize baktı.

Dünkü Ebru'yla şu anki Ebru arasındaki fark beni öylesine şaşırtıyordu ki giysileri denerken aynaya bakıp bambaşka birini görüyordum.

Akşam onu göreceğim.

Aslında bundan başka birşey yoktu aklımda.

Mağazadan elimizde paketlerle çıktık, yürürken, birden,

"Birşey var ama," dedi, "nasıl söylesem..."

"Hayır," dedim, "söyleme, duymak istemiyorum..."

Çünkü ne söyleyeceğini biliyordum.

O kadar aptal değildim. Ama şu an o kadar aptal olmak istiyordum.

Ferhat'ın bunu bir tek benim için yaptığına inanmak istiyordum.

Ve başka ne yaptığı, neler yaşadığı, kaç sevgilisi olduğu, çapkının biri olup olmadığı umurumda bile değildi.

Bunu bir tek benim için yapmıştı.

Yapmasa da bundan sonra öyle olacaktı.

Dönüp baktım, eliyle ağzına fermuar yaptı, güldük.

Saçlarımı açık bıraktım. Giyindim. Annem geldi, bana baktı, anladım laf geliyor, "Üff bu etek de biraz garip oldu ama Tolga aldırdı zorla, son modaymış," dedim, "Biraz fazla olmuş," dedi, "Yabancı yere gitmiyorum anne," dedim. Bana şöyle bir baktı, "Yemek hazır," dedi sadece...

Anneannemin sofrasına oturmadan önce annemle yemek yerdim. Çünkü o aşağıya, kalabalık sofralara gelmezdi. Onun evde tek başına yemesini istemezdim.

Fırında tavukla püre vardı yemekte.

"Sanki bir günde büyüdün," dedi, "dün gece sana bakarken gurur duydum..."

Aslında benimle böyle konuşmazdı pek. Şaşırdım.

"Gurur mu duydun?"

"Evet, bütün olan bitenlere rağmen iyi dereceyle okulunu bitirdin, güzel bir gelecek için hazırsın ama daha önemlisi artık çocuk değilsin..." sonra durdu, "gerçi ne zaman çocuk oldun ki?.." dedi.

Lokmamı yuttum. Suyumdan bir yudum aldım. Böyleydi değil mi?

Ben hiç çocuk olamamıştım.

Herşey öyle istediğiniz gibi olmuyor ki hayatta. Tıpkı o geceki gibi, pırıl pırıl ay gözlerinizi mutluluğa boyuyor ama sonra birden bir bulut geliyor.

Kendime aynada baktım. Eteği giymeye cesaret edemedim. Yine pantolon giydim.

Aşağı indim. Çerkes tavuğu, vişneli yaprak sarma, patates salatası, enginar, pancar, közde patlıcan, domates dolması, pastırmalı humus, kavun, peynir, küçük tabaklarda istavrit, tarama, ançuez, fava, kabak çiçeği dolması… Saniye'ye masayı kurarken yardım ettim.

Kristal avizeler yanıyordu.

Misafirler yavaş yavaş gelmeye başladı.

Sohbet koyulaştı. Konuşmalar sürerken, o en sevdiğim şairin dizelerini dinlerken sanki anlatılanların hepsini üstüme alınıyordum.

"Gözlerine bakıp sanki mavi diyeceğim / sanki çocuk diyeceğim.."

Kapı her çalındığında yerimden fırlamak istiyordum.

Geç kalmıştı.

Kalın gözlüklü sinema eleştirmeni İtalyan filmlerinin yeni sinemamız üzerindeki etkisini anlatıyordu. Kimileri söylediklerine katılırken bazıları itiraz etti. İnsan film üzerine konuşurken bile en sıkıcı kısmıyla neden ilgilenir bilmem.

Benim aklımda o filmlerdeki mutlu sonlar vardı. Hep ayrılık için bir neden... Savaş... Yanlış anlamalar... Ya biri evlidir, ya biri çok yaşlıdır... Hep imkansız birşey vardır... Araya giren birileri... Sonra biri kaçar... Biri onu izler... Onlar da biz de doğrunun bu olmadığını düşünsek de yine de vazgeçmeyiz... Bir mucize bekler gibi bekleriz... Bekleyişler vardır hep... Aptalca rastlantılar yüzünden birbirinin yanından geçip giden insanlar... Bir an gelip ikisi de vazgeçer ve seyirci hayal kırıklığına uğrar...

Ama sonunda tam adam trene binip giderken kadın koşarak gelir, peronda yüzlerce insanın arasında tedirgin halde onu görmeye çalışır... Adam bavullarını yerleştirmektedir, pencereden dışarı bakmaz. Tren kapılarını kapatır, ilerlemeye başlar, kadın koşmaktadır çaresizce, fonda birbirlerine ilk rastladıkları salaş meyhanedeki müzik çalmaktadır, kadın çaresizlikle trenin gidişine bakar, ağlamaktadır, adamın onu görüp görmediğini bilemeyiz, sonra tren giderken kadın tek başına peronda öylece durur, trenin son vagonu da geçer ve karşıda elinde bavuluyla adamın trenden indiğini görürüz.

Evet, ben böyle sonları severim.

Ünlü şairin "Sen bu şiiri biliyor musun küçük hanım," demesiyle kendime geldim. "Benim şiirlerim okullarda okutulmaz pek..."

"Evet," dedim, "daha çok kafiyeli şeyler okutuluyor ama ben biliyorum..."

"İşte buna memnun oldum," dedi, "peki sevdiğin bir şiir mi?"

"Evet," dedim, biraz utanarak, "*insan kendisine rağmen yaşayamaz / kalbimiz siyah derken biz beyaz diyemeyiz...*"

Güldü...

"Tebrikler... Ama şöyle olacak, kalbimiz beyaz derken biz siyah diyemeyiz.."

Kıpkırmızı oldum. Elbette ezbere biliyordum ama heyecandan onun karşısında yanlış okumuştum.

Sonra kadeh kaldırdı, "İşte buna içerim, gençler şiir okuyorsa gelecekten korkmaya gerek yoktur..."

Ve tabii bu söz üzerine yeni bir tartışma başladı. O sıralar, kimse şiir okumuyor, roman bitti gibi laflar dolaşıyordu ortalarda. Dergiler bu konularda dosyalar hazırlıyordu.

Ama aklım orada değildi ki... Hatta ben bu masada bile değildim.

Gelmedi.

Bir ara anneannem, "Ferhat gelecekti ama gelmedi," dedi.

Nazlı Hanım, "Canım genç, yakışıklı adam, kimbilir nerededir, söylenenlere göre pek çapkınmış..."

Bir bardak soğuk suyu kafama diktim.

"Yahu bizimle oturup ne yapsın, bekar adamın çapkın olmasında beis yok, nasılsa bizim yaşımıza gelince böyle oturup masada çene çalacak..."

Gelmedi.

Sanki ben o trenin peşinden koşan kadınmışım gibi kalbim çarpıyordu, içimde tarif edemeyeceğim bir kasılma, sanki midem yukarı doğru yükselirmiş gibi garip bir his, tren yavaş yavaş gidiyordu, gece geç saatlere geliyordu artık, ben trenin peşinden koşmuyordum, olduğum yerde duruyordum ama gelmedi.

Saat geç oldu.

Herkes yavaş yavaş kalktı.

Gecenin başında şölen sofrası gibi parlayan masa dağınık, yorgun, terkedilmiş bir hale döndü.

Sare Hanım koltuğuna oturdu, kahvesini istedi, ben de yanına geçtim.

"Bak görüyor musun," dedi, "Selim yine çok güzel çiçekler getirmiş, ne zarif çocuk, getirsene, bak şurada..."

Getirdim.

"Biliyor musun ismini?"

"Hayır," dedim "ama çok güzeller..."

"Unutmabeni bunlar, eh romancıya da böyle çiçekler yakışır..."

Unutma beni...

Gelmemişti.

Belki de yalnızca basit bir rastlantı olmuştu. Belki bir yere gitmiş ve oradan çıkamamıştı. Belki bir resme dalmıştı.

Ama ya dün geceden sonra benimle karşılaşmak istemediyse?

Kimbilir, belki de düşününce pişman olmuştu yaptığına...

Bana ümit vermekten korkmuş ya da olanların anlaşılacağından çekinmişti.

Tanımıyor ki seni, dedim kendi kendime yatakta dönüp dururken...

Nereden bilsin ne yapacağını, ya herkesin ortasında olmadık birşey söylersen?

Ya dün geceden bahsettiysen?

İyi ama onu ben çağırmamıştım ki? Neden geleceğini söylemişti o zaman?

Anneanneme hayır diyemediği için mi?

Olabilir.

Belki de birdenbire böyle davranacağımı düşünmemişti. Çok mu hızlı gelmişti ona olanlar?

Yalnızken, ayışığında, denizin ortasında, sallanıp duran bir teknede öpüşmek güzeldir ama sonra herkesin içinde kimlikler değişir değil mi?

Ben dün gece başka biriydim.

Bunları sahiden düşünmüş olabilir miydi yoksa hiç umurunda bile değil miydi? Nazlı Hanım'ın söylediği gibi bu gece de başka bir heyecanın peşinden mi gitmişti?

Ben de onu tanımıyordum ama her nedense böyle yapmadığına inanıyordum.

Hatta emindim.

Belki de bütün gece karşımda rol yapmak istemedi. Hiç birşey olmamış gibi davranmak belki ona göre değil.

Zaten gelse de karşılıklı konuşamayacaktık ki... Ama ben gözlerine bakacaktım kaçamak... Belki bir gülümseme yakalayacaktım belli belirsiz. Belki ben o dizeleri okurken ne düşündüğü belli olacaktı.

Sonuçta ben kendimi çok büyümüş saysam da onsekiz yaşındaki kızla, kendisinden çok küçük bir kızla, hem de tanıdığı bir ailenin kızıyla, üstelik hakkında bunca dedikodu varken....

Evet evet... Bence onu öpeceğimi, böyle birdenbire aklıma estiği gibi davranacağımı düşünmemişti. Şimdi de ona kapıldığımdan, aşık olduğumdan ve başına bela olacağımdan korkuyordu.

Asıl korkması gereken ben değil miydim? Garip ama ben korkmuyordum.

Şimdi burada yatağın içinde kuşkular içimi kemirirken, binbir soruyla uğraşıp dururken bir günde nasıl bu hale geldiğimi anlamaya çalışıyordum aynı zamanda.

Gelmediyse gelmedi.

Ne olmuş seni öptüyse? Evlilik teklif etmedi ya... Sen de kalktın koşa koşa gittin peşinden. İnsan, üzerinde mezuniyet elbisesi, topuklu ayakkabılarla bu balıkçı sandalında gece vakti ne sallanıyorum diye sormaz mı?

Sormadın.

Üstelik hayatında ilk kez sarhoş olmuşken...

Yok öyle kendimi kullanılmış, kandırılmış filan hissetmiyordum. Yalnızca anlamaya çalışıyordum çünkü eğer içimdeki duygu bu kadar büyükse ondan gelenin bu kadar farklı olması mümkün değildi bence.

Ama eğer öyleyse de bir daha görüşmezdik olur biterdi. Madem pişman olmuştu ben de onu arayacak değildim.

Sonuçta okulun yakışıklılarından biriyle de öpüşmüş olabilirdim karanlık bir köşede dansederken ve o da beni bugün aramayabilirdi...

Ne yapalım ki, herşey her zaman bizim anladığımız gibi olmuyor.

Bir oraya bir buraya dönüp uykuya dalmadan önce verdiğim cevaplar beni hiç mutlu etmemişti.

Tren gitmişti ve peronda kimse yoktu.

Pazartesi, salı, çarşamba, perşembe…

Geçti.

Gerçi artık günlerin fazla anlamı yoktu çünkü tatildeydik.

Bitmek bilmeyen pazartesi, sıkıcı salı, dilbilgisi çarşambası değildi.

Ondan ses çıkmadı.

İki duygu arasında gidip geliyordum aslında. Kapısını çalıp neler oluyor diye sormakla beni öpüp sonra ortadan kaybolan adamı bir daha aramamak arasında kalmıştım.

Tolga, "Adam korktu, biliyorum ben, başına iş açılacak diye düşünüyor, ama şunu da söylemeliyim ki bu iş zaten yürümez…" diye konuşup duruyordu.

"Bu konuyu kapatalım ve artık konuşmayalım olur mu?" dedim.

"Tamam," dedi, "ben yalnızca senin üzülmenden korkarım…"

Seda, Tolga, Gülgün, Tolgaların teknesiyle tatile gitmeye karar verdik.

Tabii benim yanımda ne düşünsem de kafamdan atamadığım biri daha vardı ama onu kimse görmüyordu.

Bodrum o sıralar henüz bir cehenneme dönüşmemişti. Tatilin bu ilk günlerinde çok kalabalık değildi.

Su beni her zaman mutlu eder. Ilık çarşaf gibi suda yüzerken, güneşe yüzümü dönüp kendimi bırakırken, mutluydum. Gülgün bir öne bir arkaya dönüp bütün gün güneşlendiği için hemen kapkara oldu. Okul günleri, gelecekte yapılacaklar, çoktan unutulmuş sandığımız anılar, öyle çok gülüyorduk ki...

İlk kez o ıssız, sakin koylarda kendi başımızaydık. Oraya gitme, fazla açılma, dikkat et, erken yat diyen yoktu.

Tolga teknenin kaptanı gibi herşeyi idare etmekle uğraşıyordu. Kahvaltı, yemek, akşamüstü meyvaları, kendi hazırladığı kokteyller... Emektar kaptan da arada sohbete katılıyor, sonra birden ortadan kaybolup bizi yalnız bırakıyordu.

Akşamüzeri gün batarken sudan çıkıyor, hazırlanıyorduk. Onun mutlaka bir planı vardı. Sanki dört arkadaş, ıssız adaya düşmüştük ve ne istersek yapmakta özgürdük.

Gülgün'ün hazırlanması biraz uzun sürüyordu. O kokoş haliyle sahilde yürüdüğümüz zaman hemen kendimizi bir yere atmak istiyorduk çünkü herkes ona bakıyordu.

Tolga hem kendi derdindeydi hem de bize sahip çıkması gerektiğini hissediyor, yanımıza gelenleri püskürtmek için elinden geleni yapıyordu.

Ama bunu söylemeliyim ki, Gülgün'den beklerken asıl hareket Seda'dan geldi bir akşam.

Bir köşede durup kendi kendimize eğleniyorduk.

Gecenin ilerleyen saatlerinde artık tekneye dönecekken bir ara Seda'nın ortadan kaybolduğunu farkettik.

Tolga gidip onu aramaya koyuldu.

Sonra telaş içinde yanımıza döndü. Kaygılı bir halde, "Kumsaldaki şezlongların birinde oğlanın biriyle oturuyor," dedi, "hem de elele..."

"Ee gitmedin mi yanlarına?"

"Gittim, gitmez olur muyum, siz gidin ben sonra gelirim," dedi...

"Nasıl gelecek ki sonra?"

"Soramadım ki..."

"Olmaz öyle şey," dedi Gülgün, "onu bırakıp gidemeyiz, kimdir, nedir bilmediğimiz adamla..."

Gülmeye başladım. Bunu söyleyen Gülgün müydü?

"Ne olacak adam seri katil mi çıkacak?"

"İyi ama tekneye dönemez ki sonra..." dedi Tolga...

"Döner döner," dedim, "tabii isterse, şurada sandallar var, biriyle konuş, istediği zaman ona biner gelir..."

Ertesi sabah uyandığımızda Seda yoktu. Önce biraz meraklandık ama öğlene doğru geldi.

Söylediğine göre çocuğun arkadaşları gelmiş, hep birlikte sessiz bir kumsala gitmişler, orada gitar çalıp şarkılar söylemişler sonra da uyuyakalmışlardı.

Gözlerine baktım. Belki de onu tanıdığımdan beri ilk kez mutlu ve sakin görünüyordu.

Ötesini sormadım.

Kaptan karpuz, peynir, üzüm getirdi. Tombalak pembemsi üzümler buzların içinde parlıyordu.

Ben suya atladım.

Dibe, daha koyu bir yeşile doğru giderken hayat aslında hep böyle olsa diye düşündüm.

Derinleştikçe güzelleşse...

Dört, beş günlük tatil bana çok iyi gelmişti. Tabii ki Ferhat hiç aklımdan çıkmamıştı ama şimdi ne yapacağımı biliyordum. Üç ay sonra gitmiş olacaktım. Benim zamanım azdı. Öyle mi oldu, böyle mi dedi, ne düşündülerle geçirecek vaktim yoktu.

En başta kalkıp ona giderken nasıl kendim karar verdiysem şimdi de öyle yapacaktım.

Sonra?

Sonrasını hiç düşünmek istemiyordum.

Kendi kendine hayaller kurmazsan onlar gerçekleşmeyince üzülmezsin.

Ama aradan zaman geçmişti. Belki o da benim yaptığıma pişman olduğumu ya da vazgeçtiğimi düşünmüştü. Hem o da bir yerlere gitmiş olabilirdi.

Eski otelin salonunda yine aynı köşede aynı saatte onu elimle koymuş gibi buldum.

Üç beş turist uzun, şemsiyeli bardaklarda renkli koteyller içiyordu.

Garson beni tanıdı. "Hoşgeldiniz, beyefendi burada, buyurun," diye bana yol gösterdi. Şaşırdım ama ses çıkarmadan onu izledim.

Beni gördü. Başını kaldırdı, gülümsedi. Önündeki defteri kapatıp ayağa kalktı.

"Tatil yaramış," dedi.

"Demek buralardasın," dedim, "tatilde olduğumu nasıl anladın o kadar mı yanmışım?"

"Biraz ama aslında Sare Hanım'dan öğrendim," dedi.

Demek aramıştı.

"Oturmaz mısın?"

"Evet kahve içebilirim, zamanım var," dedim. Sanki buraya onun için geldiğim belli değilmiş gibi…

Olsun bozmayalım.

"Çalışıyorsan…"

"Yok yok her zamanki gibi karalıyorum sadece…"

Öylece bana bakıyordu. Gözlerimi kaçırdım, turistlere baktım. Yüksek sesle gülüp konuşuyorlardı.

"Ve," dedi, "seni gördüğüme çok sevindim…"

Hayır, bu sefer biraz mesafe olacaktı.

Hiç duymamış gibi, "Eee, neler çiziyorsun, bakabilir miyim?" dedim.

"Bazen yalnızca eşyaların farklı hallerini çizerim, farklı açılardan nasıl göründüklerini, bir tür el alıştırması…"

Defteri açtı. Aslında bu bir defter değildi, içinde kalınca kağıtlar olan büyük bir dosyaydı. Sandalye, şamdan, avize, salondaki akvaryum, bunları çizmişti, o sırada garson kahvelerimizi getirdi, ama alırken eline çarptı ve kahve dökülmesin diye dosyayı hızla çekti, çekince içinden birkaç sayfa düştü, yere eğilip aldım.

Garson özür dileyerek kahveleri bırakıp gitti.

Ben elimdeki kağıda bakıyordum.

"Eyvah fena yakalandım," dedi...

Benim resimlerimdi. Büyükçe bir sayfada beş, altı resim vardı. Hepsi farklı açılardan çizilmiş ama gözlerim nedense hep çok büyük.

"Ben miyim bu?" dedim, başka laf bulamayıp.

"Aklımda kalan sen..."

"Ben böyle mi bakıyorum?"

"Hayır," dedi, "aklımdaki sen böyle bakıyor.."

"Biri ilk kez resmimi çiziyor da," dedim "şaşırdım biraz.."

"Bunların arasındaki farkı görebildin mi?" dedi.

Yeniden baktım.

"Sanki ayrı zamanlarda çizilmiş gibi..."

"Çünkü seni gördüğüm ayrı zamanları çizmeye çalıştım..."

Şu yandan çizilmiş olan Tolga'yla evine ilk gittiğimiz gün... Şu biraz daha gülümsermiş gibi ve şaşkın bakışlı ikinci gün... Biri burada karşılaştığımız öğledensonra ve son ikisi teknedeki gece...

"Evet," dedim, "ne garip insan baktıkça başka şeyler farkediyor..."

Ben onun beni hiç aklına getirip getirmediğini düşünürken o her günü unutulmaz kılmıştı bile...

Utandım, ürperdim, şaşırdım, ne düşüneceğimi, ne söyleyeceğimi bilemedim.

"Peki ama," dedim, "bunda neden gözlerim görünmüyor..."

Baktı, "Çünkü o akşamüzeri yukarı çıkmıştık ve güneş gözlerini kamaştırmıştı, gözünde yalnızca parlak bir ışık vardı..." dedi.

Ne garip, güneşe bakıp gözlerim kamaşmıştı ve gerçekten de gözlerimde o ışık kalmıştı ama bu, dışarıdan görünen birşey olamaz değil mi?

"Her zaman yapar mısın bunu?" diye sordum.

"Neyi?"

"Yani böyle günleri, anları hep çizer misin?"

Biraz ileride oturan turistler eşyaların, akvaryumun, avizelerin hatta tavanların bile fotoğraflarını çekiyordu.

Kahkaha attı, "Onlar gibi mi? Hayır..."

Ya, demek öyle. Demek bardaki içki şişeleri, şamdan, avize, sandalye gibi değil.

"Ama anları çizmek sözünü çok sevdim. Belki de gerçekte yapmak istediğim budur. O an'ı ölümsüzleştirmek ama benim gözümdeki haliyle..."

"Peki bugünü de çizecek misin?"

"Hayır ama eğer yarın bana gelirsen aklımdakini değil de karşımdakini çizerim istersen..."

Onun aklındakini bilmem de benim aklımdakini okuduğuna kuşku yoktu.

Yine de bazen biraz durmak gerekebilir... Kızlar böyle yapar değil mi? Niyeyse?

"Olabilir ama yarın değil. Yarın biraz işim var. Belki öbürgün eğer sana da uygunsa..."

"Evet," dedi, "bana da uygun... Bir de telefonumu al istersen çünkü ben seni arayamıyorum, belki aramak istersin..."

Kahvemden bir yudum aldım. Arkama yaslandım. İçimden güldüm. Evet artık sohbete başlayabiliriz Ferhat Bey...

Tatil nasıl geçti diye mi sormuştu az önce?

Evet böyleydi. Bazı şeyleri konuşmaya gerek yoktu. Akşam olurken kalktım, resmi istemeye utandığım için biraz kızdım sonra kendime... Aslında kalkmaya niyetim de yoktu ama Seda bana gelecekti.

Tabii ki Bodrum'daki o geceyi dinlemek zorunda kalacaktım. Neler söyleyeceğini, soracağını şimdiden biliyordum ama çare yoktu.

Aynı beklediğim gibi oldu. Annemle yemek yedik. Sonra benim odaya geçtik.

Bana müzik açtırdı annem belki duyar diye.

Fısıltıyla konuşmaya başladı.

"N'apıyorsun?" dedim, "annemin işi gücü yok kapıyı mı dinleyecek? Ne yaptın birini mi öldürdün?"

"Aman sana göre kolay. Bilmiyorsun neler olduğunu..."

Biliyorum. Hatta adım gibi eminim. Öpüştünüz, çocuk biraz üstündekileri sıyırıp oranı buranı karıştırdı sen izin vermedin, bu böyle sabaha kadar sürdü ve sen çocuğun sana aşık olduğunu sanıyorsun.

Bunları söylemedim tabii...

"Oğlanın arkadaşlarının filan gelmediğini biliyorum en azından..."

"Off tamam n'apiym, yalan attım."

"Emin ol kaptan bile inanmadı..."

Şu an o havadaydım ki aslında sıkılacağım bu konuşma beni eğlendiriyordu.

Aynen dediğim gibi olmuştu. Tabii oğlan arada bizimkinin uzun konuşmalarını dinlemek zorunda kalmıştı. Şimdi ben de aynı durumdaydım. Ve ona, "Hayatında tanımadığın biriyle sabaha kadar öpüşmek hem saçma hem de sıradan, bunun için kendini suçlamana gerek yok, bunu süsleyip özel bir duruma çevirmene de gerek yok, oldu bitti, geçti," diyemezdim.

Döneli çok olmamıştı.

"Geldiğimden beri aramadı," dedi.

"Arayacak mıydı?"

"Evet telefonumu aldı. Gelince görüşürüz dedik. Teknik üniversitede okuyormuş. Benden üç yaş büyük. Yeşilköy'de doğup büyümüş. Hala da orada oturuyorlarmış. Biliyor musun çok akıllı çocuk. Hem de efendi. Yani öyle zorla üstüme filan saldırmadı."

Tolga'yı özledim. Şimdi burada olsa, "Niye ki? Sen saldırsaydın?" deyiverirdi.

Ne garip. Aslında belki de çok farklı durumda değildik. En azından ikimizin de aklında biri vardı ve ikimiz de aklımızdakini pek fazla tanımıyorduk.

"Sence birlikte olacağın biri mi yoksa o gece biraz da oradaki durumun etkisiyle fazla abartıyor olabilir misin?"

"Bilmiyorum," dedi, "ilk kez geliyor başıma sen de biliyorsun..."

"Neden onu tekneye getirmedin?" diye sordum.

"Çekindim.. Aklıma gelmedi değil ama Tolga'yla Gülgün ne yapar bilemedim..."

Aslında öyle değil. Onunla yalnız olmak istedin. Onun seni, olduğun gibi değil, senin istediğin gibi tanımasını istedin. Ona hayat hikayeni, nasıl biri olduğunu belki bizim bilemeyeceğimiz biçimde anlattın. Ve bundan utanmana gerek yok.

Üstelik bunu yapmanın nedeni, hepimizin bildiği gibi, yıllardır ayılıp bayıldığın ama asla senin farkında olmayan Can'ın, mezuniyet gecesi her nedense seninle danslar edip sonra da ortadan kaybolmasından duyduğun öfke, hayal kırıklığı ya da her neyse oydu.

Tabii ki bunları da söylemedim.

"Aman canım," dedim, "o aramadıysa sen ara, ne var bunda?"

"Yani sen şaşırmadın mı?" dedi.

Ben sen miyim Seda? Ben sana anlatsam kimbilir şimdi bana neler söylersin. Ama işte beklenmeyen şey senin başına geldi.

"Biraz şaşırdım doğrusunu istersen ama bu bizim okul yıllarından beri ilk tatilimiz, başımızda kimse olmadan... Hem galiba biraz sarhoş olmuştun..."

"Hayır, hayır," dedi, "yani çok az..."

"Bence," dedim, "üstünde çok fazla düşünme, oluruna bırak, ya da bir iki gün sonra sen ara, sonuçta tanımadığın biri, hakkında ne düşüneceğinden sana ne...."

"Ama," dedi, "o kadar güzel bir geceden sonra hiç ses çıkmaması garip değil mi? Sence ne düşünüyordur?"

Biliyordum başıma geleceği... Şimdi bu soruları hiç durmadan sorup duracak, aldığı cevapları da beğenmeyecek, böyle günlerce uğraşacaktı.

Birden kızardım. Benim durumum sanki çok mu farklıydı? Ben de bana her zaman komik gelen bu hale düşmemiş miydim?

Aradı mı, aramadı mı, geldi mi gelecek mi, ne düşünüyor, ne hissediyor diye yatakta habire dönüp durmuyor muydum?

Kendime kızdım.

Hayır, ben bütün hayatım boyunca bu saçmalıklarla uğraşmayacaktım.

"Ne düşünürse düşünsün herhalde hayatında bir kere gördüğün adama birdenbire deli gibi aşık olmadın."

Aslında onun ne duymak istediğini biliyordum.

"Hem," dedim, "belki o tatiline devam ediyordur, dönünce arar, yaptığından utanmayı da bırak, çocuk değilsin, eğer saçmalık yaptığını düşünseydim gelip seni oradan kaldırırdım..."

Bir gün sonra sözleştiğimiz gibi kapısını çaldım. Sanki tüm bunlar olmamış gibi, her zaman buluşan iki dost gibi yine karşılıklı oturup sohbete daldık. Burası her nedense bütün bu karmaşasına, benim yaşadığım yerlerden tümüyle farklı olmasına rağmen bana huzur veriyordu.

Her keresinde yeni keşfettiğim şeyler, minicik biblolar, neye yaradığını anlamadığım garip eski makinalar, kurgulu oyuncaklar, yokolup gitmiş geçmiş zaman parçaları...

Sanki o dünyanın her yerinden ve zamanın farklı dönemlerinden öyküleri toplamış ve burada kendine özel bir gezegen kurmuştu.

Hem de kapının hemen önünde sıradan mahalle hayatı sürerken...

İnsan yalnızca bir kapıyı açıp birdenbire başka bir evrene geçebilir mi?

Bahçeden çiçeklerin kokusu geliyordu. Serin ve loş. Hep o güzel, uzaklardan gelen müzikler çalıyordu. Sanki kentin dışında, bambaşka bir yere, belki bir tatil kasabasına gelmiş gibi hissediyordum kendimi.

Deniz yakınlardaydı, martıların bağırışması hiç kesilmiyordu. Ve o her seferinde utangaç bir çocuk gibi karşımda oturuyor, yanıma gelip beni öpmeye bile çekiniyordu.

Oysa ikimiz de biliyorduk buraya neden geldiğimi...

Mavili, yeşilli neredeyse şeffaf, incecik bir bluz vardı üstümde... Kısacık etek ve annemin gençlik yıllarından kalma mantar topuklu ayakkabılar. Bir de yine ondan yürüttüğüm hippi dönemi kocaman taşlı bir kolye... Biliyorum bunların zamanı çoktan geçmişti ama benim hoşuma gidiyordu. Zaten artık benden başka kimse o uzun saçlı dört adamın çaldığı aşk şarkılarına, gökyüzünde elmaslarla uçan kıza da bayılmıyordu.

Bu an'ı düşünerek sabahı ettiğim için sersem gibiydim. Hatta sabah aynada yüzüme tokat attım ki beyazlığım gitsin... Saçlarımı toplamıştım ama öylesine... Neden bilmem, biraz dağınık görünmek hep hoşuma gider...

Nelerden sözediyorduk hatırlamıyorum, çünkü aslında dinlemiyordum... Bir ara içecek birşeyler getirdi ve sonra elimden tuttu. Ayağa kalktım. Yürüdü. Yalnızca elimi tuttu ve ben de peşinden gittim.

Perdeleri kapalı, karanlık odada, kocaman yatak, duvarlarda pek göremediğim resimler, köşede üzerine giysiler atılmış bir koltuk... Yatağın hemen yanında sehpanın üzerinde büyükçe bir abajur.

Bir an kapıda durdum. Ben onu ellerinden çektim ve yere yatağın yanına oturdum. Karşımda diz çöktü. Ya sıcaktan ya çarpıntıdan bayılacağımı sandım. Hem bu anın durmasını istiyordum hem devamını görmek.

Ama bu durdurup sonra izleyeceğiniz bir film ya da masaya bırakıp sonra devamını okuyacağınız bir roman değildi.

Bu hayattı.

Beni öperken gözlerimi kapadım ve ona sarıldım.

Sanırım ilk hissettiğim gitme duygusuydu. Hayır buradan gitmek, kaçmak değil, onunla birlikte gitmek... Sanki o an birlikte yolculuğa çıkmışız gibi...

Bu bir ilkti. Ama belki de son. Belki birşeyin başlangıcı olduğu için böylesine güzeldi, belki hiç bitmeyecek birşeydi.

Derine dalmış gibi dingin ve herşeyden uzak... yüksekten atlayıp uçarmış gibi hafif, heyecanlı... rüyanın en güzel anında sebepsiz yere korkmak gibi telaşlı... gizemli bir mağaraya girmiş gibi ürkütücü...

Arkadaki aynada görüntülerimizin çoğalması gibi birbirimize dokundukça o tanımlayamadığım şey, o benzersiz heyecan, o başka hiçbir yerde duymadığım zevk de çoğalıyordu.

Kendimi ona bırakmıştım aslında, çünkü zaten ne yapacağımı bilmiyordum ki, yalnızca onu öpmeye dokunmaya devam ediyordum.

Hayır gerçekten de bu kadar mutlu olacağımı düşünmemiştim.

Sanki bütün bedenim baştan aşağı dalgaya kapılmıştı ve onunla yükselip indikçe hani arabayla büyük kasislerden geçerken içimizde oluşan o garip duyguyla kasılıyordum.

Başım dönüyordu ama korkmuyordum.

Elinden tutmuştum ve şimdi benim gizli bahçemde birlikte dolaşıyorduk. Hayallerden bir bahçenin kapısı açılmıştı. Ben kendi bahçemde çok zaman geçirmiştim ama yanımda kimse yoktu. Orası benim en derin yalnızlığımdı. Bu dünyadan, istemediğim şeylerden, bütün o hastalıklardan, korkulardan, üzüntülerden kaçtığım yerdi.

Ve şimdi orada, içimde bir yerde bir başkası dolaşıyordu.

İnsan sevişirken böyle şeyler düşünür mü? Ben düşünüyordum işte.

Korkutucuydu aslında, içimde dolaşan bir canlı varmış gibi, kulağımda garip sesler, inlemeler...

Komikti bir yanıyla...

Ama aynı anda ne tuhaf, ağlamak da geliyordu içimden.

Gözlerimi açmıyordum, karanlıkta, içerden gelen müzikten başka ses yokmuş gibi ve o da konuşmuyordu...

İkimiz de o kadar sıcaktık ki sanki kumsalda kızgın kumların üzerinde sevişiyormuşuz gibiydi.

Uzun saçlarına yapışıp öperken dudaklarını ısırıyordum.

Yuvarlandığımızı, bir yerlere çarptığımızı hissediyordum, direnmiyordum sadece ona tutunmuştum, bu duyduğum her neyse öylesine yükseliyordu ki bağırmamak için zor tutuyordum kendimi, o zaman tırnaklarımı sırtına saplıyordum durması için ama durmadı, ben de bağırdım, titriyordum ve ne yapacağımı bilemiyordum, sonunda ona tümüyle yapışmış halde ağlarken durdu.

Gözlerimi açtım. Biraz şaşırmış, biraz korkmuş bana bakıyordu.

Titreyip hıçkırıyordum ama sonra gülmeye başladım.

Bu kendiliğinden olmuştu. Ağlamak ya da gülmekle, mutluluk ya da hüzünle ilgili değildi.

O an orada onun kucağındaydım, çıplak, sıcak, ürkek ama aslında aynı anda çok uzaklardaydım. Neredeyse bütün dünyayı yukarıdan görebileceğim kadar uzakta...

Titrerken renkler görmüştüm, hiç görmediğim güzellikte, parlaklıkta, birbirine karışmış, kendiliğinden desenler oluşturmuş renkler... Keşke bunları birine anlatabilsem, keşke ona anlatabilsem ve o da çizebilse diye düşünmüştüm.

Mutluluğun resmi işte böyleydi.

Anlamsız ama eşsiz.

İnsanın hayat boyu içinde kalmak isteyeceği bir an'dı.

O benim yazımdı.
Her iki anlamda da...

Evet ben onun yüzüne, gülüşüne, konuşmasına, sesine, bakışlarına, yakın gözlüğünü takıp çıkartmasına, sigarayı tutuşuna, içkisini yudumlamasına, kokusuna, saçlarını eliyle karıştırmasına, suratını astığı, dalıp gittiği anlara aşık olmuştum.

Heyecanla yeni yaptığı resmi anlatmasına, gözlerinin dolduğu dokunaklı anılara, bazen iki çocuk gibi bazen iki koca insan gibi konuşmalarımıza...

Küçücük bir salonda o güne kadar görmediğim filmler izlemeye giderdik. Sonra o film üstüne saatlerce konuşurduk. Çoğu zaman anlamadığım şeyler anlatırdı, bilmediğim kavramlar, tanımlamalar... Bazen sorardım, bazen utanırdım.

Ben ondan sıkılmamaya da aşık olmuştum.

Beni okşamasına, yüzümü iki eliyle tutup gözlerime bakıp susmasına, kucağında kendimi kaybetmeye, onunla buluşmaya giderken titremeye, onu düşündüğüm zamanlar olur olmaz gülümseyişime, onun için ne giyeceğimi düşünmeye, günlük konuşmaların içinde gizlice kendimi herkesten farklı hissetmeye de aşık olmuştum.

Ama aslında bütün bunların dışında, onun yaptıklarına, dışarıdan görmenin, anlatmanın mümkün olmadığı içinde gizlenmiş Ferhat'a aşıktım.

Onu tanıdıkça sanki karmaşık bir yapbozun parçalarını biraraya getirip yeni yeni resimler ortaya çıkartır gibi şaşırıyordum.

O aslında kocaman bir adamdı. Benden çok büyüktü. Ama bana öyle geliyordu ki hala küçük bir çocuktu.

Sanki o bu dünyaya yanlışlıkla gelmiş, kimsenin formülünü bilmediği incecik camdan yapılmış bir canlının tek örneğiydi ve bu yüzden onu tüm kötülüklerden korumak istiyordum.

Bu gerçek mi yoksa benim kurduğum, inandığım bir hayal mi diye düşünmekten kendimi alamıyordum.

Ve açık söylemem gerekirse çok da umurumda değildi.

Duygularla gerçeklerin birbirini tutmadığını söylerler.

Duygular gerçek midir diye çok düşündüm. Evet gerçek olduğunu biliyorum. Çünkü içimde hissettiğim böylesine güçlü birşeyin gerçek olmaması imkansız.

Ama o tümüylc bana ait olan gerçek.

Hayatın gerçeğiyle ilgisi yok.

Bir akşam yemek yiyorduk. O yine anlatıyordu ama dinlemiyordum. Onu o kadar çok öpmek istiyordum ki ne dediği umurumda bile değildi.

"Ellerimi yıkayıp geleceğim," dedim ve kalkıp gittim.

Girdim, ellerimi yıkadım. Biraz sonra kapı açıldı ve içeri girdi. Kabinlerden birine beni soktu ve öpüşmeye başladık. Sonra içeri bir kadın girdi. Bekledik. Bana eliyle sus işareti yaptı. Sonra ben çıktım. Gelip masaya oturdum. Biraz sonra yanıma geldi. Kaldığımız yerden konuşmaya devam ettik.

Kimsenin bilmediği bir dünyada gizemli bir mutluluk...

Küçük, benzersiz anlar...

O kadar güzeldi ki...

Olup bitenleri kimseye söylememeye karar vermiştim. Tolga'ya bile...

İlk kez herkesten birşey saklıyordum aslında.

O bana böyle birşey söylememişti. Bunu hiç konuşmamıştık.

Evet itiraf edeyim ki herkese anlatmak istiyordum. Ama yapmadım.

Bu benim gizli hayatımdı, gizli bahçemdi ve oraya başkalarının girmesini, bir budalanın bile düşünebileceği şeyleri söyleyip kafamı karıştırmasını, bu büyüyü bozmasını istemiyordum.

O kadar iyi biliyordum ki neler söyleyeceklerini...

Hayır, dinlemek istemiyordum.

Eğer onu ilk gördüğüm gün hissettiğim doğru çıktıysa herhalde bunda bir sihir vardı.

Ben o sihri kimsenin bozmasına izin vermeyecektim.

Galiba o yaz yalan söylemeyi öğrendim.

Annem, bütün bu giyinip kuşanıp ortadan kaybolmalarımı, mezuniyet gecesinden beri beni arayıp duran Murat'a bağlıyordu. Evet aslında dansetmiştik ve kulağıma beni çok beğendiğini, görüşmek istediğini söylemişti.

Hoşuma gitmedi desem yalan olur çünkü okulda bütün kızların bayıldığı, yüzme şampiyonu, yakışıklı, zengin, okula babasının son model arabasıyla gelen, öğretmenlerin gözdesi...

Tolga işleri bozmasa ve gecenin bir saati Ferhat çıkıp gelmese ne olurdu açıkçası emin değilim.

Bir de tabii dans ederken babasının mezuniyet için hediye ettiği saatin ne kadar pahalı olduğunu iki saat anlatmasa...

Ama ne olmuşsa olmuş, çocuk o geceden beri sürekli aramaya başlamıştı.

Ne garip, bunca yıl aynı okulda yüzüme bakmayan oğlan, o gece gözlükler çıkınca, kendi çizdiğim giysiyle, biraz makyajla birdenbire beni farketmişti... Küçük budala...

O akşam Ferhat'ın yanından eve döndüğümde tümüyle başka biriydim.

Ama kimse bunu bilmiyordu.

Yemekten sonra odama çıktım, o günü düşündüm, benim bir sırrım vardı, beni mutlu eden, bana istemediklerimi unutturan bir sır.

Ama kuşkuluydum. O ne düşünüyordu, ne hissediyordu, bilmiyordum.

Bütün akşam annemlerle otururken aklımda o vardı ama çaktırmadım.

Üstümü başımı çıkardım, aynada kendime baktım, değişiklik var mıydı, bence vardı...

Bu bir ilk ve son muydu?

Belki de artık beni hiç aramayacaktı.

Zaten hiç aramamıştı ki...

Omuz silktim kendi kendime. Aramazsa aramasın. Ben ne istiyorsam onu yaptım. Bundan sonra ne olacaksa olur...

Ceketimi asarken cebinden küçük, katlanmış bir kağıt parçası düştü.

"Yarın bir arkadaşım adaya davet etti, benimle gelir misin?"

Elimde olmadan gülümsedim.

Bu ilkti ama son değildi öyleyse...

Gider miyim?

Giderim...

Doğrusu yeniden görüşüp görüşmeyeceğimizi, tümüyle ortadan kaybolup kaybolmayacağını bilmiyordum.

Çünkü evden çıkmadan önce kahvelerimizi içerken yine her zamanki gibi konuşmuştuk. Hatta beni uğurlarken yine yanaklarımdan öpmüştü.

Ve eğer aramazsa, bugünün hayatımda özel bir gün olarak kalacağına, bundan asla pişman olmayacağıma ama o zaman onu asla aramayacağıma kendi kendime söz vermiştim.

Tabii ki içimden bir ses ondan birşey geleceğini söylüyordu.

Ve geldi de...

O yüzden yatağın üstünde yarı çıplak oturmuş elimde küçük kağıt parçası, onun kargacık burgacık yazısı, kendi kendime gülümsüyordum.

Bunun nereye varacağını bilmiyorum.

Bildiğim nereye çağırsa gideceğim...

Ama ona bunu söylemeyeceğim...

Korktuğunu biliyorum çünkü.

Evet, faytona binmek istiyorum, hem de arabacının yanına oturup çıngırağı çalmak...

Vapurun saati ve iskelenin adı vardı notun altında...

Kuşlara simit atıyorum.

Vapurun güvertesinde rüzgar saçlarımı savururken...

Bugün onunla dışarıda ilk günümüz.

Martılar bizi izliyor. Deniz durgun ama rüzgar esiyor.

Biraz ürperiyorum, bana yine ceketini veriyor.

İskeleye iniyoruz. Kimseler yok.

Faytonun yanında küçük tay bizimle yürüyor. Tepeye çıkıyoruz. Faytoncu çıngırağı çalıp duruyor.

Beyaz kocaman köşkün önünde duruyoruz.

Siyah büyük bir köpekle, saçlarını kalemle toplamış sarışın bir kadın kapıyı açıyor.

Büyük dağınık bahçedeki sofraya oturuyoruz.

Köpek beni kokluyor. "Meraklanma ısırmaz, cüssesine bakma," diyor kadın...

Sakallı, şişman bir adam geliyor. Onu tanıyorum. Ünlü bir oyuncu... Ferhat'la kucaklaşıyorlar. Bana ondan sözetmemişti...

Yan gözle beni süzdüklerini hissediyorum. Benden haberleri olmadığı belli. Buraya başka kadınlarla da geldi mi? Gelmiştir.

Ben de onlardan biri olmalıyım. Belki de onun için böyle bakıyorlar. Fazla mı küçüğüm onlar için?

Elimi ayağımı nereye koyacağımı bilemiyorum.

Sarışın kadın huzursuzluğumu anlamış gibi benimle konuşuyor, ne kadar eski arkadaş olduklarını anlatıyor.

Yeni sahneleyeceği oyundan sözediyor adam. Kadın rollerini erkeklerin, erkek rollerini kadınların oynayacağı bir oyun.

Bir rulo kağıt getiriyor. Üzerinde çizimler var. "Dekor için bana akıl vermen lazım," diyor Ferhat'a, "kendimce çiziktirdim ama istediğim gibi olmadı..."

Önümdeki peynirlerle oyalanıyorum onları dinlerken...

Sonra birden, "Biliyor musun," diyor Ferhat, "Ebru çok güzel kostümler çiziyor, bu yıl Londra'ya tasarım eğitimi görmeye gidecek..."

Kızarıyorum.

Adam piposunu yakıyor. O an'a kadar benimle hiç konuşmadı. Göz göze bile gelmedi.

"Öyle mi?" diyor bana dönüp, "tiyatroyu sever misiniz?"

"Evet," diyorum, "severim..."

"Peki piyes okur musunuz?"

Bütün ünlü oyuncular gibi etkileyici ama sahte bir sesi var.

Herkes bana bakıyor. Çayımdan bir yudum alacaktım, vazgeçiyorum, bardağı tabağa bırakıyorum.

"Aslında," diyorum, "piyes okumayı daha çok severim."

Piposunu çakmakla yeniden ateşliyor.

"Öyle mi? Niye?"

"Çünkü o zaman sahneyi, giysileri, dekoru, karakterleri gözümde istediğim gibi canlandırabiliyorum..."

Elindeki aletle tütünü bastırıyor..

"İşte bu hoşuma gitti, o zaman belki bizim oyunun kostümlerini de gözünüzde canlandırabilirsiniz...."

Ben aslında sarışın kadınla konuşurken onları dinliyordum.

Bunu yalnızca nezaketen söylediğine emindim. O çok ünlü bir oyuncu ve yönetmen. Ama yine de dayanamadım.

"Buna cesaret edebilir miyim bilmem," dedim, "ama erkeklerin kadın, kadınların erkek rolü oynayacağı bir oyunun kostümlerini çizmek gerçekten de çok güzel olurdu..." durdum, kızardım, "Keşke yapabilseydim..."

Ferhat bana baktı. Gülümsedi.

"Neden olmasın," dedi, "en azından denemelisin..."

"Ama," dedim, "ben hiç böyle birşey yapmadım, nasıl olacağını da bilmiyorum..."

Adam piposunu tablaya bıraktı, gülerek, "Aslına bakarsanız, ben de ilk kez yapıyorum ve nasıl olacağını bilmiyorum..." dedi.

Şaşkın şaşkın baktım. Bu gerçek miydi?

Adam masadan kalktı, içeri gitti ve elinde şarapla geri döndü.

"Öyleyse," dedi, "kutlamalar için asla erken sayılmaz, değil mi Hümeyra Hanım..."

Kadın gidip içerden kadehleri getirdi.

"O zaman yeni kostüm tasarımcımıza kadeh kaldıralım..."

Akşamüstü yürüyüşe çıktığımızda artık ben de onlarla aynı yaştaydım. Geldiğimden beri yanımdan ayrılmayan Papi'yle beraber adanın en tepesinden aşağıya bakıyorduk.

Ben buraya Ferhat'la bir gün geçirmek için gelmiştim. Faytona binmek, elele gezmek, eski filmlerdeki gibi ağaçların arasında koşturmak için...

Komik mi?

Ama öyleydi.

Şimdiyse bambaşka bir yerde bulmuştum kendimi…

Bütün günü yeni sahnelenecek oyunla ilgili konuşurken…

Ve o oyunun giysilerini ben tasarlayacaktım.

İskeleye geldik. Yaşlı adam niyet çekiyordu. Küçük tavşanın gösterdiği kağıt parçasını alıp bize verdi. "Bir hazine var seni bekleyen/ uzaktan sana seslenen/ aç kulağını dinle/ içindeki sesi izle…"

"Aa ne güzelmiş," dedim.

"Unutma sakın bunu," dedi niyetçi.

"Unutmam," dedim.

Vapur karanlıkta geri dönerken başımı omuzuna koydum.

"Ne o?" dedi, "yoruldun mu? Yoksa hazineyi mi düşünüyorsun?"

Hayır, yorulmadım. Sana bütün bunlar gerçek mi diye sormak istiyorum ama sormayacağım.

Çünkü gerçek olmamasından çok korkuyorum.

Ve kimbilir belki de hazineyi bulmaktan çok onu aramak güzeldir…

Bu aslında beklenmedik birşey oldu. Çünkü bu sayede Ferhat'la rahatlıkla görüşebilecektim. O, oyunun dekorlarını yaparken ben de kostümlerini tasarlayacaktım.

Anneanneme, rastlantı eseri ünlü oyuncu ve karısıyla tanıştığımı, onların bana böyle bir teklif yaptığını, Ferhat'ın da işin içinde olduğunu söyledim.

"Selçuk Bey sana böyle bir teklifte mi bulundu? Bak şimdi gözüme iyice girdi, her zaman gençlerle çalışmak lazım derim..."

Sare Hanım buna sandığımdan çok sevindi. Onları eve de çağırdı ama adada oturdukları için fırsat bulup gelemediler.

Derken provalar başladı. Oyun, birbirini tanımayan iki çiftle ilgiliydi. Kayağa gittikleri küçük dağ kasabasındaki otelin barında karşılaşıyorlar. Geldikleri kentten, çocukluklarından, ortak tanıdıklardan sözederlerken sohbet derinleşiyor. İlişkiler, aldatma, evlilik üzerine zaman zaman tartışmanın şiddetlendiği, zaman zaman sırların ortaya saçıldığı bir konuşmaya dönüşüyor. Birlikte geçen uzun yılların içinde unutulmuş anılar, gizlenmiş kırgınlıklar, sırlar ortaya çıkıyor.

Oyundaki erkekler kadın giysileri giyiyor, kadınlarsa erkek...

Oyunu okuyup işin içine girince biraz paniğe kapıldım. Neyse ki Selçuk Bey'in kafasında herşey yerli yerindeydi. Benim işim aslında yepyeni kostümler çizmek değil de, oyunculara ne giydireceğimi bulmaktı.

Eh bunun için Tolga'dan iyi yardımcı olur mu? Gezmediğimiz yer kalmadı tabii... Tiyatronun deposundan Sare Hanım'ın gardırobuna kadar her yeri talan ettik.

Galiba birini tanımanın en iyi yollarından biri onunla çalışmakmış.

Kafamdakileri kağıtlara aktarıp, örnekler getirip heyecanla anlatırken Ferhat beni dinliyor, bu olmaz, o olmaz demiyor, ama saatler sonra bakıyordum ki ilk anlattıklarımla son geldiğimiz yer arasında dağlar kadar fark var.

Ama sanki o bunları söylememiş de hepsini ben bulmuşum gibi hissediyordum.

"Acaba" diyordu örneğin, "bu iki renk biraz fazla mı olur? Tabii özellikle seçmediysen..."

Birisi benimle konuşmasını görse, yıllardır bu işi yaptığıma inanabilirdi.

O kadar rahat ve sakindi ki, bütün gerginliğim on dakikada gidiveriyordu.

Bazen saatlerce orada oturup kitap karıştırıyordum.

"Bak ne buldum dün akşam, belki ilgini çeker," diye bir kitap getiriyordu.

Bazen kahvesini içerken başımı çeviriyordum ki öylece dalmış bana bakıyor.

Ama tabii ki her gidişimde ona söyleyeceklerimi filan unutuyor ve onu görür görmez üstüne atlıyordum.

Birdenbire bütün o yabancılık, ürkeklik, çekingenlik uçup gitmişti.

Sonra gün geldi ve şaşkınlıkla farkettim.

Eve dönmüştüm, yatağın üzerinde dergi karıştırıyordum. Dergide okuduğum yazıya güldüm ve dönüp sanki oradaymış gibi ona anlatmak istedim.

Bu kadar kısa sürede nasıl olduysa ona alışmıştım.

Konuşmasına, gülmesine, saçlarımı okşamasına, bana sarılmasına, öpmesine, yanımda öylece oturmasına, dalıp gitmesine, eliyle saçlarını geri atışına, uzun, ince, güzel parmaklarına...

Sanki yıllardır tanırmış gibi...

Oysa daha yeni başlamıştı. Hatta başlayan neydi ondan bile emin değildim ama o gece ilk kez "peki sonra ne olacak?" diye düşündüm, korktum.

Bunu bu kadar erken düşündüğüm için korktum.

Çünkü bazen biri sıradan bir rastlantıyla hayatınıza girer ama hayatınızdan çıktığı zaman geriye kalanın ne olacağını bilemezsiniz.

Yok canım bunu şimdi uyduruyorum. Yoksa o sıralar bunlar aklımın ucundan bile geçmiyordu.

Küçük kasabada duruyor tren. Çay söylüyorum kendime. Keşke tüm bunları yazabilseydim. Anlatılamayacak ayrıntıları, unutulmaz saatleri, rüyayla gerçeğin arasındaki gelgitlerimi…

Ama en çok da ne hissettiğimi… Galiba asıl imkansız olan bu…

Yalnızca birkaç durak kaldı.

Düşünmeyi unutmuşum. Belki de üzüleceğim için hep yaptığım gibi bütün bunları hatırlamayı bırakmışım.

Şimdi böyle hepsini yeniden hatırlamak, belki de gerçek kimliğimi bulmak için çok az zamanım var…

İnsan hayatında sevmediği, istemediği ayrıntıları gizleyerek, unutarak, belleğin tavanarasına tıkıştırarak mutlu olabilir mi?

Başkalarını belki ama bir hayat boyu kendini kandırabilir mi?

Ben öyle olacağını sanıyordum.

Şimdi böyle bir anda, bu dönüm noktasında ansızın bütün bu karşılaşmalar, yüzleşmeler yalnızca rastlantı olabilir mi?

Bu bir başlangıç mı? Yoksa son mu?

Çayımı içerken, evi, annemi, anneannemi ne çok özlediğimi anlıyorum. Bizim çaylara hiç benzemiyor.

Karşımda oturan adamın sorularına kısa cevaplar veriyorum. Benim yaşlarımda bir kızı olduğunu, evlenip uzak bir kente yerleştiğini, torunlarını görmek için bunca yolu geldiğini anlatıyor. Bütün hayatını birlikte geçirdiği eşini geçen yıl kaybetmiş. Onu, belki de yıllarca çalışıp edindiği, küçük, bahçeli evinde tek başına yemeğini hazırlarken, yerken, televizyon izlerken düşünüyorum. Yeni bir hayat kurması için çok mu geç?

"Karımın da senin gibi yeşil gözleri vardı ve sabahları ona bakınca işe gitmek bana hiç ağır gelmezdi..." diyor.

Neden mutluluk anları hep hüzünle gölgeleniyor?

Yaz sabahı parlayan güneşle kendimi denize atmak isterken birdenbire bulutun ışıkları kapatması gibi...

O anlatırken beni burada sanıyor ama değilim. Ben şu anda çok uzakta, bambaşka bir yerdeyim ve orada olmaktan mutluyum.

O yaza dönmek ve hep orada kalmak istiyorum.

Ferhat bir resim çizmişti. Cennet gibi bir yerde sayısız insan denize giriyor, çocuklar rengarenk deniz toplarıyla oynuyor, tam keşmeşkeş ama yukarıda kara bir bulut bütün ışığı değiştirmiş, herkesin mutlu olduğu an, kasvetli bir havaya bürünmüş.

Bana resmi gösterdiği zaman elimle bulutu kenara çekmek istediğimi söyledim.

Eline fırçayı alıp bulutu kenara çekti.

Sonra baktı ve güldü.

"Galiba bu benim en neşeli resmim oldu," dedi.

Yalnızca resimde değil gerçekte de o bulutu kenara çektiğini biliyor muydu benim için?

Ne tuhaf, onunla hiç ikimiz hakkında konuşmadık. Ne yaptığımızı, bunun nasıl bir ilişki olduğunu, nereye varacağını...

Bunları hiç konuşmadık. Herşey nasıl kendiliğinden olduysa öylece sürüp gidiyordu. Sanki incecik bir ipin üstünde yürür gibi... O da benim gibi her an düşünüyor muydu? Yanında olmadığım zamanlarda beni özlüyor muydu? Gözlerime baktığı zamanlar duyduklarımı her zaman hissediyor muydu?

Sormazdım.

Zaman geçiyordu ve belki hayatta en çok istediğim şey gerçekleşecekken, ben zamanı durdurmak, ertelemek, burada daha fazla kalmak istiyordum.

O zamana kadar hiç birşeye, hiç kimseye bağlandığımı hissetmediğim için başıma gelenin ne olduğunu anlamıyordum.

Bir arkadaşımın sevgilisi bir akşam ortadan kaybolmuştu. Kız onu her yerde aramış ama bulamamıştı. Ertesi gün çocuk ortaya çıktığında kıyametleri kopartmıştı. Tek düşündüğü oğlanın onu aldattığıydı.

Başına birşey gelmiş olabileceğini düşünmemişti bile.

Ferhat ortadan kaybolduğunda ben korkardım. Ona birşey olmasından, başına bir kötülük gelmesinden...

Hakkında söylenenler umurumda bile değildi.

Ve ona çok fazla şey söylemezdim. Çünkü o da benim gözlerime bakarken, beni öperken, ona yapışmışken ne hissettiğimi anlamıyorsa sözcükler daha fazlasını anlatamaz...

Benim şimdi gizli bir hayatım vardı. En yakın arkadaşlarımın bile bilmediği...

Tabii farkındaydım. Bu benim hayatımın en güzel zamanıydı ama o kimbilir kaç kadınla benzer şeyler yaşamıştı.

Bazen onun tümüyle bana ait olduğunu düşünürdüm bazen de bütün bunların yalnızca benim hayalim olduğunu.

Bir resmi vardı. Öyle bir boyayla boyamıştı ki zaman içinde resim yokolup gidecek belki yalnızca desenlerin izi kalacaktı.

Belki bizimki de böyleydi.

Uçup gidecek ve yalnızca izleri kalacak...

Onunla sevişmek...

Mutluluktu...

Beni oradan, şimdiye kadar yaşadığım yerden, bütün bağlılıklardan, yerçekiminden bile koparıp alan, uçan halının üstünde gidermiş gibi bambaşka ülkelere götüren birşeydi.

Öyle güzeldi ki manzara... Kimsenin ulaşamayacağı kadar yukarıdan herşey ne kadar da küçük, önemsiz görünüyordu.

Heyecandı...

Belki de hayatımda duymadığım kadar büyük bir heyecan. Daha evden ona gitmek üzere çıkarken ya da aynanın karşısında hazırlanırken boğluyan o çarpıntı.

Korkuydu…
Dünyanın en güzel sevişmelerinin adı neden korku olsun ki?
Kaybedecek olmaktan mı?
Bunun bir gün biteceği korkusu mu?
Başkasıyla asla böyle olmayacağını düşünmenin korkusu mu?
Onun benim gibi hissetmediğini düşünmenin korkusu mu?
Belki de hepsi.

Huzurdu…
Ait olduğun, kimsenin sana dokunamayacağı, güvenli bir yatakta uyumak gibi… Bütün büyüklerin yanlarında olduğu bahçede, yaz akşamüstü öylesine dolaşan dertsiz çocuklar gibi…

Gizemdi…
Çünkü bilmediğim kapılardan geçerken sonra neler olacağını bilmiyordum. Bu biriyle değil de sanki orada olmayan birşeyle, tanımlanmaz, elle tutulmaz, görülmez bir varlıkla sevişmek gibiydi.

Oyundu…
Tümüyle yetişkinlere ait gibi görünse de, belki başka kimselere söylenmeyecek sözcükler içerse de, herkesten gizlediklerimizi ortaya döküversek de aslında çocukça, oyunsu bir yanı vardı bütün bu hareketlerin. Ve o kapılar açıldıkça merakla sonrakine ulaşmak için gitmekten kendimi alamıyordum.

Bağlılıktı…
Belki bazı erkekler içinize yalnızca girip çıkar. Bazense orada sonsuza dek kalır.
Ben o hep içimde kalsın istiyordum.

Yalnızlıktı...

Bütün o coşku anları, yükseliş, kopuş, çığlıklar, kendinden geçmeler, baş dönmesi, titremeler, kasılmalar bittiğinde gelen yalnızlık.

Özgürlüktü...

Belki yalnızca kendi hayatım boyunca değil, geçmişten, binlerce yıl ötesinden gelen kalıpların, yargıların, utancın, cezalandırılma korkusunun uçup gittiği anlardı çünkü. Kendinle tümüyle çıplak kaldığın ve beğensen de beğenmesen de kim olduğunu gördüğün bir aynaydı.

Oyunun ilk sahnelendiği gece kalbim yerinden fırlayacak gibiydi.

Son provayı izlediğim halde sanki ilk kez görüyormuş gibi nefesimi tutarak izledim oyunu.

Işıklar yandı ve alkış koptu.

Oyuncular tek tek ve birlikte gelip selam verdiler.

Sonra ismimi duydum. Ferhat elimden tutup kaldırmasa ne olduğunu anlamayacaktım.

Bizi de çağırıyorlardı sahneye...

Hayatımda ilk ve herhalde son kez sahnede alkışların arasında çiçek aldım.

Hem de yanımda Ferhat'la...

Oyuncularla birlikte selam verirken seyirci ayakta alkışlıyordu.

Elini sımsıkı tutuyordum.

Annem, anneannem, Yıldız Teyze, Saniye, tam karşımda en önde...

Niye ağladığımı bilmiyorum.

Ama onlar da ağlıyordu.

Eve elimde rengarenk çiçeklerle döndüm.

Neredeyse herkes bizimle gelmişti.

Tabii ki kutlama anneannemde yapılacaktı.

Ferhat'a bakıyordum ve gidip ona sarılıp öpmek istiyordum.

Bunu o kadar çok istiyordum ki anlatamam.

Ama yapamadım. Annem, anneannem, Tolga herkes oradaydı.

Sakallı, gözlüklü bir adam gitar çalıp şarkı söylüyordu.

Yıllar sonra ünlü olacak bir şarkı. Kimsenin bilmediği bir şarkı.

Ben hala büyünün içindeydim.

"Ne güzelmiş, adı ne bu şarkının?" diye sordu biri...

Kimse bilmiyordu.

Yalnız ikimiz biliyorduk.

Bütün o konuşmaların, bütün o bakışların içinde kimse farketmeden gözgöze geldiğimizde ne olduğunu biliyorduk.

İlk kez herkesin içinde sabaha kadar birlikteydik.

Birlikte birşey yapmıştık. Elele sahneye çıkıp selam vermiştik. Birlikte alkışlanmıştık.

Hayatın içinde, beklenmedik bir anda sizi mutlu eden ve hiç unutulmayacak o yaz esintilerinden biriydi.

O esintiyle içimden birşey uçuyormuş gibi geldi bana o gece.

Tam da o eski filmlerdeki dış sesin söylediği gibi "günler günleri kovaladı..."

Bütün yerlere yaz bir gün gibi geçip gitti gerçekten de...

Hiç bilmediğim yerlere, geleceğe doğru yola çıkıyordum ama aynı zamanda içimde bir burukluk vardı.

Onunla ilgili düşündüklerimi ona hiç söylemedim. Aklıma eseni anlatırken yüzüne bakışımı kim görse anlamaz mıydı?

Ama ben yine de belli etmemek için elimden geleni yapmıştım.

O son buluşmamızda, yola çıkmadan önce birdenbire neredeyse herşeyi anlatacaktım ama yapmadım.

Bunun bir yaz aşkı olmadığını biliyordum. Ama onun ne düşündüğünü bilmiyordum. Çünkü o da söylemezdi. Sanki ne varsa böyle kendiliğinden olmuş, kendiliğinden bu yola girmiş, anlatmaya, konuşmaya gerek kalmamış gibiydi.

Zaten bilmezdim ki bunları. Ne yapmak gerekir, ne söylemek gerekir, nasıl davranmak gerekir...

Yalnızca içimden geldiği gibi davranmıştım.

Belki de çok hızlı olmuştu. Araya zaman ve uzaklık girince tüm bunlar değişecekti belki.

O gün daha çok orada neler yapacağımdan, yeni hayatımdan sözettik. Ben aslında fazla konuşmadım. Daha çok ona bakıyordum. Sanki bu anları belleğime yerleştirmek ister gibi.

Her nedense o gün bütün terslikler üstüste gelmiş, iki ayağımız her zaman olduğu gibi son gün bir pabuca girmiş ve yalnızca kısa süre görüşebilmiştik.

Eve geldiğimde herkes nereye kaybolduğumu soruyordu.

Ne garip, oysa gitmeden önce onunla bu son görüşmeyi çok farklı düşünmüştüm.

O da birşey söylemiyordu. Belki bu gizli kalmış aşk hikayesi, yıllar sonra hatırlayınca gülümseyeceği bir anı olarak kalacaktı.

Kimbilir belki o da benim gibi konuşmaya başlarsak bunun bir vedaya dönüşebileceğinden korkuyordu. Oysa şimdi herşey olduğu gibi kalmış olacaktı. Herhangi bir söz vermeden. Bir karar vermeden. Gelecek için plan yapmadan.

Ve biz bir gün, kısa süre sonra, ("Zaten konuşuruz, hem sen tatilde gelirsin," diyordu) kaldığımız yerden yeniden başlayabilirdik.

İçimdeki ses belki de böyle olmayacağını, gider gitmez beni unutacağını, kısa süre içinde başkasını bulacağını söylüyor ama ben o sesi o an hiç duymak istemiyordum.

Zaten o aptal filmlerde günler günleri kovalayınca ondan sonra hiç de iyi şeyler olmazdı.

Kapıdan çıkarken sarılıp öptü ve bana küçük, kadife bir kese verdi.

"Bunu yanından ayırma, seni koruyacak küçük bir tılsım..."

O minicik çok eski bir heykelcikti. Yeşim taşından çok güzel küçücük bir kedi. Gözlerinde iki parlak taş vardı.

"Demek bu benim küçük muhafızım..." dedim gülerek.

"Evet, zamanında bir prensesi korumuş, seni de koruyacak..."

"Peki," dedim, "onu yanımdan ayırmayacağım..." Tam giderken döndüm, "eğer onu ovalarsam, çıkıp gelir misin yanıma?"

"Eğer çok istersen, gelirim," dedi.

Taksiye bindim. Kediciği okşadım, gülümsedim.

Hayır ağlamayacağım.

Bazı şeyleri ille de söylemek gerekmez.

Biliyorum ben.

Sabahın erken saatinde evden çıkışımız bile tam hengameydi. Neredeyse üç gündür bavul yapmakla uğraşan annem yine de son anda ne unuttum acaba diye söylenip dolaştıkça anneannem de sinirleniyordu.

Tolga gelip bizi aldı, tabii ki hepimiz ağlıyorduk, Saniye arkamızdan su dökmeyi unutmadı.

Tolga'nın annesiyle babası havaalanına geldi.

Birşeyleri geride bırakmak nedense beni hep korkutur. O yüzden tatile gitmeyi, uzak yerleri sevmem.

Tolga yerinde duramıyordu ama ben uçağın penceresinden aşağıda giderek küçülen evlere bakarken ağlamak istiyordum.

Annem de bizimle geldi.

Kimse bunu söylemiyordu ama ben onun neden geldiğini, aslında neden korktuğunu biliyordum.

Uzun süredir daha doğrusu yaz boyunca hastalığım nüksetmemişti. Yine birkaç kez gece ter içinde uyanmıştım. Yine ayaklarım, başım, ellerim ağrıyordu ama ben bunlara artık alışmıştım. Ve kulağımda hiç bitmeyen o derin uğultu...

Güneşli bir İstanbul gününden karanlık Londra akşamüstüne geldik.

Daha yaz yeni bitiyordu ama hava karanlık ve yağmurluydu.

Eve girerken güldüm. İngilizce kitaplarımızdaki merdivenle çıkılan, küçük, iki katlı, kırmızı tuğladan yapılmış eski evlerden biriydi.

Sanki Mrs. Brown kapıyı açıp bize merhaba diyecek gibiydi.

Biraz daha küçük olsak tavanarasında kimbilir ne oyunlar kurardık.

Eşyalarımızı yerleştirip dolaşmaya çıktık.

Ev eski ve küçüktü ama hem okula hem de merkeze çok yakındı.

Şimdi birdenbire bambaşka bir dünyadaydım.

İlk kez başka bir ülkede, yağmurun ışıkları bozduğu bu akşamda, kentin kalabalığında, içimde ayrılık, hüzün, mutluluk, yeniden başlamanın heyecanı, karmakarışık duygular içinde yürüyordum.

Meydandaki atlıkarınca koca kente çocuksu bir görünüm veriyordu.

Çok uzun zaman sonra ilk kez annemi de heyecanlı gördüm. Sanki o çocukluk yıllarımdaki hali birden geri gelmiş gibiydi.

Yemek boyunca ertesi gün neler yapılması gerektiğini, neler alınacağını anlatıp durdu.

Elindeki küçük fotoğraf makinesiyle habire fotoğraf çekiyor, bize de poz verdiriyordu.

Tolga, babasının tüm söylenmelerine karşın edebiyat sosyolojisi diye ne olduğunu bilmediğimiz bir bölüme kaydını yaptırmıştı.

"Hem içinde edebiyat var hem de havalı, tam benlik," diye gülüyordu.

Tabii ki babası onun işletme, ekonomi gibi bir bölüm okuyup geri döndüğünde işlerin başına geçmesini istiyordu ama Tolga'nın bunu yapmayacağını hepimiz bilyorduk.

Daha birkaç yıl önce, bana, "Babamın bütün hesaplarını, yatırımlarını buldum, eğer o ölünce bütün işleri batırsam bile hayatımın sonuna kadar bir elim yağda bir elim balda yaşayabilirim..." demişti.

"Seni evlatlıktan reddederse görürsün," diye dalga geçtim.

"O ancak filmlerde oluyor, Hulusi Kentmen Tarık Akan'ı evlatlıktan reddediyor ama onu da öğrendim bizde öyle bir yasa yokmuş..."

Tabii o sırada buna gülüp geçmiştim. İnsan lise yıllarında böyle planlar yapar da hayat bunlara pek izin vermez. Bir anda kendini bambaşka bir yerde buluverirsin. Ama Tolga'nın fikri pek değişmiş gibi değildi. Asıl derdi burada özgür olmak, yazılarını yazmak, müzelere, sergilere, konserlere gitmekti.

Aklım İstanbul'da, Ferhat'ta olsa da bu yabancı kentin sokaklarında yürürken keyfim yerine gelmişti. Çocukken ikimize ait evimiz olsa, keşke kardeş olsak ve aynı evde otursak diye konuşurduk. Belki artık çocuk değildik ama hayalimiz gerçekleşmişti işte.

Yeni insanlar tanıyacaktık, yeni yerler keşfedecektik, belki kendimizle ilgili bilmediğimiz şeyler öğrenecektik...

Tolga'nın daha önce kitaplardan gösterdiği görkemli eski yapıların, sarayın, müzelerin, heykellerin arasından yürürken yeni hayatın ilk gününe adım attığımı biliyordum.

İçimde tuhaf bir duygu vardı.

Tolga'ya sarıldım yolun ortasında.

"Evet," dedim, "işte yaptık... Buradayız..."

Annem şaşkın şaşkın biz birbirimize sarılmış dönerken şemsiyeyi üstümüze tutmaya çalışıyordu.

Henüz bilmiyordum ama galiba bu kentten en çok hatırlayacağım şey yağmur olacaktı.

İnsan ne zaman geçmişi düşünür?

Geleceği düşünmek istemediği zaman mı?

An'da olmak acı verdiği zaman mı?

Belki de onun için şimdi bütün bunları yeniden sanki roman yazar gibi hatırlamaya çalışıyorum.

Korktuğumu biliyorum ama korkmamış gibi yapıyorum.

Hep böyle yaptım. Hayatım boyunca.

Ferhat'la yeni tanıştığım, evine gittiğim ilk günlerde rüyamda çok garip bir yer görmüştüm. Tümüyle biçimsiz, bildiklerimize benzemeyen bir evdi.

Birbirine tam bağlanmayan katlardan oluşan, duvarları olmayan bir ev.

Hiç tanımadığım garip bir adam oturuyordu orada. Niye orada olduğumu bilmiyorum. Bazı insanlar yemek yiyor, bazıları oyun oynuyor, ev sahibi herkese emirler yağdırıyordu. Canlı köpekler, oyuncak trenler sanki yerçekimi yokmuş gibi havada uçuyordu.

O adamdan da o evden de korkup gitmek istedim ama yapamadım. Onun üst kattaki odasını görmek istiyordum. O başkalarıyla ilgilenirken oraya girdim.

Büyük ağaçlar vardı odada. Aynı zamanda sanki akvaryumdaymışız, suyun içindeymişiz gibi ama su yoktu. Yalnızca suyu hissediyordum.

Gerçeküstü bir resmin içinde gibiydim ama gerçekti. Şaşkınlıkla eşyaların arasında dolaşırken ev sahibi zorla sürüklediği kocaman, eski bir bavulla geldi. "Ben de sizi arıyordum, bavulunuzu getirdim, bundan sonra burada kalacaksınız..." dedi ve nefes nefese çıkıp gitti.

Kapıları, duvarları olmayan bir ev. Sanki sonsuz boşluktaki uzay istasyonu gibi... Burada ne işim var, bu tanımadığım adam kim, neden burada kalmam gerekiyor diye düşünüyordum ama öte yandan da tüy gibi hafif hissediyordum kendimi. Bütün bunları düşünmek, kaygılanmak istemiyordum.

Tanıdık birşeyler, tanıdık birilerini arıyordum ama yoktu.

Burada tek başımaydım.

Bir an öldüğümü düşündüm.

Rüyamın içinde öldüğümü...

Öldüğümü ve yanımda tanıdığım kimse olmadığını...

Uyandığımda uzun süre bu rüyanın etkisinden kurtulamadım. Ama korkmamıştım. Aksine yeniden uykuya dalıp neler olacağını görmek istiyordum ama tabii ki yapamadım.

Garip olan şu ki, Londra'ya gittiğimiz o gece biraz yorgun uykuya daldığımda aynı evi yine gördüm.

Ama o rüyayı daha önce gördüğümü hatırlamadım. Yalnızca bu evi nereden tanıyorum diye düşündüm.

Tren ilerliyor. Biraz uykum var. O, kimseye, doktorlara bile anlatamadığım uyuşma başladı yine her yerimde. Başımdan ayaklarıma kadar. Kulağımı sanki incecik bir matkapla deliyorlarmış gibi ince bir sızı ve kesilmeyen ses...

Bileklerimde yine o morluklar var.

Birkaç ilacın saati geldi, onları içiyorum.

Hepsi gerçekten geçecek mi?

Buraya gelme kararını verirken çok kısa süre içinde hiç beklenmedik şeyler olacağını bilmiyordum. Onun için de kendi kendime ya hepsi geçecek ya da o garip ev gibi yerler göreceğim uzun, sonsuz bir uykuya dalacağım, diyordum.

Ama şimdi...

Yolun sonuna geliyoruz ama ben bu yolculuğun bitmesini istemiyorum.

Tıpkı o rüyanın bitmesini istemediğim gibi...

Yapamaz mıyım? Son istasyonda inip başka bir trene binip tüm bunları unutup geri dönemez miyim?

O yalnızca birkaç saat uzakta... Nereye gittiğimi bilmiyor.

Yeniden yanına dönmek, yeniden yıllar öncesine, o ilk tanıştığımız günlere dönmek istiyorum. Bir zaman hatasını geriye almak neden imkansız olsun?

Sarışın, tulum giymiş çocuk bahçeli küçük bir evin önünde bisikletine binmiş bize el sallıyor.

Kimbilir kaç kez önünden geçip giden tanımadığı hayatlara böyle el salladı, sallayacak.

Ama sonra nereye gittiğini, ne yaptığını bilmediği o insanları unutup yoksul, eski evine geri dönecek.

Küçük çocuk hızla küçülüyor, kaybolup gidiyor.

Gözümü kapıyorum ve yalnızca üzerindeki lacivert tulumu görüyorum.

Neden korkuyorum, ölümden mi?

Aslında hayattan da hep korkmadım mı?

İnsanın başına gelecek en güzel şey ne olabilir?

Belki bir hastalıktan kurtulmak…

Tabii bir süreliğine…

Bir sabah uyanamayacağınızı bilirsiniz. Ama bir sabah birdenbire yirmi yaş genç uyanacağınızı düşünemezsiniz.

Herkes günün birinde deprem olacağını, kaza geçirebileceğini, ya da aklını kaybedebileceğini bilir ve aynı zamanda mucizeler olmayacağını da…

Ama dünya tıpkı benim rüyamdaki gibi öylesine renkli ve bilinmezlerle dolu ki herkes hayatın sonu olduğunu bilmiyormuş gibi yaşıyor.

Zamanın içinden geçiyorum. Hayatların içinden.

Mutluluk ancak anlarda var diye düşünüyorum. Kısa, geçip giden zamanlarda…

Hep öyle düşündüm.

Hayat, güneşin doğuşuyla başlayıp batışıyla biten, yorucu, zor, çileli bir uğraşın sonunda toplanan kuçücük çiçeklerin kokusunu aldığında hissettiğin kadar aslında…

Hepsi bu.

Rüyamdaki o ev belki asla gerçek bir ev kuramayacağımızı anlatıyordu. O adam Ferhat'a hiç benzemese de belki o ev onun eviydi.

Onu düşünüyorum.

Olmak istediğim tek yer onun yanı şu an.

Neden söylemedim peki?
Bunca yıl sonra bütün bunlar sıradan rastlantılar olabilir mi?

Doktor, "Yanınızda kimse olacak mı?" diye sormuştu. "Hayır", dedim. Bütün belgeleri imzaladım.

Bu benim hayatım.

Benim ölümüm.

Belki de uzaklıklar aşkı daha yakına getirir.

Yeni bir hayatın içinde, tanımadığım bu kentte yabancıyken kimi zaman çok neşeli kimi zaman hüzünlü dolaşırken, olur olmaz yerlerde aklıma o gelince gözlerim dolarken kendi kendime dedim ki, bunda üzülecek ne var, pek çok insan yanında biri varken bile böyle bir çarpıntı hissetmiyor, içinde bu duygu varken o uzakta olmuş olmamış ne farkeder?

Bazı insanların gözlerinde tam olarak adlandıramadığınız birşey vardır. Farklı birşey. Sanki içinizi görüyormuş gibi bir bakış. Sanki gözlerinizin içine bakarken o an ne düşündüğünüzü hissedermiş gibi... Sizi bazen üzebilen, bazen ne olursa olsun mutlu eden, bazen kuşkuya sürükleyen... Sizinle ilgili sizin bile bilmediklerimizi bilen...

Bazen sizi kendine çeken bir erkek gibi, bazen kendi içine kapanıp uzaklara gitmiş biri gibi, bazen şaşkın, küçük bir çocuk gibi...

Ama her zaman anlamı olan bir bakış.

Bir keresinde heyecanla konuşurken birden durdu ve "Beni dinlemiyorsun değil mi, ne oldu?" diye sordu.

Evet dinlemiyordum. Daha doğrusu dinlediğimi sanıyordum ama ne söylediğinin farkında bile değildim.

Dedim ki: "Gözlerinin içine girdim ve sanki içindeki gizli geçitlerde kayboldum."

Bu kez düşünceli, ürkek baktı.

"Hayır hayır, öyle değil, orada kaybolmaktan çok memnunum..." durdum, daha alçak sesle içimden geleni söyledim: "hatta galiba orası kendimi en iyi hissettiğim yer..."

Böyle konuştuğum zaman yüzümü okşar ya da bana sarılırdı.

Şimdi düşünüyorum da bana bildik sevgi sözleri söyler miydi, iltifat eder miydi, ara sıra cesaret edip bunları söylediğimde cevap verir miydi?

Hayır, pek sanmıyorum.

Ama sanki o konuşmadan da bana herşeyi anlatırdı. Kimbilir belki de bana öyle gelirdi.

Ama ne önemi var ki?

Asıl olan birinin size söylediklerinden çok hissettirdiği değil midir?

Hem doğrusunu söylemek gerekirse, daha önce güya bana güzel sözler söylemeye çalışan hatta bunu abartan insanlar da tanımıştım ve bazen gerçekten boğazım sıkılıyormuş gibi olup nasıl kaçsam diyc düşünmüştüm.

Bazen derler ya sevgi emektir diye...

Hangi sevgi? Belki çocuk sevgisi, anne sevgisi...

Aşk emek filan değildir.

İnsan birine aşık değilse sırf size çok iyi davranıyor diye ona aşık olamazsınız. Evet belki seversiniz, o kadar.

Adamın biri beni el üstünde tutuyor diye ona kalbim çarpacak değil.

En azından benim için bu böyle.

Onun yanında hiç, aşkıma karşılık veriyor mu, benim gibi mi hissediyor, benim gibi her an görmek istiyor mu diye düşünmedim.

Yok yalan söylemeyeyim, tabii düşündüm ama bu pek umurumda olmadı.

Bunları kurup üzülmedim.

Bazen uzun zaman ortadan kaybolduğunda kaygılandım, bazen söylediklerinden, anlattıklarından kendime pay çıkartıp gitmemi mi istiyor diye üzüldüm, kimi zaman artık gitmem gerektiğini düşündüm ama bunlar hep anlık şeylerdi.

Yeniden görüştüğümüzde aklımdaki kuşkuların hepsi o an uçup giderdi.

Genç bir kızın duygularından, ona olan aşkından çok mu gururlanıyordu?

E n'olmuş? Suç muydu bu?

Hatta denilebilir ki onu ayartan bendim.

Bana söz vermiş miydi, bana yalanlar mı uydurmuştu, gitmek istemiştim de gitme diye yalvarmış mıydı? Hayır.

Onun kendine göre hayatı vardı, nasıl istiyorsa öyle yaşıyordu. Ama daha önemlisi, bazıları gibi, herkesin onun düşüncelerine, hayat biçimine uymasını, öyle davranmasını beklemiyordu.

O gözlerde ne vardı? Belki kimsenin belki kendisinin bile bilmediği birşey. Kendi gözlerini görmemişti ki zaten... Benim için böyleydi. Başka bir yerden gelmiş gibi... Uzaktan, hiç görmediğimiz yerlerden... Çok eskiden, belki hayatlarımızdan daha uzun zaman öncesinden...

Evinde olduğumuz bir gün ellerim titremeye başladığında ve anlayacak, hastalığımı farkedecek diye korku içinde bir an önce oradan gitmek istediğimde beni yatağa yüzüstü yatırdı.

Gözlerimi kapatmamı istedi.

Yanıma oturdu. Bana dokunmuyordu ama ellerini üzerimde gezdirdiğini hissediyordum. Başıma doğru geldiğinde sıcaklık arttı. Şaşırdım. Şaşırdım ama gözlerimi açıp bakamadım. Bir süre hiç kıpırdamadan öylece elleri başımın üzerinde durdu. Oradaydı elleri çünkü giderek artan sıcaklığı hissediyordum. Ama dokunmuyordu. Derin derin nefes aldı yalnızca.

Çok kısa sürdü, belki beş, belki on dakika...

Sonra durdu.

"Yavaşça kalkabilirsin," dedi.

Sanki doktorun söylediklerini dinler gibi dediğini yaptım şaşkın şaşkın.

Yatağın kenarına oturdum.

"Bu senin için çok büyük ağırlık," dedi, "en azından şimdilik ondan kurtuldun..."

Ne dediğini anlamadım.

Ayağa kalktım. Koltuğa geçip oturdum. Başım ağrımıyordu ve ellerim de titremiyordu.

Ürpererek ona baktım. Gözlerinde yine o uzaktan, derinlerden gelen bakış vardı.

Bu neydi?

"Ne yaptın?" dedim.

Birden bakışları değişti, gülümsedi, "Birşey yapmadım," dedi, "şimdi başının ağrısı geçti mi?"

Başka yerlerden gelen enerjiler, bilinmeyen boyuta geçebilen insanlar, kozmik bağlar, bilinmeyenden alınan haberler...

Hayır bunlara asla inanmadım.

Yalnız bir keresinde anneannem, "Biz hayatı çok iyi bildiğimizi sanırız ama küçük beynimiz ancak birkaç sözcükle kurabildiğimiz cümleleri anlayacak kadardır, geri kalanları asla bilemeyiz," demişti.

Başımın ağrısının aniden geçmesini anlayamadığım o gün birşey daha oldu. Köşede duran bir teknenin yanına götürdü beni. "Bak," dedi, "sana ismine uygun bir uğraş buldum.." Baktım ama anlamadım. "Bu bir ebru teknesi, bunu sana göndereceğim, annenlere kendin aldığını söylersin, şurada biraz daha büyüğü var, bir dahaki gelişinde sana nasıl yapıldığını gösteririm, çok hoşuna gideceğini ve sana çok iyi geleceğini düşünüyorum..."

Eve döndüğüm zaman başımın yeniden ağrıyacağını düşündüm ama ağrımadı. Huzurlu, gülümsediğim bir uykuya daldım.

Evet, hayatımda ilk kez beni rüyamda bile gülümseten biri vardı.

Önceleri ilk başladığımda ne yaptığımın farkında değildim. Öylesine suyun içine boyaları bırakıyor ve kendiliğinden biçim kazanmalarını sonra da bozulmalarını izliyordum.

Sonra yavaş yavaş renklerin içiçe geçip oluşturduğu ve küçük dokunuşlarınıza direndiği, sanki sizin değil de doğanın istediği biçimlerin ortaya çıkmasını, anların, saniyelerin bile yakalamaya çalıştığınız deseni birdenbire bambaşka birşeye dönüştürdüğü ya da bozup yokettiği inanılmaz bir süreçle karşılaştım.

Resim yapmak gibi değildi. Sürekli devinim, sürekli bir değişim, küçük teknenin içinde sonsuz formlar yaratmak. Ve zamanla orada canlı bir organizmanın farklı biçimlerle bana kendini gösterdiğini benimse yalnızca ona aracılık ettiğimi farkettim.

Bazen yaptıklarım, çiçeğe, göze, kuşa benziyordu bazense varolmayan, yalnızca orada o an için bana kendini gösteren sanki neşeyle göz kırpıp ortadan kaybolan canlılara...

Tıpkı hayata benziyordu. Siz hayal kuruyordunuz ve düzen oluşturmaya çalışıyordunuz ama su canlı gibi kımıldıyor, o mükemmel biçim bozuluyor, kayboluyor, yakalayamıyordunuz yeniden, belki yalnızca o an görüyordunuz ve değişiyordu.

Böylece aslında aynı resmin içinde binlerce resim görüyordunuz. Zamanla anladım ki bunu bana yalnızca ismim yüzünden vermemişti. O suyun içindeki resimlerle uğraşırken istemediğim şeyleri unutacağımı ya da aksine hatırlayacağımı ve kimi zaman gözyaşıyla, kimi zaman neşeyle o teknenin başında saatler geçireceğimi çok iyi biliyordu.

Aklımdaki deseni çalışıyordum ve az sonra bakıyordum ki bambaşka renkler çıkmış ortaya ve gerçekte akıl edemeyeceğim kadar mükemmel figürler oluşmuş.

Bazen öyle hissederim ki uzaktan bir el dokunuyor bana, o anları yeniden yaratıyor, zamanın geçişini benimle birlikte anlamlandırıyor.

Sonra onları kağıtların üzerine alıyordum ve ertesi gün yeniden baktığımda şaşırıp kalıyordum çünkü çoğunu hatırlamıyordum bile...

Bir keresinde biri bana bunun nasıl bir süreç olduğunu sordu. Tabii ona söyleyemedim ama bence Ferhat'la seviştiğimde hissettiğim şeyle aynıydı. Kaybolmak, unutmak, buradan sonsuzluğa gittiğini, belki de varolmayan birine ait olduğunu hissetmek ve yalnızca mutlu olmak.

Onun için ilk açtığım serginin adını da "Benim Gizli Rüyalarım" koymuştum.

Ama bunlar çok sonra oldu.

Bütün bunların olması için zamanın geçmesi, benim büyümem (büyüdüm mü gerçekten?) pek çok şeyi unutmak ve bazılarını yeniden ilk günkü gibi hatırlamak istemem gerekiyordu belki de...

Kokular, renkler ve desenler çocukluğumdan beri hayatımdı belki ama günün birinde tüm bunların biraraya geleceğini, benim için bambaşka bir dünya oluşturacağını o zamanlar hiç düşünmemiştim.

O küçük teknenin zamanla büyüyeceğini, desenlerin artık kağıtlara değil kumaşlara basılacağını, dünyanın dört bir yanında ipek fularlara, şallara, eşarplara, mendillere hatta elbiselere hayat vereceğini kim bilebilirdi ki?

Oldu işte.

Londra'daki okul benim bildiğim okullara benzemiyordu. Daha çok atölyede öğretmenlerin gözetiminde çalışıyorduk ve kimse bizden kendi söylediklerini yapmamızı istemiyordu. Yalnızca arada gelip düzeltmeler yapıyor ya da önerilerde bulunuyorlardı. Bazen de pek fazla konuşmadan çizdiklerinizi buruşturup atıyorlardı.

Zaman zaman ünlü modacıların, terzilerin atölyelerine gidiyor ve işlerin nasıl yürüdüğünü öğrenmeye çalışıyorduk.

Herkes şimdiden birbirine rakipmiş gibi görünüyordu ama bir yandan da birbirimizin yaptıklarını izliyor ya da aramızda tartışıyorduk.

Farklı yerlerden gelen genç insanların farklı fikirleri, farklı yetenekleri, farklı renkleri, desenleri vardı. Adeta bütün dünya orada ülkelerinin tınılarını, duygularını getiren müzisyenlerden oluşan bir orkestra gibiydik ama aynı zamanda hepimiz yalnızdık.

Temel derslerin dışında eğlenceli görünüyordu ama aynı zamanda kimse size ne yapacağınızı söylemediği için tek başınıza kalakalıyordunuz. Belki de biz böyle alışmadığımız için bu beni biraz zorluyordu.

Bulabildiğim bütün kitapları alıyor, alamazsam kütüphanede onları inceliyor, müzeleri geziyor ve her geçen gün ne kadar az şey bildiğimin ama çok bildiğimi sandığımın farkına varıyordum.

Annem tabii ki evi hemen düzene sokmuş, her gün nereden buluyorsa alıştığımız yemekleri pişiriyor, bazen gündüz gezse de akşam mutlaka bizi evde karşılıyordu.

Sonra bir akşam birdenbire artık geri dönmeye karar verdiğini söyledi.

Tolga'nın buna benden çok sevindiğine eminim. Artık kendi başımıza kalacaktık. Onun için neden böyle ani bir kararla geri döndüğünü sorgulamadım. Geldiğimizden beri hastalanmamıştım, nöbet geçirmemiştim, keyfim yerindeydi, herşey tam da düşündüğümüz gibi gidiyordu. Herhalde artık beni yalnız bırakmasının zamanı geldiğini anladı diye düşündüm.

Tolga doğrusu biraz dağıtmıştı. Annem gittikten sonra bunun daha da kötüye gideceğini biliyordum. Öyle de oldu. Okula gidiyor, derslerine çalışıyordu ama aklı fikri gezmekteydi.

Yıllar sonra ilk kez kimsenin onu yargılamayacağı bir yerdeydi ve üstündeki o büyük baskı ortadan kalkmıştı.

Ama belki de şimdi buradan, uzaktan bakınca, bu yılların getirdiği sınırlamanın kalkması onun için taşınması ağır bir yük olmuştu.

Ferhat'la birkaç kez telefonla konuştuk. Ben ona mektuplar yazdım ama ondan küçük kartlar üzerine çizilmiş resimler ve birkaç satır dışında pek birşey gelmedi.

Aslında yeni şeyler öğrenirken, yeni insanlarla tanışırken, alışamadığım bir kentte hala konuşmakta zorlanırken (trafik bile tersten akıyordu) çok düşünecek zaman kalmıyordu.

Akşamları bütün gün okulda anlatılanları, gösterilenleri yeniden gözden geçiriyor, anlamadıklarımı başka kitaplardan bulmaya çalışıyordum.

Bu benim için büyük şanstı ve yalnızca okula gidip gelerek birkaç yıl geçirmek, sonra elimde diplomayla İstanbul'a dönüp modaevi açmak gibi bir niyetim yoktu. Bu okuldan mezun olan ve ara sokaklarda küçücük, ancak meraklıların geldiği dükkanlar açan genç kadınlara hayrandım. Bambaşka, alışılmamış şeyler tasarlıyorlardı. O yılın moda kumaşlarını, renklerini filan umursamadan... Tümüyle kendi istedikleri gibi...

Zaman buldukça oralara gidiyor, onlarla tanışıyor, yaptıklarını anlamaya çalışıyordum..

Ve tabii haftasonları Tolga'yla küçük eski sinemada izlediğimiz filmler...

Kimi olağanüstü fotoğraflardan oluşan, kimi yalnızca bir kadının bilinç akışını anlatan, kimi karmakarışık bir kentte sizi anlaşılması güç maceralara sürükleyen özel filmlerdi bunlar.

Sanki insan belleğinin sınırlarını zorlayan, onun kısıtlanmış çılgınlığını göstermeye çalışan, belki hepimizin gördüğü yaşadığı şeyleri bambaşka bir biçime sokup sizi şaşırtan acayip filmler.

Aslında tüm bunlar bana heyecan veriyordu. Sinema, konserler, ben fazla içmesem de kalabalık, soğuk barlar... Sergilere gidiyordum ve Ferhat'ı düşünüyordum. Acaba günün birinde o da böylesine ünlü olacak mıydı? Buralarda sergileri açılacak mıydı? Hatta kimbilir eserleri müzelere konulacak mıydı?

Kimi zaman yolda yürürken, kimi zaman uykuya dalarken tabii ki hep aklımdaydı.

Bazen kalkıp ona mektup yazmaya koyuluyor sonra okuyunca yollamaktan vazgeçiyordum. "Bize ne olacak şimdi, biz birlikte miyiz, sen benim sevgilim misin?" gibi şeyler vardı aklımda ama bunları yazınca kendime kızıyor, yırtıp atıyordum.

Bir iki kez telefonlaştık ama telefonda konuşmayı bilmez. Sanki herhangi bir arkadaşımı aramışım gibi okulu, dersleri, neler yaptığımı, hangi sergiye gittiğimi soruyordu. Birden yalnızca gerçek anlamda değil ikimizin arasında da bir mesafe belirmişti.

İnsan bazı şeyleri düşünmek istemese de aklına gelmesini engelleyemiyor. O da böyle sanki gittiğim her yerde bir biçimde, yanımdan hiç ayırmadığım o küçük kediciğin içindeymiş gibi benimleydi.

Göz görmeyince gönül unutur derler.

Hayır unutmuyor aslında. Ama araya başka görüntüler giriyor.

Tolga kısa süre sonra sanatçıların gittiği bir pub'a takılmaya başladı. Ve sonra da genç, çok yakışıklı bir bale öğrencisiyle tanıştı.

Artık birbirimizden gizleyecek birşeyimiz yoktu.

Kıskançlığın ne olduğunu gerçekte ilk kez onlardan öğrenecektim.

Bir gece birlikte gittikleri davetten çıkınca kıyametler kopmuş, Tolga başka biriyle biraz samimi olduğu için yolda kavgaya tutuşmuşlar ve karakolluk olmuşlardı.

Çocuk da onu terkedip gitmişti.

Geç kalmasına alışıktım ama içime doğmuş gibi o gece uyuyamadım. Sabaha karşı geldiğinde hala sarhoştu ve deliler gibi ağlıyordu. Sakinleştirip uyutmam epey zaman aldı.

O hafta evden çıkmayıp yazılar yazdı, ağladı, müzik dinledi.

Neyse ki sonunda cumartesi sabahı çocuk kapıda belirdi.

Onu içeri alırken Tolga, "Hayır, defolup gitsin, onu görmek istemiyorum," diye bağırıyordu. Hemen üstüme yağmurluğumu geçirip kendimi dışarı attım.

Niye hepimiz gerçekte o anda ondan başkasını görmek istemediğimiz halde böyle yaparız?

Yolda yürürken bile bağırışları geliyordu.

Ben kimseyle kavga edemem. Birbirine bağıran insanların yanında durmak istemem. Şuralarda bir yerde tahta var mı diye baktım, benim başıma bunlar gelmesin diye tahtaya vurdum.

Neyse ki işler tatlıya bağlandı ve ertesi cumartesi kendimizi kentin iki saat uzağında harika bir eski zaman kasabasında bulduk.

Andrew'nun ailesinden kalma evde onun özenle hazırladığı yemekleri yiyip uçsuz bucaksız kırlarda dolaştık. "Dikkatli basın bu gördüğünüz yeşillikler, dağlar, tepeler hep kraliçenin mülküdür," diye dalga geçiyordu.

Yıllar sonra onu dünyaca ünlü bir balenin ilk gösteriminde alkışlarken bu haftasonunu hatırlayacağımı bilmiyordum tabii.

Nedenini bilmiyorum, belki de o ikisinin ben uzun koltukta uyuklarken klasik müzik eşliğinde şaraplarını içip uzun uzun kitaplardan, şiirden sözetmelerini, kalkıp dans etmelerini görünce, Ferhat'a mektup yazdım.

Ama bu kez bu haftasonunu, evi ama daha önemlisi bütün duvarları süsleyen yüzlerce yıllık tabloları anlatırken birdenbire, ona biriyle tanıştığımı yazdım. Evet benden hoşlanan ve ara sıra buluştuğumuz bir çocuk vardı ama öyle ciddiye alınacak türden değildi. Bunu neden ona yazdım bilmiyorum.

Belki de biliyorum da söylemek istemiyorum.

Bu mektuptan sonra ondan uzun süre ses çıkmadı. Telefon etmeye de çekindim. Kızmış mıydı? Bunları duyunca artık görüşmemenin daha doğru olacağını, ona bunu ima ettiğimi mi düşünmüştü?

Yoksa zaten istediği buydu da bana söyleyememiş, şimdi hazır bahane bulmuşken rahata mı ermişti?

Ne diye durup dururken böyle bir saçmalık yaptım diye kendime kızıyordum tabii.

Kendim yapıp sonra giderek ona kızmaya başladım. İnsan en azından arayıp sormaz mıydı? "Sen ne biçim kızsın, gider gitmez birini mi buldun?" demez miydi?

Ah tabii kendi yeni sevgili bulmadıysa!

Aklıma bunlar geliyor, iyice deliriyordum. Her gün telefon çalacak mı, mektup gelecek mi diye beklemeye başladım. Kendime inanamıyordum. Aklımca onu denemeye mi kalkışmıştım? Biriyle tanıştım diye deliye dönüp koşa koşa buraya gelecek filan mı sanıyordum acaba?

Ne budalayım!

Dayanamayıp Tolga'ya ne yaptığımı anlattım.

"Erkek milleti değil mi hepsi aynı," diye beni güldürdü ama aynı zamanda kızdı. "Deli misin kızım sen, koskoca adama böyle şey söylersen ne yapacak, emin ol karalar bağlamış oturuyordur evinde... Genç aşık iki ay geçmeden yenisini bulmuş! Sence ne düşünüyordur?"

"Zaten sana söyleyende kabahat..."

"Tabii adamı durup dururken kıskandırmaya çalışacak kadar ezik olanda hiç kabahat yok," diye beni iyice çıldırttı.

Şimdi yeniden yazıp durumu düzeltebilir miydim?

Yok ona da elim gitmiyordu.

Anlaşılmaz biçimde tam kendime kızmışken birden ona kızmaya başlıyordum çünkü.

Böyle epey zaman geçti. Sessizlik uzadıkça uzadı. Ne kart, ne mektup, ne telefon...

Demek böyle bitecekmiş dedim kendi kendime yolda yürürken, ağlıyordum ama inadım tutmuştu. Eve gelince kediyi aldım, tam çekmeceye kaldıracaktım ki aklıma geldi. Komik ama ovaladım.

Sihirli lambadan çıkan cin gibi gerçekten gelecek miydi?

Bana öyle söz vermemiş miydi?

Kıyamadım yine çantama koydum.

Oyılbaşı kendimi hiç iyi hissetmiyordum. Tolga beni neşelendirmek için evde parti vermek niyetindeydi. Andrew'yla oturup kostüm partisi mi yapsalar dönem partisi mi yapsalar tartışırken bile kavga çıkmış, çocuk yine evden kovulmuştu.

Artık onların bu haline alışmıştım. Çünkü pek neşeli, güzel başlayan akşam birden bir sözle değişiyor, kıyametler kopuyor, bardaklar havada uçuşuyor ve sonunda her zaman Andrew evden çıkıp gidiyordu.

Ama bu fazla uzun sürmüyor, birkaç güne kalmadan yine buluşuyorlar, hiçbirşey olmamış gibi kaldıkları yerden yeniden başlıyorlardı.

Ben hiç yeni yıl havasına girememiştim. Zaten burada kar da yağmıyordu ki...

Mağazaların vitrinleri, sokak ışıklandırmaları, meydanlarda dolaşan Noel Babalar beni pek etkilememişti.

Kendime itiraf edemiyordum ama uzakta da olsa Ferhat'ın varlığı bana neşe veriyordu. Şimdi durup dururken yaptığım saçmalık yüzünden onu kaybettiğime hem inanamıyordum hem de hala ona dargındım.

Hem ona hem kendime...

Tolga iki gün öncesinden evi süslemeye başladı. Sonunda 70'li yıllar partisi yapmaya karar vermişlerdi. Müzikler, giysiler ayarlandı, yemek ve içki alındı... Hatta nereden bulmuşlarsa garip bir alet almışlardı, karanlıkta duvarda dönüp duran renkli desenler oluşturuyordu.

Bir gece önce Andrew'yla ikisi sabaha kadar uğraştılar. Ben yatıp uyudum.

Sabah erken kalktım. İkisi yeniden geri kalan ufak tefek şeyleri almak için alışverişe gittiler. Ben de köşedeki kafede kahvaltı ettim. Sonra da onlara hediye almaya gittim.

Zaten benim çağırdığım okuldan üç beş kişi ve bir öğretmenle eşiydi. Onların da geleceğine emin değildim.

Yağmurlu, karanlık bir gündü. Bu havada bile çiçekçiler yerindeydi. Dönerken çiçek almayı unutmayayım dedim. Birkaç mağaza dolaştım. İkinci el dükkanlarından birinde istemediğim kadar çok şey vardı.

Sanki gerçekten 70'lere dönmüş gibiydim. Mağazada çalışanlar bile o günlerden kalmıştı sanki. İçeride deli gibi rock çalıyor, gelenler üstüste atılmış yüzlerce elbisenin, pantolonun, gömleğin içinden birini çekiştirip duruyordu.

Tolga'ya rengarenk kocaman bir şapka beğendim. Satıcı kadın bunun ünlü zenci şarkıcının şapkası olduğunu söyledi ve hatta fotoğraf gösterdi ama adamı tanımıyordum.

Andrew için de kocaman, ağır tokası olan yılan derisi bir kemer aldım. Bu akşam giyeceği üstüne yapışan kırmızı pantolonla güzel duracaktı.

Sonra çiçekleri aldım ama taksi bulamadığım için epeyce yürüyüp epeyce ıslandım.

Eve geldiğimde her yerimden sular akıyordu. Neyse ki çiçeklerle hediyeleri iyi sarmalamıştım.

Titriyordum soğuktan.

Kapının önünde rüzgar yağmur damlalarını yüzüme öyle sert vuruyordu ki çantamdan anahtarı çıkartamıyordum.

Tek istediğim hemen eve girmek ve kendimi sıcak suya atmaktı. Ayaklarım donmuş gibiydi çünkü.

Anahtarı çıkartmak için elimdekileri merdivene bırakırken kafamı kaldırdım.

Ve öylece kalakaldım.

Merdivene oturmuş, sigara içiyordu.

Başında eski moda kasket, üstünde yakalarını kaldırdığı uzun balıksırtı palto, sigarayı avucunun içinde tutmuş bana bakıyordu gülerek...

Bazı anlar vardır ya ağlamakla gülmek arasında kalırsınız. Aslında mutlusunuzdur ama aynı zamanda içinizden ağlamak gelir. Hani çok güzel filmlerin acıklı biteceğini düşünürken beklenmedik bir rastlantı olur ve aslında herşey yoluna girdiği halde ağlarsınız ya işte onun gibi...

Ama tuhaf olan bu benim için yalnızca o an değil orada onunla geçirdiğimiz üç gün boyunca böyle oldu. Yüzüne bakıyordum ve gülerken birden gözlerim doluyordu.

Sanki hayatta en çok istediğini bulmak ama onu kaybedeceğini bilmek gibiydi bu.

Londra'nın hiç gitmediğim çok güzel, sakin bir semtinde, kısa süreliğine Paris'e giden bir ressam arkadaşının evini ayarlamıştı.

Tabii ki yılbaşı partisine katılamadım. Üstümüzü başımızı kurulayıp eşyaları bıraktıktan sonra yanıma birkaç şey aldım ve Tolga'ya not bıraktım. Hayır, bunca zaman sonra kalkıp gelmişken onu tanımadığı insanlarla paylaşmaya, belki de hayatımın en özel yılbaşı gecesini, ilerleyen saatlerde tamamen kafayı bulup saçmalayacaklarına emin olduğum bir sürü deliyle mahvetmeye hiç niyetim yoktu.

Yağmurun altında sarılıp yürüdük. Bir yılbaşı akşamüstüydü. İnsanlar evlerine yetişmeye çalışıyordu. Bütün taksiler doluydu. Her yer ışıl ışıldı. Sanki benim için özel bir kutlama yapılıyormuş gibiydi. Dağılıyordu ışıklar yağmurda. Ne kalabalık, ne yağmur, ne birbirine çarpan telaşlı insanlar umurumdaydı. Ben kendimi benim için bu geceye özel hazırlanmış kentte onunla yalnız hissediyordum.

Sonunda taksi bulup eve geldik.

Ama içimde bir tedirginlik vardı. Ne zamandır görüşmüyorduk. Üstelik son yazdığım mektuptan sonra bana kızdığını, kırıldığını düşünüyordum. Şimdi ne olacağını, herşeyin istediğim gibi olup olmayacağını bilemiyordum. Burada ilk kez onunla gerçekten yalnızdık. Onun evinde değil. Kendi şehrimizde değil. Üç günlüğüne gelmişti.

Yalnızca o ve ben.

Ev soğuktu.

Şömineye birkaç odun atıp tutuşturdu.

"Bu gerçek mi?'" diye sordum, "Yani burada olman…"

Daha bu akşamüzeri ansızın kendimi hiç bilmediğim bu semtte hiç bilmediğim bir evde onunla şöminenin önünde bulacağım aklımın ucundan bile geçmemişti.

"Umarım geldiğime sevinmişsindir, belki de sormam gerekirdi ama bir anda karar verdim…"

Sevinmek mi?

Delirmiş.

İçimdeki duygunun adı sevinçle, mutlulukla, böyle tek bir sözcükle tanımlanamazdı. Eğer bir yazar ya da şair böyle bir sözcük bulmuşsa da ben onu bilmiyordum.

"İyi ki geldin," dedim yalnızca.

Öpüşürken ağlamak üzereydim ve kendimi tutmaya çalışıyordum.

Ama o böyle duygusal konuşmaları sürdüremez. Hemen bana komik hikayeler anlatmaya başladı. Yalnızca yarım saat sonra sanki hep buradaymış, daha dün birlikteymişiz gibi çene çalıyorduk.

Bana sormasından korkuyordum ama bir yandan da yaptığım saçmalığı anlatmak, aslında böyle birşey olmadığını söylemek istiyordum ama sanki o mektubu okumamış gibiydi.

Bu hep böyle olmamış mıydı? Bana dokunduğunda, beni öptüğünde kendimi ona bırakmak isterken birden öylesine anlatmaya başlar, ben de ne yapacağımı şaşırırdım...

"Hadi kalk bakalım,"dedi, "bu gece yılbaşı..."

Camları, kapıları ışıklarla süslenmiş evlerin önünden geçip eski, küçük pub'a geldik. Arkadaşının adını söyleyince hemen yer buldular. Geçmiş zamandan kalma bir yer gibiydi. Gibi değil de bence zaten öyleydi. Sanki burada zaman donmuş, dışarıdaki dünyadan farklı bir biçimde birileri burada kendi istedikleri zamanı yaşamaya devam ediyordu.

Biz atıştırırken içerisi yavaş yavaş dolmaya başladı. Zaten gelenlerin hepsi birbirini tanıyor gibiydi. Şu para atıp istediğiniz şarkıyı çaldığınız müzik kutularından vardı. Epeyce bozukluk aldık ve aklımıza gelen bütün şarkıları üstüste çalmaya başladık.

Önceleri belki aslında yalnızca meraktı. O güne dek hiç tanımadığım, rastlamadığım bir dünyaydı çünkü. Dünya derken gülümserdim kendi kendime... Bir odanın içinde nasıl bir dünya olabilirdi ki?

Ama olmuştu işte.

O atölyeye gittiğim ilk günden sonra hep sanki gizemli bir masalı okurken birdenbire kendimi masalın içinde bulmuş gibi hissetmiştim.

Her yerde sanki antika dükkanındaymışsınız gibi garip eşyalar vardı. Bunları nereden bulmuş, neden almış bilmek zordu. Çünkü hemen hemen hepsi işlevsizdi.

Çalışmayan radyolardan eski daktilolara, kırık dökük kristal takımlardan kurmalı oyuncaklara kadar binlerce irili ufaklı eşya vardı her yerde.

Tıpkı resimleri gibi...

Sanatçılar kendilerine bu dünyanın içinde yeni bir dünya yaratabilirler ama o bence bütün bu resimlerle heykellerle uğraşırken aslında kendisini yeniden yaratmaya çalışmıştı. Tıpkı mermer bloktan bir insan figürü yapıp sonra onun canlanmasını beklemek gibi...

Bu mümkün müydü?

Neden kimi zaman çok güzel yüzler, figürler çizdiği halde daha çok karmakarışık, çirkin insanları, açılmış yaraları, bir yerinde bir sakatlık olanları, cüceleri, garip kılıklara bürünmüş kadın mı erkek mi belirsiz insanları çizdiğini anlamak zordu.

İnatla bunları çizmesinin ve bu nedenle de insanların bu resimlere bakmak bile istememesinin nedenini uzun zaman anlamamıştım.

Şimdi bunca zaman sonra belki anlayabiliyorum...

O, insanların birbirine olan düşmanlığını, başkalarına olan öfkemizi, bize benzemeyenleri nasıl sevmediğimizi anlatmaya çalışmıştı belki de...

Ve neden en küçük kağıt parçalarına, yanından ayırmadığı defterinin sayfalarına bile onca insan yüzü çizerdi?

İçiçe geçmiş bu yüzler farklı açılardan baktığınızda farklı biçimlere dönüşürdü.

Önce hep küçük bir kağıtla başlar sonra giderek büyütür ve bazıları dev birer yağlıboya tabloya dönüşürdü.

Aynı şeyi o tahta top için de yapmıştı. Önce küçük misket kadar olanlarıyla başlamış sonra giderek büyütmüştü.

Hem çok gerçekti bütün bu insanlar, yüzler, çocuklar, hayvanlar hem de sanki bir hayalin içinde silinip gidecekmiş gibi görünüyordu.

Farklı zamanlardan eşyaların, olur olmaz bitkilerin, meyvelerin ne olduğunu ancak şimdi yıllar sonra anlayabiliyorum.

Evet o aslında insan belleğini çiziyordu. Farklı zamanlardan, karmakarışık anılarla, bilgilerle, görüntülerle dolu belleğin o inanılmaz eriyiğini resmediyordu. Ve öylesine deliceydi ki bakarken huzursuz oluyordu insan.

Birdenbire onca insanın, onca eşyanın, renklerin arasından zincirinden kopmuş bir atlıkarıncanın atları üzerinize geliyordu örneğin.

Belki de rüyalarıydı bunlar onun ya da bir eleştirmenin yazdığı gibi bilinçaltına yapılan yolculuk...

Sayısız kez baktığınız bir resimde bile bir gün o ana kadar göremediğiniz bir ayrıntıyla karşılaşabilirdiniz.

Kimileri resmin içindeki bütün bu parçaları birbirine bağlamaya, bundan öyküler çıkartmaya uğraşmışlardı. Ama eski zamanlardan kalma bir çalgıyla bir konser biletinin, küçük böceklerle Bremen Mızıkacılarının, kurşuna dizilen bir adamla birbirine geçmiş sevişen insanların, yüzü yaşlı kırışık bebekle yarım yamalak bir aşk mektubunun ve buna benzer sayısız şeyin biraraya geldiği tablodan nasıl bir öykü çıkartılabilirdi ki...

Kimbilir belki de herkes kendi öyküsünü çıkartıyordu...

Ama o bunları konuşmayı sevmezdi. Resimleri hakkında hiç konuşmazdı.

O hayatın tümüyle bir rastlantılar zincirinden oluştuğuna inanırdı. Belki de resimlerindeki bu birbiriyle ilgisiz görünen ayrıntıların nedeni buydu.

Elbette o gece, o eski püskü tavernada otururken bütün bunları düşünmüyordum. Ona söylemesem de aklıma gelen tek şey hayatımda nedensiz biçimde kendimi ondan başka kimseye ait hissetmediğimdi.

Oturduğumuz duvarın önünde çok eski büyükçe bir duvar saati vardı. Şu sarkaçlı olanlardan. Kurt yenikleriyle dolu, antika, anneannemin evindekine benzer bir saat. Ben ona pencereli saat derdim. Çünkü camını açıp kurma görevi benimdi.

Eğer saatin kadranını ayarlayabildiğimiz gibi gerçek zamanı da ayarlayabilsek, ileri, geri alabilsek ya da durdurabilsek hayat ne kadar başka olurdu.

O üç gün biterken bana bıraktığı mektup hala yanımda. Sabah uyandığım zaman başucumda bulduğum mektup.

"Biliyorum birlikte çok az zaman geçirdik. Birbirimizi tanıdığımızı bile söyleyemeyiz değil mi? Tıpkı isminle anılan o sanattaki gibi seni düşününce değişen renkler, biçimler, elle tutulamayan şeyler geliyor aklıma. Çok güzel ama belirsiz. Belki senin için de böyledir. Heyecan verici ama aynı zamanda kaybolup gideceği için ürkütücü...

Gerçek mi hayal mi belli olmayan birşey.

Kimbilir belki asıl güzel olan, bütün bu kısa anları benzersiz kılan, içimde yıllar sonra ilk kez böyle bir duygu uyandıran da bu.

Senin o güzel yüzünü tutmak sanki suya renk bırakmak gibi... Onun gözlerinde dağılışını izlemek... Bakışlarındaki derin ama bilinmez düşünceleri okumaya çalışmak... Başka dünyada buyumuş bir kız... Başka bir dünyadan gelmiş koskoca bir adam... Hala rüyasının içinde kalmayı başarmış küçük bir çocuk...

Benim için başından beri sevmekle korku birarada oldu. Seni incitmek mi? Üzmek mi? Hayatının daha başında canını yakmak mı? Bilmiyorum.

Sen bana bunları hiç söylemedin. Hatta umursamazmış gibi davrandın.

Ama biliyor musun, insan büyüdükçe, yaşlandıkça, birinin hayatına girmenin çok kolay ama çıkmanın çok zor olduğunu anlıyor.

Eğer ilişkiye başlarken yıllar sonrasını görebilseydik belki de çoğumuz daha en baştan vazgeçerdik.

Ama kimbilir belki de en iyisi geleceği hiç düşünmemektir.

İlişki dedim ve derken bile birdenbire elim durdu. Bizimkine ilişki denebilir mi? İkimiz de birbirimizin hayatından ancak anlattığımız kadar haberdarız. Ne kadar yalan ne kadar doğru söylediğimiz, yaşadıklarımızı nasıl değiştirdiğimiz, anıları bile nasıl anlattığımız belli değil.

Sen şimdi hayatının başındasın. Yapacağın çok şey var ve eminim en güzelini yapacaksın. Bense şimdiden çok yorgunum. Yapmak istediklerimi yapabilecek miyim onu bile bilmiyorum.

Seni görmek inan ki uzun zamandır bana en iyi gelen şeydi. Hatta belki de hep aklımda olan ama bir türlü başlayamadığım resimleri yapmam için bana yeniden ilham verdi.

Biz hiç bundan sonra ne olacak demedik birbirimize... Aslında galiba ben kendi hayatımda da bundan sonra ne olacak, hiç bilemedim. Şimdi de bilmiyorum.

Uzakta olduğunda da seni düşündüğüm zaman hep gülümsüyorum. Bazı sabahlar uyandığımda aklımda senin yüzün oluyor. Garip bir biçimde senin yüzünü, bakışlarını, dalmış, uzaklara gitmiş halini, içtenlikle gülümsemeni, saçların yüzüne dökülmüş hüzünlü duruşunu çizmek istiyorum. Çiziyorum da...

Bazı şeyleri konuşmamamızın nedeni galiba gerçek olmasa da ikimizin arasında bir dünyada buluşuyor olmamız. Belki de söylemediklerim söylediklerimden, söyleyebildiklerimden daha çok.

O bazı şeyler bu dünyayı bozacak ve aniden renkleri, ışığı, eşyayı sıradanlaştırıp bizim onlara yüklediğimiz anlamdan, verdiğimiz biçimden uzaklaştıracak gibi geldi belki de ...

Sabah uyandığımda Londra'nın puslu ışığında uzun uzun seni seyrettim. Rüyanda nerelerde olduğunu düşündüm. İstediğim, böyle tanımadığımız bir evde, uzak bir kentte, kimseler yokken yanında uyumaya devam etmek ve günleri hep böyle aldırışsız, dışarıda dünya yokmuş gibi geçirebilmekti.

Yazık ki hayat buna izin vermez.

Onun için çalınmış zamanlarımız çok güzeldi.

Dışarısı soğuk, yağmurlu, karanlık... Bu satırları yazıp kalın kazağımı, yağmurluğumu giyip havaalanına doğru yola çıkıyorum.

Seni uyandırmadım.

Vedaları sevmem.

Kucağımda kulağıma fısıldadığın son sözcüklerin güzelliğinde, mutluluğunda, huzurunda kalmanı istedim.

Hep böyle kal."

Sonraları çok düşündüm. Herşey bir zaman sorunu mu? Bir arkadaşım üç yıllık ilişkisi sürerken ama o ilişkiden aslında çok mutsuzken biriyle tanışmıştı. Gizli saklı onunla birlikte olmuştu.

Ama nişanlısı ondan ayrılmak istemiyordu ve o da kızı üzmemek için mi yoksa söz verdiği için mi bilmem bu ilişkiye son veremiyordu. Öte yandan gizli ilişkisi onu mutlu ettiği için de hayatına devam ediyordu.

Belki onunla tanışmasa nişanlısından ayrılacaktı. Belki de evlenecekti. Sonunda bir gün kıza herşeyi anlatıp ayrılmaya karar verdi. Ama bu konuşmalar biraz uzun sürdü ve o arada gizli sevgilisiyle görüşmedi. İlişkisini bitirip sonra onunla konuşmayı ve artık onunla birlikte olmayı hatta evlenmeyi düşünüyordu.

Gözyaşları, kavgalar uzayıp gitti ama sonunda kızcağız durumu kabullendi ve herşey bitti.

Ama bilmediği şuydu. Gizli sevgili bu arada başkasıyla tanışmış ve onunla bir yola girmişti. Aradığı zaman artık bu ilişkinin onu mutlu etmediğini ve bitirmeleri gerektiğini söyledi.

Ne yaptıysa, ona ilişkisini bitirdiğini ve artık yalnızca onu istediğini söylese de geç kalmıştı. Belki yalnızca birkaç hafta...

O mektubu yazdığı gece dışarda biraz üşümüş kahve içerken ellerimi tutup bana baktı. Önemli birşey söyleyeceğini düşündüm. Yoksa ona yazdığım mektubu, uydurma sevgilimi mi soracaktı? Sormadı. Her ne söyleyecekse dilinin ucuna kadar gelmişti ama söylemedi.

"Hadi eve gidelim, üşüdün sen, burnun kızarmış," dedi yalnızca.

Sabah yüzümde gülümsemeyle uyandım ama sonra yanımda olmadığını farkettim. Seslendim, yoktu. Belki de yiyecek birşey almaya gitti kahvaltı için diye düşündüm. Ama kalkıp biraz kendime gelince farkettim ki eşyaları yok.

Sonra masanın üzerinde mektubu buldum.

Evet vedaları sevmezsin biliyorum. Ama keşke izin verseydin de en azından havaalanına kadar yanında kalsaydım.

Okudum, yeniden okudum, pek anlamadım aslında. Bu veda mektubu muydu? Öylesine yazılmış bir mektup muydu? Yoksa böylece devam edeceğimizi mi anlatıyordu?

Bir tek uyanıp yüzüme baktığı cümlesi kaldı aklımda. Çünkü sabah uyanıp yanınızdaki insana bakarken mutlu olmaktır aşk.

Başından beri olduğu gibi yaşananlar sis bulutunun ardındaydı. Tam elle tutacağınızı sandığınız an kaybolan tanımlanamaz birşey gibiydi.

Hem çok mutluydum hem de hüzünlü.

Eşyaları topladım, mektubun sonunda yazdığı gibi her tarafı kilitleyip anahtarı söylediği yere gizledim.

Keskin hava insanın yüzüne çarpıyordu ama bana iyi geldi. Biraz yürüdüm. En azından bu sokakları, bu evleri, bu güzel semti o günkü haliyle belleğime kazımak için.

Tıpkı yılbaşı akşamüstü merdivenlerde belirdiği gibi üç gün sonra aynı biçimde kaybolup gitmişti.

Kediyi ovalamıştım değil mi?

Öyle anlar, o anlara ait duygular, renkler, akılda kalan resimler, kokular var ki hayatın içinden onları çıkartmak, tıpkı bir tablodaki gibi dondurmak ve sonsuza dek korumak istiyor insan.

Ama olmuyor.

Bir keresinde Ferhat benim fotoğrafımı çekerken, "Yazık ki bazı şeyler fotoğrafa çıkmıyor, bazı insanlar da..." demişti. Buna çok gülmüştüm.

"Ben fotoğrafa çıkmıyor muyum?"

"Evet," dedi, "bazen gördüğün derinlik, gördüğün şeyin arkasındakiler, belki de ona bakarken içinden gelenler fotoğrafa çıkmıyor, yalnızca herkesin görebildiği suret beliriyor, galiba bu nedenle resim çiziyorum..."

Ama resimler de fotoğraflar gibi o anların bellekteki algısını tam olarak yansıtamaz.

Ben o sabah yolda yürürken, yağmur yüzüme çarparken, o üç günün içindeki anları, kokuyu, dokunuşları, onun sesini, kendine özgü vurgularını, bakışını kaçırmasını, elinin üzerindeki damarları, kulağıma karanlıkta fısıldayışını, yerçekimsiz bir ortamdaymış gibi kucağında yuvarlanışımı, titreyişleri, sıcaklığı, kendi içimden çıkıp uzaktan kendime bakarmış gibi hafiflediğimi, ayak parmaklarımın bile uyuşmasını, gülmekle ağlamak arasında gidip gelişimi, ürpertiyi, korkuyu, direnmeyi ve kendini tümüyle bırakışı, öpmek sevmek ve canını yakmanın aynı anda nasıl istenebileceğini, bilincimden geçen ve hiç anlam veremediğim sayısız düşüncenin, görüntünün biraz sonra yalnızca kendi başıma dolaştığım kişisel bir sirke dönüşmesini, orada bulduğum şeylerle yaşadığım anın karışmasındaki inanılmaz uyumu belleğimde taşıyordum.

Ama onu resmetmek hatta sözcüklere dökmek imkansızdı.

İşte deniyorum ama olmuyor.

Kimbilir belki de asıl önemli olan yaşananlar değil yaşadıklarımızı nasıl algıladığımızdır.

Hepimiz annemizin kucağındaydık ama hiçbirimiz aynı kokuyu duymadık ve sorsak hiçbirimiz o kokuyu anlatamayız.

Onun bir resmi vardı.

Yukarıda, kağıttan kesilmiş yüzlerce küçük beyaz kuş uçuyor, aşağıda insanlar panayırda geziniyorlardı. Ayrıntılara bakarsanız kimileri oyuncak ayı için atış yapıyor, kimileri hilkat garibesini izliyor, kimileri halka atıyor, kimi yalnızca dondurma yiyerek dolaşıyordu. Küçücük insanların yüzlerine yakından bakınca güldüklerini, öylesine bir yerlere baktıklarını, yorgun olduklarını bile görebilirdiniz.

Resmin üstünde bir ışık vardı. O ışıkta kuşlar dalgalanıyor ve uçuyormuş gibi görünüyorlardı.

Sonra tabloyu kenara çekince bir başka resim ortaya çıkıyordu. Aslında ilk anda aynı tablo gibiydi. Ama bu kez kuşlar savaş uçaklarına, aşağıdakiler de kaçışan, çocuklarını kurtarmaya çalışan, yerlerde sürüklenen, kanlar içinde yatan insanlara dönüşüyordu.

İkinci resim açılıp da bunları görünce irkildim. Çok etkileyiciydi ama aynı zamanda çok üzücü...

Dayanamayıp, "Neden bunun tersini yapmadın?" diye sordum.

"Çünkü hep böyle olur..." dedi.

Nedense yolda yürürken aklıma o tablo geldi yine. Sonra unuttum. Şimdi uçakta olmalıydı. Acaba neler düşünüyordu? Benim gibi mutlu muydu? Kuşkulu muydu? Uçakta yine bu üç günün resimlerini çiziyor muydu?

İnsanların pardesülerine, yağmurluklarına sarılıp üşüyerek hızlı hızlı yürüdüğü soğuk, puslu Londra sabahı... Neredeyse önümü zor görüyordum.

Ve o çocuk müzikallerinden birindeymiş gibi neredeyse zıplayarak yürüyordum.

Gerçekten hep öyle mi olur?

Neden sonra donmak üzere olduğumu farkettim ve kendimi taksiye zor attım.

Şimdi gel de olup bitenleri Tolga'ya anlat.

Herhalde meraktan delirmiş halde beni bekliyordu. Üstüste sorularla beni delirtecekti.

Yok tabii ki anlatmayacaktım. Ki anlatmak için de delirmiyor değildim. Taksi de inadına her kırmızı ışığa yakalanıyordu.

Ama zaten o değil herhangi biri yüzüme baksa ne hissettiğimi, neler olup bittiğini anlayabilirdi.

Herhalde buraya geldiğimden beri beni ilk kez böyle sıçrayarak yürürken görecekti.

Tıpkı eski günlerdeki gibi hemen onun yanına gitmek istiyordum.

Tabii okula gitmeye kalkmadıysa... Yok benim bu sabah eve geleceğimi biliyorken kesinlikle gitmemiştir.

Bir yandan da saate bakıyordum. Ferhat ne zaman varacaktı İstanbul'a? Hesabım da o kadar kötüdür ki saat farkını bile tutturamıyordum. Bu akşam beni arayacak mıydı? Aramazsa ben aramalı mıydım?

Aman neyse, şimdi gidip sıcak suya girecektim ve uzun uzun orada kalacaktım. Sonra sandviç ve çay alıp meraktan çıldırmış arkadaşımla sohbete dalacaktım. Bugünü tembelliğe ayırdım. Kulağımdaki ağrı bile şu an umurumda değil.

Eski Londra taksisi büyük sarayın önünden geçiyor, sincapların dolaştığı parkın, heykellerin, turistlerin, yağmurda hızlı hızlı yürüyen insanların, şemsiyelerin arasından geçiyor.

Şoför dikkatle radyodaki maçı dinliyor. Arkada ayaklarımı uzatmış etrafı seyrediyorum.

Parkta şık giysileriyle iki genç kız at biniyor. Yaşlı çöpçü imkansız bir çabayla yerdeki sarı yaprakları süpürmeye çalışıyor. Kendi kendime o şarkıyı mırıldanıyorum, "Sonbahar Yaprakları"...

Galiba buraya geldiğim günden beri ilk kez kenti böyle turist gibi geziyorum.

Öyle puslu ki, gerçeküstü bir resim gibi.

Sanki az sonra her yer sisin içine gömülecek ve biz kentin dolambacında kaybolacağız.

Dickens romanları gibi...

Yolu kaçırmamak için dikkat kesiliyorum.

"Evet, buradan sağa lütfen."

İlk kez başını çevirip bana bakıyor, gülümsüyor, "Biliyorum," diyor. "Meraklanma biz alışığız," der gibi.

Eski otelin önündeki kapıcı melon şapkasını çıkartıp büyük, lüks arabadan inen şık hanımı karşılıyor. Çinçilla kürkünün içindeki kadın da ona selam veriyor.

Geçtik.

Rüzgarda uçuşan eteklerini kapatmaya çalışan kız şemsiyesini düşürüyor.

Geçtik.

Bastonuyla aniden kendini yola atan yaşlı beyefendi yüzünden fren yapıyoruz. Adam yalnızca dönüp bize şöyle bir bakıyor ve istifini bozmadan ağır adımlarla karşıya geçiyor. Şoför garip bir aksanla küfrediyor ama anlamıyorum.

Geçtik.

Silecekler daha hızlı çalışıyor.

Camları silmeye çalışan, kırmızı ışıkta durunca dilenen çocuklar yok henüz.

Belki de bizim göremediğimiz yerlerdeler.

Yüksek topuklu ayakkabıları, kırmızı paltosu, kocaman şapkasıyla bir kadın minik, tüylü köpeğini gezdirirken yağmurun altında iskeleye çelik borular taşıyan mavi tulumlu iki işçi ona ıslık çalıp gülüşüyor.

Geçtik.

Bir kenti yalnızca böyle taksinin içinde geçerek izlemek bile bir film gibi. Elimde kamera olsa, sislerin içinde olup bitenleri, sanki bir hayalin içinde geçen sıradan bir günün sıradan hikayeleri gibi çekebilsem...

Çünkü tüm bunlar hayalle gerçek arasında...

Hayatımda gördüğüm en büyük atın üstündeki polis etrafı izliyor. Bir an gözgöze geliyoruz.

Geçtik.

Şoför birden çığlık atıyor. Dalgınlığımdan uyanıyorum korkarak. Herhalde takımı gol attı.

Gülümsüyorum sadece.

Köşeyi dönüyoruz ve evin önünde duruyor.

Evet tam da düşündüğüm gibi. Ev hep loş olduğundan sabah bile ışık yaktığı için Tolga'nın evde olduğunu anlıyorum ve seviniyorum.

Şimdi hem zaman hem de mekan olarak çok uzakta, o unutulmaz günün yıllar sonrasında, böyle trende giderken bir kentin değil, kasabaların, uçsuz bucaksız ormanların, insanın burada ne işi var diyeceği ıssız yerlerdeki tek tük evlerin, soğuk istasyonların –ellerinde bavullarıyla yolcular biniyor, yolcular iniyor– arasından geçerken o puslu Londra sabahını hatırlıyorum.

Hayatınızın bir sabahı herşeyi değiştirebilir.

Burada puslu bir hava yok. Aksine herşey özel bir gözlük takmışım gibi parlak.

Tren yavaşlıyor.

Karşımdaki adam kalkıp bavulunu alıyor, "Size iyi yolculuklar," diyor ve koridora çıkıyor. Tren sallanarak duruyor.

Burada mıyım şimdi yoksa o Londra sabahında mı?

Tolga kapıyı açtı. Heyecanla sarılıp öptüm.

Küçük bavulumu içeriye atıp hemen banyoya gireceğimi, bana sandviç yapmasını, sonra olanları anlatacağımı söyledim. Bütün bunları anlatırken onun hiç konuşmadığını farkettim.

Döndüm.

Yüzünde garip bir ifade vardı.

Eyvah, dedim, mutlaka kavga çıktı, yine ayrıldılar, bizimki bozuk...

"Dur, dinlemeden önce bana on dakika ver," dedim.

"Birşey oldu," dedi.

Dışarıya bakan pencerelerden yağmur süzülüyordu.

Yüzüne baktım ve sevgilisiyle kavga çıkmadığını o an anladım.

"Ne oldu?" dedim.

"Gel şuraya otur, anlatacağım," dedi.

Oturdum.

"Az önce annen aradı, okula gittiğini söyledim, akşamüstü yeniden arayacak ama istersen sen şimdi ara..."

Yılbaşı akşamı annemi aramıştım. Tolga ve arkadaşlarımızla beraber olduğumuzu söylemiştim.

Gülmüyordu.

Garip, tedirgin bir hali vardı.

"Kahve yapmıştım, üşümüşsündür, dur sana da getireyim," dedi.

"Ne oluyor Tolga?" dedim.

Onu o kadar iyi tanıyorum ki...

Yüzünden bile belli...

"Ne oldu, çabuk söyle..."

Geri döndü, yanıma oturdu.

"Dün gece anneannen rahatsızlanmış, telaşlanmışlar, e ben de okula gitti dedim, sen şimdi ararsın, herhalde önemli değildir..."

Biri size boş boş bakıp, önemli değildir diyorsa önemlidir.

Bunu bilecek kadar büyüğüm.

Babam o kapıdan çıkıp gittiğinde anneme ne olduğunu sorduğumda da "Birşey yok," demişti.

Koltuğa yığıldım.

"Bana doğru söyle," dedim, "ne oldu?"

"Söylüyorum ya canım, herhalde fenalık geçirmiş, doktor gelmiş, annen de seni aramak istemiş..."

Zaman…

Daha demin mutluluktan uçarken… Ayaklarım yerden kesilmişken… Belki de hayatımın en güzel günlerinden birini, bu puslu kentte masal alemindeymiş gibi yaşarken…

Bir bıçak saplandı.

Ne olur, dedim, ne olur, bu kez, hiç değilse bu kez kötü birşey olmasın. Hiç değilse bu sabah olmasın.

Ama oldu.

Öyle dememiş miydi Ferhat, "Çünkü hep böyle olur."

Yılbaşı akşamı tabii ki anneannemin evinde yine herkes toplanmıştı. Sabaha kadar süren sohbetlerden, şarkılardan sonra ertesi gün Sare Hanım biraz geç kalkmıştı. Başı ağrıyordu, çarpıntısı vardı. Pek umursamamıştı. Annemin ısrarına rağmen doktor çağırmak da istememişti.

"E sabaha kadar oturduk, bu yaşta bunlar olacak tabii, siz de herşeyi izam ediyorsunuz, başım ağrıdı doktor, sırtım kasıldı doktor, böyle hayat geçmez, akşama kalmaz toparlarım," demiş ama akşama doğru odasına çekilip uyumuştu.

Öyle gün içinde pek uyumazdı.

Ertesi gün daha iyi hissetmiş, yine kahvesini, sigarasını içmiş ama pek keyfi yokmuş.

Hiç adeti olmasa da hasta çorbası dediği tavuksuyu çorba istemiş, başına, "Sanki başım kaşınıyor, gıdıklanıyor, anlayamadım," diyerek buz torbası koydurmuş.

Annem bütün bunlardan hoşlanmadığı için doktor çağırmış. Anneannem her ne kadar buna kızsa da tansiyonu biraz yüksek çıkmış, çarpıntısı varmış, yatıştırıcı vermiş doktor, çok yorulduğunu, dinlenmesi gerektiğini söyleyip gitmiş.

Gece vakti Saniye, garip bir sesle yerinden fırlamış. Yanına gelince onun kendinde olmadığını, hırıldadığını, yüzünün bir yarısının kaydığını farketmiş.

"Rabbim affetsin, bir gözü başka yere bakıyordu," diye ağlamış sonra.

Bulabildiğim ilk uçakla İstanbul'a geldim.

Yol boyunca mucize olacak ve ben eve gittiğimde anneannem yine beni her zamanki gibi karşılayıp şaka yaptığını söyleyecek diye düşünüyordum. Böyle düşünüyordum ama ağlıyordum.

Elimde, okurmuş gibi yaptığım ama aslında tek satırını bile anlamadığım bir kitap vardı. Yanımda oturan kadın, "Çok mu acıklı kitap? Okumayın kızım, ben acıklı kitapları sevmem, zaten hayat yeterince acıklı," dedi.

Yalan mı?

Eve gelirken kendi kendime dedim ki, bu ne acayip yolculuk, daha dün bambaşka bir yerde, sisler içindeki eski zaman kentinde kendini masal kahramanı sanıyordun, şimdi yine bir eski zaman kentinde taksinin içinde bambaşka duygudasın.

Bangır bangır arabesk şarkı çalıyordu. Taksinin naylonla kaplanmış arka koltuğunda sallanıyordum, benimle birlikte arka camdaki oyuncak köpek de başını sallıyordu.

Yıkık dökük binlerce yıllık surların önünden geçiyorduk. Çok yaşlı, kambur bir adam sırtındaki çuvalla topladığı çöpleri arkasından sürüklemeye çalışıyordu.

Binlerce yıllık surlar... Dünyanın en büyük imparatorluklarından birinin meydan okumasının simgesi olarak yapılmış... Hemen önünde çöpleri taşıyarak yaşamaya çalışan yaşlı bir adam...

Sanki bütün bu imparatorlukların çöplüğünü taşırmış gibi bir ifade var yüzünde.

Dün hiç bilmeden geçtiğim sokaklarla, hayatımı geçirdiğimi sandığım ama aslında farkında bile olmadığım ülkemin sokakları arasında gerçekle rüya arasında incecik bir çatlak bulmuş gibi dolaşıyorum.

Yanımızda çalan çıngırakla kendime geliyorum, sebze yüklenmiş bir atlı araba yanımızdan geçiyor.

Aynı anda gürültüyle solumuzda dev gemiler...

Sağımızda kırık dökük evler... Pencerelere asılmış çamaşırlar... Neredeyse çökmek üzere olan ahşap eski zaman konakları...

Deniz fenerinin yanından geçiyoruz.

Ve bir tren geçiyor o eski mahallelerin arasından...

Trenler, gemiler, arabalar, faytonlar, uçaklar...

Hep bir yere mi gitmek istiyoruz?

Ne bulacağımızı düşündüysek...

Rengarenk çamaşırlar uçuşuyor, çocuklar küçük kağıttan topun peşinde koşuşuyor, gemilerin ne olduğunu anlamadığım düdükleri, martıların sanki çok ciddi şeyler anlatırmış gibi bağırışları...

Eski takside sallanarak gidiyorum ve dünyalar birbirine karışıyor...

Ben kimim?

Dün neredeydim? Şimdi neredeyim?

Puslu bir günün içinden çıkıp geldim.

Kimbilir ne zaman burayı korumak için yapılan surların önünden gidiyoruz. Eskiden düşmanı korkutsa da şimdi yıkık dökük, yosun tutmuş perişan taş parçaları...

Herşeye rağmen koruyamamışlar.

Ve koku...

Kömür kokusu, deri kokusu, çöplerin kokusu, lodosla gelen yosun kokusu, kentin atıklarının kokusu, taksideki keskin vanilya kokusu, şoförden gelen tütün kokusu, balık kokusu…

Yoksulluğun kokusu…

Buradayım.

Kendi ülkemde.

Evet, bu benim ülkemin kokusu, benim kokum.

Nereye gidersem gideyim benimle gelecek.

Benim evim burası.

Aslında neyle karşılaşacağımı bilmiyordum. Annem telefonda gevelemişti ama ona inanmıyordum. Beni evde Saniye'yle Seda karşıladı.

Doğruca hastaneye gittik. Sare Hanım yoğunbakımdaydı. Beynine pıhtı gitmiş ama doktorlar henüz ne yapacaklarına karar verememişler.

Seda kem küm anlatıyordu...

"Hayır, ona birşey olmaz, o atlatır," diyordum ağlamamak için takside.

Ama annem beni görür görmez ağlamaya başladı. Bekleme odası kalabalıktı. Daha birkaç akşam önce her zamanki gibi gülüp eğlenirken şimdi burada kaygılı, asık yüzlerle bekliyor, alçak sesle konuşuyorlardı.

Yanına girmeme izin verdiler. Her yerine borular bağlanmış, yanında garip sesler çıkartan makinalar, oksijen maskesi, öylece yatıyordu. Gözleri kapalı. Uyur gibi...

İncelmiş damarlarına iğne takılmış. Elini tuttum. Sanki elimi sıktığını hissettim.

"Ben geldim," dedim.

Kopmak üzere olan gergin bir tel gibi hissediyordum kendimi.

Sakın ağlama.

Bir keresinde ben fenalaştığımda yanıma gelmişti. "Ölecek miyim anneanne?" diye sormuştum. "Kimse ölmüyor, daha uzun zaman buralarda olmanı istiyoruz, hem insan öyle kolay kolay ölmez merak etme, olsa olsa çile çeker, hem dur bakalım ben dururken sen nereye gidiyorsun," diye güldürmüştü beni.

"Hatırladın mı anneanne," dedim, "daha uzun süre buralarda olmanı istiyoruz, uzun, güzel bir uyku çekip sonra yanımıza geleceksin..."

Çıktım, insanlarla konuşuyordum, annemle konuşuyordum ama sanki hala o sisin içinde gibiydim. Sürekli birileri gelip gidiyordu. Ne konuşmaları tam anlıyordum ne de elimden birşey geliyordu. Kulağımdaki ağrı dayanılmaz hale gelmişti.

Yürürken bir ara ayağımı boşa atıyormuşum gibi oldu, az daha düşüyordum, duvara tutundum belli etmeden, su alıp bir yere oturdum.

Sonra Taner Amca geldi. "Şu anda yapabileceğimiz hiçbir şey yok, doktoruyla konuştum, beklemek zorundayız, Sare Hanım güçlüdür, siz de güçlü olacaksınız," dedi.

Evet o güçlüdür. Her zaman herşeyin üstesinden gelir. Ama şimdi kıpırdamadan yatıyor. Çaresiz. Aklından birşey geçiyor da söyleyemiyor mu? Neler olduğunun farkında mı? Yoksa yalnızca derin, sessiz bir uykuda mı?

Hayır ben değilim. Ben güçlü filan değilim. Olmak da istemiyorum artık. Bunca zaman yalnızca güçlü olmayı oynadım.

Yıllardır en yorgun olduğum zamanlarda bile kulağımdaki o ağrıyla, derinlerden, çok uzaktan gelen sesle yaşamaya alıştım. Çocukken kendi kendime bunu geçirmenin mutlaka bir yolu olduğuna inanırdım. Kafamı sıkmak, ellerimle alnımı ovuşturmak, kulaklarımı kapamak, yastığın altına girmek, soğuk suyun altında durmak, dua etmek...

Ama öyle olmuyor.

Taner Amca yanıma geldi, oturdu, "Sen iyi misin?" dedi.

O benim yalnızca doktorum değil. Benim şansım. Ona hep güvendim. Ne söylerse yaptım. Acıdan ağlarken, artık düşünemezken, herşeyden vazgeçerken beni azarlamasına bile alışığım. Ama şimdi o da çaresiz görünüyor.

Boş boş yüzüne baktım. İyi miyim? Düne kadar o kadar iyiydim ki... Yollarda çizgi film kahramanları gibi sıçrayarak yürüyordum.

"Yarını bekleyeceğiz. Sabah yeniden gelirim. Seni içeri alacaklar. Yanına gidip elini tut. Onunla konuş. Seni duyacağını biliyorum."

Neden ağlamamaya çalışıyorum?

Binlerce yıldır varoluşla yokoluşu kimse çözebildi mi?

O eski uygarlıkların, ölüm ülkesine giderken neler yapmamız gerektiğini anlatan kitaplarını hatırlıyorum burada, ayaklarını sürüyerek dolaşan, artık gerçek hayatlarındaki alışkanlıklarını umursamayan, bıkkın, asık yüzlü insanların arasında...

İşte şimdi oradayız. Yaşamla ölüm arasında.

Asla çözemediğimiz o incecik sınırda.

Hep biri öldüğünde ne derdi gülerek, "E canım buraya kazık kakacak halimiz yok ya, elbet bir gün uykuya dalacağız ve kimbilir belki de bu en güzel uykumuz olacak..."

Aklımda daha birkaç gece önce dinlediğimiz o güzel şarkı var.

Ferhat geçiyor aklımdan, neden burada olmadığını hatırlıyorum. Londra dönüşü Van'a gideceğini, orada çocuklarla çalışma yapacağını...

Yoğunbakımın bekleme odası geceyarısı bile dolu. "Ne çok seveni varmış," diyorlar. Gidip pencereden bakıyorum. Başka hastalarla birlikte öylece yatıyor. Onların yakınları da kaygılı...

"Elini tuttum ve o da elimi sıktı," diyorum doktora, "Bazen istemsizce yaparlar, şu an bilincinin açık olduğunu söyleyemem," diyor ve işine geri dönüyor.

Onun için, hayatla ölüm, bilinenle bilinmeyen arasındaki sınır sıradan... Kimbilir kaç kişinin oradan oraya geçtiğini görüyor her gün.

Ama ben elini tuttum. Eli sıcaktı. Elimi sıktı.

Ben biliyorum.

En azından...

Bilmek istiyorum.

Neden hiçbirimiz, her gün herkesin başına gelenlerin sonunda bizim de başımıza geleceğini düşünmeyiz?

O benim bütün hayatımı değiştiren kadın.

Belki bana hayatı öğreten kadın.

Doktorların söylediklerini hiç dinlemedi ki... Hep gülüp geçti.

"İnsan ya kendisine hayatı yasaklar ya da hayatını yaşar," derdi hep.

Çünkü uzun yıllar o yasaklarla yaşamıştı. Doğru olanı yapmaya, yapılması gerekenleri düşünmeye çalışmıştı.

"Hayatın bütün bilgisine sahip olduğuna inanan ve bize ne yapmamız gerektiğini söyleyip duranlardan kaçı sonsuza dek yaşadı, var mı etrafta öyle bir tanıdığınız?" diye kahkahayı patlatmıştı bir keresinde.

Bunca yılda onu nadiren başında buz torbasıyla yatarken görmüştüm.

Hastalık sözünü bile sevmezdi.

Bir kış, ciğerleri sökülür gibi öksürürken doktor ona sigarayı tamamen yasaklamıştı. O gider girmez, ünlü bir yazarın hediye ettiği uzun ağızlığı çekmeceden çıkarttı, "Ne yapalım bundan sonra bununla içeceğiz," deyip yaktı.

Sabaha karşı hastanede, kirli, yer yer döşemesi sökülmüş kanepede oturuyorum. Annem ağlamaktan bitap düşmüş kucağıma uzanıyor. Yorgun. Saçlarını okşuyorum ve ona acıyorum.

Neden bu inanılmaz insanın, torunuyla kurduğu ilişkiyi kızıyla kuramadığını düşünüyorum.

Hiç konuşmadık bunları.

Her zaman annesinden uzak durduğunu, ondan çekindiğini, ona içten içe gizli bir öfke duyduğunu ama onu çok sevdiğini biliyorum.

Saniye sanki evdeymişiz gibi hastaneyi ezber etmiş, bize yiyecek içecek getiriyor, hastabakıcılar etrafımızda pervane olmuş, onlara emirler yağdırıyor.

Seda şaşkın, ne yapacağını bilmez halde beni rahatlatmak için durmadan konuşuyor.

Dinlemiyorum.

Çok yorgunum.

Yine rüyayla gerçek arasındaki o buğulu alandayım.

Daha birkaç gün önce tümüyle kaybettiğimi sandığım insanı yeniden bulmuştum.

Bütün kenti kaplayan sis onu görünce silinip gitti.

İnsanın içindeki duygunun, gerçek bir duygunun, siz istediniz diye öylesine kaybolup gitmeyeceğini anladım.

Mutsuzluktan mutluluğa geçiş yalnızca bir andı.

Ve birkaç gün sonra tam tersi de yalnızca bir an...

Artık biliyorum, mutluluk sürüp giden birşey değil.

Mutsuzluk da öyle.

Ara ara kapalı kapının camından içeri bakıyorum. Öylece yatıyor. Uzun, derin bir rüyada gibi...

Eğer konuşabilseydi, "Şu kordonları sök ve beni buradan çıkarıp eve götür," derdi. Onun tonlamasıyla...

Garip ama gülümsüyorum.

Dedim ya rüyayla gerçek arasındaki buğulu alandayım diye...

Peki gerçeklerle yüzleşmeye hazır mıyım?

Tabii ki hayır.

Galiba sabaha karşı uyuyakalmışım. Saniye, çayla simit getirip beni uyandırdı. Doktor gelmişti ama değişiklik yoktu.

Bir iki saat sonra birkaç doktor biraraya gelip ne yapacaklarına karar vereceklerdi.

Anladığım kadarıyla ameliyat yapmak istiyorlar ama yaşı nedeniyle buna cesaret edemiyorlardı.

Rüyamda Ferhat'ın, bir şiirin dizelerini dev bir tuvale resmettiğini görmüştüm. Yere yaydığı kocaman tuvalin üzerinde harflerle oynuyordu.

Sonra kendimi uzaklarda, deniz kıyısında görüyorum, neden anneannemin yanında değilim diye suçluluk duyuyorum, birilerine geri dönmek istediğimi anlatıyorum ama yanımda kimliğim yok ve nerede olduğumu bilmiyorum. Size yardım edemeyiz diyorlar. Dillerini bilmediğim insanların arasındayım, neden orada olduğumu, ne yapacağımı bilmiyorum ve paniğe kapılıyorum.

Uyandım ama rüyanın etkisi hala üzerimde.

Bir türlü kendime gelemiyorum.

Başımda garip bir uyuşukluk, kulağımda yine o uğultu...

Kendini topla.

Çayımı içerken birden kapı açıldı ve o içeri girdi.

Üzerinde yine o eski balıksırtı palto, saçlar dağınık, sakalları biraz uzamış...

Bu şimdi gerçek mi?

Gelip bana sarılınca gerçek olduğunu anlıyorum.

"Sen... Van'da değil miydin?"

"Bir arkadaşım aradı, atlayıp geldim," diyor.

Annem, Seda, herkes bize bakıyor.

Bu adamın kim olduğunu biliyorlar ama neden buraya geldiğini, neden bana böyle sarıldığını kimse bilmiyor.

Daha neye uğradığımı şaşırmışken hemşire içeriden çıkıp doktora sesleniyor. Genç doktor koşarak yoğunbakıma giriyor.

Birşeyler oluyor.

Hepimiz yoğunbakımın kapısına gidiyoruz.

Sare Hanım yüzündeki oksijen maskesini çıkarıp atmış, damarlarındaki iğneleri sökmeye çalışıyor.

Rüyadan uyanıyorum.

İçeri girmek istiyorum, bırakmıyorlar.

Son durağa geliyoruz. Az kaldı. Aslında çok da uzun olmayan bir yolculukta bugüne kadar sanki vakit bulamamışım gibi bütün hayatımı yeniden düşünüyorum.

Ne garip, unutulmuş anılar çıkıp geliyor, hiç üstünde durmadığım ayrıntılar beliriyor, bazı şeylerin hatırladığım gibi olmadığını anlıyorum, bazılarını ne kadar zorlasam da hatırlamakta güçlük çekiyorum.

Belki de bazılarını şimdi böyle geriye bakarken yeniden anlamlandırıyorum.

Belki de onlara olmayan anlamlar yüklüyorum.

Ama öyle olmamış mıydı?

O sabah daha tam uyanamamışken, hiç aklımda yokken o kapıdan girmiş ve aynı anda anneannem kendine gelmişti.

Yalnızca rastlantı mı?

O zamana kadar kendimi tutmuştum ama artık daha fazla dayanamadım ve Ferhat'a sarılıp deli gibi ağlamaya başladım.

Yaşlı doktor geldi, içeri girdi. Annemle Saniye dualar okuyordu.

"Geri döndü," dedim Ferhat'a, "döndü değil mi?"

"Buraya gelirken içimden geçtiği gibi..." dedi.

Bir keresinde Taner Amca'yla benim hastalığımdan konuşurken, "Belki gökyüzü hakkında bile çok şey biliyoruz ama kendi beynimiz hakkında pek az şey..." demişti.

Şimdi yaşlı doktor da benzer şeyler söylüyordu. O bilinçsizlik hali geçmişti ama ne zaman ne olacağını bilmiyorlardı. Bir tarafı tutmuyordu. Yüzü kaymış gibi, ağzı uyuşuk, güçlükle konuşuyor, dediklerinin ancak bir kısmı anlaşılıyordu.

Bunun da kalıcı olup olmadığı belli değildi.

Yine de hepimiz mutluyduk. En azından geri gelmişti. Eve gitmek istiyordu ama doktor izin vermedi. "Biraz daha elimizin altında olsun, her an müdahale etmek gerekebilir, böyle zamanlarda dakikalar bile çok önemli," dedi.

Tabii onu ikna etmek de bana düştü.

Ertesi gün odaya çıkartma sözü verdik. O soğuk odada, iki dünya arasındaki bekleme odasında öylece kıpırdamadan yatmak istemiyordu.

Sonra Taner Amca geldi, doktoruyla birlikte yeniden yanına girdiler. "Bu gece bizim için önemli," dedi sonra, "bu geceyi yoğunbakımda geçirsin, ani birşey olmasını istemiyoruz, bazı ilaçlar veriyoruz, heyecan ya da panik yeni bir duruma yol açabilir, yanına girebilirsiniz ama fazla kalmayın ve mümkünse ağlamayın. Ben yarın daha iyi haberler vereceğimi düşünüyorum..."

"Durumunun farkında mı?" diye sordum.

"Az çok," dedi, "şu anda aslında yarı uyur durumda, kriz geçirdiğini ve düzeleceğini, kontrol altında olduğunu söylüyoruz, bu gece uyuyacak, konuşurken saçmalarsa korkmayın..."

Üşüdüm. Akşam oluyor. Çayla kurabiye yiyorum. Neden bütün bunları yazmadım diye kızıyorum kendime.

Sanki yazmak hayatı saklamaya yetermiş gibi...

Sanki hayatımın romanını yazarmış gibi yolculuk bitmeden tüm bunları hatırlamaya çalışıyorum.

Neden?

Bir anlam bulmak için mi?

Gerçekten de bir anlamı var mı?

Bütün bu görüntülerin, rüyaların, bunca yılda yaşanan, hiç nedensiz biçimde kimileri unutulmazken kimileri yitip giden anların, beklenmedik bir karşılaşmayla bütün hayatımızı değiştiren insanların, onca çalışmanın, mutluluğun, ilk karşılaşmadan sonra bizi hep kaygılandıran korkuların, hastalıkların, ölümlerin, ölümü unutabilmek için bunca çabalamanın, taşınılan evlerin, kurulan hayatların, bütün bu eşyanın, uzaklara gitmenin, geri dönmenin, aşkların, sevgilerin, ayrılıkların, kavgaların, peşinden gidilen sözlerin, tutmaktan vazgeçilen sözlerin, bizim yalnızca kısa bir zaman diliminde içinden geçip gittiğimiz ama yine de değiştireceğimize inandığımız hayatın gerçekten anlamı var mı?

O gün Ferhat'ın telaşlı ve düşünceli bir hali olduğunu sanırım farketmedim. Zaten o anda neyin farkındaydım ki...

Gitmesi gerektiğini söyledi.

"Senin gelmeni hiç beklemiyordum," dediğimde, yüzüme gülümseyerek bakıp, "Hayır, bekliyordun..." dedi.

Sonra bana sıkıca sarıldı.

Vedalaştık.

Anneannem görmese de yoğunbakımın penceresinden içeri baktı ve ona el salladı.

Birkaç gün sonra eve döndük.

Sonunda kurtulduğu için mutluyduk. Ama artık eskisi gibi değildi.

İşte bir bulut gelmiş ve bütün resmi, renkleri, ışığı, müziği değiştirmişti.

Sare Hanım büyük koltuğunda oturuyor, boşluğa bakıyor, yüzünde bambaşka bir ifade var artık. Bir yanı tutmuyor. Artık istediğini yapamıyor. Aslında yapmak da istemiyor.

İstekleri dışında pek konuşmuyor. Her gün alması gereken sürüyle ilaç var.

Biz sanki hayat eskisi gibi oyunu oynuyoruz ama tabii ki beceremiyoruz.

İlk günler gelen giden eksik olmuyor.

Ama sonra onlar da yavaş yavaş azalıyor. Zaten onların gelmesinden çok memnun görünmüyor. Çoğu zaman konuşan insanlara değil de uzaktaki bir noktaya bakıyor.

Çocukken anneme kızdığım zaman kendimce böyle bir oyun oynardım. Saatlerce dalıp gider, hiç konuşmazdım. Deli olurdu annem.

Şimdi o da sanki böyle yapıyor. Küsmüş çocuk gibi...

Sanki bir yanı o hiçbirimizin bilmediği ama onun gördüğü dünyada kalmış gibi...

Eve ilk geldiğimizde ayna istedi. Eski el aynasını getirdim. Kendine baktı, baktı, iç geçirdi. Bir daha da istemedi.

Onu böylece bırakıp gidemezdim. Neredeyse gittiğim için kendimi suçluyordum zaten.

Kaydımı dondurmaya karar verdim.

Taner Amca, ona her gün çeşitli hareketler yaptıracak birini buldu. O ne yaparsa yapsın eskisi gibi davranmamızı, konuşmamızı istedi.

"Şu andaki durumu aslında beynindeki sıkıntıdan çok kendisini bu durumda görmek istememekten kaynaklanan bir depresyon ama ağır bir depresyon... Bunun için de bir doktor arkadaşımı göndereceğim. Durumunu kabullenmesi ve yeniden yaşamaya başlaması lazım. Şu an yaşamayı durdurmuş halde."

Yaşamayı durdurmak...

Öyle iyi biliyordum ki bu duyguyu...

Kimbilir kaç gece artık vazgeçmek, durdurmak değil, sonlandırmak bile istememiş miydim?

Şimdi tıpkı onun yaptığı gibi sürekli uyumak, karanlıkta kalmak, yorganın içinden çıkmamak...

O bir sürü ilacı artık içmemek...

Taner Amca'yı geçirirken kolumu tuttu, "Bence okuluna dönsen daha iyi edersin ama senin kararın yine de... Pek çok hasta bu durumda böyle tepki verir ama zamanla geçer. En azından sizinle burada... Sen kendini çok üzme, çok fazla düşünme, bunların geçeceğine inan. Bu arada seninle konuşmam gerekenler var ama yalnız. Bir ara bana uğra..." dedi.

Meraklandım ama çok üstünde durmadım.

O ışıltılı geceler, o güzel sabahlar, o evin neşesi kaybolup gitti. Sessizlik, hüzün, sıkıntı geldi yerine. Alışmadığımız, bilmediğimiz bir hayat başladı.

Eskiden buraya nadiren inen annem artık hep aşağıdaydı ve annesine bakmaktan sanki memnun gibiydi. Bunca yıl sonra Sare Hanım ilk kez ona muhtaçtı.

Ne demişti bana bir akşam:

"Çok şey bilince hiç birşey bilmiyormuş gibi olursun... çok şey yaşayınca hiç yaşamamış gibi olursun… çok yaşlanırsan çocuk gibi olursun…"

Şimdi o çocuk gibiydi ve annem de onun annesi gibi...

Yalnızca birkaç ay önce buradan giderken "yeni bir hayat" demiştim.

Çok kısa süre sonra böyle geri döneceğim ve yeni hayatın bambaşka bir biçim alacağı aklımın ucundan bile geçmemişti.

Hastaneye geldiği o sabahtan sonra Ferhat'tan ses çıkmamıştı. Birkaç kez telefon ettim ama telefon açılmıyordu.

Yeniden Van'a döndüğünü düşündüm.

Ama dönmemişti.

Herhalde birkaç hafta sonraydı. Anneannemi ziyarete gelen yaşlı gazeteci onun yurtdışına kaçtığını söyledi.

Kaçmak mı?

Şaşkın şaşkın baktım.

O kadar habersizdim ki olup bitenlerden.

Londra'ya geldiğinde bana Van'da çocuklar için yapacağı atölye çalışmasını uzun uzun anlatmıştı. İnanılmaz heyecan içindeydi.

İstanbul'da bunca konuşulan bir ressamken yeni sergi açmak yerine oraya gitmesi beni çok etkilemişti. Sergileri çok konuşuluyor ama resimleri satılmıyordu.

Galericiler ondan, daha küçük boyutta, evlere, işyerlerine asılacak, "karamsar olmayan" resimler çizmesini istiyorlardı.

"İçimden gelmeyenleri nasıl çizebilirim ki?" diyordu.

Sanırım uzun zaman yapmak istediğiyle yapması gerekenler arasında kalmaktan çok sıkılmıştı. Öte yandan para kazanması gerekiyordu. Sonra ünlü bir galericiyle anlaşmış, ona sergi sözü vermiş ve çocuklarla yapacağı bu çalışma için para almış.

Londra'ya da o parayla gelmiş olmalıydı. Gözlerinin parladığını farketmiştim yapacaklarını anlatırken... Sanki kendi doğup büyüdüğü topraklara geri dönerek aslında yaptıklarının anlamını yeniden bulmaya çalışıyordu. Bütün bu para konuşmalarının, pazarlama çabalarının, onu biçimlendirme isteklerinin dışına çıkmak istiyordu belki de...

Ama onbeş günlük kamp sırasında gözaltına alınmış, terör örgütüyle ilişkisi olduğu, çocukları buna alet ettiği gibi suçlamalarla sorgulanmıştı.

Gazeteci bunları anlatırken ne hissettiğimi bugün gibi hatırlıyorum.

Korku, büyük bir çarpıntı, şaşkınlık...

Böyle birşey olmadığına, asla olamayacağına emindim ama onun o kapalı hayatı nedeniyle daha önce başka konularda hakkında ne kadar çok söylenti varsa şimdi bundan da pek çoklarının kuşkulanacağını hatta inanacağını biliyordum.

Öyle bir zamandı ki akla gelmedik insanlara akla gelmedik suçlar atılıyor ve onlar kendilerini savunamadan birileri televizyonda, gazetelerde onları hemen mahkum ediveriyor, geçmişe dönüp, söylediklerinden, yazdıklarından kendilerince deliller buluyor, daha sorguları bile bitmeden cezayı kesiyorlardı.

Kimse tam olarak neler olduğunu anlamıyordu.

Herkes komplodan, kumpastan sözediyordu ama kimin kime komplo yaptığını, hangisinin doğru olduğunu kimse tam olarak anlayamıyordu.

Öyle çok ses çıkıyordu ki sesiniz o seslerin içinde boğulup gidiyor, aylar, yıllar süren davalar sırasında hapislere atılan insanların söyledikleri artık duyulmaz oluyordu.

Üstelik bu duruma herkes alışmaya başlamış, artık en olmadık insanlar hakkındaki en garip suçlamalar bile normal hale gelmişti.

Kimse kimseye inanmıyor, insanlar yakından tanıdıkları hakkında söylenenlere bile itiraz etmek yerine "acaba olabilir mi" diye düşünmeye başlıyordu.

Belki de asıl korkunç olan buydu.

En yakınlarından, yıllarca tanıdığın insanlardan hatta en sonunda kendinden bile kuşkuya düşmek...

Sare Hanım bunları dinlerken baktığı o boşluktan gözlerini çevirdi, bize döndü, "Nerede?" diye sordu.

Uzun zaman sonra ilk kez bir konuşmayla ilgilenmişti.

Gazeteci, "Gözaltında epeyce eziyet görmüş ama sonra bırakmışlar, galiba izlendiğini ve yeniden tutuklanacağını anlamış, yurtdışına kaçmış, şimdi nerede olduğunu kimse bilmiyor..." dedi.

Sıradan bir haberi anlatır gibiydi.

Birden o sabaha döndüm.

Yüzündeki o garip, düşünceli, kaygılı, yorgun ifade buydu demek ki...

Yine de oraya gelmişti.

Veda etmeye mi?

Belki de telaşla gitmesinin nedeni buydu.

Belki de oradan çıkıp bilinmeyen bir yere gidiyordu.

Belki de bana söylemek isteyip de söyleyemediğini düşündüğüm buydu.

"İşin kötüsü," diye devam etti gazeteci, "yakalama kararı çıkartmışlar, kaçmasaydı şu anda hapiste olacaktı..."

Kalktım. İçeri gittim. Karanlıkta duvara yaslanıp yere oturdum. Kulaklarımdaki çınlama neredeyse çığlığa dönüştü. Ellerimle kulaklarımı kapadım.

Ama işe yaramadı.

Çığlık dışarıdan gelmiyordu çünkü.

Çığlık benim içimdeydi.

Belki ancak şimdi aradan zaman geçince anlayabiliyorum bazı şeyleri.

Anneannemin hep güçlü, canlı, neşeli görünmesi aslında onun en büyük korkusuna karşı oluşturduğu bir kalkandı.

Ölüm.

Dedemin uzun ve acılı ölüm sürecini gün gün yaşamıştı. Onun artık bedeninin neredeyse tükendiği, her yerinde yaralar açıldığı günlerin ardından bilincini kaybetmesi, olur olmaz konuşması, kimseyi tanımaması Sare Hanım'da büyük bir korku yaratmıştı.

Ama sonuna kadar ona bakmış, her zaman başkalarının onu görmek istediği gibi güçlü, dirayetli, cesur bir kadın olmanın ağırlığını taşımak zorunda kalmıştı.

Onu kaybettikten sonra bambaşka bir hayat kurması, sürekli ışıkları yanan evde hiç yalnız kalmak istememesi, her akşam toplanan insanlar, eğlenceler, müzik aslında hepsi bu korkuyla ilgiliydi.

Doktorların tüm uyarılarına rağmen ne en küçük bir hastalığı ne de yaşlandığını kabul etmişti.

"İlaçlarımı alıyorum işte daha ne istiyorlar, sigara yok, kahve yok, o yok, bu yok, böyle de yaşanmaz ki canım," diye kestirip atardı.

Benim hastalığımı kabullenmeyişi, neredeyse görmezden gelmesi, beni de hep güçlü durmaya, olup bitenlerle başa çıkmaya zorlaması da bundandı.

Oysa aslında birçok doktorla konuşmuş, neler olup bittiğini ayrıntılarıyla öğrenmişti.

Belki de sonunda onların da gerçekte ne yapacaklarını bilmediğini, bir çare olmadığını anlayıp yapılacak tek şeyin bu hastalıkla yaşamak olduğunu düşünmüştü.

Ya da hep yaptığı gibi kötü şeyleri kapının dışında tutmak istemişti. Hep kızmaz mıydı bize, "Ölümden sözetmeyin çünkü o hep buralarda bir yerlerdedir, duyar, gelir," diye...

Annemle ilişkisinin bozulmasına, son yıllarında bütün enerjisini dedeme vermek zorunda kalıp kızıyla yeterince ilgilenemeyişinin neden olduğunu (bunu hiç söylemese de) bence biliyordu.

Hatta babamı seçmesine karşı çıktığı halde annemin onu dinlemeyişinde bile kendisini suçluyordu. Belki de gerçekten bu annemin ondan öç alma yoluydu.

Üstüne üstlük babamın gitmesinden sonra bir de bizimle ilgilenmesi gerekmişti.

Hayır, bundan şikayetçi değildi. Aksine bizim burada olmamızdan çok memnundu. Beni her gördüğünde "İşte benim küçük mutluluğum, neşem," derdi.

Bazen onun hayatını düşünürken, belki de ölümün bir gün birdenbire çıkageleceğini ve o zamana kadar istediği gibi yaşaması gerektiğini düşünüyordum.

Sanırım, bizlerin, çevresindeki insanların onunla ilgili algısına, sanki her zaman burada kalacağı, başına birşey gelmeyeceği yanılsamasına bir zaman sonra kendisi de inanmıştı.

Ve sonra en büyük korkusuyla yüzleşmişti.

O bekleme odasında yatarken aslında uzak ve geri dönülmez ülkenin kapısındaydı.

Ama eğer böyleyse ve o korkuyu yaşayıp geri geldikten sonra neden kaldığı yerden devam edemiyordu?

Başımı okşarken ona bakıyordum. Onu böyle görmek beni çok üzüyordu. Sanki gerçekten de çok uzaklardan gelmiş gibi yorgundu. Sanki artık o sırrı öğrenmiş ama söyleyemiyor gibi bir hali vardı.

Hayır, kötü düşünmeyecektim. Zaman geçecek ve o yeniden eski Sare Hanım olacaktı. Yine buraya insanlar gelecek, yine müzik çalacak, danslar edilecek, kahkahalar geceyarısından sonra bile etraftan duyulacaktı.

"Sen ne zaman okuluna dönüyorsun?" diye sordu bir akşam.

Onunla kalmak ve onu yeniden eski haliyle görmek istiyordum. O anda tek istediğim buydu.

"Ben o okulu sevmedim, burada okuyacağım," dedim.

İnanacak sanki...

Yüzümü okşadı, gülümsemeye çalıştı.

İlk kez bu evde dört kadın yalnız başımızaydık. Saniye sanki bu sayede tüm bunlar düzelecekmiş gibi durmadan yiyecek birşeyler getiriyordu. Şimdi de onun çok sevdiği meyve şekerlemelerinden getirmişti.

Annem her nedense vazgeçemediği Barbara Cartland romanlarından birini okuyordu.

Kalktım, ışıkların hepsini yaktım. Müzik dolabından onun sevdiği plaklardan birini alıp çalmaya başladım.

"Kimse bir yere gitmiyor Sare Hanım," dedim, "hepimiz burada yanındayız..."

Zoraki gülümsedi.

Hepimiz...

Ama sanki o artık burada değildi.

Belki de hayatımızın en sessiz, en uzun kışıydı.

Kendimi içinde bulunduğum garip ruh halinden kurtarmak için ne yapacağımı bulmaya çalışıyordum. En çok da ebru. Neredeyse her gün...

Kağıdın üzerine aldıktan ve kuruttuktan sonra getirip anneanneme gösteriyordum. Bu ona çok iyi geldi. Garip bir biçimde onları görünce heyecanlanıyor, biraz geciksem sesleniyor, bitmedi mi hala diye soruyordu.

Ara sıra Seda'yla dışarı çıkıyor, dertleşiyorduk.

Belli etmiyordum ama başımdaki uyuşukluk, kulağımdaki ağrı ve sesler giderek artıyordu.

Birşeyin geldiğini biliyor ve çok korkuyordum.

Hiç sırası değildi.

Ne olur şimdi olmasın diye dua ediyordum her gece.

Yürürken sarhoş gibi birden ayağım boşluğa basıyor, bir yerlere, birine tutunmak zorunda kalıyordum ve bu giderek daha da sıklaşmıştı.

Bir yere uzun süre bakınca orada sanki boşluktaki ekranda film izler gibi başka görüntüler beliriyordu. Uyanıkken rüya görüyordum.

Sabahları erken saatte çarpıntıyla uyanıyor, yeniden uyumaya çalışırken başımdaki uyuşma yüzünden bir türlü dalamıyor ve böyle saatler geçiriyordum.

O kış ne çok kar yağdı.

Sare Hanım koltuğunu pencerenin önüne aldırdı. Oradan lapa lapa yağan kara bakar ve gülümserdi.

Denizin üstüne yağan kar, her iki kıyıdaki koruları kaplayan beyazlık, çok üşümemize rağmen iyi geldi bize.

Fazla iyileşme yoktu ama aylar geçtikçe daha çok konuşmaya başladı. Söylediklerini biz alıştığımız için anlıyorduk ama misafirler zorlanıyordu. Bu da onun canını sıkıyor, sonra yorulduğunu söyleyip başka kimseyi istemiyordu. Tek elini kullanmaya alıştı. Önceleri kahvesini eli titrediği için dökerken hemen her gün gelen terapist sayesinde güçlendi.

Hatta en baştan kesinlikle reddettiği tekerlekli iskemleyle onu birkaç kez dışarı da çıkardık. Çok sevdiği köşedeki balıkçıda Yorgo Amca ona harika bir buğulama yaptı.

Ferhat'tan hiç ses yoktu. Nereye gittiğini, ne yaptığını kimse bilmiyordu. Hakkındaki dava devam ediyor, herkes iddiaların çok kötü olduğunu, çok büyük bir ceza geleceğini söylüyordu. Onunla bağlantılı tanıdığım kimse yoktu. Mecbur kalmasa böyle yapmayacağını, en azından bana haber ulaştıracağını düşünüyordum ama yine de kızıyordum ona.

Selçuk Bey'i aradım, başkalarını buldum ama sanki herkes bir sırrı saklar gibi suspus olmuştu.

Sonra biri geldi ve onun Almanya'ya gittiğini, orada eski sevgilisinin evine yerleştiğini söyledi.

Boğazımda birşey düğümlendi. Başım döndü. Daha fazla soramadım. Doğru mu, yalan mı? Bilemedim. Ama öyledir ya, insan hep kötüsüne inanır.

Bu kader mi? Babam gibi aynı ülkeye mi gitti?

Kırgındım.

Ona, hayata hatta anneanneme bile...

Ne yapalım ki benimki de böyle bir hayattı.

Bir gün Seniha Teyze yaptığım ebrulara bakarken, "Bak aklıma ne geldi," dedi, "bunları kumaşlara basalım... İpek fularlar, eşarplar yapalım."

"Olur mu ki?" dedim.

"Neden olmasın, pek güzel olur ama önce küçük bir sergi açalım, herkes görsün, basında çıksın, ne yapacağımızı anlatalım..."

Tam da artık karların hemen ardından beyaz bahar çiçekleri açmaya başlamıştı.

Daha çok çalışmaya başladım. Artık kocaman bir teknem vardı. Küçük kağıtlar yerine büyük kartonlara alıyordum ebruları.

Ne tuhaf! Beni bırakıp gitmişti. Ama bana birşey bırakmıştı ve o benim bütün hayatımı belirleyecekti. Suyun içinde küçük dokunuşlarla değişen renklerle oluşan bir dünya.

Elinizden kayıp giden rüyalar gibi.

Demişti ki, "Ressam, her zaman yaptığı esere hakimdir, istediğini değiştirir, istediği rengi bozar, yeniden yapar, ama ebru sanatçısı görünmez bir elle birliktedir, bazen yakaladığı deseni, rengi yeniden bulamaz, bazen aklından geçeni yaparken hiç beklenmedik bambaşka bir desenle karşılaşır. Ve belki de asıl yapması gereken odur..."

Kayıp giden rüyalar.

Evet, renklere bakıyordum, desenlere ve onu düşünüyordum aslında, o benim kayıp giden rüyamdı.

Ve evet doğru, benim elimi tutan görünmez bir el vardı.

İşte öyle garip birşey.

Onu hatırlıyordum. Hep içimde bir yerde. Burukluk mu? Mutluluk mu? Özlem mi? Umut mu?

Çünkü günün birinde sanki onu yeniden bulacakmışım gibi, bir yerlerden çıkıp gelecekmiş gibi...

Yapmamış mıydı?

Ama gün günden yaşananlar siliniyor. Unutuluyor. Belki öyle istediğimiz için... Ara sıra kış ortasında yazdan kalma bir gün gibi bulutların arasından güneş parlayıp sönüyor.

Saklambaç oynar gibi...

Tam da öyle değil miydi?

Gözlerimi kapatıp sayarken ortadan yokolmuştu ve onu bulamıyordum.

Aylardan nisan mı? Mayıs mı?

Bilmiyorum.

Çünkü günler bizim için artık başkaları için olduğundan farklıydı. Günler, bu evin içinde yaşananlardı. Perşembe mi, pazartesi mi çok da umurumuzda değildi.

Birşeylerin yeniden değiştiği bir gün olduğunu biliyorum yalnızca.

O eski kulenin yanında daracık arnavut kaldırımı yokuşun üzerindeki galeride sergim açılıyor.

Ebrular çerçevelendi. Hepsine isimler verildi.

Son gece sabaha kadar onları asmakla uğraşırken bakıyorum ve kendi kendime "Bunları ben mi yaptım," diyorum. Yoksa gizemli bir el mi yaptırdı hepsini?

Kapıda fotoğrafım var. Turuncu, yeşil, mavi renklerle dolu bir ebrunun önünde boşluğa bakar gibi duruyorum.

Ben.

Ebru.

Sare Hanım herkesten önce sergiyi geziyor tekerlekli iskemlesinde. Elimi sıkıyor, ağlıyor. Sonra insanlar geliyor. Kalabalık. Gazeteciler sorular soruyor. Cevaplamaya çalışıyorum. Nasıl başladım? Neden başladım? Bundan sonra ne yapacağım?

Kem küm ediyorum. Neyse ki Seniha Teyze var yanımda. Ne söylenmesi gerekiyorsa söylüyor.

Tanıdıklar var, yazarlar, ressamlar, yönetmenler, akşam yemeklerinde birlikte olduğumuz pek çok insan...

Fotoğraflar çekiliyor. Gülümsüyorum.

Tolga, rengarenk çiçekler yollamış, "Sen herşeyin en güzelini yaparsın, orada olamadığım için deliriyorum ama yaza az kaldı, bu ilk sergin ama son olmayacak, sakın hepsini satma, en güzeli benim..." yazmış.

Aklıma mezuniyet gecesi geliyor.

Ferhat yine aniden çıkıp gelir mi?

Buradan, bu kalabalıktan beni çıkartıp nereye kaçtıysa beni de oraya götürür mü?

Hayır, gelmeyeceğini biliyorum.

Ama bu an'ı en çok onun görmesini isterdim.

İlk ebrunun ismi, "Gizli El".

Her neredeyse belki de neden o ismi koyduğumu bilir, hisseder.

Seniha Teyze çok mutlu. "Sana öyle bir koleksiyon yapacağım ki inanamayacaksın, bu fularlar, eşarplar efsane olacak," diye anlatıyor sürekli.

Annem bana sarılıyor. Sare Hanım'la kadeh kaldırıyoruz. Seda yanımdan ayrılmıyor.

Galiba bahar geldi.

Anneannem yoruldu. Annem onu eve götürdü.

İnsanlar içiyor, kendi aralarında konuşuyor ve artık sergiyle ilgilenmiyordu.

Genç kemancı eski çağlardan şarkılar çalıyordu. Başka çağlardan ama yine de bizi içine alıp hüzünlendiren, eski bir zamana taşıyan, yeniden buraya getiren...

Seda'yla bir köşede oturduk.

Ben de yorulmuştum.

Dün gece sabaha kadar düzenlemelerle uğraşmıştım ve heyecandan pek uyuyamıştım.

Kısa, kırlaşmış saçlı, kirli sakallı, ince yünden çok şık koyu yeşil takım giymiş biri geldi yanımıza.

Seda ayaklandı.

Adam ona değil bana bakıyordu.

"Aaa, Onur Bey hoşgeldiniz," dedi.

Sonra benimle tanıştırdı.

Ünlü bir mimardı ama ben tanımıyordum.

"Sizi tebrik etmek istedim, ebrunun bu kadar ilgimi çekeceğini düşünmezdim, uzun zamandır bu kadar hoşuma giden eserler görmedim," dedi.

"Hangi ebrunun?" diye manasız bir espri yaptı Seda.

Zoraki gülümsedim.

Doğruyu söylemem gerekirse hayatımda gördüğüm en yakışıklı adamdı.

Espriyi duymamış gibi yaptı.

Belki şu sakallarını da kesse daha iyi olacaktı.

Yeni restore ettiği bir yalı için ebrulardan bazılarını almak istiyordu.

"Bu yalnızca sergi," dedim, "bunlar satılık değil.."

"Biliyorum,"dedi, "ama eğer gelip yalıyı görürseniz, bunların orada olmasını istersiniz bence, cumartesi sabah işiniz yoksa birlikte gidelim mi?"

Şaşkın şaşkın baktım.

Nereye?

Seda, "Boğazın en güzel yalılarından biri," dedi, "beraber gideriz, en azından görmen lazım çünkü Onur Bey çok güzel şeyler yaptı.."

Bir an gözgöze geldik, gözlerini kaçırdı.

Ne zamandır bana, "Artık biriyle tanışman lazım, bu adamı unutman lazım," deyip duruyordu.

"Aslında biliyor musunuz, evde bunlardan daha çok var, bir ara onları da görmeye gelin, sergi için aralarından zor seçtik," dedi.

O sırada bilmiyordum.

Seda'nın evli bir adamla birlikte olduğunu, Onur'un adamın en yakın arkadaşı olduğunu, bu nedenle tanıştıklarını ve onu o gece benimle tanıştırmak için çağırdığını...

Yalan söylemeyeceğim.

Çok yakışıklı, havalı, güzel konuşan, espriler yapan, etkileyici biriydi.

Sohbet devam ederken birdenbire kalktı, "Bu sizin geceniz, galiba fazla meşgul ettim, cumartesi sabah buluşuyoruz, yeniden tebrik ediyorum," dedi ve elimi sıkıp gitti.

Cumartesi sabah buluşuyor muyuz?

"Bu neydi böyle?" diye sordum Seda'ya.

Muzipçe gülümsedi, "Bilmem, sence?" dedi.

Gerçekten de hayatın bizi nereye sürükleyeceğini, hiç beklenmedik rastlantılarla dünyanın birdenbire değişebileceğini düşünmüyoruz.

Ama öyle oluyor.

Evet itiraf ediyorum ki o gece serginin heyecanıyla, yorgunluğuyla eve geldiğimde, belki de aylardır ilk kez güzel bir uykuya dalarken uzun zaman sonra birinin ilgimi çektiğini düşündüm.

Düşündüm ve bu yüzden utandım.

Öyle derin uyumuşum ki sabah beni uyandırmaya kıyamamışlar. Kendime geldiğimde neredeyse öğle olmuştu.

Sare Hanım bile bunca zaman sonra ilk kez keyifliydi.

Annem herkesin benim yaptıklarımla ilgili söylediklerini anlatıyordu heyecanla.

Kendime gelmek için kahvemi içerken annem, masanın üstüne dizdiği çiçekleri gösterdi.

Biri galeri sahibinden, biri Seniha Teyze'den gelmişti. Ve rengarenk lalelerden kocaman bir buket daha vardı. Küçük zarfın içindeki kartı çıkardım. "Laleler ebrulara yakışır diye düşündüm, görüşmek üzere, tebrikler... Onur..." yazıyordu.

Birden durdum.

Galiba Tolga'dan başka bir erkekten ilk kez çiçek alıyordum.

İyi ama adresi nereden bulmuştu? Galeriye mi bırakmıştı? Annem gözucuyla bana bakıyordu. Tabii ki sormadım.

İlk kez bir erkekten çiçek alıyordum, ilk kez bir erkeği aldattığımı düşünüyordum.

Ne saçmalıyorum ben? Belli ki çapkının biri. Benimle niye ilgilendi bilmem ama ilgilendiği belli. Hoş , zarif bir adam. Hepsi bu. Çok fazla düşünmeye, üstünde durmaya gerek yok.

Kendi kendime bunları söylerken cumartesi sabahını düşünüyor muydum?

Evet, düşünüyordum.

Bir iki gün sonra gazetelerde sergiyle ilgili yazılar çıktı. İlk kez kendi fotoğrafımı gazetede gördüm. Annem hepsini kesip dosyaladı.

Seniha Teyze'yle buluştuk ve neler yapacağımızı konuştuk. Doğrusu şaşkındım. O günlerde bunun yıllar sonra bambaşka birşeye dönüşeceğini, birçok ülkede tanınacağımı ve geçimimi böyle sağlayacağımı hiç düşünmüyordum.

Yalnızca o fularların, eşarpların üzerinde kendi desenlerimi, renklerimi, rüyalarımı görecek olmanın heyecanı içindeydim.

Seda bana herşeyi anlattı. Onun böyle bir ilişkiye girmesine çok şaşırdım. Gizli patikada yürüyordu ve sonuçlarına katlanacaktı. En azından çok uzun zaman sonra mutlu görünmesinin nedeni buydu ve bunu yargılamaya hiç niyetim yoktu. Bazen başkalarının hayatı için susmak en doğrusudur.

Adamın karısından ayrılacağını, zaten çok uzun zamandır mutsuz olduğunu, çok iyi biri olduğunu anlatıp duruyordu. Hem yaptığından utanıyor, hem de vazgeçemiyordu.

Şimdi olsa belki ona, kaçamak zamanların, çalınmış saatlerin, yalnızca keyifli geçirilen günlerin hep yarım kalacağını, sonunda hiç sandığı gibi olmayacağını söylerdim.

Yalnızca Onur'la beni tanıştırmak için planlar yapmasına kızdım. Ama biliyordum ki benim iyiliğimi düşünüyor, kayıp bir aşkın ardından gözyaşı dökmemi, boşu boşuna gelmeyecek birini beklememi istemiyor, içinde bulunduğum durumdan çıkmam için yeni heyecanlar yaşamam gerektiğine inanıyordu.

"O senin eserlerini istiyor, gerisi sana kalmış," dedi.

"Eserlerimi mi?" diye kahkaha attım.

Gece gitsem mi gitmesem mi diye düşünmekten uyuyamadım. Aslında galiba gideceğimi biliyordum ama her nedense içimdeki ses gitmemem gerektiğini söylüyordu.

Gittim.

Sabah Seda gelip beni aldı, bahar sabahı, denizin üstünde ışıklar titrerken sanırım hayatımda gördüğüm en güzel eve girdim.

Ev sahibesiyle Onur bizi kapıda karşıladı.

Zayıf, orta boylu, sade ama bakımlı bir kadın... Herhalde otuzlu yaşlarının sonunda. Yanındaki köpek bile özel seçilmiş. Kızıl kahve renkli uzun tüylü afgan tazısı. Bu ev ona büyük dedesinden kalmış. O zamandan kalan ağaçlarla dolu dev bir bahçe... İnsanın neredeyse bütün gününü yalnızca bakarak geçirebileceği bir manzara... Uzaktan geçen gemiler...

Onur'a baktım gözucuyla. Erkek için fazla şık ve bakımlı diye geçirdim aklımdan.

Öyleydi gerçekten de.

Fazla yakışıklı, fazla bakımlı, fazla düşünceli, fazla esprili.

Belki de bazı insanlar için en başta hissettiğimiz doğrudur.

Garip ama Ferhat'ın neredeyse tam tersiydi.

Ferhat başkalarının ona bakışını ne kadar umursamıyorsa Onur tümüyle başkaları için yaşayan biriydi.

Ama aynı zamanda aralarında benzerlik de vardı. Onur da onun gibi kendisini yaratmış biriydi. Yani aslında kendi hayatının mimarıydı.

Elbette bütün bunları o gün değil, ardından gelen aylar içinde anlayacaktım.

Ama o aylar içinde bir biçimde ona alıştım. Hatta diyebilirim ki ben de ona uymaya başladım.

İnsanları alıp götürebilen, masadaki herkesin ilgi odağı olan, anlatacak pek çok hikayesi olan biriydi.

Belki asıl etkileyiciliği de bundandı.

İstanbul'da okumuş sonra yurtdışına gitmiş, ünlü bir mimarlık şirketinde çalıştıktan sonra geri dönünce yıldızı parlamıştı.

Hem işini iyi yapıyordu hem de gerçekten zevkliydi. Bir evi restore ederken öyle ayrıntılar buluyordu ki eve sihirli değnek girmiş gibi bambaşka bir hale getiriyordu.

O sabah bahçede dolaşırken ağaçların arasında duvar dibine dayanmış eski mermer çeşme dikkatimi çekti.

"Dayımların evinin bahçesindeydi. Erenköy'de küçük, orta halli, sobalı bir evdi. Şimdi tabii yıkıldı ve yerine apartman dikildi. Oradan ancak bu çeşmeyi kurtarabildim," dedi.

Onu dayısıyla yengesi büyütmüştü.

"Bana onlardan kalan tek şey bu. Onu görmek beni hem mutlu ediyor hem de üzüyor."

"O yüzden mi evinize değil de buraya koydunuz?" diye sordum. Bu bana biraz garip gelmişti aslında.

"Evet," dedi, "hani insan birini çok sever ama onun kendisine zarar verdiğini, üzdüğünü bilir, hem onu görmek hem de ayrılmak ister, aynı bunun gibi..."

Galiba ondan asıl etkilendiğim, bunu anlatırken gerçekten karşı kıyıya bakıp dalması olmuştu.

Her nedense aslında pek de önemli görünmeyen bu anı beni çok şaşırtmıştı. Belki onu anlatma biçimi...

Sanki o çeşmeye dokunurken benim bilmediğim gizemli bir geçmişe, çocukluğun karmaşık, üstüne tül örtülmüş dünyasına geri dönmüş ve yüzüne baktığımda hiç tanımadığım o küçük oğlanı bir an için gördüğümü sanmıştım.

O zaman onu ilk kez merak ettim. Bütün bu fazlalıkların içindeki adamı...

Ebruların nereye asılacağını gösterdi sonra bize... Üstelik tek tek anlatıyordu renkleriyle... Pırıl pırıl bir cumartesi sabahı. Seniha Teyze'ye sormam lazımdı.

"Ben sordum bile," dedi...

"Öyle mi?"

"Evet, o da sana sormamı söyledi..."

Ne diyeceğimi bilemedim ve "Peki o zaman," dedim.

"O zaman bunu kutlayalım," dedi Jülide Hanım.

Kendimizi bahçede özenle hazırlanmış masada bulduk. Üstelik yalnızca beş, on dakikalığına geldiğimiz bu evde, peynirlerle, kurutulmuş etler ve meyvelerle dolu masada saatlerce oturduk.

Bunca zaman sonra ilk kez birileriyle oturup konuşmak, neredeyse hayatın tek resmiymiş gibi belleğime kazınan koltuklardan, tablolardan, biblolardan başka bir yerde, uzun, üzücü, korkutucu kışın ardından ilk güzel bahar sabahında bana çok iyi geldi.

Kısa süre sonra sanki hepimiz eskiden beri tanışıyormuşuz gibi çene çalıyorduk.

İnsanın aklında, yüreğinde biri varken onu başkasıyla unutması imkansızdır.

Bunu biliyordum.

Ama Onur sanki bunu anlamış gibi, başlarda benimle yalnızca flört eder gibi göründü hatta arkadaşlarından biriymişim gibi davrandı.

Okulu bırakmıştım ama Seniha Teyze'nin yanına gidiyor, haftada birkaç gün oradaki ustalardan bilmediklerimi öğrenmeye çalışıyordum.

Ve tabii çizimlere de devam ediyordum.

Sare Hanım artık daha iyiydi. O da benim bir an önce okula dönmemi istiyor, onun yüzünden gidemediğimi düşünüp üzülüyordu.

Annem yeni biriyle tanışmamdan, dışarı çıkmamdan memnundu.

Seda bu sayede gizli sevgilisini benimle tanıştırabilmiş, hep birlikte bir yerlere gidebildiğimiz için de rahatlamıştı.

Ben Onur'u hep Ferhat'la kıyaslıyordum.

Aramızda mesafe vardı ve ne gariptir ki o mesafe hiç kapanmayacaktı.

Ben kendimi geri çekiyordum ama o da sanki tam yakınlaşacağımız zaman beni durduruyordu.

Yoksa fısıltılar başlamıştı.

Zaten hep birileriyle birlikteydik. Onun hayatı böyleydi. Evini bile ilk kez kalabalık bir partide görebilmiştim.

Camlar, aynalar, altın varaklar, modern tasarımlarla Osmanlı zevki birleşmiş ama bana kalırsa garip bir tarz çıkmıştı ortaya.

Yemek salonunun duvarları simsiyah boyanmış, büyük, ağır antika masa ve siyah kadife sandalyeler... Tavandaki süslemelerle, meyve resimleri biraz kırıyordu bu karanlığı...

Uzun koridor boyunca duvara eski bir savaş sahnesi resmedilmişti.

Bir odada yıpranmış, çatlamış kahverengi deri koltuklar ve büyük bir kütüphane vardı.

Belki binlerce kitap... Oraya girip ışığı yaktığınız anda hep aynı müzik çalmaya başlıyordu.

Uzak bir ülkeden ve eski zamandan gelen bir müzik.

Sonradan neden hep bu müzik çalıyor diye sormuştum.

Çok genç yaşta uyuşturucudan ölen bir arkadaşının bestesi olduğunu söylemişti.

İnsan başkalarından korkar.

Hepimiz en yakınlarımıza karşı bile zırha bürünürüz. Bizi yoran bir zırh. Büyümek belki de budur. Anne kucağından çıktıktan sonra, birileriyle karşılaşmaya başladığın anda, sonra okulda, sonra işte, sonra sokakta hep birilerinden korunmaya çalışmak...

Eğer Tolga'yı saymazsam bir tek Ferhat'ın yanında böyle hissetmemiştim. Garip bir biçimde onun yanında inanılmaz derecede rahattım. Oysa erkeklerin yanında kendimi hiç rahat hissetmem.

Nedenini bilmiyordum ama Onur'un yanında da rahat değildim. Çok bilmiş halinden mi? Kesin yargılarla konuşmasından, emir verir gibi cümleler kurmasından mı?

Çevresindekilere, çalışanlara, gittiğimiz yerlerdeki garsonlara sanki hepsi onun için dünyaya gelmiş ve istediğini anında yapmalıymış gibi davranmasından mı?

Bunları kabaca yapmıyordu. Aksine gördüğüm en nazik insanlardan biriydi ama yapıyordu işte.

Kızdığı zaman bile gülerek espriyle öyle bir cümle kurardı ki karşısındaki öylece kalırdı. Sonra sanki laf olsun diye söylemiş gibi başka bir konuyla devam ederdi.

Bazen söylediğini beğenmezse şöyle bakar ve konuyu değiştirirdi.

Galiba içinden tam olarak ne geçtiğini anlayamadığım o bakış beni rahatsız ediyordu.

Zaten o başkalarını dinleyen biri değildi.

Daha çok kendisi konuşurdu. Ağaçlardan oyuncaklara, kitaplardan müziğe, bilmemneredeki kayıp adadan türü tükenen böceklere kadar bilmediği yoktu. Bir konuşmada sıkılırsa öyle bir konu açardı ki kimse o konuda birşey bilmediği için dinlemek zorunda kalırdı.

İşin garip yanı bu durumdan kimse sıkılmıyordu. Her yere davet ediliyor, insanlar onunla olmak istiyor, çoğu zaman ondan hayranlıkla sözediliyordu.

Aslında belki de bütün bunları sonraları düşündüm. O günlerde pek üstünde durmuyordum. Yavaş yavaş onun haline tavrına alıştım. Iki günlüğüne bir yere gitse özlemeye bile başladım.

Anneanneme onu tanıştırmadan önce anlatmıştım. Dinledi dinledi sonra elimi tuttu, "İyi biri mi?" diye sordu.

Bütün bu anlattıklarım ona birşey ifade etmemişti.

"Bilmem ki," dedim, "iyi biri bence..."

O yaz üç, dört günlüğüne kalabalık bir tatile gittik.

Ama teklifini kabul ederken birşeyler olacağını artık biliyordum.

Dans ettik, öpüştük, gece sabahlara kadar deniz kenarında konuştuk. Benim anlatacağım ne vardı ki? Her zamanki gibi o anlattı. Ben dinledim. Benim anlatacaklarım hiç de iç açıcı değildi çünkü.

Anlattıklarımı da biraz değiştirip biraz süsleyerek anlattım.

Herkes öyle yapmaz mı?

Odamda yalnız kaldığımda hala içimde suçluluk vardı.

Ya Ferhat zordaysa? Ya çıkar gelirse? O savaş filmlerindeki gibi hissediyordum. Öldü denilen asker geri döner ve sevgilisini evlenmiş bulur...

Ama neden suçluluk duyuyordum ki?

Asıl olan ne hissettiğim değil miydi?

Duyuyordum çünkü aslında hala onu seviyordum.

Onur'a aşık değildim.

Herhalde o da değildi.

Kendi kendime "O zaman fazla düşünmeye de gerek yok," dedim.

Çünkü çok yorgundum. Üzgündüm. Onun neşesi, beni getirdiği bu yeni hayat, yeni insanlar uzun zaman sonra kendimi iyi hissetmemi sağlamıştı.

O tatil bana iyi geldi.

Belki onun da herkesin üstünde taşıdığı zırhı biraz olsun çıkardığını farkettim.

Evden uzaklaşmak, bambaşka bir ortamda birkaç gün geçirmek, denize girmek güzeldi... Unutmak için... Yeniden başlamak için... Hayatın hep sıkıntıyla, kuşkularla, kaygılarla kurulmadığına inanmak için...

Belki de Seda haklıydı. "Adam sana deli oluyor, bütün kadınlar peşindeyken senden başkasıyla ilgilenmiyor, bunca zaman ne bekliyorsun anlamıyorum, fazla naz aşık usandırır benden söylemesi..."

Tatilden döndüğümüzde beni eve bırakırken sarılıp uzun uzun öptü beni.

Artık kafam karışık değildi.

Ya da öyle olduğuna inanmak istiyordum.

Ne yapalım ki böyle.

Biri seni elinden tutup bir yerlere taşıyor, biriniyse oturup bekliyorsun gelsin diye, gelmiyor.

Tatilden döndüm ve karşımda Tolga'yı buldum.

Anneannemin dizinin dibine oturmuş, ona Londra hikayeleri anlatıyor.

Büyük olasılıkla yarısını uyduruyor.

Sarıldık. Ne çok özlemişim onu.

"Arkadaşlarla" gittiğim tatili anlattım ben de...

Annem yüzüme renk geldiğini söylüyordu.

Tolga bir ara kulağıma, "Ben senin yüzüne niye renk geldiğini biliyorum merak etme tek tek anlatacaksın biraz sonra," diye kıkırdadı.

Hiç ona anlatmadan olur mu?

Birkaç kez telefonla konuşmuştuk ve ona şöyle hafiften sözetmiştim ama Seda'dan da ayrıntıları aldığına şüphem yoktu.

Ayağında leopar desenli ayakkabılar, daracık neredeyse üstüne yapışmış pantolon, üstünde rengarenk gömlek bir de karışık taşlardan kocaman kolye...

Her zamanki gibi farklı...

Yemeğe oturduk hep birlikte. Saniye bile Tolga'yı gördüğüne pek sevinmiş, habire ona yedirmeye çalışıyor, "Sen oralarda özlemişsindir bak enginar var, börek var, kısır da yaptım," diye çocuğu bunaltıyordu.

İlk kez onu bu kadar zamandır görmüyordum.

En son konuşmamızda baletten ayrılmıştı. Ama tabii onun işi belli olmaz yeniden buluşmuş ya da başkasını bulmuş olabilir. Yüzünden anlaşılmıyor. Mutlu mu, değil mi? Gizli sıtma. Belli etmez.

Anneanneme neşelensin diye hikayeler anlatıp dururken ona baktım.

Şeytan çekici dedikleri oydu herhalde.

Kendi içinde ne yaşarsa yaşasın işte böyle hemen girdiği yerin havasını değiştirir, insanı en kötü havadan bile çıkartıp güldürmeyi başarırdı.

"Aa ne bu haliniz canım, cenazeye mi geldik," dediği an herkesin keyfi yerine gelirdi.

Ama ne tuhaf onun keyfi yerinde değildi...

İçinde çok başka şeyler olduğunu ben biliyordum.

Keşke olmasaydı, keşke biz birlikte olsaydık, evlenseydik diye geçti içimden.

Kimbilir ne eğlenirdik...

İşin komiği ikimiz birlikteyken başkalarıyla olduğumuzdan daha çok eğlendik her zaman.

Söylesem ne güler buna şimdi.

O günlerde bilgisayar oyunları yeni çıkmıştı. Sonra yüzlercesini yaptılar.

Ama kendi hayatımızı yeniden kurmak için bir oyun yapsalar ne güzel olurdu.

Geri dönüp kimi günleri silmenin, kimi günleri yeniden oluşturmanın, şu yola girerken vazgeçip başka yoldan gitmenin mümkün olduğu bir oyun...

Şu yıkılan evi yeniden yapmanın, o kapanan kahveyi açmanın, bizi durup dururken bırakıp giden bir dostla yeniden buluşmanın... Hatta söylenmiş sözleri geri almanın mümkün olduğu...

Tabii biliyorum, olmuyor.

Hayat bizim istediğimiz gibi kurulmuyor.

Olsun, en azından hayal kurabilirim...

Hep öyle yapmadım mı?

Kendimi tavandaki aynada görüyorum. Ona ışıkları kapatmasını söylüyorum. İlk kez onunla yalnızım. Onun evinde. Onun aynalarla kaplı odasında. Hayır ne olacağını bilmiyorum. İstediğimin ne olduğunu bilmiyorum.

Sanki kendimi olacakların akışına bırakmış gibiyim.

İlk gençlik günlerinde aşktı sevişmek...

Birini okşamak, dokunmak, öpüşmek, yüzüne, gözlerine bakmaktan kendini alamamaktı. Kendiliğinden gelen sıcaklığın sizi yakması, durduramadığınız çarpıntının çekimiydi...

Korkuyla daha ileri gitmemek için, kendini bırakmamak için o yükselen sıcaklığı, adlandıramadığınız heyecanı durdurmaya çalışmaktı.

Şimdi yıllar sonra ilk öpüştüğüm sarışın oğlanı, saf, komik haliyle üstüme atlamaya çalışıp durduğunu ama yine de saatlerce oturup benim konuşmalarımı, şiir okumalarımı dinleyip umudunu kaybedene kadar beklemesini hatırlıyorum.

Zaman geçince artık o öpüşmenin devamının gelip gelmeyeceğini anlamak, ne istediğini öğrenmek, belki artık bunun aşk değil yalnızca istek olduğunu farketmekti...

Ancak Ferhat'la ikisini birarada yaşadığım zaman, birini gerçekten istemenin, seviştikten günler sonra bile onu içinde hissetmenin, nereye giderse gitsin aklına geldiğin an yeniden istemenin gerçek aşkla sevişmek olduğunu anlayabildim.

O yanımda yokken bile ona sarılmadım mı hep geceleri...

Kendi içindeki bir tünele girmek gibiydi çünkü. Orada kendi gizemini bulmak, gizlenmiş, örtülmüş, yasaklanmış şeyleri sanki içiçe geçmiş kutuları açıp içlerinden tek tek çıkartmak...

Hayır şimdi başka yerdeyim. Başka biriyle birlikteyim ve bunları artık düşünmemeliyim.

Onur bana bütün bunları unutturacak ve bu duyguların hayatta yalnızca birine ait olmadığını, kimsenin vazgeçilmez olmadığını gösterecek.

Onun için kendimi ona bırakıyorum.

Ama bu koku, bu dokunuş... İlk kez olduğu için mi... Beni sürekli yönetmesi, saçlarımı çekmesi, ağzımı kapaması... Kendimi bırakıyorum ama huzursuzum.

Onu tanıdıkça alışacağımı düşünüyorum.

Ama öyle olmuyor. Aradan geçen zamanda düşünmemeliyim dediğim şeyleri düşünüyorum hep. Karanlıkta, müziğin sesini açıp sevişirken aklımda, yanımızda birisi daha var.

Önceleri bundan utanırken, derin bir suçluluk duyarken giderek alışıyorum. Çünkü ancak onu düşünerek mutlu olabiliyorum.

O ilk günlerde, gecelerde bunun üzerinde çok fazla durmadım. Hayat yalnızca mutlu sevişmelerden ibaret değildi.

Yalnızca birkaç ay sonra bir akşam sakin sakin "Artık gelip burada benimle oturmanı istiyorum," dedi.

"Burada mı?" dedim şaşkın şaşkın.

Önce bunun evlenme teklifi olduğunu anlamadım.

Bunu bu kadar rahat söylemesine anlam veremedim.

Sonra gülerek, "Tabii gelip seni annenden istedikten sonra," dedi.

Herhalde hiç kimse, hatta başımın etini yiyen Seda bile bunu yapacağımı düşünmüyordu.

Aslında teklifi bile sanki teklif değil de emir gibiydi. O karar vermiş ve başka türlü olamazmış gibi...

O gece benim evet demeyişime, hatta cevap vermeyişime şaşırmadı.

Sanki evet demişim gibi, düğünün nasıl olacağını anlatıyor, evde istediğim değişiklikler varsa onları hemen söylememi istiyor, balayı için nerelere gidebileceğimizden sözediyordu.

Bizim eve bir kere gelmiş, dışarı yemeğe çıkacağımız bir akşam elinde çiçeklerle yarım saat oturmuştu.

Annem tabii ki onu pek beğenmiş, Sare Hanım'sa yorum yapmamıştı.

Aslında kafasından neler geçtiğini merak ediyordum ama nedense sormak istemedim. Belki de duyacaklarımı az çok kestirdiğim için...

Yalnız Tolga, "Bu ne acele, biraz daha bekleseydin, daha ne kadar tanıyorsun ki bu adamı, okula geri dönersin diye umuyordum ama anlaşılan sen çoktan vazgeçmişsin," diye bozuldu.

Doğrusu ben evlilik konusunu neredeyse hiç düşünmemiştim ama öyle çok kafamda büyüttüğüm bir mesele de değildi.

Hem anneannemin hem de annemin evliliklerine bakınca öyle bir yastıkta kocanacak mutlu evlilik hayalleri filan da kurmamıştım.

Ne kız bebeklerini giydirdim ne bana aldıkları küçük evlerin içini eşyalarla doldurdum.

Mutsuz olursam boşanırım olur biter diye düşünüyordum.

Çünkü ne ona deliler gibi aşıktım ne de ondan büyük bir beklentim vardı.

Bildiğim şuydu ki biriyle evlenmenin nasıl olacağını evlenmeden anlamak imkansızdır.

Onur'la mutluydum. Onunla oturup konuşmaktan, gezip eğlenmekten, tatile gitmekten keyif alıyordum. Bana böyle davranan ilk erkek de oydu.

Onur'un geldiği akşam annem, "Böyle alelacele düğün olmaz, yakışık almaz, insanlar ne düşünür, önce nişan yapıp biraz beklemek lazım..." dedi.

O da buna fazla direnmedi. "Gerçi artık tanışmak için süreye ihtiyaç yok, bunlar eski adetler ama madem istiyorsunuz aile arasında nişan takalım, bir iki ay içinde de hazırlıkları bitirip nikah tarihi alalım, ben işlerin uzamasını sevmem..." dedi.

İşlerin?

Evet ona göre bu da bir işti. Bir işe karar verdiğinde nasıl davranıyorsa bunda da öyle yapacaktı.

Benim o akşam biraz içim sıkıldı. Çünkü aklıma gelmeyen bir sürü saçmalıkla uğraşmak zorunda kalacağımı, annemin tutturmalarını savuşturmak için ne yapacağımı, gelinlikmiş, çeyizmiş, düğün yeriymiş, davetli listesiymiş gibi zırvalarla bunalacağımı o akşam farkettim.

Sare Hanım uzun uzun Onur'u inceledi. Yalnızca birkaç soru sordu. Yaşlı dayısını kaybettikten sonra kimsesi kalmadığını öğrendi. Oturacağımız evin yakın olmasına sevindi. Eski günlerinde olsa kimbilir neler sorar, sonra bana neler anlatırdı ama artık hiç keyfi yoktu. Zaten günün büyük bölümünü uyuyarak ya da koltuğunda uyuklayarak geçiriyor, misafir istemiyor, biraz fazla konuşan oldu mu huysuzlanıyordu.

"İyi bir adama benziyor, madem sen seviyorsun..."

Madem sen seviyorsun cümlesini öyle bir söyledi ki aslında sanki "Seviyor musun gerçekten?" der gibiydi.

Neyse ki annem daha Onur kapıdan çıkar çıkmaz nişanın nasıl olacağını, nerede olacağını, kimlerin gelmesi gerektiğini anlatmaya başladığı için söz ortada kaldı.

Belki de bilinçaltımda bu evden de artık kurtulmak istiyordum. Anneannemin bu hali beni çok üzüyordu. Aynı zamanda evin o çok sevdiğim, neşeli, canlı hali gitmiş, kasvetli, sessiz garip bir hal almıştı.

Onur'un teklifini olsa olsa birkaç ay erteleyebilirdim. Ama sonunda istediği olmazsa benden ayrılırdı, bunu biliyordum.

Artık 40'lı yaşlarının ortalarındaydı ve çocuk istiyordu.

Doğrusu onunla tanışana kadar çevremde dolaşan, benimle görüşmek isteyen erkekler de beni hiç etkilememiş hatta kendi kendime bu insanlarla hayat geçiren kadınlar mı var, ben buna yemek süresince zor katlanıyorum diye düşünmüştüm.

Tabii Seda'nın sürekli "Adamın etrafı güzel kadınlarla dolu, senin bu saflığına çarpıldı, sakın bunu uzatma," deyip durması da ayrı.

Bir keresinde, "Hala aklında o deli ressam varsa unut, ondan insana hayır gelmez, kaçıp gitmiş, üstelik de yaşlı..." deyince kızdım, "Bir daha bu konuyu açma," dedim, sustu.

Ama aklımda birşey daha vardı.

Onur'la nişanı nerede yapalım, evde, bahçede küçük bir davet mi olsun diye konuşuyorduk.

Bu konulardan benim gibi sıkılmış değil aksine heyecanlanmış görünüyordu.

Hatta evi nasıl değiştireceğini, benim için çalışma odası hazırlayacağını anlatırken kağıt üzerinde çizip gösteriyordu.

Bir türlü lafa giremiyordum. Sonunda, "Sana söylemem gereken birşey var," dedim.

Durdu, yüzüme baktı.

"Benim de vardır mutlaka ama şimdi söylemenin zamanı değil, ben insanları kendim tanımak isterim, onların ya da başkalarının anlattıklarıyla değil," dedi.

Belki geçmişimden sözedeceğimi düşünmüştü. Belki de Ferhat'ı duymuştu.

"Benden önceki hayatın seni ilgilendirir, benim için önemli olan bundan sonrası..."

"Ama bu öyle birşey değil," dedim ve ona hastalığımdan ilk kez sözettim. Tabii oldukça hafifleterek.

Pek üzerinde durmadı. Elimi tuttu, okşadı. Belki de korktuğu şeyi söylemediğime sevinmişti.

"Gördüğüm kadarıyla hasta bir halin yok. Doktorların merakı bunlar hep. Gereken ne varsa birlikte araştırır buluruz. Herşeyin çaresi vardır..."

Evet o öyle düşünürdü. Herşeyin çaresi vardır.

O an böyle söylemesi beni çok mutlu etti hatta evlenme kararını verdiğim için kendimi ilk kez iyi hissettim ama tıpkı annem gibi onun da görmek istemediği şeylerden kaçtığını, belki de bu yüzden hayatını sürekli güzelleştirmeye çalıştığını, üzücü, tatsız anıları bile silip yokettiğini anlamamıştım.

Evliliğimizin ilk yazında bir deniz yolculuğuna çıktık. Üstümde bana son hediyesi renkli, uçuşan bir yazlık elbise, kafamda kocaman şapka, genç gelin olarak kaptanın masasında yenen yemek, yemekten sonra güvertede ayışığında içilen içki...

Onur her zamanki şıklığı ve havalı haliyle tanımadığı yabancı insanlarla sohbet ediyor, gemiler hakkındaki bilgisiyle kaptanı bile hayretler içinde bırakıyordu.

Herşey tam da filmlerdeki gibiydi.

Tam Onur'a yakışır cinsten.

E, o Cary Grant'sa ben de Grace Kelly olmalıydım tabii. Zaten neredeyse bütün gardırobumu baştan aşağı yenilemiş, en iyi modaevlerinden daha balayından önce yığınla şey alınmıştı.

Hoşuma da gitti. Bir tek son moda topuklu ayakkabılar ayağımı sıkıyordu o kadar.

Ama biraz sonra hava bozdu.

Vapur dalgaların üzerinde inip kalkmaya başladı.

Kamaraya geldik ve birden fenalaştım. Başım dönüyor, midem bulanıyor, titriyordum.

Üstümü başımı bile zor çıkardım.

"Deniz tutmuştur, belki de fazla şarap içtin, uyuyunca geçer," diyordu ama ben yatamıyordum. Yatınca daha beter başım dönüyordu ve paniklemeye başladım. Çünkü ne olduğunu anlamamıştım. Böyle vapurla yolculuk etmediğim için gerçekten deniz mi tuttu, zehirlendim mi yoksa yine atak mı geldi bilemiyordum.

Derin derin nefes almaya çalışıyordum ama sanki alamıyormuşum gibi geliyordu.

Ter içinde kusuyordum ama midemin bulantısı geçmiyordu.

Ona doktoru getirmesi için yalvarıyordum ama nedense "Birşeyin yok, geçer," diye inat ediyordu.

Ağlamaya başladım.

Sonunda gidip doktoru kaldırdı.

Tansiyonum ölçüldü, ateşime bakıldı, kalbim dinlendi.

"Korkacak birşey değil muhtemelen yemek dokundu ve hava da böyle olunca... Alıştığımız şeyler, merak etmeyin..."

Yaşlı doktor bana ilaç verdi ve sabah yeniden gelip göreceğini söyleyerek gitti.

"Gördün mü," dedi, "benim dediğim gibi, boşu boşuna kaldırdık adamı bu saatte, deniz tuttu işte..."

Zangır zangır titriyordum, hem üşüyordum hem ter içindeydim, bayılmamak için kendimi tutmaya çalışıyordum ama kulaklarımdaki ağrı dayanılmaz hale gelmişti.

Birden bana kızdığını anladım.

Doktoru uyandırdığım için mi?

Hayır, onun söylediğine inanmadığım için...

Ve daha da kötüsü, ertesi gün ve daha sonraki gün kamarada neredeyse bembeyaz olmuş yatarken, ne olur bir yerde inip geri dönelim diye yalvarırken öfkesi giderek arttı.

Bana özel haşlanmış patates, lapa getirtiyor, yiyemeyince daha çok sinirleniyordu.

"Herkesi deniz tutuyor, şımarıklığın lüzumu yok, doğru dürüst yemek ye, ilacını al kendine gelirsin..." diyordu.

Onunla tartışacak, "Sen ne biçim adamsın, ben burada ölüyorum, sen hala tatilin bozuldu diye söyleniyorsun," diyecek halim bile yoktu.

Farkettim ki onunla ilk kez yalnızız.

Yanımızda her zamanki gibi tanıdıklar, arkadaşlar yok.

Vapurun belki de en lüks, en havalı kamarasında yorganın altına girmiş yatıyordum.

Arada titreme geliyor, terliyorum, yüzüm gözüm şişmiş.. Benimle biraz oturuyor, sonra mavi beyaz çizgili gömleği, beyaz pantolonuyla yukarıya güverteye çıkıyor, saatler sonra geri geliyordu.

Kendimi zorluyordum ama ellerim ayaklarım tutmuyordu. Doktor bunun alerjik olabileceğini söyleyip başka ilaçlar vermişti ama onları değil gizlice kendi ilaçlarımı içtim.

Galiba asıl kızdığı, hastalanmam değildi. Ona göre ne olursa olsun söyledikleri yapılacak, böylece düzelecektim.

Onunla ilk kez yalnızdık.

Ama anladım ki asıl ben yalnızım.

Ve onunla hep yalnız olacağım.

Sonra yavaş yavaş anlamaya başladım. Aslında evlilik ona göre değildi. Bir yaşta yapılması gerekiyordu o kadar. Orada, o deniz yolculuğunda ilk kez karşılaştığım yüzünü gittikçe daha sık görmeye başladım.

Hastalığımın gerçekten ne kadar ciddi olduğunu anladığında işler daha da kötüye gitti.

Aslında onu anlıyordum.

Hayatına devam edecek, ben yanında olsam da olmasam da eskisi gibi gezip eğlenecekti.

Durup dururken başına sorumluluk aldığına pişman olmuştu ama açıkça söyleyemiyordu.

Korkuyordu ve bu onun için katlanılamaz birşeydi.

Erkekler korkaktır. Kendilerini kahraman gibi görürler ama en küçük acıya bile katlanamazlar.

Bense artık bambaşka biriydim. O bana kötü davrandıkça kendini ona beğendirmek için uğraşan, onun istediklerini giyen, onun istediği gibi konuşan hatta onun istediği gibi susan birine dönüşmüştüm.

Eskiden benimle oturup kafasındaki projeleri anlatırken, yapacaklarımı dinlerken, filmlerden, şarkılardan konuşurken keyfi yerindeydi.

Ama şimdi ya her akşam dışarı çıkmak istiyor ya birilerini çağırıyor, olmadı odasına çekilip çizim yapıyor, ben uykuya daldıktan sonra gelip yatıyordu.

Ona göre herkes beni kıskanırken ben mutlu olmayı bilmiyordum.

Aslında bir kadının bir erkeğe kendisini kötü hissettirmesi çok kolaydır. Ama bunu yapmak istemiyordum. O da yaptıklarından memnun değildi. Zaman zaman böyle davrandığı için üzüldüğünü, suçluluk duyduğunu farkediyordum.

Şimdi en başta görmemeye çalıştığım ne varsa artık gözüme batıyordu.

Başkalarını etkilemek için yaptıkları, anlattıkları artık bana ilginç gelmiyordu. Çünkü nasıl söze gireceğini, ne anlatacağını, hatta el kol hareketlerini bile artık biliyordum.

O görüntülerin prensiydi.

Çizdiği evler gibi, kendisini de çizmişti ve o kabuğu kırmanız imkansızdı.

Kimbilir belki de haklıydı. Kendi istediği hayatı kurmuş ve böyle devam etmek istiyor, bunu kabul etmeyenleri de hayatından çıkartıyordu.

Ama birşey daha vardı.

Tanıştığımız zaman herkes gibi o da içki içiyor ve çocukluğumdan beri anneannemin misafirlerini tanıdığım için bu bana doğal geliyordu.

Ama sonra giderek çok fazla içtiğini farkettim.

Başkalarının yanında kendisini kontrol ediyordu. Hatta sarhoş olunca çok neşeleniyordu. Ama eve gelip biraz daha içince birden değişiyordu.

O kibar adam gidiyor, yerine saldırgan, aşağılayıcı, kendisinden başka herkesi küçümseyen bambaşka biri geliyordu.

Bazen hiç olmadık bir konuda öylesine bir fikir söylediğimde birden çıldırıyor, bana etmedik hakaret bırakmıyordu.

Önceleri bunu çok önemsememiştim. Çünkü bu kadar çok içmenin hastalık olduğunu bilmiyordum.

Sarhoş oldu ve saçmaladı diyordum.

Zaten sabah uyanınca, "Dün ben zırvaladım mı, galiba yine fazla kaçırdım," diye gönlümü alıyordu.

Ama aslında ben iki ayrı insanla birlikteydim.

Ve bu gerçeği yalnız ben bildiğim için giderek daha çok kızıyordu.

Bir keresinde yeni yaptığı binayla ilgili konuşurken bana da ne düşündüğümü sordu. Ben de beğenmediğim birkaç ayrıntı söyledim.

Birden fırladı, içeri gitti, yeni yaptığım ebruları yerlere atıp bana hakaretler yağdırdı. Yeni aldığım büyük tekneyi devirdi. Sonra da çıkıp gitti.

İlk kez ondan korktum.

Birşey yapmam gerektiğini biliyordum ama ne?

Dedim ya iki ayrı insan vardı.

Ertesi sabah yüzlerce gülle uyandım. Karta "Senin gibi özel bir insanla birlikteyim ve bunu mahvediyorum, ne olur bana yardım et, bir daha olmayacak, söz veriyorum ve seni çok seviyorum..." yazmıştı.

Yazık ki bunların işe yaramayacağını bilmem gerekirdi.

Bir bahaneyle kavga çıkartıp nereye gittiğini, sabahın körü sarhoş nereden döndüğünü bilmiyordum ve sormak da istemiyordum.

Ne onunla konuşabiliyordum ne de başkasıyla.

Zaten kısa süre sonra Seda'nın sevgilisiyle araları açıldığı için onunla bile görüşemiyordum. Tolga'yla bir kez biraraya gelmişlerdi ama ondan da hiç hoşlanmamıştı.

Neredeyse annemlere gidip gelmeme bile söylenir hale geldi sonunda.

Bu oyunu neden oynuyordum bilmem.

Belki de yeni bir başarısızlığı daha kaldıramayacağımı düşündüğüm için...

Belki annem için söylediklerimin benim başıma gelmesine katlanamadığım için...

Belki ne olursa olsun aramızı düzeltebileceğime inanmak istediğim için...

Belki çaresizlikten...

Evet galiba bu daha doğru.

Hayatımdaki bütün erkekler beni bırakıp gidecek diye düşünmemin daha doğrusu derinde bir yerde böyle hissetmemin nedeni açıktı tabii…

O yüzden Onur'dan ayrılmak istemiyordum. Belki de o yüzden gözlerimi kapadım. Belki de başka bir kadının çoktan farkedeceği birçok ayrıntıyı görmezden geldim.

Gerçi görsem ne olacaktı ki?

Anneannem demez miydi hep, "Bizim ev kadınları kendisini ya hafiye ya yargıç sanır ve sonunda kapının önünde tek başına kalakalır," diye…

Gördüm sonunda…

Ama öyle her zaman olduğu gibi bir yerde onlara rastlamadım. Birilerinden de duymadım. Kadın da gelip bana itiraf etmedi, Onur da…

Ama ben gördüm.

Ve ne garip, gerçekle ötesinin karıştığı yerde hem de..

O akşam yine arkadaşlarıyla dışarı çıkmıştı. Lise yıllarından kalma alışkanlıkla en yakın arkadaşlarının doğumgünü ya da bilmemne gününün anısı olan gecelerde çıkar, sabaha kadar gezer ve genellikle zil zurna eve dönerdi.

Bir çizimle uğraşıyordum ama bilgisayarımda program kilitlendi ve ne kadar uğraşsam da açamadım.

Gidip onun bilgisayarından kendime mail atsam işe yarar mı diye düşündüm. Bunu niye düşündüm bugün de anlamış değilim çünkü gerçekten çok saçma...

Sanırım bazı şeyler böyle saçmalıklarla oluyor. Bazen birşey hiç beklenmedik bir anda karşınıza çıksın diye belki...

Çalışma odasına gittim, ona hediye aldığım antika masasına oturdum, bilgisayarının kapağını açtım.

Bilgisayarını kapamamıştı.

Uydurma birşeyler yazıp kendime yolladım. Tam kapamak üzereydim ki birden ekranın altında küçük bir kutu açıldı.

"Uyuyor musun?" yazıyordu.

Önce sanki gizli kapaklı birşey yapıyormuş da yakalanmış gibi korktum. Sonra şaşkınlıkla kutuya baktım.

"Orda mısın? Değilsen belki de daha iyi..." yazdı.

Kutuyu açtım. Büyüdü. Üstünde, yabancı bir kız ismi çıktı.

Ama herhangi bir isim değil. Benim bildiğim bir isim. Hayır tanıdığım değil. Bir film kahramanının, Onur'un en sevdiği filmdeki kadın karakterin ismi: Holly Golightly...

Bu da neydi böyle... Bir arkadaşı mı? Kim? Benim tanıdığım biri mi?

Ellerim titremeye başladı.

Bekledim.

"Belki daha iyi, çünkü sana anlatacaklarım var ve bunlara cevap vermek istemeyeceğini de artık çok iyi biliyorum," yazdı.

Bu bir arkadaşı değildi.

Arkama yaslandım. Koltuğun gıcırdaması bile beni korkuttu sanki duyulurmuş gibi...

"Uzun zaman oldu, biliyorum sen hiç söz vermemiştin, benim seçimimdi. Bunların hepsini biliyorum korkma..."

Ne yapacağımı şaşırmış ekranın karşısında büyülenmiş gibi yazılanları okuyordum.

Biri şu an bir yerde Onur'a birşeyler yazıyordu. Biri değil bir kadın.

Önce bilgisayarı kapatıp oradan kaçmak geldi aklıma. Tabii ki yapmadım. Kim yapar ki...

Bilgisayarın kilitleneceği tutmuştu, Onur'un arkadaşlarıyla çıkacağı geceye denk gelmişti, ben asla yapmadığım birşey yapıp onun bilgisayarını açmıştım, üstelik bilgisayar açıktı ve tam kapatacağım anda bu mesaj gelmişti. Tam on saniye sonra gelse görmeyecektim.

Bunların hepsi rastlantı mıydı?

"Bunları biliyorum ama senin bilmediklerin var ve sana onları anlatmak istiyorum."

İçimden "Kimsin sen," yazmak ve bu acayip durumu sona erdirmek geliyordu ama yapamıyordum.

Saate baktım daha geceyarısı bile değildi.

Önce Onur'un da pek çok erkek gibi sanal ortamda kırıştırdığını düşündüm tabii...

"Bütün bunlar, seninle ikimizin kurduğu bu özel tarikat, gizli yazışmalar, şifreler, başka isimlerle telefona kaydetmeler, herşeyi silme zorunluluğu beni, dünyayı ele geçireceğini sanan o delilerden birine dönüştürmedi ama uzun uzun düşündüm ve artık çocuk olmadığımızı, bütün bunların delilik olduğunu anladım."

Bacaklarımdan boynuma sanki sıcak su akar gibi hissediyordum. Tek korktuğum paniklemek ve yeni bir atakla burada bu durumda bayılmaktı. Sakinleşmek için birşey içmek istedim. Büfesinde içki vardı ama su ya da buz yoktu. Biraz konyak doldurup geri geldim.

Kalbim o kadar hızlı atıyordu ki yerinden çıkacak sanıyordum.

O devam etti,

"Güzeldi. Çok güzeldi. Hayatı belki anlamlı kılan, belki bütün kötülüklerden bizi uzak tutan şey: Mutluluk. Ve ben belki ilk kez mutluydum. Bir saat, iki saat, bir gece, bir kahve içimi, bir yemek süresi... Mutluydum. Hepsi için hazırlanırdım biliyor musun? Farkında bile değilsindir. Üstelik son saniye haber verirsin hep. Olsun. O kadar alıştım ki o anda giyinmeye, makyaj yapmaya, saçlarımı düzeltmeye..."

Başparmağımı emiyorum, ekrana bakıyorum ve bunların gerçek olup olmadığını yine bilmiyorum, kendi kendime, "Hayır bunlar yine senin rüyaların olmalı," diyorum.

"Ve biliyor musun, senin için hazırlanmaya bayılırım. Ne renk giysem, ne giysem, bunu mu beğenir yoksa bunu mu... Sonra birden mesaj gelir ve sen gelmekten vazgeçersin, birşey çıkmıştır, aslında yalan söylediğini bilirim, karından sözetmek istemezsin, işin vardır, toplantı uzamıştır, dünya kurulalı beri erkeklerin karılarına, sevgililerine, metreslerine söyledikleri yalanlar..."

Komik ama gerçekten o an gülümsedim. Sahiden de bunca yılda daha iyi yalan bulamamıştı hiçbiri...

Sessizlik oldu. Bir süre yazmadı. Sigara yaktığını ya da içki aldığını düşündüm. Konyaktan bir yudum aldım, boğazım yandı. "Yavaş iç, sakın sarhoş olma," dedim, kendi kendime.

"Sen gelemediğinde belki hemen yatıp uyursun ve unutursun ama ben üstümde evde giyilmeyecek giysilerle, topuklu ayakkabılarla, içimde garip çamaşırlarla, saçlarım yapılmış, makyajlı halde, masanın üstünde, orda burda yaktığım mumların ışığında oturup ne yapmalıyım diye düşünürüm. Aslında belki artık onu bile düşünmüyorum. Sadece oturuyorum ve gelemedi, aslında benimle olmak isterdi ama olmadı diye kendimce senin yerine bahaneler buluyorum. İşin tuhafı şu ki, senin bulmadığın bahaneler bunlar..."

Öyle garip bir duygu içindeydim ki kızgın mıyım, delirdim mi, üzgün müyüm, ağlamak mı istiyorum, gülmek mi, Onur'u arayıp bağırıp çağırıp buradan gitmeli miyim, yoksa sonuna kadar dinlemeli miyim bilmiyordum ve bilgisayarım gibi kendimi de kilitlenmiş hissediyordum.

"Sana bunları ilk kez anlatıyorum. Sen benim duygularımı sorar mısın? Ben seninkileri sorar mıyım? Hayır. Biz sanki bütün bunlar hiç yokmuş, buluştuğumuz anlarda dünyada yalnız biz varmışız gibi hissediyorduk ve belki de bunca zaman bunu sürdürebilmemizin nedeni buydu... Dedim ya aynı gizli tarikatlar gibi...

Çünkü konuşmaya kalkışınca herşeyin bir anda bizi sarmalayan o sihirden çıkıp çıplak, sıradan, alelade bir gerçek halinde karşımıza çıkacağını biliyorduk değil mi?

Onca konuşma arasında aldatma sözcüğü hiç geçmedi aramızda örneğin.

Ama yaptığımız buydu.

İki yalancı, bir başkasını aldatıyorduk. Sen ayrıca beni de aldatıyordun. Ben de belki bir anlamda seni, onu ve kendimi...

Biliyorum, sana sorsam, bunun neden bu denli önemsendiğini, insanların bu nedenle niye bu kadar mutsuz olduğunu, eğer biri seni aldatıyor ve sen buna katlanamıyorsan çekip gitmen gerektiğini söylerdin.

Ama sen karına onu aldattığını söyledin mi hiç?

Bunu doğrusu hala merak ediyorum. Belki de söylemişsindir. Belki de o hiç sormamıştır cevabını duymak istemediği için. Belki de yalan söylemişsindir.

İtiraf etmeliyim ki hiç tanımadığım bu kadın için bütün bu zamanda hiç de öyle büyük bir vicdan azabı duymadım. Ama senin duyduğunu biliyorum.

Zaten kimi zaman karından değil de sırtında taşıdığın o suçluluk duygusundan niye ayrılamadığını düşündüm."

Bir an Ferhat'ı düşündüm. Onunla yaşadıklarımı...

"Sen kötü bir insan mısın? Hayır. Kötü insan bana göre başkaları için kötülük düşünenlerdir. Sen öyle değilsin. Bütün bunlara aslında üzüldüğünü, karın ya da benim ya da ikimiz için vicdan azabı duyduğunu düşünüyorum. Bazen de umurunda olmadığını... Gerçekten belki de bu sorunun cevabını bilmiyorum. Bu senin için kaçış mıydı? Beni sevdiğini biliyorum. Çok kez ayrılmak isteyip ayrılamadığını, bir nedenle bana bağlandığını... Ama nedenini? Hayır."

Bağlanmak mı? Çok kez ayrılmak mı?

"İnsan bazen hiç aklına gelmeyen, kendisinin yaşamayacağını sandığı bir durumun içinde kalıyor ve anlaşılmaz biçimde o durumu sürdürüyor.

Bu aldatma hikayelerini ne çok dinlemişizdir hepimiz.

Kadınlar için neredeyse ölümcül olan bu durum erkekler için yumuşatılıyor. Hepimizin bildiği gibi onların yaptıklarına kendimizce isimler takıyoruz, bahaneler uyduruyoruz. Çapkın, hovarda, zampara sözcüklerini aşağılamak için değil de sanki afacan, yaramaz der gibi şımartma sözcükleri olarak kullanıyoruz.

Çocukken annemin arkadaşları geldiğinde konu açılır, kimi zaman orada olmayan birinin kocasının yaptıklarını sağır sultan duymuş olur, kimi zaman ağlayarak gelen kadın başına gelen felaketi anlatır ve onu sakinleştirmek, evliliğini kurtarmak, olayları yeniden yoluna koymak, o bilmemne kadının eline adamı bırakmamak, çocukları düşünmek gibi bin türlü neden bulunarak kadın sonunda ikna edilirdi.

Oysa aynısını kadın yapsa, o zaman bambaşka olur, herkesçe dışlanır, başına gelmedik kalmaz, artık hakkında tümüyle farklı sözcüklerle konuşulurdu.

Bütün bunların nedeni, kadınların aldatma dedikleri şeyin çok farklı olmasıyla mı ilgili yoksa?

Kocasını sırf eğlence olsun diye aldatan ya da iki günlük geziye gittiği anda bile hemen birini bulan kadın pek duymadım.

Kadınların çoğu iflah olmaz romantikler çünkü. Belki gerçekte nedenleri farklı bile olsa bir başkasına gittiklerinde ona aşık olduklarına inanıyorlar.

Ve hatta çoğu zaman gerçekten de oluyorlar.

Çünkü belki de senin söylediğin gibi, aşk kendimizi ve elbette karşımızdakini kandırmaktır."

Şaşkın şaşkın ekrana bakıyorum, ders dinler gibi... Komik ama bir an bu kadınla tanışıp karşılıklı konuşmak istiyorum. O devam ediyor.

"Sen belki karını aldattın bense kendimi...

Ama merak etme, bunu acıklı film cümlesi olarak söylemiyorum. Hayatımı senin yüzünden mahvettim, yıllarımı sana verdim anlamında değil.

Sen bana yalan söyledin mi? Evet söyledin. Ama onlar ufak tefek yalanlardı. Örneğin yılbaşında, örneğin doğumgününde bir yerlere gitmen gerektiği gibi... Elbette biliyordum karınla olacağını...

Ama bana ne söz verdin, ne gelecekle ilgili birşey söyledin, ne de bensiz yapamayacağını...

Sadece bazı geceler aramızdaki büyünün bize gerçekleri unutturduğu saatlerde ve tabii biraz içmişken, "Lütfen hayatımdan çıkma," derdin.

Keşke bunu söylerken gözlerimin içine öyle bakmasaydın... Galiba erkekler anlık tutkularda kayboluyor, kadınlarsa o tutkunun sonsuza dek süreceğine inanmak istiyor. Masallardaki gibi... Ama size o masalları okutmadılar değil mi?"

Bir aşk hikayesinin tam ortasında mıydım yoksa sonunda mı? Kocam sıradan bir çapkın mıydı yoksa gerçekten gizli aşkın kahramanı mı?

"Benimleyken ne kadar mutlu olduğunu, sarhoş olduğunda bana ne güzel şeyler söylediğini ama sonra birdenbire bambaşka birine dönüştüğünü, sabah uyanınca pişman olduğunu da biliyorum. Ne garip ama bütün bunlar aslında çok sahici... Öyle de olmalıydı. Çünkü benle mutluydun ama aslında yapmaman gereken birşey yapıyordun. Eğer hiç umurunda olmasa belki de seni bu kadar sevmezdim."

Birden afalladım. Bu kadın alelade bir metres değildi. Onur'a aşıktı. Bu sözler bir metresin değil aşığın ağzından çıkacak sözlerdi. Ve bu yeni değildi. Öylesine basit birkaçamak da değildi.

"Ebru..."

Birden irkildim. Yakalanmış gibi. Sanki bana sesleniyormuş benim burada olduğumu, bunları okuduğumu anlamış gibi....

"Birçok kadının senin peşinde olduğunu biliyordu, başından beri... Ve eminim ki onu aldattığını da düşünüyordur. Ama benden başka kimseyle olmadığını ben biliyorum. Yoksa bu kadar gelgitler yaşamazdın. Yalnızca daha çok kadınla yatarak başarılı olduğunu sanan erkekleri de tanıyorum çünkü, sen onlardan değilsin."

Bir yudum daha aldım. Bu kez daha büyükçe ve gerçekten boğazım yandı.

"Şimdi düşünüyorum da senin de kadınsı bir yönün var. Sen de iflah olmaz bir romantiksin. Seni ilgilendiren aslında kaçamak da olsa bir kadınla yaşadığın o an'ın duygusu... O duygu kaybolduğunda sen de kayboluyorsun.

Merak ettiğim ve cevabını hala bulamadığım birşey daha var. Ne zamandı bilmiyorum ama bir akşam bana, hayatımda ne yapmak istediğimi sormuştun? Önce anlamadım. Sonra, evlilikten, çocuklardan sözettiğini anladım. Bir anlamda benimle zaman geçiriyorsun ama hayatın da geçiyor demek istiyordun. O gece bunu benden artık kurtulmak istediğine yordum. Sonra vicdanını rahatlatmak için yaptığına inandım. İnsan kendisini her gördüğünde titreyen bir kadına gidip başka bir hayat kurmasını öğütler mi?

Gerçekte sen herkesi düşünen, herkesin hayatını hisseden biri miydin yoksa doğuştan taşıdığın bu garip suçluluk duygusu muydu sana bunları yaptıran bunu hiç anlayamadım."

İnsan kocasının aşk mektuplarını bulabilir, ona atılan mesajları yakalayabilir, karşılıklı konuşmaları sonradan okuyabilir ama böyle canlı olarak bir sevgilinin kocasına olan duygularını saniye saniye izleyebilir mi?

Anneannem olsa "Tam senin başına gelecek şey," derdi. Kalp atışlarım biraz yavaşlamıştı. Her nedense gülmek geliyordu içimden, kahkahalarla hem de... Bu da gelecekti başıma değil mi? Gelmiş işte...

Başka türlü olsa neler söylerdim de... Kıza bak, hazırlanıyormuş o gelecek diye... Beyefendinin hangi gömlekle hangi kravatı takacağına bile karar veren kim diye sormadın ama...

Ve hala yazıyor...

"Eminim gün içinde benim seni düşündüğüm gibi beni düşünmemişindir. Bense öyle çok düşündüm ki seni... Her gece uyurken bile sanki sana sarılırmış gibi uyudum."

Hayatımda hiç küfür etmedim. Bilmem bile... Ama doğrusu şimdi bu kıza küfretmek isterdim. Aslına bakarsanız garip bir durumdaydım. Hem kızıyordum hem dinlemek istiyordum hem de budalanın birine aşık olmuş bu kıza acıyordum.

Onur mu bütün bunları düşünecekti? "Gönül eğlendirmek," der geçerdi sorsam. Ama insan belki de en yakınlarındakini tanıyamıyor Ferhat'ın dediği gibi. Belki de onları hiç ilgisiz biri bizden daha iyi tanıyor.

Birden ayrıntıları merak ettiğimi farkettim. Neydi onu bu kıza götüren şey? Böyle gizli saklı, birkaç saate, bir geceye, belki bir tatil zamanına sıkışan? Aşksa, beni bırakıp gidebilirdi. Çocuğumuz da yok. Benden mi sıkılmıştı? Eh buna hayır diyemem. Ben de ondan sıkılmıştım aslında. Uzun zamandır sevişmediğimizi de düşünürsem...

"Belki de biz yalnızca hayatın güzel anlarını yaşadığımız için, yalnızca tutkuyu yaşadığımız için bu kadar uzun sürdü. İnsan bir evde birlikte oturduğu biriyle bunları hissedemez. Bazen gelirdin ve kravatını gevşetip ilgisiz şeyler anlatırdın, sanki seni başka kimse dinlemiyormuş ve o yüzden bana anlatıyorsun gibi gelirdi. Ben dinlerdim ama aslında ne anlattığını pek farketmezdim. Senin konuşmana, ellerine, dudaklarına bakardım. Sonra şarkılar dinlerdik. Eski, artık kimselerin bilmediği Türkçe şarkıları seversin. Bana da sevdirdin sonunda. Oysa annemler dinlerken nasıl sıkılırdım."

Yalnız ben de biraz sıkılmaya başlamıştım. Bir an aklıma birşey geldi. Galiba bu üçüncü ya da dördüncü yudumdan sonra oldu. İkircikteydim ama sonra neden olmasın dedim.

"Sonra beni öperdin ve o an çoktan başka bir dünyaya geçmiş olurdum. Buna ten uyumu mu deniyor bilmiyorum. Sanki artık orada değildim ve rüya görüyordum."

"Ben geldim" yazdım.

Sessizlik oldu.

Yalnızca gülümseme işareti geldi.

"Aslında kendi kendime konuşuyordum, istersen devam edeyim," yazdı.

"Biraz izin ver okuyayayım yazdıklarını," dedim.

"Oku ama cevap verme, seninle tartışmak için yazmıyorum bunları, bittiğini biliyorum, sakın hayır deme, sadece sana bunları söylemek istedim, belki de içimden çıksın istedim, yoksa yoluma devam edemem..."

"Bekle..." dedim.

Ne kadar sürerdi ki bütün bunları okumak. Başından beri okumaya çalıştım. Bittiğini biliyorum ne demek? Bir de ayrılık hikayesi dinleyecektim anlaşılan. Ne şans ama? Tam da bitirmişken yakalanmak.

Şimdi ben Onur olacaktım. Onun ağzından konuşacaktım. Ama nasıl? Acaba ne olmuştu? Ne konuşmuşlardı ki şimdi bitti diyordu. Kimdi bu kız? Kadın? Eski sevgililerinden biri mi? Kopamayan şu garip ilişkilerden mi? Hayır öyle olsa bu kadar uzak konuşmazdı.

"Evet asıl söylemem gerekeni geciktirdim yine. Hayatımın en mutlu günlerini yaşadım senle. Herşeye rağmen. Garip olan da buydu zaten. Bütün bunları düşünsem de kimi akşamlar sabahlara kadar kursam da aslında bambaşka bir havadaydım. İlk aşkını yaşayan genç kız gibiydim.

Kimi zaman haftada bir, kimi zaman onbeş günde bir, kimi zaman tatile denk gelirse ayda bir de görüşsek farketmiyordu. Her seferinde sanki düğüne gidecek gibi hazırlığa sabahtan başlıyordum.

Mantıklı açıklamalarla çözülecek, üstesinden gelinecek birşey değildi. Bu duygu beni esir almıştı ve onunla boğuşmamın anlamı yoktu. Seninle ilgili bile değildi aslında... Bu benim hayatımdı. Benim duygumdu.

Evet o duyguyu bana sen verdin ve beni değiştirdi.

Hiç bilmediğim yanlarımı ortaya çıkardı, yeniden kadın olmayı, yeniden aşık olmayı, yeniden sevmeyi, yeniden ağlamayı, yeniden kahkahalarla gülmeyi öğrendim o duyguyla..."

Ne tuhaf, demek sizin anlayamadığınız şeyleri bir başkası anlayabiliyor, belki sizin onda göremediğiniz özelliklerini görüyor, sizin sevemediğiniz adamı böylesine sevebiliyor.

"Aslında düşündüm ki birini aldatmak, hayatın içinde gizli bir hayat daha sürdürmek sanıldığı gibi eğlenceli değil.

Benim yanımda herşeyi unuttuğunu biliyorum. Ama aslında unutmuyordun. Yalnızca o an derinlere saklıyordun. Ama şimdi eminim ki bu seni giderek mutsuz etti.

Peki neydi o zaman?

Yalnızca bir zaaf mı?

Benden vageçememek ki?

Gün gelip hayatını değiştireceğini düşünmek ama birçok nedenle bunu sürekli ertelemek mi?

Eksik kalan birşeyleri tamamlamak mı?

Hala çocukluktaki gibi özgür olduğuna inanma isteği mi?

Ama çocuklar da özgür değildir ki…"

Evet doğru tesbit! Çocuk… Sorumluluk almak istemez hiçbir zaman. En küçük bir zorunluluktan bile kaçar. İleriye dönük planlar onu mutsuz eder. Belki de yalnızca anları yaşayarak, belki de yalnızca hayatın güzel bölümünü yaşayarak, hazların peşinden giderek mutlu olmak isteyen biri o...

Ama hayat buna izin verir mi?

Şimdi bu tanımadığım kadının Onur hakkında yazdıklarını okudukça aslında onu hiç böyle değerlendirmediğimi hatta hakkında hiç böyle derinlemesine düşünmediğimi farkediyorum.

İçimden, umarım ayrıntılara girmez, diyorum. Çünkü en çok ayrıntılar acıtır.

"Kimse bilemez," yazıyorum, "herkes bütün bunların nedeni olduğuna inanır ama aslında yoktur, bir gün bir şey olur, bir gün, bir koku, dokunuş, gülümseyiş seni başka bir yere çeker ve bazen gitmek istersin, hepsi bu.."

Yazıyorum ve şu anda gerçekten böyle düşünebildiğime, ağzımdan bu sözlerin döküldüğüne, böylesine sakin kalabildiğime ben de şaşırıyorum. Sadece yazarken ellerim titriyor ve bazı harfler karışıyor.

Bir Fransız arkadaşım bir gün, "Aldatmak yoktur, yakalanmak vardır," demişti. Kocasını kendi yatak odasında bir kadınla yakalamış, kıyameti kopartırken kadın sessizce giyinip çıkıp gitmişti.

Belki çok komik ama kocası onun hayal gördüğünü, aldığı sakinleştirici ilaç yüzünden böyle olduğunu, aslında orada kimse olmadığını söylemişti.

"Biliyor musun buna daha çok delirmem gerekirken gülmeye başladım. Ve şimdi de gördüğün gibi gülerek anlatıyorum."

"Peki ne yaptın sonra?" dedim.

"Aslına bakarsan hiç birşey. Çünkü iki yıl önce ben de onu aldatmıştım ve o bunu asla öğrenemedi. Ama ben öğrendim. Bu olaydan sonra yazlık evi üzerime geçirdi ve ben de madem benden önce de ilişkisi olmuştu şimdi ne değişti diye düşündüm."

"Yani böylece artık ona kızgın değil misin?"

"Hayır, bazı adamlar çapkındır, aslında bence bütün adamlar öyledir ama bazıları bunu yapmaya cesaret edemez."

"İyi ama" diye itiraz ettim, "seni aptal yerine koymuş.."

"Hayır, hayır aksine kendisini aptal yerine koydu, kimsenin bu zırvaya inanmayacağını elbette biliyordu, bana o an, ayrılalım ben bu kadını seviyorum da diyebilirdi..."

"Bu daha dürüstçe olmaz mıydı?"

"Olurdu elbette ama ben onu gerçekten seviyorum ve onunla çok eğleniyorum, beni bırakıp gitmesi beni çok üzerdi, o zamandan beri artık bunlara cesaret edemiyor. Dürüst ama beni boğan bir kocayı tercih eder miydim diye sorarsan, ki ben kendime çok sordum, etmem..."

Evet o böyle söylemişti ve şimdi aslında dürüst olması gereken belki de bendim.

Ferhat'ı düşünmediğim tek gün bile olmuş muydu?

Sevişirken bile aklımdakinin o olduğunu söylememin zamanı gelmedi mi artık?

Ben zaten Onur'u sevmemiştim ki... Sevmek nedir biliyordum çünkü. Ben Ferhat'ı sevmiştim. Sevmek öyle birşeydi. Sürekli aklına gelmek, sürekli aklında olmak, uzaktayken de onu hatırlamak, alışveriş yaparken bile şu renk ona yakışır, bu gömlek ne güzel olur demek...

O aklıma geldiğinde yüzümde gülümseme belirir, içimde bilinmez bir duygu yükselirdi sanki.

Ama Onur'a doğumgününde hediye alırken bile iki saat dolaşırdım ve yine de bulamazdım.

Çoğu akşamlar yatsa ya da odasına geçip çalışsa da yalnız kalsam diye düşünürdüm.

Yatağa geç gitmek için sürekli bahaneler bulurdum.

Arkadaşlarıyla buluşmasına, iş gezilerine hiç sesimi çıkartmazdım.

Belki de bu yüzden aslında çok kızmadım.

Olmayacak bir işe kalkışıp onu da mahvetmemden daha doğal ne olabilirdi ki...

Tolga evleneceğimi duyduğunda deliye dönmemiş miydi?

Sare Hanım bana, "Birini yanında hep isteyecek kadar sevdiğine emin değilsen sakın evlenme sonra çok mutsuz olursun," demişti.

Bu evliliğin fazla sürmeyeceğinden herkes emindi aslında.

Bense kendimce oyun oynuyordum ve istersem yapabilirim diye düşünüyordum.

Belki de o güne kadar aslında kimse bana Onur gibi davranmadığı için aklımı çelmeyi başarmıştı.

Ferhat bana kadın gibi davranmazdı. Sevişmelerimiz dışında tabii. Yüzüme bile bakarken sanki çok sevdiği bir çocuğa bakar gibi bakardı.

O bana insan gibi davranırdı.

Onur bana ilk kez kadın gibi davranmıştı. İtiraf etmeliyim ki bu konuda oldukça başarılıdır.

"Evet," yazdım, "devam et..."

Onur'dum ya şimdi...

"İstersen yatabilirsin eminim yorgunsundur yine… Yarın hepsini okursun…"

"Hayır, dinliyorum," yazdım.

"En son Paris'teki otelde telefonda karınla konuştuğunda kendimi nedense ilk kez çok kötü hissettim. Orada hiç değilse tümüyle ikimize ait ilk tatilde, yalnızca benim olduğunu düşündüğüm anda telefonu alıp sakin sakin işlerinden sözedip onu sevdiğini söylediğinde macera bir anda bitti. O anda başı dönmüş, bayılacak gibi olmuş, korkmuş ve sana ne yapacağını soruyor, o saatte doktoru aramasını tavsiye ediyordun ve birkaç dakika sonra onu sakinleştirip beni öpecektin. Ama yapmadın. Sabah ilk uçakla dönmeye karar verdin, telefonu kapadıktan sonra sigara yaktın, kahve aldın ve benden özür diledin. Böyleydi. Gerçek, üstünü böyle tüllerle örterek gizleyebileceğimiz türden birşey değildi."

Gözlerimden kendiliğinden yaşlar akmaya başladı. O geceyi hatırladım. Çok uzak değil daha onbeş, yirmi gün önceydi.

Birden sırtıma bıçak saplanmıştı ve korkmuştum. O yüzden aramıştım Onur'u…

Hatta birden işleri iptal edip ertesi gün döneceğini söylemesine de şaşırmıştım. Benim ataklarıma yabancı değildi çünkü.

Şimdi bunları okurken o bıçak yeniden saplandı.

"Sen uçağı ayarlayıp bavulunu toplarken aslında onu çok merak ettiğin için değil kendi suçluluk duygundan yola çıktığını biliyordum artık. Bavulu toplayan sen değildin, vicdanındı."

Gözlerimi sildim. Aldatılan kadın, aldatan adam, vicdan, suçluluk... Ne çok dinlemiştik bu hikayeleri... Hiç boşuna bu havaya girme dedim kendi kendime. Her zaman alay ederdin bunlarla. Şimdi kendini bu duruma düşürmeyeceksin.

O devam etti yazmaya...

"Orada tek başıma iki gün geçirdikten sonra döneceğim akşam küçük kalabalık bir lokantada yemek yedim. Aklıma ne geldi biliyor musun? Bütün o geceler, sevişmeler, mutluluklar değil... Bir akşam beni sinemaya götürmüştün, patlamış mısırlarımızı alıp arka sırada oturmuştuk, karanlıkta elimi tutmuştun, lise yıllarımdaki gibi... Hüzünlü bir filmdi, sonunda kız ölüyordu ama ben ağlamadım, belki de seninle bunca zaman yaşadığım en güzel andı çünkü..."

Sinema mı? Bunca yıl beni hiç sinemaya götürmemişti. Her zaman sinemayı sevmediğini söylerdi çünkü. Ne garip, belki de bütün duyduklarımdan çok bu bana dokundu.

O yazıyordu:

"Yan masamda oturan adam bana kadeh kaldırıp birkaç şey sordu. Biraz sohbet ettik. Eşini kaybettikten sonra akşam yemeklerini artık bu küçük, şirin lokantada yediğini söyledi. Bana kısaca hayatından bahsetti, karısıyla en azından son yıllarda çok güzel tatiller yaptığını ve onu yıllarca ihmal ettikten sonra daha iyi tanıdığını ama geç kaldığını itiraf etti. Kalkarken onu öptüm ve teşekkür ettim. Neden teşekkür ettiğimi sordu.

Bilmiyorsunuz ama hayatımı artık tümüyle değiştirmeye karar verdim bu yemek sırasında, dedim. Elinizdeyken, yapabiliyorken yapın küçük hanım, yoksa sonra üzülürsünüz diye cevap verdi.

O yüzden bana açıklama yapmana gerek yok. Sana ne kızgınım, ne kırgınım, ne de artık bir beklentim var. Zaten olmamalıydı. Her zaman benim eski dostum, yakınım olarak kalacaksın, bunu silmek imkansız. Ve benim için vicdan azabı duyma, eğer merak ediyorsan, hiç beklenmedik birşey yapacağımı söyleyebilirim, yeniden Paris'e gidiyorum yarın ve bazen bir rastlantının hayatımı değiştirebileceğine yeniden inanmak istiyorum. Hoşçakal..." yazdı ve kayboldu.

Öylece biraz oturdum bilgisayarın başında. Sonra saate baktım. Onur birazdan gelirdi. Bu yaptığımı kendime yediremiyordum aslında. Hayatımda hiç böyle birşey yapmamıştım ve yapan kızlara da acırdım. İnsan büyük konuşmamalı dedikleri bu mu acaba?

Açıkçası içimden öfkeli olsam da bana bunu nasıl yapar diye düşünmedim. Konyağımı aldım, salona geçtim, koltuğa oturup sigara yaktım.

Demek Paris'e gidiyormuş.

Hem de aniden karar vererek.

Doğru mu, değil mi, Onur'u kışkırtmak için mi söyledi bilmiyorum ama bütün yazdıklarından sonra ona inanıyordum.

Henüz ne yapacağımı düşünmek için erkendi. Henüz yalnızca okuduklarımı düşünüyordum. Birçok ayrıntı şimdi aklıma geliyor, taşlar yavaş yavaş yerine oturuyordu ama bunu sürdürmek istemiyordum. Çünkü o zaman daha çok öfkelenecektim.

Ne gariptir ki üzgün değildim.

Hatta içimden bir ses bu senin kurtuluşun olacak diyordu.

Arkama yaslandım ve geçen yılları düşündüm.

O gelmeden gidip yattım. Geldiğinde uyumuş olmak istiyordum. Çünkü aslında o son kadehi içerken ne yapacağıma karar vermiştim.

Bu çok acayip gece benim için bitmişti.

Yalnızca bu gece değil, bu üç yıl da bitmişti.

Şimdi bunu ona nasıl söyleyeceğimi düşünmeliydim.

Tabii ki olan bitenden haberi yoktu ve hayatın kimbilir ne zamandır olduğu gibi sürüp gittiğini sanıyordu.

Aslında yarın hem sevgilisini hem karısını kaybedeceğinden de haberi yoktu.

Gerçi konuşmaya bakılırsa kadın bu ilişkiyi bitirmeye kalkışmıştı ama ben pek emin değildim. Biliyorum ki böyle ilişkiler kolay kolay bitmez. Sürüklenip gider. Kadın da bunu bildiği için hiç tanımadığı bir adamın yanına gidiyordu. Yoksa onun hala Onur'a aşık olduğundan adım gibi emindim.

Kimbilir Onur bunu öğrenince onun yanına koşacak ve belki beni de bırakacaktı.

Ama şimdi sıra bendeydi.

Kapının açıldığını duydum. Gözlerimi kapadım. Geldi, benim uyuduğumu gördü, banyoya girdi.

Her zamanki gibi üstünü çıkartmasını, pijamalarını giymesini, yanıma gelmesini duydum. Arkasını dönüp yattı.

Bunca yıldır sana arkasını dönüp yatan bir adamla yaşamanın suçu kimde olabilir ki?

Bir kere bile söyledin mi?

Sordun mu?

Evet ağlamak istiyordum hem de deli gibi…

Kendimi tutuyordum.

Hastaneye yattığım zaman bile bir an önce oradan kaçıp sevgilisinin yanına giden bir adamla yaşıyorum.

"Sen git, ben iyiyim," dediğim zaman "peki o zaman" diyen bir adamla..

Sabah kahvaltısında istediği peynir olmazsa, domatesleri istediği gibi dilimlenmemişse, yumurtası tam kayısı olmamışsa surat asan bir adamla…

Aynı tonda bin tane gömleğinden birini giymek istediğinde yakası güzel ütülenmemişse söylenen bir adamla…

Saçımı boyattığımda, kestirdiğimde, yaptırdığımda farketmeyen bir adamla…

Bana iki yıl üstüste doğum günümde aynı kolyeyi alan adamla…

Benden başka herkese iyi, nazik olan bir adamla…

"El iyisi" derdi Sare Hanım böylelerine…

"Aynanın karşısında bir kadından daha çok zaman geçiren adamlardan uzak dur," demişti Tolga…

Ağlamak mı, gülmek mi, onu uyandırıp kıyameti kopartmak mı, içimden gelenleri bilemiyorum artık.

Ne aşağılık olduğunu yüzüne söylesem mi?

Yoksa ne budala olduğumu kendime mi söylesem?

Horlamaya başladı bile. Tabii ki sarhoş...

Kalktım.

Salona gittim. Hayır bir kadeh daha içmeyecektim. Sarhoş olup onu uyandırıp kavga etmek istemiyordum.

Bütün bu karışık duygulara rağmen garip bir biçimde aslında kendimi iyi hissediyordum.

Bitmişti.

Biz birbirimizi sevememiştik.

Hepsi buydu.

Bu başıma gelen felaket değildi. Aksine bana hayatımı kurtarmam için verilmiş bir şanstı.

O kadına kızmam değil teşekkür etmem gerekiyordu.

Belki anlaması zor. Onur da niye bana katlanmıştı ki? Neden, sevdiği ya da yanında mutlu olduğu bir başkası varken hem de....

Sorumluluk mu? Düzen isteği mi?

Ama biz aile değildik ki? Bizim çocuğumuz bile yoktu.

O kadını da sevmiyordu aslında. Kendinden başka kimseyi sevmiyordu ki...

Eğer sevişmenin ne olduğunu bilmeseydim, kadın olmanın nasıl birşey olduğunu bilmeseydim şimdi o kadını çok kıskanırdım.

Ama biliyordum. Kimseye söylemesem de çok iyi biliyordum hem de...

Garip, beklenmedik bir geceydi. Sıradan gecelerden birinde birdenbire bunlar olmuştu işte. Belki de sıradan binlerce sıkıcı gecenin böylece sürüp gitmesini engelleyecek birşey.

Şimdi bütün bunları kafamdan silip atmalıydım. Babamın gidişinden ben sorumlu değildim. Onur'un bunları yapmasının nedeni de ben değildim.

Neredeyse gün doğuyordu.

Hayır yüzyüze konuşmak istemiyordum.

Bir kağıt aldım ve yazmaya başladım.

"Sevgili Onur, nedense bazı insanlar birbirleriyle herşeyi konuşamazlar. İkisi de içlerinden farklı şeyler düşündükleri halde bunu söyleyemezler. Hatta başkalarıyla konuşur, doktorlara gider ama yine de karşısındakine gerçeği anlatamazlar.

Seninle kimi zaman konuşmak istedim ama yapamadım. Belki de sen bu tür konuşmaları sevmediğin için... Belki de hep geçiştirdiğin için…

Geriye dönüp bakınca, beni ilk gördüğü andan itibaren peşimde koşan, ilgisiyle beni şaşırtan birini görüyorum. Kibar, sevecen, düşünceli, anlayışlı…

Yalnızca bir yıl sonra, beni neredeyse görmeyen, ilgilenmeyen, olur olmaz tersleyen, kabalaşan bir başka adam...

Evden sürekli kaçmaya, yalnız kaldığımız anları olabildiğince azaltmaya çalışan, başkalarının yanında yine eski eğlenceli, neşeli adamken benim yanımda somurtan…

Evlenmeye karar verdiğimizde sana pek çok insanın bilmediği şeyleri, hastalığımı anlatmıştım.

Kabul etmeliyim ki çoğu zaman, beklenmedik nöbetler geldiğinde, gecenin yarısı beni hastanelere taşımak zorunda kaldığında, bayıldığımda gerçekten öldüğümü sanıp deliye döndüğünde hep yanımda oldun.

Ama insan birbirine ağır gelir derdi anneannem. Zaman geçince bunlara katlanmak güç geliyor biliyorum. Bir çekmece dolusu ilaç içen, her gittiğimiz yerde yediklerine, içtiklerine dikkat etmesi gereken, vücut kokusu bile değişen, çoğu zaman yorgun, korkudan evden çıkmak istemeyecek kadar yorgun, vaktinden önce yaşlanmış bir kadını kim ister ki?

Tabii ki seninle evlenirken bunların düzeleceğine, iyiye gideceğine inanıyordum. Doktorlar anne olmanın bana iyi geleceğini söylüyorlardı. Ama ne yazık ki o da olmadı.

Aslında çoğu zaman en kötü anlarda bile sana yük olmamaya, gözlerimden yaşlar gelecek kadar acı çektiğimde bile senden gizlemeye çalıştım.

Ama artık itiraf etmenin zamanı geldi.

Birlikte mutlu değiliz. Ve senin bunu belki de yalnızca vicdan azabın nedeniyle sürdürdüğüne artık hiç kuşkum yok.

En yakın arkadaşının sana söylediği gibi belki de karşılaştıklarının arasında en düzgün, en iyi kız olduğum içindir.

Ama sana birşey söyleyeyim mi, ben iyi, düzgün bir kız olmak istemiyorum.

Yapmak istediklerimi, belki de beni bütün bu hastalıklardan, sıkıntılardan uzaklaştıracak, belki bana çok iyi gelecek şeyleri bile bu üç yılda erteledim durdum. Eve geldiğinde yüzünün gülmesi için, bana sarıldığın zaman mutlu olman için, açıkçası ne hazin ama beni sevmen için kendimi bir yana bıraktım. Arkadaşlarımdan bile uzaklaştım. Seninle olmak için yapayalnız kaldım.

Hayır, aşk emek vermekle ilgili değil. Bunu artık biliyorum. O, ne senin, ne benim kafese kapatıp zaman zaman seveceğimiz gizemli bir kuş değil.

Kimseye sormadan geliyor ve yine bir gün kimseye sormadan çıkıp gidiyor.

Seninle oturup bütün bunları konuşmak, hayatı yeniden yoluna koymak, belki birilerinden yardım istemek... Hayır bütün bunlar için çok geç.

Eğer her zaman içimdeki sesi dinleseydim, gerçek duygularıma inansaydım, onları düzenlemeye, hayata uydurmaya, bir biçime sokmaya çalışmasaydım daha mutlu olurdum.

Kimbilir belki bunu farketmem için de bu zamanın geçmesi gerekiyormuş."

Bunları yazdım, biraz durdum. Güneş doğuyordu. Kafam hem hiç olmadığı kadar karışık hem de aslında bu sabah gibi berraktı.

"Sana birşey daha itiraf edeceğim. Ben başkasına aşığım. Onun için de senden ayrılıyorum. Bir an önce boşanma işlerini halledersen beni çok mutlu edersin."

Yazdıklarıma yeniden baktım.

Evet böylesi daha iyi olacaktı.

Bu saatten sonra oturup da onun neler yaptığını yüzüne vurmaya, inkarlarını dinlemeye, iyice canımı acıtacak ayrıntıları duymaya hiç niyetim yoktu. Halim de... Zaten artık neye yarardı ki?

"Senden hiçbirşey istemiyorum. Her zaman benim için yaptıklarını, iyiliğini hatırlayacağım. Hoşçakal."

Tabii ki ağladım. Ellerim titredi yeniden okurken. Bunca zamanın özeti bu muydu?

Okulda koskoca romanların ana fikrini çıkartın dedikleri zaman yaptığımız gibi yazarın belki yıllarca en küçük ayrıntılarıyla uğraşarak yazdığı kitabı birkaç satırda özetleyivermek.

Evet böyleydi.

Mektubu masanın üzerine koydum.

Yalnızca çantamı ceketimi aldım ve çıktım.

Nereye gideceğimi, ne yapacağımı, şu an bile neler olacağını bilmeden, içimde hüzün, aynı zamanda beklenmedik bir heyecan vardı.

Yollar boştu. Ne zamandır bu saatte sokağa çıkmadığım için garip geldi bana. Pırıl pırıl güneş, hafif bir esinti vardı. Ürperdim ama yürüdükçe alıştım.

Yavru bir köpek peşime takılıp benimle oynamaya çalıştı.

Neden olmasın, dedim kendi kendime, bu belki de gerçekte olması gereken şeydir, yeni bir hayattır, senin yeni bir hayata ihtiyacın var.

Evet vardı. Bunca zaman sanki karanlıkta, bodrumda yaşamış gibi bu sabah ışığında gözlerimin kamaşması bundandı.

İşte yeni hayat önümde boş, uzun bir yoldu.

Bizim eve geldiğim o sabah aslında kendimi iyi hissettiğimi düşünüyordum ama sonra artık takatim kalmadı ve birdenbire kapının önünde yığılıp kaldım.

Tıpkı babam gittikten sonra olduğu gibi...

Sonra hatırladıklarım uyku gibi...

Daha doğrusu rüyadayken rüyada olduğunu bilmek gibi...

Sesleri duyuyorum. Annemle Seda konuşuyorlar. Fısıltıyla...

"Duymuyor," diyor Seda.

Sahi rüyaların sesi var mıdır?

Ama duyuyorum. Garip bir biçimde tıpkı rüyada bağırmak isteyip bağıramamak gibi duyuyorum demek istiyorum ama sesim çıkmıyor. Yine de bu beni korkutmuyor. Yalnızca inanılmaz yorgunken uyumak gibi...

Neredeyim? Hastanede mi? Evde mi? Bilmiyorum.

Bazen üstüste hızla görüntüler geçiyor, yüzler, televizyon görüntüleri, hayvanlar, geçmişe ait fotoğraflar, anılar, koşan bir çocuk... Sonra yeniden yavaşlıyor.

"Taner Bey gelecek mi?" diye soruyor annem. "Gelsin, ne olur gelsin," demek istiyorum.

"Evet bir saate kadar uğrarım dedi," diyor Seda, "isterseniz siz yiyin ben buradayım nasıl olsa..."

"Yok istemem kızım, doktor gelsin de... Onur nerede, kavga mı ettiler acaba?"

Bana birşey olmuş. Ne oldu ki?

Çiçeklerin arasında dolaşıyorum, evet hatırladığım bir yer burası, anneannemlerin evinin bahçesi, rengarenk güller var, uzakta çilek bahçeleri, kiraz ağaçları var.

"Merak etmeyin," diyor Seda, "bunu da atlatacak, üzmeyin kendinizi artık..."

"Artık benim de takatim kalmadı," diyor annem.

Benim de kalmadı anne.

Galiba bu kez benim de kalmadı...

Hiç kimseye asla söylemediğim birşey var, nedense aklıma o geliyor, ölmekten korkmadım hiç ama ölmeye yatmaktan korktum, kıpırdayamamaktan, ses çıkartamamaktan, gidememekten, orada kimsenin bilmediği bir yerde arada kalmaktan...

Hayır bu rüya olmalı, çok yorgundum çünkü hatırlıyorum, o kadar yorgunum ki yalnızca uyumak istiyorum, ellerimi bile kaldıramıyorum yorgunluktan...

Burada bir rüyanın içine hapsolup sonsuza dek kalmayacağım değil mi?

Ağlamaya başlıyorum. "Ama ben kimseye birşey yapmadım, ben hiç kötülük yapmadım, neden bütün bunlar bana oldu?" diyorum.

Sonra anneanneme çiçekler götürüyorum. Öylece yatıyor, elini tutmaya çalışıyorum ama kıpırdamıyor, bembeyaz kesilmiş, elinin damarları kaybolmuş, yalnızca kahverengi lekeler vardı ellerinde ve soğuk...

Odamın duvarına elimi sürüyorum ve jöle gibi yumuşadığını farkediyorum, sonra elimi içine sokabildiğimi...

Duvarın içinden geçiyorum ve gökyüzünden yere uzanan rengarenk çiçeklerle, sarmaşıklarla dolu bir tür ormana giriyorum.

Bütün o çiçeklerin kokusu, ormanın serinliği, o çiçeklere dokunurken hissettiklerim öylesine gerçek ki bunun rüya olmadığına inanıyorum.

Çocukken gördüğüm ve neredeyse tüm ayrıntılarıyla anlattığım rüyaları dinlerken herkes hayalgücümün ne kadar güçlü olduğunu söyler, bense benden başka kimsenin böyle rüyalar görmediğini düşünerek sevinirdim.

Büyüdüm ve bu hiç değişmedi.

Rüyalarım hala böylesine gerçek ve ben hala rüyayla gerçeği karıştırıyorum.

Şimdi bunca zaman sonra birdenbire bugün mü?

Onca şeye dayanmışken, onca şeyin üstesinden gelmeyi başarmışken, bütün bu acılarla, hep evet artık bitti derken yeniden başlamışken, neden şimdi?

İşte yine geldi... ellerim titriyor, kafam kayarmış gibi, belleğin içinde sanki birşey bütün anıları bir anda hızla sürüklüyor, sonra ağırlaşıyor, bütün bunları yıllarca anlattım ama kimse anlamadı, ne doktorlar ne başkaları, işte o küçükken gördüğüm rüyadaki gibi hep o uçurumun kenarından aşağı bakarken duyduğum his ve uyanmaya çalışmak, ama uyumuyorum, uyumadığımı, bunun rüya olmadığını biliyorum, keşke olsa, keşke hepsi, bütün bu hayat öyle olsaydı ve şimdi uyansaydım, ama değil, geri döndü biliyorum, adını bilmediğim şey, beni yoketmeye karar veren öteki ben mi, sebebini asla bilemediğim o uğursuz şeytan mı, yok yok yalnızca genetik bir bozukluk, sakin ol, paniğe kapılma, binlerce kez kendi kendime söyledim bunları, ama insan bedenini denetleyemediği zaman paniğe kapılır, sen biliyorsun, başkaları başına bir kez geldiğinde korkar ama sen biliyorsun, yürüyemediğin, yürümeyi unuttuğun anları düşün, çay fincanını tutmaya çalışıp düşürdüğün anları düşün, sen biliyorsun, gelen yabancı ama aslında senin için çok tanıdık, onu kaç kez yendin, bu oyunu kaç kez oynadın, yeniden oynayabilirsin, yeniden kazanabilirsin....

Evet bir oyun.

Yıllar önce birdenbire kendimi içinde bulduğum, hiç beklenmedik bir anda başlayan ve giderek korkunçlaşan bir oyun bu.

Ama zaten hayat da böyle değil mi? Sonunda, ne yaparsanız yapın kaybedeceğiniz bir oyun değil mi? Üstelik oyunlardaki gibi sizin yaptığınız hatalara bağlı değil.

Herşeyi doğru yapsanız da kaybedeceğiniz başından belli bir oyun.

İyi ama bazıları için en azından oynarken eğlenceli...

Son zamanlarda yaşadığım en güçlü ataktı ve kendime geldiğimde her yerim karıncalanıyor, bana neler olduğunu hatırlamaya çalışıyor ama hatırlamıyordum.

Önce çok korktular ama sonra yavaş yavaş kendime geldim.

Eve döndüğümüzde herkes Onur'u merak ediyordu ama ona haber vermemelerini söyledim. Gerçi zaten ortada yoktu ve beni aramayı bile düşünmemişti.

Onlara kavga ettiğimizi, Onur'un da iş gezisine gittiğini söyledim.

Tek istediğim sıcak suya girmekti.

Çocukluğumdan beri beni en çok rahatlatan şeyin su olması ve sonunda suyun içine yazılar yazmaya, resimler çizmeye kalkışmam ne garip...

Suya iz bırakılmaz derler. Ama işte bırakıyorum.

Anneanneme sorarsanız Ebru'nun bir anlamı bulut olduğu için, Seda'ya sorarsanız su burcunda doğduğum için...

Ama en kötü günlerimde, en hasta olduğum zamanlarda bile beni rahatlatan tek şey su...

O gün de sıcak suda uzandım.

Onur'la yeniden konuşmama gerek yoktu.

Bilirsiniz, Amerikan filmlerinin çoğunda bir yüzleşme sahnesi vardır.

Başına gelenlerin suçlusu olarak anne ya da babasını gören adam onlarla yüzleşir.

Kadın, hayatını mahvettiğini düşündüğü kocasıyla yüzleşir.

Gerçekte bir sır nedeniyle araları açılan iki eski dost yüzleşirler...

Ben kimseyle yüzleşmek istemem.

Beni daha da fazla üzecek gerçeği öğrenmek de istemem.

Sanki bütün hayat bir aldanma değilmiş gibi, çoğumuz gerçeği öğrenmek isteriz.

Ne yani, o astronotlar aya gerçekten gitmedilerse bunu öğrenip mutlu mu olacağım?

Zaten artık öğrenmem gereken ne vardı ki? Belki bana yalanlar söyleyecek, belki kadının delinin biri olduğuna ikna etmeye kalkışacaktı.

Gerçi o anda tam olarak neler olduğunu, kadının tüm yazdıklarını, benim verdiğim cevapları sonra ona bıraktığım mektubu da doğru dürüst hatırlamıyordum.

Daha geçen hafta Taner Amca'yla konuşmuştum.

Bana uzun zaman önce sözettiği o deneysel ameliyatın artık çok geliştiğini ve bunu düşünmem gerektiğini söylemişti.

Sanki arınması gereken benmişim gibi sıcak suyun içinde uzandım.

Su herşeyi taşır, alıp götürür ama onda birşey kalmaz.

Su unutmaktır aynı zamanda.

Ben de unutmak istiyordum.

Artık tüm bunları idare etmeye çalışmaktan, ataklarımı gizlemeye çalışmaktan, Onur hastalığımı öğrendikten sonra sanki suçluymuşum gibi ona belli etmemeye uğraşmaktan, bu evliliği aslında çok sıkıldığım halde yürütmekten, giderek anneme dönüşmekten çok yorgundum.

Evet ben bu değildim.

Olmak da istemiyordum artık.

Hayat anneannemin dediği gibi ya kendine yasaklayıp çile çektiğin ya da her ne olursa olsun, başına ne gelirse gelsin istediğin gibi yaşaman gereken birşeydi.

Demek öyleymiş, demek böyleymiş diye bir akşam önceki yazışmaları hatırlayıp kendimi daha fazla yıpratmayacaktım. Ona kızgın filan da değildim.

Ben de belki babam gibi günün birinde hayatımı değiştirecektim ama geç kalmadan ve onun gibi başkalarının hayatını bozmadan.

Yazdığım mektuptan sonra arasa da onunla konuşmayacaktım.

O gece ilaçlardan mı, yorgunluktan mı yoksa üzerimden aslında yük kalktığı için mi bilmem çok güzel uyudum.

Ertesi sabah tanıdık bir avukattan boşanma davası için neler yapmam gerektiğini öğrendim.

Sonra Taner Amca'yı aradım ve ameliyata gireceğimi ama annem dahil hiç kimsenin haberinin olmasını istemediğimi söyledim.

Telefonda sessizlik oldu.

"Birkaç gün sonra gidiyorum, gitmeden yüzyüze konuşalım, sen de biraz daha düşün, birlikte karara varırız," dedi.

Ama ben çoktan kararımı vermiştim.

Annem tabii ki çıldırdı. "Bir kavga yüzünden yuva yıkılır mı, biraz bekle elbet çıkıp gelecek, özür dileyecektir," deyip duruyordu.

Tabii ki onlara gerçekte neler olduğunu anlatmadım.

"İnsan sürekli mutsuzluğunu gizleyerek yaşayamaz anne," dedim sonunda, "herkes senin gibi değil..."

Yüzüme ters cevap verecekmiş gibi baktı ama vermedi.

Seda da merak içindeydi ama korkudan soramıyordu.

Annem, "Hiç değilse etrafa söylemeyelim, biraz bekleyelim, anneannene belli etme," gibi tam ona uygun lafları sırayla söylüyordu ama hiç umurumda değildi. Tabii ki anneanneme söyledim.

Belki biraz da vazgeçememek için yaptım bunu.

Zaten o sanıldığı gibi tepki vermedi.

"Sen kendin için iyi olanı bilirsin, bazen direnmek olsa olsa zaman kaybıdır," dedi.

Neyse ki annem yanımızda değildi.

Onur direnmedi. Gelip özür de dilemedi. Herhalde artık bunun yürümeyeceğinin farkındaydı ya da kimbilir belki benden sandığımdan çok sıkılmıştı ve söyleyemiyordu.

Boşanma işlemleri bitti, biraz zaman geçti. Artık kafamda tek şey vardı o da bir an önce ameliyata girmek.

Ama bir akşam eve geldiğimde annemi ağlarken buldum.
Anneannemle oturuyorlardı.
Acaba ameliyat olayını mı öğrendi diye düşündüm.
"Baban aradı..." dedi.
Çantamı yere bırakıp koltuğa yığıldım.
Babam mı?
Ne bu şimdi?
"Çok ağır hastaymış, seni görmek istiyormuş..."
Boşluğa baktım.
Benim babam var mı ki beni görmek istiyormuş?
Daldım gittim.
Bir keresinde Ferhat'a babamdan sözetmiştim. Neler anlattım şimdi hatırlamıyorum. Ama hiç ses çıkarmadan dinledi.

Sonra, o insanı sakinleştiren, yatıştıran, iyi hissetmesini sağlayan konuşma biçimiyle, "Biliyor musun," dedi, "bazen hayat hatta çoğu zaman bizim kurguladığımız gibi olmuyor, insan bazen verdiği sözleri tutamıyor, olan bitenlerle başedemiyor, zaaflarına yeniliyor..."

Babamın başına birşey gelmedi, onun başedeceği bir zorluk da yoktu yalnızca evet belki zaaflarına yenildi...

"Sana anlatmıştım," dedi, "babam sanki doğaya, bilime isyan etmiş gibi çocuklarının öleceğini ya da sakat kalacağını bildiği halde inat etti. Bunun için onu hiç affedemedim. Ama ne gariptir ki böyle yapmasaydı ben burada şimdi senin karşında oturuyor olmayacaktım. Ve hiç kuşku yok ki onlar için herkesten çok o acı çekti. Belki de savaşa giden bir komutan gibi bir mucize için o acılara katlanmayı seçti."

Gerçekten böyle düşünebiliyor muydu?

"Böyle düşününce ona daha farklı bakmaya başladım. Ve aldığı onca katlanılmaz cezadan sonra onu bir de benim cezalandırmaya kalkışmamın ne kadar saçma olduğunu farkettim."

Evet aslında onun anlattığı çok daha korkunçtu. Ölen kardeşler, yaşayan ama hayat boyu başkalarına muhtaç bir kardeş, mutsuzluklar, ayrılıklar, yalnızlıklar... Ve bütün bunları yaşayan anne...

"Tabii bunları düşünmemişti bence. Eğer düşünseydi benden sonra kardeşimin dünyaya gelmesini istemezdi. Belki de hayatı öylesine kabullenmiş, kadere inanmış, tüm bunların yaradandan geldiğine ve böyle olması gerektiğine inanmış biriydi. Yüzüne düşündüklerimi söylemedim. Ama çok zaman sanki karşımdaymış gibi kendi kendime konuştum."

Ne söyleyeceğini biliyordum.

Ve söyledi.

"Belki de günün birinde onunla karşılaşman, söyleyeceklerini o ölüp gitmeden söylemen iyi olur..."

Evet ben de onunla sanki karşımdaymış gibi ne çok konuşmuştum. Kimi zaman ben ölürken gelmiş ve yanımdaymış gibi ya da kimi zaman o ölürken...

Sanki bir gün bunun olacağını bilirmiş gibi anlatmıştı bana...

Ve şimdi babam ölüm döşeğinde beni görmek istiyordu.

O konuşma şimdi uzaklardan çıkıp gelmişti ve sanki yine orada onun evinde oturmuş konuşur gibi hatırlıyordum.

"O benim için çoktan öldü," dedim, "onun ölümünün yasını öyle uzun zaman tuttum ki yeniden o ölümü yaşamak istemem..."

"Belki de hala tutuyorsun," dedi...

Böyle söylüyordum ama doğru muydu? Gülümseyerek anlamış gibi bakıyordu yüzüme…

Yalandı çünkü babamın Seda'yla beni hayvanat bahçesine götürdüğü o günü, her yerimiz pamuk şeker ve dondurma olmuş halde eve geldiğimizde annemin söylenmelerini, eve gelirken babamın, bak şimdi annen neler söyleyecek, ne eğleneceğiz deyişini, çok istediğim konsere bana sürpriz yapıp en önden yer ayırmasını, Ajda'nın kulisine bizi sokup Tolga'ya imza attırmasını, şimdi yerinde gökdelenlerin yükseldiği dev çayırlıkta yaptığımız piknikleri, benim için yaptığı küçük tahta evi, geceleri mutlaka kısa da olsa yanımda oturup alnımdan öperek 'Allah rahatlık versin' deyişini, annemin dırdırları sırasında bana bakıp çaktırmadan aldırma der gibi göz kırpışını, maç izlerken söylenip heyecanlanmasını, bazen dalıp gidişlerini, 'her sabah kahvaltıda yedi zeytin yemek lazım,' demesini, saçını hep ceket cebinden çıkardığı metal tarakla taramasını, yolda yürürken boynumdan tutmasını, hemen her hafta bana aldığı kitapları…

Bunların hiçbirini unutmamıştım ki…

İnsan öyle her istediğini silemiyor. Bellek kendi bildiği bir oyunla istediğini istediği yere koyuyor, sizin o karmaşık tavanarasını yeniden düzenlemenize izin vermiyor.

Ferhat'ın uzaktan gelen sesiyle dalgınlığımdan sıyrıldım.

"İnsan çocukluğundan ayrılamaz, birçok şeyle vedalaşırız da onunla vedalaşamayız."

Kimbilir belki de haklıydı. Onun babası böyle davranmasa, benim babam çekip gitmese o an orada onunla olmayacaktım. Hayatım tümüyle farklı olacaktı.

İyi mi, kötü mü, artık bunu bilmek imkansız. Ama böyle olmuştu işte.

İçimde sanki iki Ebru vardı. Biri ne olursa olsun beş dakikalığına bile olsa gidip onu görmemi söyleyen, öteki kendi kendine yıllardır verdiğin sözü tut, gitme, o senin baban değil, diyen...

Ben onu mahkemeye çıkartmış, yargılamış ve mahkum etmiştim.

Buna hakkım var mıydı?

Üstelik savunmasını dinlememiştim.

Bir keresinde Sare Hanım, "bu konuyu fazla kafana takma, de ki baban kaza geçirdi, öldü," demişti.

Ama öyle değildi işte. Öyle olsa çok daha kolay olurdu.

Babam koca bir kamyonu üzerimize sürmüştü ve biz oraya buraya savrulup yine de hayatta kalmayı başarmıştık.

Ben Ferhat gibi düşünemiyordum. O bunların bir nedeni olduğunu düşünüyor, bunu yapanın aslında çok daha fazla acı çektiğine inanıyordu.

"Hayatı belirleyen şey ölümdür," demişti. "Ve ölüm herşeyi anlamsız kılar. Bütün bu konuştuklarımızı, suçlamaları, ihanetleri, kavgaları..."

Ona baktım, ellerini tuttum. Yanına oturdum.

"Ben şimdi buradayım, sen de burada mısın?" diye sordum.

"Artık hep tam da burada olacağım," dedi.

Eğilip beni öptü ve bütün bunların bizi getirdiği yerin burası olduğundan başka aklımda birşey kalmadı. Silindi gitti.

Ama herkes verdiği sözleri tutamıyor değil mi?

Şimdi tam da hayatımın bu en garip zamanında hiç beklenmedik biçimde babamın ortaya çıkıvermesi neyin işaretiydi?

O gece sabaha kadar yatakta dönüp durdum. Ne kaybedecektim? Çok mu üzülecektim onu görünce? Zaten yeterince üzülmemiş miydim? O kendi kendime yaptığım konuşmalarda neredeyse ezberlediğim cümleleri yüzüne söyleyebilecek miydim?

Hayatımın belki de en önemli kararını verdiğim bir anda ne değişecekti ki?

Küçük, eski, ahşap bir kutu.

Belki anneannemin çocukluğundan kalmış... İncecik solmuş renkli desenlerle bezeli...

Onu bana anneannem vermişti. Demişti ki verirken, "Bunun içine sence en değerli şeyleri koy, yıllar sonra büyüdüğün zaman onlara bakınca o kutunun içinde kendini göreceksin..."

Bu sözler o zaman bana sanki bir masalda, birden belirip kaybolan yaşlı bilgenin küçük kıza söylediği sözler gibi büyülü gelmişti. Ve o kutuyu büyülü bir hediye gibi saklamıştım.

Neler koymuştum içine?

Annemin bebekken kesip sakladığı bir tutam saç. Bebek patiklerim. Gümüş mama kaşığım. Çizdiğim ilk resimler. Seda'nın, Tolga'nın bana aldığı hediyeler. Küçük bir müzik kutusu, minicik bir hatıra defteri, birkaç fotoğraf, babamın en yakışıklı fotoğrafı (arkasında uçsuz bucaksız denizin göründüğü, bir geminin güvertesinde pipo içerken yüzünde düşünceli ama hafif mutlu bir gülümseme, daha çok genç...), annemin eteğine tutunmuş, evin kapısında herhalde babamın çektiği fotoğrafım, ilk gittiğim konserin bileti, mektuplar, annemle babama yazdığım ama hiç göstermediğim mektuplar, Tolga'nın bana yazdığı mektuplar, Sare Hanım'ın bana verdiği zümrüt küpeler, en sevdiğim, kurunca zıplayan küçük sincap, babamın bana ortaokula başlarken verdiği yeşil çizgili dolmakalem, zaman içinde anlamını, önemini yitiren ufak tefek şeyler...

O kutuyu yıllarca aradım ama bulamadım.

Sonunda kendi kendime dedim ki, okulunu bırakıp ülkene döndün, evliliğini bitirdin, yeni bir hayata başlamaya karar verdin. Kimsenin bilmediği, senin de sonunun ne olacağını bilmediğin bir ameliyata gidiyorsun.

Belki de o filmlerdeki gibi bir yüzleşme sahnesinin zamanı gelmiştir.

Gittim.

Berlin'e yakın bir hastaneye...

Babamın ölüm döşeğinin yanında sandalyede oturdum. Ne yapmam gerektiğini, ne söylemem gerektiğini bilemiyordum. Bunca yıl ne düşündüysem unutmuş gibi öylece oturdum.

Aslında yabancı gibiydi. Hatırladığım, çocukluğumdaki babaya benzemiyor. Çok kilo almış, saçları dökülmüş, bıyıklarını kesmiş.

Gündüz ama beyaz tavandan sarkan çıplak lamba yanıyor. Büyükçe ama hasta yatağı ve iki sandalye dışında birşey olmayan çıplak bir oda.

Yalnızca hüzün veriyor.

Dışarda yağmur.

Zorlukla konuşuyor. Çünkü boğazında birşey var. Boğazına delik açıp oraya birşey yerleştirmişler. Metalik bir sesle konuşuyor. "Geldiğin için teşekkür ederim," diyor ve ağlıyor. Gözlerinden yaşlar akıyor ama ağladığı bile zor anlaşılıyor.

Ve o ses, artık onun kendi sesi bile yok. Sanki robot konuşuyormuş gibi...

Odaya geldiğimde yüzünde oksijen maskesi vardı, onu çıkartmalarını istedi.

Kulaklarım ağrıyor. Başım dönüyor. Ne hissettiğimi kestiremiyorum.

Bütün düşündüklerim, gelirken yolda bile ona söylemeyi düşündüğüm cümleler anlamını yitiriyor.

Ben şu an ölmekte olan ve acı çcken bir adamın yanında oturuyorum.

Eğer bunca yılı birlikte geçirseydik ve şu an yine burada olsaydım ne değişirdi bilemiyorum.

Eminim daha çok üzülürdüm.

"Beni neden çağırdın?"

"Seni görmek için" diyor kesik kesik, "çok güzel olmuşsun, çok büyümüşsün..."

Sanki dışardan bir ses onun yerine konuşurmuş gibi…

Asıl bunun için ağlamak istiyorum. Neden daha önce çağırmadın? Neden bana ne olduğunu anlatmadın. Belki de anneme değil sana hak verirdim. Belki de aslında bütün bunlar bu kadar büyütülecek şeyler değildi... Belki kocamın daha üç yıllık evlilikte bana yaptıklarından beter değildi.

"Ben ölüyorum, bilmen gerekenler var..."

Buraya gelirken onunla konuşacaklarımı, yıllarca düşünüp durduğum şeyleri, soruları, cevapları kafamda canlandırmıştım ve onu affetmediğimi söyleyecektim değil mi?

Eliyle yanındaki dolabın çekmecesini gösteriyor. "Orayı aç," diyor... İlaç istiyor sanıyorum. Açıyorum ve kutuyu görüyorum. Bir an öylece kalakalıyorum.

Ne demişti Sare Hanım, "Bir gün, yıllar sonra büyüdüğünde o kutuya bakacaksın ve orada kendini göreceksin..."

Ne düşüneceğimi bilemedim. Sanki benim hayatımı alıp götürdüğü gibi kutudaki hayatımı da çalmıştı.

Ama yanına birkaç eşya alıp o evden bir akşam birdenbire çıkıp giden adam benim küçük kutumu yanında götürüp yıllarca saklamış mıydı?

Ne diyebilirdim ki?

"Onu senden gizlice almıştım, şimdi sana geri verme zamanı..."

Benden yalnızca özel büyülü kutumu aldığı için mi özür dileyecekti yoksa?

Sen benden yıllarımı aldın mı deseydim?

O yalnızca bir kutu. Büyülü filan değil. İçine küçük bir kızın mutsuzluklarını, küçük sevinçlerini, anlamsız üzüntülerini, anmalıklarını doldurduğu bir kutu.

Ona baktım. Yüzü çökmüş, zayıf, belki yalnızca gözlerinde ufak bir hayat kırıntısı kalmış bu adam benim babamdı.

Ve belki de o an, o kutuyu gördüğüm an ona olan tüm kızgınlığım geçti.

Çocuk gibi onu yıllarca saklaması acıklı değil komikti çünkü. Ben onun ölen kızı değildim. Ben yaşıyordum. Beni istediği an arayıp bulabilirdi. Ama onun yerine benden gizlice kaçırdığı çocukluk hatıralarımı saklamış ve kimbilir belki zaman zaman onları açıp ağlamıştı.

Bütün erkekler böyle korkak mı?

Ama ben şimdi ağlamayacaktım. Ona sormak istediğim tüm sorular artık anlamsız geliyordu. Uzak bir ülkede, kendi doğduğu, büyüdüğü yerlerden uzakta, bu eski püskü hastanede, sıvalar dökülmüş, eşyalar eskimiş, ölüyordu.

Belki bütün bu yaptıklarından pişmandı. Belki mutsuzdu. Kimbilir belki de gerçekte istediği hayatı sonunda yaşamayı başarmıştı...

Hayatta en çok korktuğum şey öldükten sonra sorguya çekilmek değil miydi? Şimdi onu ölmek üzereyken ben mi sorguya çekecektim. Ferhat'ın dediği gibi, "Kimin böyle bir hakkı olabilir ki?"

Nasıl böyle oluyor? Hayat birdenbire şu kırışmış ellerden, kemikleri çıkmış yüzden, belki daha birkaç gün önce gülerek bakan gözlerden çıkıp gidiyor ve sizi en yakın dostuna, ölüme teslim ediyor.

Ağlamayacak mıydım? Birdenbire gözlerimden yaşlar boşanıyor. Hayır o ölüm değil, o benim babam, kokusunu, buradaki bütün bu garip kokulara rağmen aldığım babam, ne yapmış olursa olsun onun şimdi benim kutumdaki yakışıklı resminden bu hale dönüşmesini istemiyorum.

Giderken nasıl elimden hiçbir şey gelmediyse şimdi de gelmediği için üzgünüm.

Elini tutmak için elimi uzatıyorum.

O sırada kapı açılıyor. Dönüp bakıyorum. Yaşlıca, iyi giyimli, bakımlı bir hanım elinden tuttuğu kız çocuğuyla içeri giriyor. Sarı saçları iki yandan örülmüş.

O an buraya neden çağırıldığımı anlıyorum.

"Beni," diyor, o garip metalik sesle, "affedebilecek misin?"

Ona, sonra kapıda ne yapacağını bilmeden duran o kadınla kıza, hiç tanımadığım küçük kızkardeşime bakıyorum.

Ve bilmiyorum neden, artık ağlamıyorum.

"Hayır," diyorum, "seni asla affetmeyeceğim..."

Başaramadım.

Onu bunca yıl sonra o halde gördüğüm için mi, birden karşıma çıkan o kadın ve küçük kız yüzünden mi, annemi düşündüğüm için mi?

Yaşadığım bütün bu hastalıkların, sıkıntıların, korkuların, yalnızlığın nedeni olarak onu gördüğüm için mi?

Ölmeden önce geride kalanlara birşeyler ayarlamaya çalıştığı ve beni yalnızca bu yüzden çağırdığı için mi?

Bilmiyordum.

Yalnızca bir tek söz söyleyecektim aslında.

Onlar o an kapıdan içeri girmese, elini tutup, "Bütün bunları unutalım artık, geçti, gitti," diyebilirdim.

Filmlerde, romanlarda kendi hayatını kurmak için çılgınca şeyler yapan insanları kahraman olarak görüp sevmemiş miydik?

Yazık ki insanın içindeki duygu, ona uzaktan bakarak verdiği anlamla bağdaşmıyor her zaman.

Neredeyse yeniden geri dönüp ona sarılmak ve "Hayır, affettim, tabii ki affettim," demek istiyordum.

İnsan ölmek üzere olan birine, düşmanına bile bunu söyleyemez mi?

Yalan bile olsa söyleyemez mi?

Kucağımdaki kutuya baktım. Sanki açmaya korkuyordum.

Sanki çok derinlere gizlenmiş, herkesten saklanmış, unutulmuş ne varsa oradan çıkıp üzerime gelecekti.

Açtım.

Hüzün de verse, canımı da yaksa o benim hayatım.

Kendime kızmayacaktım. İçimden ne geliyorsa onu söyledim. Belki asıl söyleyeceklerimi söylemedim. Ne kadar kendimi kandırsam da onu affetmemişim.

Sonra annemi düşündüm.

O bile böyle yapmazdı.

Bana, gitme demedi.

Bunca yıl onunla ilgili kötü söz söylemedi.

Ama tabii o anda, aslında babamın ona mektuplar yolladığını, bütün bunlardan haberi olduğunu ama bana söylemediğini bilmiyordum.

Ne derdi anneannem, "Hayatta hiçbir şey için geç değildir, sözler söylenir ve unutulur, yeter ki onları yeniden söylemeyi bilelim... Başkasına duyduğun öfke seni mutsuz eder, taşıması en zor yüktür..."

Ne yapalım ki başaramadım.

Berlin'deki o hastaneden çıkıp trene bindim.

Kısa bir süre için bir arınma kliniğine gittiğimi söyledim.

Annem tabii yine kıyametleri kopardı. Son başıma gelenlerden sonra tek başıma asla gidemeyeceğimi söyledi, beni ikna edemeyeceğini anlayınca kendisi de gelmek istedi ama sonunda pes etti.

Taner Amca'nın evinde kalacağımı söyleyince biraz rahatladı.

Aslında daha önce konuşmuştuk. Neler olacak, neler yapılacak, ameliyat nasıl geçecek, sonrası... Pek fazla dinlediğimi söyleyemem. Kafama bir delik açacaklardı işte. Sonrasını onların da bildiğinden emin değildim.

"Annenlerden bunu gizlemek bana hiç doğru gelmiyor, bunu söylemek istiyorum," dedi.

"Eğer intihar etmeye karar verseydim, bunu onlara söyleyecek birine benziyor muyum sizce?" diye sordum.

"Hiç güzel bir benzetme olmadı ama peki, artık küçük Ebru değilsin, sen böyle istiyorsan böyle olsun, ben yanında olacağım..."

Bir sürü acıya katlandım. Artık sabah uyandığımda ağzımdaki o metal tadı istemiyorum. Her an birşey olacak korkusuyla yaşamak istemiyorum.

Nereye varacağını tam olarak bilemeyen eski zaman kaşifleri gibi bilinmez bir yolculuğa çıktım ve bundan sonra ne olacaksa olacak...

İlk kez gördüğüm, eski evlerle dolu sokakta yürüyorum. Bu sabah biraz soğuk ama yine de güneşli. Taner Amca hastaneye giderken beni kasabanın merkezine bıraktı. Boynumdaki atkıyı iyice sarıyorum.

Evde oturmak yerine üşüsem de biraz dolaşmak, yeni yerler görmek daha iyi.

Paçalı atların çektiği arabalar, şık giysiler içindeki sürücüler, yüzyıllar öncesinden kalma gelenekleri yaşatmaya çalışan insanlar...

Beyaz, iki katlı bir evin önünden geçerken duruyorum. Bahçede minyatür bir ev var. Uzakdoğuda yaptıkları türden. Küçük figürler, azizler, rengarenk küçücük bir ev.

Ferhat'ın yaptığı o garip apartmanı hatırlıyorum.

Bundan biraz daha büyüktü. Belki iki ya da üç metre uzunluğunda beş, altı katlı bir apartman... Ama garip olan, her daireyi tek tek yapmasıydı. Kiminde bir adam tek başına televizyon izliyor, kiminde bir aile yemek yiyor, kiminde bir kadın pencerenin önünde sigara içiyor...

Hani gece bazı apartmanların önünden geçerken içlerindeki hayatı merak edersiniz ya, ışıkları yakınca öyle bir hisse kapılıyordunuz.

Böyle birşeyle ne kadar çok uğraştığına şaşırmıştım.

Dalmış bunları düşünürken bir kadın geliyor yanıma, bahçe kapısını iterken, gözlerimin içine bakarak, "Bana mı geldiniz?" diye soruyor.

Şaşkın şaşkın kadına bakıyorum.

"Yo, hayır, ben yalnızca..."

"Girin girin," diyor dinlemeden, "bana geldiniz..."

Ne yapacağımı şaşırıyorum.

"Gelsenize," diyor kadın, "merak etmeyin size çay ikram edeceğim... Burnunuz kızarmış, üşümüşsünüz... Belli ki yabancısınız..."

Sanki tutulmuş gibi arkasından yürüyorum. Kapıyı açıyor, beyaz kabarık tüylü bir kedi mırıldanarak kapıda onu karşılıyor ve içeri giriyoruz.

Eski püskü eşyalar, sanki öylesine toplanıp getirilmiş gibi birbirine uymayan ıvır zıvırla dolu bir ev.

Birşeyleri itiyor, elindekileri bir yere koyuyor, beni kırmızı kadife koltuğa oturtuyor.

"Çok uzaktan geliyorsunuz değil mi?" diye soruyor.

"Evet," diyorum, "İstanbul'dan..."

Kayboluyor. Kendi kendime "Neler oluyor?" diyorum.

Elinde tepsiyle geri geliyor. Kaynayan su, minik fincanlara konulmuş çaylar... Güzel bir koku duyuluyor.

"Uzaktan gelen insanlar hep bir yerleri özler," diyor.

Çayın demlenmesini beklerken, birkaç dakika daha geç kalsa karşılaşamayacağımızı, üstelik birinin onu çarşıda lafa tuttuğunu anlatıyor.

60 yaşlarında olmalı. Gençliğindeki haliyle yaşıyor. Yalnızca biraz şişmanlamış, saçları beyazlaşmış, gözlerindeki kırışıklar artmış.

"Ben," diyorum, "aslında öylesine geziyordum ve bu sokağa girdim, ne çok falcı var burada.."

"Öyle olmalı, çoğu insan bu sokağa bunun için gelir ama ben fal bakmıyorum," diyor, sonra çayı demlerken, "yani uzun zamandır bakmıyorum..."

Portakal kokulu çaydan koyuyor küçük fincanlara...

"Kimsiniz siz?" diyorum.

"Bugün rastlaman gereken biriyim belki," diyor, "falcılar gerçekten geleceği bilselerdi bu sefil mahallede oturmazlardı diye düşünüyorsun değil mi?"

Gülümsüyorum, çaydan bir yudum alıyorum. Ilık ve çok güzel kokuyor, çok hafif, belli belirsiz tarçın tadı var.

"Çok güzelmiş, teşekkür ederim," diyorum.

"O da çok uzaklardan geldi senin gibi ve uzakta hep bizimle hiç tanımasak da benzer düşünceleri olan dostlarımız vardır."

Şimdi Seda olsa eminim bunun büyülü bir karşılaşma olduğuna inanırdı.

"O boynundakini çıkar sonra dışarıda üşüyeceksin," diyor, öyle rahat, annem gibi söylüyor ki ister istemez dediğini yapıyorum.

Karşımdaki koltukta oturmuş çayını içerken, "Sonradan anlatırsın, bir gün sefil bir mahalleye gittim ve sokaktan geçerken deli kadının biri beni evine davet etti, çay ikram etti, sonra ben uyudum ve böbreklerimi mafyaya sattı," diye... Kahkaha atıyor.

Gülümsüyorum. Aslında ne yapacağımı bilemediğim için...

"Gözlerin uzakta dedim, ama yalnızca gözlerin değil, ruhun da çok uzaklarda..." diyor.

Gerçekten delinin teki mi? Korkmalı mıyım? Hiç tanımadığım bir yerde, hiç tanımadığım bir kadının evindeyim...

"Uzakta derken kendi ülkende, şehrinde demek istemiyorum, ruhun senden uzakta..."

Birden bu garip sabahta bu garip evde içimden ağlamak geliyor. Çünkü belki de ne zamandır söylemeye çalışıp anlatamadıklarımı söylüyor.

"Ama onu sana biri geri getirecek... Hem de hiç ummadığın biri..."

Dut yemiş bülbül gibi karşısında oturuyorum. Hah, diyorum, şimdi fala başladı, birazdan bana daha da garip şeyler anlatacak ve sonra da para isteyecek...

Ama öyle olmuyor. Bana artık yapması gereken işler olduğunu ve istediğim zaman oraya yeniden gelebileceğimi söylüyor.

Sokağa çıktığımda hem şaşkınım hem de keyifli. Annemin çok eskiden benim duymadığımı düşünerek teyzeme anlattığı o kehanet hikayesi geliyor aklıma...

Ben bebekken gittiği falcının ona, Emirgan'daki evin bahçesini, bahçedeki gizli geçitleri ve yıllar önce orada yaşanan korkunç olayı anlattığı...

Annem her ne kadar etkilense de çok üzerinde durmuyor falcı kadının söylediklerinin... Ta ki birdenbire hastalandığım güne kadar... O zaman yıllar sonra gerçekten de evin olduğu yerde, tarihi köşkte çok eskiden korkunç bir olay olduğunu, bir kadının çocuklarıyla birlikte kendisini yaktığını, bunun gizlendiğini ama sonunda ortaya çıktığını ve çocuklar ölüp kadın kurtulsa da sonsuza dek lanetlendiğini öğreniyor...

Annemin bu hikayeyi benden gizlemesinin nedenini sonradan anlıyorum. Çünkü başıma gelenleri aslında bu hikayeye bağlıyor ama bunu söylemeye dili varmıyor.

Ürperiyorum.

Yetiştiğim okullarda ve evde bana hep bütün bu safsatalara inanmamam öğütlendi. Anneanneme sorulacak olsa dünya göründüğü gibidir ve olanların bir nedeni vardır. Bilinmeyenler, gizemli şeyler, başka dünyalar onu ilgilendirmez.

Ama şimdi bunca yaşantıdan sonra hiç de öyle düşünemiyorum. Kimbilir belki de başka şeylere inanmak istiyorum.

Üstelik bu benden saklanan kehanetteki gizli geçitlerde az zaman geçirmedim.

Yalnız çocukken değil büyüdüğüm zaman da gizli geçitlerde dolaşmayı hep heyecan verici buldum. Hayatımda değilse bile en azından hayalimde...

Yalnızca görünenlerin gerçek olduğu bir dünya sıkıcı değil mi zaten?

Ben, evet, gerçek hayatı rüyayla karıştırdım çoğu zaman. Hatta bunu bilerek yaptığım, öyle sanıyormuşum gibi davrandığım zamanlar da çok oldu.

Bazen birinin aslında ne yapmaya çalıştığını, ne düşündüğünü anlayıp başka şeyler anlattığında farkında değilmiş gibi yaptım. Bazen gayet iyi anlasam da anlamamış gibi davrandım.

Herşeyi bilen ve bunun kibriyle dolaşan biri olacağına biraz budala olmanın ne zararı var?

Falcıların sokağından çıkıyorum ve nereye gittiğimi bilmeden öylesine yürüyorum.

Kendimle başbaşayım ama o garip kadının söylediği gibi aslında kendimden çok uzaktayım.

Çıkarken bana ismimin ne anlama geldiğini sordu, "Bulut gibi birşey," dedim.

"Ne güzel bir isim, benimki de Juliette, hani şu ünlü aşk hikayesindeki..." dedi gülerek...

Bir yere doğru giden insanları izliyorum ve rengarenk bir sokağa giriyorum.

Festival mi, panayır mı? Karnaval mı?

Duvarları boyayan çocuklar, yerlere yayılmış tuvallere resim çizenler, sokak çalgıcıları...

Birileri isteyenin resmini çiziyor, genç müzisyenler caz çalıyor. Kafalarında kocaman şapkalar var. Önlerindeki kutuya birkaç kuruş atıyorum.

Küçük, sevimli arabada satılan kahveden alıyorum. Biraz acı ama olsun, içimi ısıtıyor.

Bir kadınla erkek tüm bedenleri altın yaldız kaplanmış, birbirlerine sarılarak farklı heykeller yaratıyor.

Elele tutuşmuş yaşlı çiftler, sarılmış gençler, elleri cebinde sanatçı görünümlü tipler, öğretmenlerinin peşinde pek de etrafa aldırmadan şakalaşan çocuklar...

Birden unutuyorum. Buraya neden geldiğimi, nerede olduğumu, kim olduğumu... Sanki hep buradaymışım ve hayat hep böyle renkli, neşeli bir festivalmiş gibi geliyor.

Oysa yalnızca birkaç gün sonra buradan biraz uzaktaki kliniğe yatacağım ve neler olacağını bilmiyorum.

Biraz yoruldum. Bizim simitimize benzeyen, tuzlu birşey satıyorlar. Ondan alıyorum ve küçük bir tabureye oturuyorum. Keşke o tombul sabah simidi olsaydı.

Tezgahlarda hepsi el yapımı yüzükler, bilezikler, boncuklar, kolyeler, küpeler satılıyor. Birileri dövme yapıyor.

Bir palyaço elindeki akordiyonla vals çalarak önümden geçiyor.

Yaşlıca, eski ama şık giysileri olan dalgalı, beyaz saçlı adam bana gül veriyor. Bana söylediklerini anlamıyorum. Simitçiyle gözgöze geliyoruz, gülüyor. Adam yalnızca gülü verip gidiyor.

Bütün ülkeler böyle olsa keşke, diye düşünüyorum.

Hep karnavalda gibi...

Bu insanların belki hiçbiri zengin değil. Hatta giysilerine bakılırsa çoğu yoksul. Ama farklı renklerden, farklı ırklardan, farklı ülkelerden, yaşlardan insanlar bu garip karnaval havasında, bu küçük kasabada biraraya gelmiş eğleniyorlar...

Kafalarında kukuletalarla, yerlere kadar uzanan bol, geometrik desenli giysileriyle üç, dört kişi geliyor, hemen karşımda oturup eskiden çok güçlü bir uygarlıkken birdenbire yokolup giden o insanların müziğini çalmaya başlıyorlar.

Ellerinde antik çalgılar...

Gizemli ormanların, kimsenin çıkmak istemeyeceği kadar yüksek dağların içinde belki de ilk büyük kentleri kuran insanlar sonra nereye gitmiş olabilir ki?

Belki de saklanmak işe yaramıyor.

Artık eve dönsem iyi olur. Kalkıyorum. Elimde, kırmızı gül, gülümsüyorum.

Kalabalığın içinde yürüyorum.

Birkaç kişi duvarı boyuyor. Ellerini başının arasına almış, dizlerini göğsüne çekmiş bir kadın, tam olarak adlandıramadığınız, tanıyamadığınız hayvanlar, her türlü yiyecekle dolu bir masada tıkınan şişman, zengin adamlar, çoktan türleri tükenmiş sürüngenler, saçları sakallarıyla ünlü bir rock topluluğu, birbirini öldüren askerler, elleri, ayakları olmayan, yerde sürünerek yürüyen çocuklar, köpeğini gezdiren çok güzel bir kadın, farklı dillerde yazılar...

Oraya toplanmış kalabalığın içinde resmi anlamlandırmaya çalışıyorum. Öyle çok ayrıntı var ki...

Resim önümüzde çizilmeye devam ediyor. Bir resmin, bu andan sonra neler olacağını bilmediğiniz bir hayatın kurulmasını izliyoruz.

Birden...

Yine mi?

Yine rüyayla gerçeği karıştırıyor muyum?

Bu benim tanıdığım bir duygu.

Ona, beyaz gömleklerinin üzerine takması için verdiğim şey.

Başım dönüyor.

Bir yerlere tutunsam...

Elinde kocaman bir fırçayla orada.

Boynunda benim ona verdiğim fular.

Herşey yanıltsa da o yanıltmaz.

Gülerek resim çizen adamlarla konuşuyor ve boşlukları dolduruyor.

Saçları iyice beyazlaşmış, kısalmış, biraz yorgun yüzü...

Bazen...

Bazen mi?

Hep hayaller kurarsın Ebru...

Burada, hiç tanımadığın bir yerde, yıllar sonra, hayatının en büyük yolculuğuna çıkmışken, öylesine sokaklarda dolaşırken...

Bu gerçek olabilir mi?

Araya birileri giriyor.
Önüme geçen şişman kadını itiyorum.
Onu görmeye çalışıyorum yeniden..
Sakın düşme!
Dönüyor.
Kısa bir an.
Beni görüyor.
Görüyor değil mi?
O palyaço akordiyonuyla neşeli bir şarkı çalıyor.
Donmuş kalıyorum orada.
O an gözgöze geliyoruz.
Elindeki fırçayı atıyor, bana doğru geliyor.
Düşeceğim.
Bu sen misin?
Yıllar önce sana verdiğim fularla...
Saçların kısalmış... Bembeyaz olmuş...
Yine o beyaz, uzun gömlek...
Yine o gülümseyiş...
Yine o içime saplanan bakış.

Sanki yavaş çekim gibi... Elindeki fırçayı atıyor...
Bana doğru geliyor.
Bayılacağımı biliyorum.
Yine rüyada mıyım onu bilmiyorum.
Kendimi onun kucağında buluyorum.
O garip sirk müziği, kalabalık, karmaşa...
Hep böyle rüyalar gördüm.
Ama bu gerçek.
Çünkü kokusunu alıyorum.
Ne demişti Juliette?

"Ruhun şimdi senden çok uzakta ama onu hiç beklenmedik biri sana geri getirecek..."

Böyle şeyler olur mu?
Oldu işte.

Ona kızgın mıyım?
Onun yüzünden mi oldu bütün bunlar?
Ona soracağım çok fazla soru var mı?
Hayır. Artık ne anneme, babama, ne Onur'a ne başka birine, hiç kimseye kızgın değilim.
"Burada ne yapıyorsun?" diyor.
"Asıl sen burada ne yapıyorsun?" diyorum.
Zayıflamış. Gözlerinin altında torbalar var. Kısa saç çok yakışmış.
Ne çok zaman geçti.
Benim sana sormam gereken sorular var.
Bu belki de pek çok insanın başına gelen, kırık bir aşk hikayesiydi. Öylece kalacak, zamanla unutulacak, yıllar sonra belki küçük bir sızı gibi hatırlayacağınız...
Şimdi bütün olanlardan sonra, bir anda biten bir evlilikten çıkıp, ani bir karar verip, uzak bir kasabaya gelip yeniden onunla karşılaşmak yalnızca rastlantı mı?
Tabii ki ona niye burada olduğumu söylemeyeceğim.
"Gel," diyor, "üşümüş gibisin, evim hemen şurada..."
Üşümüş mü?

Şu anda başıma geldiğini söyleyebileceğim en son şey bu olurdu.

Keşke o kadar basit olsaydı.

Kalabalığın içinden geçerken koluma giriyor. Belki on, onbeş dakika yürüyoruz.

Büyük, demir kapıyı açıyor. Depo gibi bir yere giriyoruz.

"Sana sıcak birşey yapayım, çay ister misin?"

Hayır, daha sert birşeye ihtiyacım var.

Bunca yıl sonra inanılmaz bir biçimde karşılaştık ve sen bana çay ister misin diye mi soruyorsun?

Yüksek tavanlı, soğuk, eski binanın içindeyiz.

Köşede tavana dayanan dev, ahşap bir top var.

Yine İstanbul'daki gibi bir sürü garip şey etrafta.

Küçük kadehe şeffaf bir içki koyuyor. Ne olduğunu bilmiyorum. Alıp kafama dikiyorum.

Sonra bir tane daha...

"Şimdi bana herşeyi anlatacaksın," diyorum.

"Neden gittiğini, neden bana hiçbir şey söylemediğini... Artık birşey söylemeyen insanlardan, birşey soramadığım insanlardan, kimseye bunları söyleyememekten çok yoruldum..."

Bunları ben mi söylüyorum?

Kimseye söyleyemediklerimi şimdi ona mı söylüyorum?

Gülümsüyor.

"Anlatırım ama uzun ve sıkıcı bir hikaye aslında," diyor.

"Kendi ülkemden sürüldüm... Sürülmek ne kelime, kaçmak zorunda kaldım. İnsan kendi ülkesinden kaçıp hiç tanımadığı bir yere neden sığınsın? Bundan daha büyük utanç olabilir mi?"

Hayır artık gülümsemiyor.

Taner Amca'yı aradım, bir arkadaşıma rastladığımı, merak etmemelerini söyledim.

Aslında ne anlatacağı umurumda bile değildi.

Uzaktan geldim. Uzağa, belki de hayatımın sonuna doğru bir yolculuğa çıkıp... Yılların içinden... Ve orada böyle bir anda en olmayacak şey gibi birden onu gördüm.

Unuttuğumu sanmışken...

Artık bütün kırgınlıklar geride kalmışken...

Daha doğrusu öyle sanırken...

İnsan bunca yıl sever mi birini?

Biliyorum ki onu düşünmeden geçen tek günüm bile olmadı. Yalnızca unutmak istedim. Derinlere gizleyip... Babamda yaptığım gibi... Alınyazısı gibi...

O da beni bırakıp gitmişti. Ne garip, hayatımı en çok etkileyen iki erkekten biri kendi isteğiyle bütün hayatını değiştirdi ötekiyse hiç istemediği halde başka bir hayata başlamak zorunda kaldı.

İnsan birini seviyor, bir başkasına belki bir süre aşık oluyor, birini yanında istiyor ama zamanın içinde bir yerdeki o duygu yalnızca size onu verene ait kalıyor.

O aslında ne kadar uzakta da olsa, kaybolmuyor. Sanki dönüp baksan orada durduğunu görecekmişsin gibi...

O duyguyu tanıdım.

Ve gerçek olduğunu biliyorum.

Onunla karşılaştığım anda yıllar öncesinde her gördüğümde ne hissettiysem o...

Biliyorum çünkü hayattaki hiçbir bilgi böylesine gerçek olamaz.

Ve yine biliyorum ki aşkın geçmiş zamanı yoktur. Çünkü gerçekten aşık olmuşsan her zaman aşıksındır.

Ben hayal bile olsa onu yanımda taşımıştım. Rüzgarı tutmak gibiydi oysa.

Ama işte şimdi o yılların içinde hep bana onun kokusunu getiren rüzgar yeniden esiyordu ve sanki kendi ülkemi, çocukluğumu da buraya taşıyordu.

Sanki güçlü olmamı sağlamak için...

Birden kendime geliyorum. Tren duruyor.

Paltomu giyiyorum. Küçük bavulumu alıyorum.

Taner Amca istasyonda beni bekliyor.

O çok sevdiğim yazarın söylediği gibi, yaşamın ucuna yolculuktayım.

"Madem merak ediyorsun," dedi Ferhat ve bana neler olduğunu anlattı.

Bir arkadaşının hem de en güvendiği yardımcısının onu ihbar ettiğini, kaçmak zorunda kaldığını, buraya gelince bilmediği bu ülkede, bilmediği bir dilde ne yapacağını şaşırdığını...

Öylesine tanıştığı bir arkadaşının sayesinde buraya gelmişti.

Bir gece barda içtikten sonra sokakta yürürken biri ona saldırmış, bacağından bıçaklamış, onunla kavga ederken iki genç gelip onu kurtarmış. Yalnızca yabancı olduğu için...

Sabah kendisini onların evinde bulmuş.

"Uyandığımda şişman, yaşlı bir kadınla karşılaştım. Bana tatlı çörekle kahve getirmişti. Hemen yanlarındaki bu döküntüye taşındığımı, ressam olduğumu biliyorlardı yalnızca... Beni kurtaran çocuklardan birinin annesiydi."

Bilmediği bir ülkede, kimsenin onu tanımadığı, kimseyi tanımadığı bir yerde, herşeyden kaçıp gizlenmeye çalışırken...

Sonra onlarla ve daha küçük çocuklarla resim çalışmaya başlamıştı. Yakınlardaki okulun müdürü ona destek olmuştu. Onlar da uzak ülkelerden gelen sığınmacılardı.

Şimdi o çocuklar için uzaktan gelmiş bir lider gibiydi.

Haftasonları hep birlikte yoksul mahallelere yemek götürüyor, atölyedeki resim çalışmalarına katılan çocuklara ne biliyorsa öğretmeye çalışıyordu.

O benim sevdiğim adamdı.

Ben babamı bile affedememiştim ama o kendisini ihbar eden arkadaşını affetmişti.

"Şimdi sen söyle," dedi, "burada ne arıyorsun?"

Doktorumu ziyarete geldiğimi söyledim.

"O zaman," dedi, "onları da al, iki gün sonra sergi açılışım var, birlikte gelin..."

Orada gördüğüm o kocaman ahşap top ünlü bir sergi salonunun önüne konacaktı.

Yalnızca ahşap bir top.

Sana artık söylemek istiyorum. Bana söylemediklerini, beni korumak için bana haber yollamadığını, hayatıma girdiğin gibi çıkıp gitmeye çalıştığını biliyorum.

Ama artık bütün bunlar umurumda bile değil.

"Hadi gel," diyor, ben bunları söyleyemeden, "seni goturеyim, yolları bilmezsin, cumartesi akşamı bekliyorum..."

Kalabalık...

Eski bir sarayın önündeyiz... Soğuk.

Avludaki kalabalığın içinde ilerliyoruz.

Binanın önünde üzeri örtülü birşey var.

Dev birşey...

Karanlıkta...

Çok şık kadınlar, erkekler...

Özel giydirilmiş garsonlar, genç kızlar ellerindeki tepsilerle içki ve kanepe dağıtıyor.

Yağmur yağdı yağacak.

Önce müzik başlıyor.

Bir köşede orkestra çalıyor.

Bu kentin simgesi olan adamın yazdığı bir şarkı.

Ve sonra renkli ışıklar yanıyor.

Örtü çekiliyor.

O ahşap top yavaş yavaş ortaya çıkıyor.

Herkes merakla bakıyor.

Bu yalnızca dev, ahşap bir top.

Birisi gelip topun içindeki kapıyı açıyor.

O yeraltına gömülmüş terakota askerler gibi, topun içinde yine ahşaptan oyulmuş askerler var.

Işık onları aydınlatıyor.

Hepsinin yüzü farklı.

Kimi kaygılı, kimi sert, kimi öfkeli, kimi boş bakıyor.

Ama aynı üniformaları giymişler.

Neredeyse topun içinden çıkacak gibi görünüyorlar.

Bunun adı "Truva Topu".

Birden hatırlıyorum.

Tam anlam veremediğim resimlerini... Heykellerini...

Bir resmini görmüştüm. Kendi portrelerini çizmişti. Aynı tuvalin içinde yüzlerce küçük portre... Hepsinde başka görünüyordu.

"Bunun ismi var mı?" diye sormuştum.

"Hayır," demişti, "benim yüzlerim..."

"Binbir Surat," koy adını demiştim. Çok gülmüştü.

Şimdi anlıyorum. Bütün o resimlerde aslında aynı şeyi anlatmaya çalışıyordu.

Renkli ışıklar yanıp söndükçe topun içindeki yüzler değişiyordu.

Herkes bir başkasıydı.

Onun evinde gördüğüm, aynaya bakan kadın resmini hatırladım.

Aynaya bakıyor ama aynada başka bir yüz görüyor.

"Artık dönelim," diyor Taner Amca, "yolumuz uzun, yarın sabah erken kalkacaksın..."

Yine o uçurumun kenarındayım.

Yine rüyayla gerçek arasında bir yerde...

Ferhat diyor ki, "Korkma düşmek yok, buradan atlayacağız ve uçar gibi bizden başka kimsenin bilmediği bir ülkeye gideceğiz..."

Ama korkuyorum.

İlaçların etkisi, rüya görüyorsun, diyorum kendi kendime...

Anneannemi, annemi görüyorum.

Hayır hiç biri burada değil.

Buraya yalnız geldim, hatırlıyorum.

"Düşmek yok..."

Çok uzun, sayısız merdiveni tırmandım ve sanki sonunda inanılmaz bir manzarayla karşılaşacağımı, bundan böyle yalnızca görmek istediklerimi göreceğimi düşündüm. Kimseye söylemeden, bütün o kırgınlıkları, üzüntüleri, kaybedişleri kendi kendime yaşadım.

Şimdi bu anda, uçurumdan, bu, hayatımın en büyük kabusundan aşağı düşemem...

Hayatında hiç uçurum görmemiş birinin uçurumlardan deli gibi korkması ne tuhaf!

Birden hafifliyorum.

Bana sayı saymamı söylediler, en son hatırladığım bu...

"Kendine geliyor," diyor biri... Taner Amca adımı söylüyor, "Geçti," diyor. Biraz yankılanır gibi sesler...

Çocukluğun bahçesi, gizli geçitler, sanki tam düşerken biri elimden tuttu...

Gözlerimi açıyorum.

Biri sahiden de elimden tutuyor.

Biri değil o!

Bu nasıl olabilir ki...

Hala rüyada mıyım?

Hem rüyamda hem burada nasıl elimi tutmuş olabilir?

Bunu yapacağımı, burada olacağımı bilmiyor ki...

O garip iki renkli gözleriyle bana bakıyor.

Evet o, şimdi eminim, şimdi rüyada değilim, çünkü kokusunu duyuyorum.

"Artık burada mısın?" diye soruyor.

Burada mıyım?

Gözlerimi iyice açıyorum. Gülümseyen yüzler var.

Gerçek olduğuna inanmak için elini sıkıyorum.

"Evet," diyorum, "ben geldim, buradayım..."

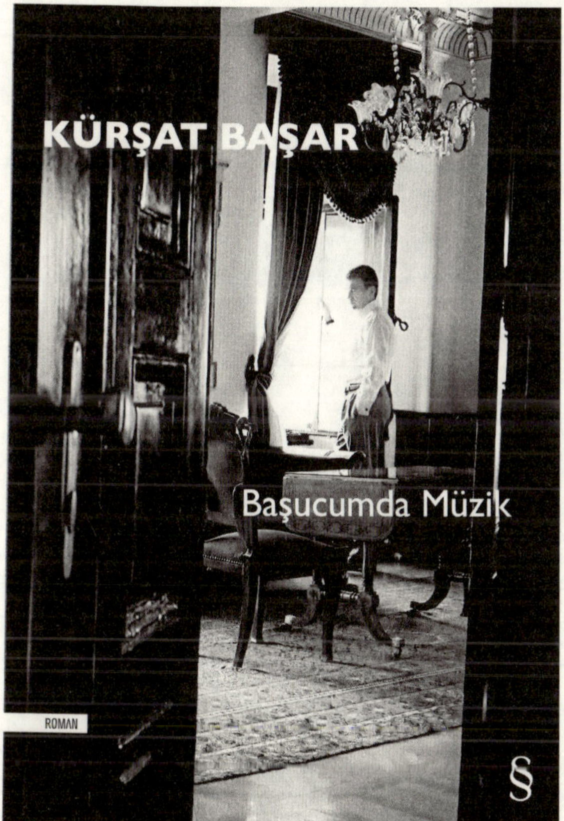
KÜRŞAT BAŞAR
Başucumda Müzik
ROMAN
§

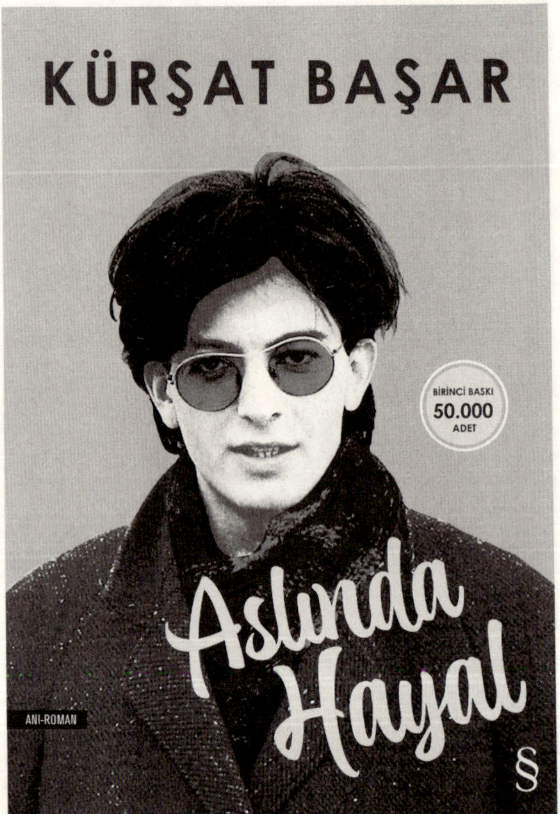
KÜRŞAT BAŞAR
BİRİNCİ BASKI
50.000
ADET
Aslında
Hayal
ANI-ROMAN
Ş

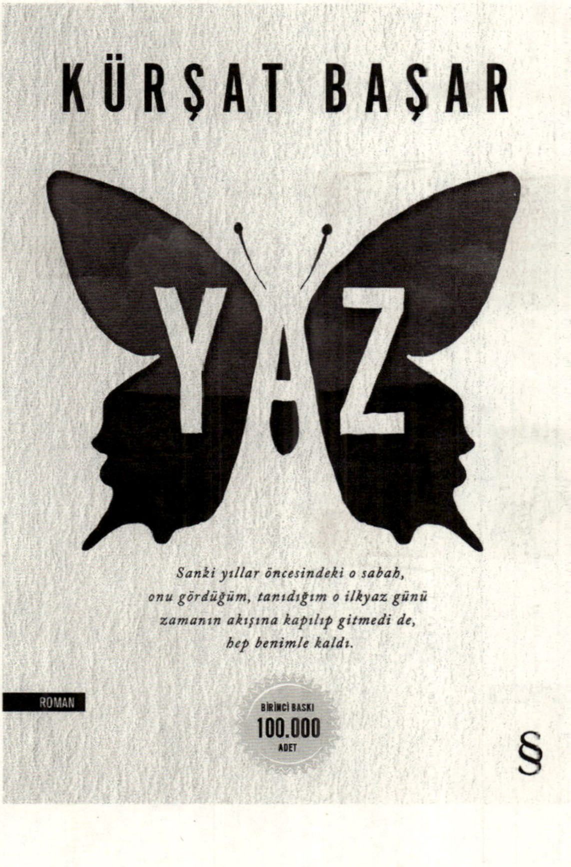
KÜRŞAT BAŞAR
YAZ
Sanki yıllar öncesindeki o sabah,
onu gördüğüm, tanıdığım o ilkyaz günü
zamanın akışına kapılıp gitmedi de,
hep benimle kaldı.
ROMAN
BİRİNCİ BASKI
100.000
ADET
§

KÜRŞAT BAŞAR

YAĞMURLAR

Bazen

YILLAR

Unutmak

SOKAKLAR

İstersin

DENEME

YARIM KALAN ŞEYLER

§